ME **4**

DISEASE CONTROL PRIORITIES • THIRD EDITION

Mental, Neurological, and Substance Use Disorders

DISEASE CONTROL PRIORITIES • THIRD EDITION

Series Editors

Dean T. Jamison
Rachel Nugent
Hellen Gelband
Susan Horton
Prabhat Jha
Ramanan Laxminarayan
Charles N. Mock

Volumes in the Series

Essential Surgery
Reproductive, Maternal, Newborn, and Child Health
Cancer
Mental, Neurological, and Substance Use Disorders
Cardiovascular, Respiratory, and Related Disorders
HIV/AIDS, STIs, Tuberculosis, and Malaria
Injury Prevention and Environmental Health
Child and Adolescent Development
Disease Control Priorities: Improving Health and Reducing Poverty

DISEASE CONTROL PRIORITIES

Budgets constrain choices. Policy analysis helps decision makers achieve the greatest value from limited available resources. In 1993, the World Bank published *Disease Control Priorities in Developing Countries* (*DCP1*), an attempt to systematically assess the cost-effectiveness (value for money) of interventions that would address the major sources of disease burden in low- and middle-income countries. The World Bank's 1993 *World Development Report* on health drew heavily on *DCP1*'s findings to conclude that specific interventions against noncommunicable diseases were cost-effective, even in environments in which substantial burdens of infection and undernutrition persisted.

DCP2, published in 2006, updated and extended *DCP1* in several aspects, including explicit consideration of the implications for health systems of expanded intervention coverage. One way that health systems expand intervention coverage is through selected platforms that deliver interventions that require similar logistics but deliver interventions from different packages of conceptually related interventions, for example, against cardiovascular disease. Platforms often provide a more natural unit for investment than do individual interventions. Analysis of the costs of packages and platforms—and of the health improvements they can generate in given epidemiological environments—can help to guide health system investments and development.

DCP3 differs importantly from *DCP1* and *DCP2* by extending and consolidating the concepts of platforms and packages and by offering explicit consideration of the financial risk protection objective of health systems. In populations lacking access to health insurance or prepaid care, medical expenses that are high relative to income can be impoverishing. Where incomes are low, seemingly inexpensive medical procedures can have catastrophic financial effects. *DCP3* offers an approach to explicitly include financial protection as well as the distribution across income groups of financial and health outcomes resulting from policies (for example, public finance) to increase intervention uptake. The task in all of the *DCP* volumes has been to combine the available science about interventions implemented in very specific locales and under very specific conditions with informed judgment to reach reasonable conclusions about the impact of intervention mixes in diverse environments. *DCP3*'s broad aim is to delineate essential intervention packages and their related delivery platforms to assist decision makers in allocating often tightly constrained budgets so that health system objectives are maximally achieved.

DCP3's nine volumes are being published in 2015 and 2016 in an environment in which serious discussion continues about quantifying the sustainable development goal (SDG) for health. *DCP3*'s analyses are well-placed to assist in choosing the means to attain the health SDG and assessing the related costs. Only when these volumes, and the analytic efforts on which they are based, are completed will we be able to explore SDG-related and other broad policy conclusions and generalizations. The final *DCP3* volume will report those conclusions. Each volume will provide valuable, specific policy analyses on the full range of interventions, packages, and policies relevant to its health topic.

More than 500 individuals and multiple institutions have contributed to *DCP3*. We convey our acknowledgments elsewhere in this volume. Here we express our particular gratitude to the Bill & Melinda Gates Foundation for its sustained financial support, to the InterAcademy Medical Panel (and its U.S. affiliate, the Institute of Medicine of the National Academy of Medicine), and to the External and Corporate Relations Publishing and Knowledge division of the World Bank. Each played a critical role in this effort.

Dean T. Jamison
Rachel Nugent
Hellen Gelband
Susan Horton
Prabhat Jha
Ramanan Laxminarayan
Charles N. Mock

VOLUME 4

DISEASE CONTROL PRIORITIES • THIRD EDITION

Mental, Neurological, and Substance Use Disorders

EDITORS

Vikram Patel
Dan Chisholm
Tarun Dua
Ramanan Laxminarayan
María Elena Medina-Mora

WORLD BANK GROUP

Softcover
ISBN (paperback): 978-1-4648-0426-7
ISBN (electronic): 978-1-4648-0428-1
DOI: 10.1596/978-1-4648-0426-7

Hardcover
ISBN (hardcover): 978-1-4648-0427-4
DOI: 10.1596/978-1-4648-0427-4

Cover photo: © Curt Carnemark / World Bank. Further permission required for reuse.
Cover design: Debra Naylor, Naylor Design, Inc., Washington, DC.

Library of Congress Cataloging-in-Publication Data

Names: Patel, Vikram, editor. | Chisholm, Dan, editor. | Dua, Tarun, editor. | Laxminarayan, Ramanan, editor. | Medina-Mora, Maria Elena, editor. | World Bank, issuing body,

Title: Mental, neurological, and substance use disorders / editors, Vikram Patel, Dan Chisholm, Tarun Dua, Ramanan Laxminarayan, Maria Elena Medina-Mora.

Other titles: Disease control priorities ; v. 4. Description: Washington, DC : International Bank for Reconstruction and Development /The World Bank, [2015] | Series: Disease control priorities ; volume 4 | Includes bibliographical references and index.

Identifiers: LCCN 2015041175 (print) | LCCN 2015041905 (ebook) | ISBN 9781464804267 (alk. paper) | ISBN 9781464804274 (alk : paper : hc) | ISBN 9781464804281 (ebook)

Subjects: | MESH: Mental Disorders. | Developing Countries. | Public Health. | Substance-Related Disorders.

Classification: LCC RA790.5 (print) | LCC RA790.5 (ebook) | NLM WA 395 | DDC
   362.19689—dc23

LC record available at http://lccn.loc.gov/2015041175

Contents

Foreword

I personally felt mental health's deep-rooted importance when I returned home to Rwanda in 1996, just after my people were traumatized by the 1994 Tutsi genocide. At a time when we needed mental health services the most, there was only one psychiatrist in the entire country. In an act to survive and rebuild, we turned to our communities for healing. Giving a voice to the people and collectively finding a solution to the mental health challenges that we faced at that time has helped Rwanda to resiliently move forward on a path toward recovery.

This volume of *Disease Control Priorities,* third edition *(DCP3),* is thus a welcome call to action for augmenting the response needed to address the growing challenge of mental, neurological, and substance use (MNS) disorders. Such illnesses lurk in the shadows. Although they account for 10 percent of the global disease burden, they are left underestimated and unsupported worldwide.

In the pages that follow, the world has in its hands a series of evidence-based approaches, cost-effective strategies, and implementation guidelines for MNS disorders. This comes at an opportune time. Changing epidemiological and social determinant health profiles show the world's readiness for sustainable development goals (SDGs) to aim for universal health coverage. We, as global leaders, have a moral obligation to advocate for comprehensive, effective services backed by human-rights-oriented legal frameworks to protect those living with MNS disorders as part of this quest toward meaningful universal health coverage. Prioritizing the *supply* of quality MNS services at the community level while also improving the *demand* for such services must come with this advocacy effort.

Although these steps may seem daunting, there is reason for hope. We can build on the lessons from the world's 15-year fight against HIV/AIDS. Across low- and middle-income countries (LMICs) in the 1990s, both supply and demand for HIV/AIDS services were absent because there were no delivery platforms. No money or support was given to create a delivery structure. No laws were written to protect the human rights of those stigmatized by HIV/AIDS.

Today, it is a drastically different story. Progress against HIV/AIDS for the past 15 years tells us that no evidence-based, multisectoral, holistic, and rights-based approach is too sophisticated for LMICs. It demonstrates that specialized referral service systems are possible, even for one of the most complicated and stigmatized of conditions. It illustrates that as bidirectional supply and demand is created, the much-needed link between patients' needs and an effective global care response will grow stronger.

I challenge global leaders to build upon these lessons learned from the HIV/AIDS response and apply it positively to the challenge of MNS disorders. We must no longer overlook the deleterious effects that the lack of quality MNS services has upon our communities. We should strive to build universal health care systems specifically recognizing MNS disorders' genetic, biological, and cultural roots. And as a global community, I implore us to create enabling environments to address the social determinants of health affecting MNS disorders.

This call to action need not be answered alone; let us work together as a global team to change the status quo and demand health equity for all.

Agnes Binagwaho, MD, MPed, PhD
Minister of Health, Rwanda

Preface

Mental, neurological, and substance use (MNS) disorders contribute approximately 10 percent of the global burden of disease. They often run a chronic course, are highly disabling, and are associated with significant premature mortality. Moreover, beyond their health consequences, the impact of these disorders on the social and economic well-being of individuals, families, and societies is enormous.

Despite this burden, MNS disorders have been systematically neglected in most of the world, particularly in low- and middle-income countries (LMICs), with pitifully small contributions to prevention and treatment by governments and development agencies. Systematically compiling the substantial evidence that already exists to address this inequity is the central goal of volume 4 of *Disease Control Priorities*, third edition (*DCP3*). The evidence presented in this volume will help to build an evidence-based perspective on which policies and interventions for addressing MNS disorders should be prioritized in resource-constrained settings. These recommendations will be of relevance to ministries of health and—given the intersectoral nature of the interventions and impacts of MNS disorders—to ministries of health and social welfare, as well as to institutions and donors concerned with sustainable development. Reaching a broader audience of academics, research organizations, and public health practitioners is another goal of this effort.

MNS disorders include a large number of discrete health conditions, each with its own epidemiological characteristics and interventions for prevention and care. These disorders, like most chronic noncommunicable diseases, are caused by complex interactions among genetic, biological, social, and psychological determinants. In this volume, we chose to address only those conditions that are associated with a significant global burden. In doing so, we address the majority of the burden associated with these disorders. We have organized these heterogeneous groups of disorders into five groups: adult mental disorders, child mental and developmental disorders, neurological disorders, alcohol use disorders, and illicit drug use disorders. The volume also addresses suicide and self-harm, which are strongly associated with MNS disorders.

In addition to providing an up-to-date synthesis of the burden, prevalence, determinants, and interventions for prevention and care of the selected disorders, the volume offers a number of novel contributions to the policy-relevant evidence on MNS disorders.

- First, we present a systematic analysis of the excess mortality associated with these disorders, enhancing our understanding of the true burden of disease attributable to them.
- Second, the discussion of interventions embraces a health system perspective, such that, after a review of the effective interventions for specific disorders, these are then organized according to how they might be delivered across three distinct and complementary platforms: population, community, and health and social care. This approach allows us not only to reflect on how interventions are planned and delivered in health systems, but also to highlight the potential opportunities, synergies, and efficiencies for resource allocation.
- Third, in addition to a review of the recent evidence for cost-effectiveness, the efforts to scale up the community-based services for mental health in selected LMICs—India and Ethiopia—have been examined through the lens of extended cost-effectiveness

analysis to consider the distribution of costs and outcomes, as well as the extent to which policies offer financial protection to households.

We thank the large international group of authors who have contributed to the development of the volume for their time, effort, and thoroughness and for presentation of the evidence succinctly. We hope readers will find that the exhaustive information the authors have synthesized is presented in a manner that is clear and engaging. We thank the Bill & Melinda Gates Foundation for providing funding support to the *DCP3*, the Institute of Medicine for coordinating the peer-review process, and the World Bank staff who coordinated the publication of the volume. We are grateful to the *DCP3* secretariat, in particular, Dean Jamison and Rachel Nugent, for their expert inputs on various chapters. In addition, we thank Brianne Adderley, Kristen Danforth, and Elizabeth Brouwer for their unstinting support, and Rachana Parikh for coordinating the volume.

The findings of this volume make an emphatic case for a substantially increased investment in the prevention of and care for MNS disorders. We document highly cost-effective strategies for the prevention of some MNS disorders and affordable models of care for the delivery of treatment interventions in routine health care platforms through nonspecialist health workers. Such investments make economic sense for two reasons: the interventions we recommend are cost-effective, and the impact of these interventions on social and economic outcomes is immense. The counterfactual situation of not doing enough, which prevails in most populations, is leading to enormous loss of human capital and will hinder the ambition of sustainable development. The evidence in this volume can be translated into practice only with strong political will and commitment from the governments and developmental agencies who now have to make the necessary investments in their scale-up.

We have the evidence to act. There is a moral case to act. The time to act is now.

Vikram Patel
Dan Chisholm
Tarun Dua
Ramanan Laxminarayan
María Elena Medina-Mora

Abbreviations

ACE	Assessing Cost-Effectiveness
ADHD	attention deficit hyperactivity disorder
AEDs	anti-epileptic drugs
AIDS	acquired immune deficiency syndrome
AIMS	Assessment Instrument for Mental Health Systems
APA	American Psychiatric Association
ATS	amphetamine-type stimulants
AUDs	alcohol use disorders
BAC	blood alcohol concentration
BBV	blood-borne virus
BMT	buprenorphine maintenance treatment
BPSD	behavioral and psychological symptoms of dementia
BZP	N-benzylpiperazine
CBI	cognitive behavioral interventions
CBT	cognitive behavioral therapy
CD	conduct disorder
CDC	Centers for Disease Control and Prevention
CEA	cost-effectiveness analysis
ChEI	cholinesterase inhibitors
CHW	community health worker
CHOICE	Choosing Interventions that are Cost-Effective
CI	confidence interval
CoD	cause of death
CRA	comparative risk assessment
CSG	Consejo de Salubridad General
DALYs	disability-adjusted life years
DARE	Drug Abuse Resistance Education
DCP2	*Disease Control Priorities in Developing Countries,* 2nd ed.
DCP	Disease Control Priorities
DOH	Department of Health
DFID	Department of International Development
DSH	deliberate self-harm
DNA	deoxyribonucleic acid
DSM-5	*Diagnostic and Statistical Manual of Mental Disorders,* 5th ed.
DW	disability weight
ECT	electroconvulsive therapy

ECEA	extended cost-effectiveness analysis
EEG	electroencephalogram
EOD	early-onset dementia
ES	effect size
FAS	Fetal Alcohol Syndrome
FASD	Fetal Alcohol Syndrome Disorders
FRP	financial risk protection
GBD	Global burden of disease
GBD 2010	Global Burden of Disease Study 2010
g/dl	grams per deciliter
GDP	gross domestic product
GHE	Global Health Estimates
GNI	gross national income
GRADE	Grading of Recommendations Assessment, Development and Evaluation
HCV	hepatitis C
HICs	high-income countries
HIV/AIDS	human immunodeficiency virus/acquired immune deficiency syndrome
HIV	human immunodeficiency virus
HMT	heroin maintenance treatment
HR	hazard ratio
IASC	Inter-Agency Standing Committee
ICD	International Classification of Diseases
ICT	information and communications technology
IHD	ischemic heart disease
IHME	Institute for Health Metrics and Evaluation
IMAI	Integrated Management of Adult and Adolescent Illness
IOM	Institute of Medicine
IQs	intelligence quotients
INCB	International Narcotics Control Board
IOM	Institute of Medicine
IQR	interquartile range
LICs	low-income countries
LMICs	low- and middle-income countries
MCH	maternal and child health
MDMA	3,4-methylenedioxy-N-methylamphetamine
MDPV	methylenedioxypyrovalerone
MHaPP	Mental Health and Poverty Project
mhGAP	Mental Health Gap Action Programme
MICs	middle-income countries
MMT	methadone maintenance treatment
MNS	mental, neurological, and substance use
MOH	medication-overuse headache
MSIC	Medically Supervised Injecting Centre
NIAAA	National Institute of Alcohol Abuse and Alcoholism
NCD	noncommunicable disease
NICE	National Institute for Health and Clinical Excellence
OCD	obsessive-compulsive disorder
ONDCP	Office of National Drug Control Policy
OOP	out-of-pocket
OR	odds ratio
OST	opioid substitution treatment
PAF	population attributable fractions
PC101	Primary Care 101

PHC	primary health care
PRIME	Programme for Improving Mental health carE
PSST	problem-solving skills therapy
PTSD	post-traumatic stress disorder
QA	quality assurance
QALYs	quality-adjusted life years
QI	quality improvement
RR	relative risk
RCT	randomized controlled trial
SAPS	South African Police Service
SAR	Special Administrative Region
SDG	sustainable development goal
SEL	social emotional learning
SHR	sustained headache relief
SIFs	supervised injecting facilities
SMART	Self-Management and Recovery Training
SMDs	severe mental disorders
SMR	standardized mortality ratio
SNRIs	serotonin-norepinephrine reuptake inhibitors
SSRIs	selective serotonin reuptake inhibitors
TC	therapeutic community
TCA	tricyclic antidepressant
TPO	Transcultural Psychosocial Organization
TTH	tension-type headache
TQ	Ten Question
UHC	universal health coverage
UI	uncertainty interval
UMICs	upper middle-income countries
UNDCP	United Nations International Drug Control Programme
UNODC	United Nations Office on Drugs and Crime
UPF	universal public finance
WHO	World Health Organization
WMH	World Mental Health
WONCA	World Organization of Family Doctors
YLDs	years lived with disability
YLLs	years of life lost

Chapter 1

Global Priorities for Addressing the Burden of Mental, Neurological, and Substance Use Disorders

Vikram Patel, Dan Chisholm, Rachana Parikh, Fiona J. Charlson,
Louisa Degenhardt, Tarun Dua, Alize J. Ferrari, Steven Hyman,
Ramanan Laxminarayan, Carol Levin, Crick Lund, María Elena
Medina-Mora, Inge Petersen, James G. Scott, Rahul Shidhaye,
Lakshmi Vijayakumar, Graham Thornicroft, and Harvey A.
Whiteford, on behalf of the DCP MNS authors group

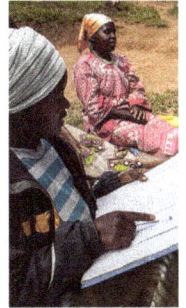

INTRODUCTION

This volume of the third edition of the Disease Control Priorities (DCP) project addresses mental, neurological, and substance use (MNS) disorders. MNS disorders are a heterogeneous range of disorders that owe their origin to a complex array of genetic, biological, psychological, and social factors. Although many health systems deliver care for these disorders through separate channels, with an emphasis on specialist services in hospitals, the disorders have been grouped together in this volume to guide policy makers, particularly in low-resource settings, as they prioritize essential health care packages and delivery platforms (box 1.1).

MNS disorders are grouped together because they share several important characteristics, notably:

- They all owe their symptoms and impairments to some degree of brain dysfunction.
- Social determinants play an important role in the etiology and symptom expression for many of these disorders (box 1.2).
- The disorders frequently co-occur in the same individual.
- Their impact on families and society is profound.
- They are strongly associated with stigma and discrimination.
- They often observe a chronic or relapsing course.
- They all share a pitifully inadequate response from health care systems in all countries, particularly in low- and middle-income countries (LMICs).

Our grouping of MNS disorders is also consistent with programs intended to address their health burden, exemplified by the Mental Health Gap Action Programme (mhGAP) (WHO 2008), and with the goals of the third edition of *Disease Control Priorities (DCP3)* of synthesizing evidence and making recommendations across diverse health conditions. As we emphasize in this volume, these shared characteristics shape the response of countries in addressing the burden of MNS disorders. For example, a strong case is made for an integrated public health response to these conditions in all countries, but particularly in LMICs because of the paucity

Corresponding author: Vikram Patel, Public Health Foundation of India, the London School of Hygiene & Tropical Medicine, and Sangath, Goa, India, vikram.patel@lshtm.ac.uk.

Box 1.1

From the Series Editors of *Disease Control Priorities,* Third Edition

Budgets constrain choices. Policy analysis helps decision makers achieve the greatest value from limited available resources. In 1993, the World Bank published *Disease Control Priorities in Developing Countries (DCP1)*, an attempt to assess the cost-effectiveness (value for money) of interventions in a systematic way that would address the major sources of disease burden in low- and middle-income countries (Jamison and others 1993). The World Bank's 1993 *World Development Report* on health drew heavily on the findings in *DCP1* to conclude that specific interventions against noncommunicable diseases were cost-effective, even in environments in which substantial burdens of infection and undernutrition persisted.

DCP2, published in 2006, updated and extended *DCP1* in several respects, including explicit consideration of the implications for health systems of expanded intervention coverage (Jamison and others 2006). One way that health systems expand intervention coverage is through selected platforms that deliver interventions that require similar logistics but address heterogeneous health problems. Platforms often provide a more natural unit for investment than do individual interventions, but conventional health economics has offered little understanding of how to make choices across platforms. Analysis of the costs of packages and platforms—and the health improvements they can generate in given epidemiological environments—can help guide health system investments and development.

DCP3 differs substantively from *DCP1* and *DCP2* by extending and consolidating the concepts of

platforms and packages, and by offering explicit consideration of the financial risk protection objective of health systems. In populations lacking access to health insurance or prepaid care, medical expenses that are high relative to income can be impoverishing. Where incomes are low, seemingly inexpensive medical procedures can have catastrophic financial effects. *DCP3* offers an approach that explicitly includes financial protection as well as the distribution across income groups of financial and health resulting from policies (for example, public finance) to increase intervention uptake (Verguet, Laxminarayan, and Jamison 2015).

The task in all *DCP* volumes has been to combine the available science about interventions implemented in very specific locales and under very specific conditions with informed judgment to reach reasonable conclusions about the impact of intervention mixes in diverse environments. The broad aim of *DCP3* is to delineate essential intervention packages—such as the package for mental, neurological, and substance use disorders, in this volume—and their related delivery platforms. This information will assist decision makers in allocating often tightly constrained budgets so that health system objectives are maximally achieved.

DCP3's nine volumes are being published in 2015 and 2016 in an environment in which serious discussion continues about quantifying the sustainable development goal (SDG) for health (UN 2015). *DCP3*'s analyses are well-placed to assist in choosing the means to attain the health SDG and assessing the related costs for scaled-up action.

of specialist services in these settings. Such services have been the hallmark of the health system response to these conditions in high-income countries (HICs).

DCP1 had only addressed a few MNS disorders: psychosis and bipolar disorder. *DCP2* had focused on the cost-effectiveness of specific interventions for burdensome disorders, organized separately for mental disorders, neurological disorders, alcohol use disorders, illicit drug use disorders, and learning and developmental disabilities. In this third edition,

we have considered interventions for five groups of disorders—adult mental disorders, child mental and developmental disorders, neurological disorders, alcohol use disorder, and illicit drug use such as opioid dependence—and suicide and self-harm-health outcomes strongly associated with MNS disorders. Within each group, we have prioritized conditions associated with high burden for which there is evidence in support of interventions that are cost-effective and scalable.

Social Determinants of Mental, Neurological, and Substance Use Disorders

A range of social determinants influences the risk and outcome of MNS disorders. In particular, the following factors have been shown to be associated with several MNS disorders (Patel and others 2009):

1. Demographic factors, such as age, gender, and ethnicity
2. Socioeconomic status: low income, unemployment, income inequality, low education, and low social support
3. Neighborhood factors: inadequate housing, overcrowding, neighborhood violence
4. Environmental events: natural disasters, war, conflict, climate change, and migration.
5. Social change associated with changes in income, urbanization, and environmental degradation

The causal mechanisms of the social determinants of MNS disorders indicate a cyclical pattern. On the one hand, socioeconomic adversities increase the risk for MNS disorders (the *social causation* pathway); on the other hand, people living with MNS disorders drift into poverty during the course of their life through increased health care expenditures, reduced economic productivity associated with the disability of their condition, and stigma and discrimination associated with these conditions (the *social drift* pathway).

Understanding the vicious cycle of social determinants and MNS disorders provides opportunities for interventions that target social causation and social drift. In relation to social causation, the evidence for the mental health benefits of poverty alleviation interventions is mixed but growing. In relation to social drift, the evidence for the individual and household economic benefits of the prevention and treatment of MNS disorders is compelling, and supports the economic argument for scaling up these interventions (Lund and others 2011).

Inevitably, such an approach does not address a significant number of conditions, for example, multiple sclerosis as a neurological disorder and anorexia nervosa as an adult mental disorder. However, the recommendations in this volume, particularly regarding the delivery of packages for care, could be extended to other conditions not expressly addressed. In addition, some important MNS disorders or concerns are covered in companion volumes of *DCP3*, notably, nicotine dependence, early childhood development, neurological infections, and stroke.

This volume addresses four overall questions and themes (box 1.3):

- First, we address the question of *why* MNS disorders deserve prioritization by pointing to and reviewing the health and economic burden of disease attributable to MNS disorders. We build on the 2010 estimates of the Global Burden of Diseases, Injuries, and Risk Factors Study (GBD 2010) in two important ways: by examining trends in the burden over time, and by estimating the additional mortality attributable to these disorders.

- Second, we address the question of *what* by reviewing the evidence on the effectiveness of specific interventions for the prevention and treatment of a selection of MNS disorders.
- Third, we consider *how* and *where* these interventions can be appropriately implemented across a range of service delivery platforms.
- Fourth, we address the question of *how much* by examining the cost of scaling up cost-effective interventions and the case for enhanced service coverage and financial protection for MNS disorders.

This chapter also considers how some countries have attempted to incorporate this body of evidence into scaled-up programs for MNS disorders. The chapter discusses lessons on barriers and strategies for how these will need to be addressed for successful scaling-up.

The primary focus of the volume—and *DCP3* as a whole—is on LMICs. We include HICs in the section on global disease burden, and we draw liberally on the concentration of available evidence on intervention effectiveness from these countries.

Box 1.3

Key Messages

This volume of the third edition of *Disease Control Priorities* addresses mental, neurological, and substance use (MNS) disorders. These heterogeneous conditions share several characteristics, not least that they are among the most neglected of diseases globally. This volume focuses on those conditions associated with the greatest burden for which there are effective and scalable interventions. The key findings and messages of the volume are presented in this overview chapter, as well as an assessment of critical health system barriers to scaling up evidence-based interventions and how to overcome them.

The following are the key messages:

1. *The burden of MNS disorders is large, growing, and underestimated.*
   The public health burden of MNS disorders, as estimated by disability-adjusted life years, is on a sharp upward trajectory; it increased by 41 percent between 1990 and 2010 and now accounts for one in every 10 years of lost health globally. Even this sobering statistic is an underestimate, because it does not explicitly take into consideration either the substantial excess mortality associated with these disorders, estimated in this volume for the first time, or the enormous social and economic consequences of MNS disorders on affected persons, their caregivers, and societies.

2. *Many MNS disorders can be prevented and treated effectively.*
   A wide variety of effective interventions can prevent and treat MNS disorders. Although some of these interventions are also supported by evidence of cost-effectiveness, significant gaps remain in the availability of evidence to support the scaling-up of many interventions. Some of these interventions can have significant impacts on other global health and development priorities. For example, the effective management of maternal depression can affect child health outcomes, and the effective management of conduct disorders in children can affect adult antisocial and criminal behavior.

3. *Best practice interventions for MNS disorders can be appropriately implemented across a range of population, community, and health care platforms.*
   - At the population-level platform of service delivery, best practices include legislative and regulatory measures to restrict access to means of self-harm/suicide and reduce the availability of and demand for alcohol.
   - At the community-level platform, best practices include life skills training in schools to build social and emotional competencies in children and adolescents.
   - At the health care platform, which covers self-care, primary health care, and hospital care delivery channels, best practices include self-management of migraine; diagnosis and management of epilepsy, headache, depression, anxiety, alcohol and illicit drug use disorders; and continuing care of schizophrenia and bipolar disorder in primary care.

4. *Public financing of scaling-up is affordable and increases financial protection.*
   The costs of providing a significantly scaled-up package of specified cost-effective interventions for prioritized MNS disorders is estimated at US$3–US$4 per capita of total population per year in low- and lower-middle-income countries, and at least double that in upper-middle-income countries. This package includes interventions at the population, community, and health care levels. Since a significant proportion of MNS disorders may run a chronic and disabling course and adversely affect household welfare, it is important that intervention costs are largely met by governments through increased resource allocation and financial protection measures. Investment of public resources in the prevention and treatment of MNS disorders addresses a large and neglected public health concern; if targeted wisely, this investment will produce substantial economic as well as health benefits in populations at an affordable cost. A policy of moving toward universal public finance can lead to a far more

box continues next page

Box 1.3 (continued)

equitable allocation of public health resources across income groups.

As many countries and the global community move toward a consensus on the need for universal health coverage, this volume provides clear recommendations about which interventions should be prioritized, how they can be delivered, and the expected cost of scaling up these interventions. We provide evidence from four countries to demonstrate how a combination of political will and increased financial commitment to support the delivery of cost-effective preventive and treatment interventions through public systems can lead to significant improvements in service coverage and health outcomes. In most countries, a range of health system barriers will need to be addressed to achieve these goals, not least the

lack of strong and technically sound leadership to guide the scaling-up effort, the relatively low levels of demand for care for some of the most common conditions, the high levels of stigma attached to many conditions, and the continuing reliance on specialized hospital-based care as the primary delivery platform.

Realizing the health gains associated with the interventions recommended in this volume will require more than financial resources. Committed and sustained efforts will be needed to address these barriers. The ultimate goal is massively increasing opportunities for persons with MNS disorders to access services without the prospect of discrimination or impoverishment, and with the hope of attaining optimal health and social outcomes.

WHY MNS DISORDERS MATTER FOR GLOBAL HEALTH

The GBD 2010 identified MNS disorders as significant causes of the world's disease burden (Whiteford and others 2013). The DCP3 series as a whole uses the Global Health Estimates of disease burden. This volume also includes data from the 2010 GBD study, which are used in the burden calculations presented in chapter 3 (Charlson and others 2015). The broad patterns conveyed are the same across the 2010 GBD study (Whiteford and others 2013), the more recent 2013 GBD data (Global Burden of Disease Study 2013 Collaborators 2015), and WHO's Global Health Estimates (WHO 2014).

In chapter 2 in this volume (Whiteford and others 2015), we investigate trends in the burden caused by MNS disorders. There was a 41 percent increase in absolute disability-adjusted life years (DALYs) caused by MNS disorders between 1990 and 2010, from 182 million to 258 million DALYs (the proportion of global disease burden increased from 7.3 to 10.4 percent). With the exception of substance use disorders, which increased because of changes in prevalence over time, this increase was largely caused by population growth and aging.

DALYs are constituted of two components: years of life lost (YLLs) and years lived with disability (YLDs). Figure 1.1 summarizes the proportion of all-cause YLLs and YLDs explained by MNS disorders in 2010. As a group, MNS disorders were the leading cause of YLDs in the world. In 2010, DALYs for MNS disorders were highest during early to mid-adulthood, explaining

18.6 percent of total DALYs for individuals aged 15 to 49 years, compared with 10.4 percent for all ages combined. Within the 15 to 49 years age group, mental and substance use disorders were the leading contributor to the total burden caused by MNS disorders. For neurological disorders, DALYs were highest in the elderly.

There are important gender differences in the burden of these disorders. Overall, males accounted for 48.1 percent and females for 51.9 percent of DALYs for MNS disorders. Males accounted for more DALYs for mental disorders occurring in childhood, schizophrenia, substance use disorders, Parkinson's disease, and epilepsy; whereas, more DALYs accrued to females for all other disorders in this group. The relative proportion of DALYs for MNS disorders to overall disease burden was estimated to be 1.6 times higher in HICs (15.5 percent of total DALYs) than in LMICs (9.4 percent of total DALYs), largely because of the relatively higher burden of other health conditions, such as infectious and perinatal diseases, in LMICs. However, because of the larger population of LMICs, absolute DALYs for MNS disorders are higher in LMICs compared with HICs.

Data from GBD 2010 on burden caused by premature mortality may incorrectly lead to the interpretation that premature death in people with MNS disorders is inconsequential. This interpretation is due to how causes of deaths are assigned in the International Classification of Diseases (ICD) death coding system used by GBD 2010. Yet, evidence shows that people with MNS disorders experience a significant reduction in life expectancy, with the risk of mortality increasing with

Figure 1.1 Proportion of Global YLDs and YLLs Attributable to Mental, Neurological, and Substance Use Disorders, 2010

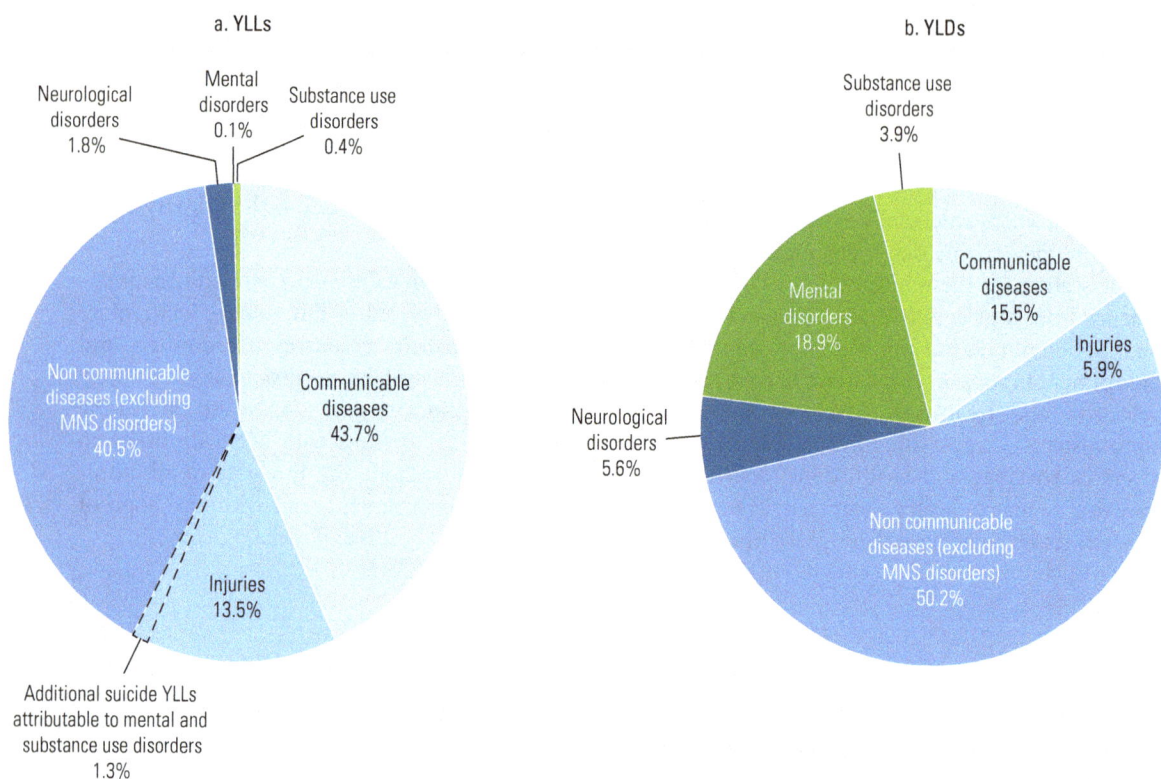

a. YLLs

Neurological disorders 1.8%
Mental disorders 0.1%
Substance use disorders 0.4%
Non communicable diseases (excluding MNS disorders) 40.5%
Communicable diseases 43.7%
Injuries 13.5%
Additional suicide YLLs attributable to mental and substance use disorders 1.3%

b. YLDs

Substance use disorders 3.9%
Mental disorders 18.9%
Neurological disorders 5.6%
Communicable diseases 15.5%
Injuries 5.9%
Non communicable diseases (excluding MNS disorders) 50.2%

Source: Whiteford and others 2015; http://vizhub.healthdata.org/gbd-compare.
Note: In GBD 2010, injuries included deaths and YLLs due to suicide. Mental and substance use disorders explained 22.5 million suicide YLLs, equivalent to 62.1 percent of suicide YLLs or .3 percent of total all-cause YLLs (Ferrari and others 2014).

the severity of the disorder (Chang and others 2011; Lawrence, Hancock, and Kisely 2013; Walker, McGee, and Druss 2015).

Therefore, chapter 3 in this volume (Charlson and others 2015) explores differences between the GBD 2010 estimates of cause-specific and excess mortality of these disorders, and potential contributors to life expectancy gaps. Although reported YLLs accounted for only 15.3 percent of MNS disorder DALYs, equivalent to 840,000 deaths, natural history models generated by DisMod-MR (a disease modeling tool) estimate that substantially more deaths are associated with these disorders. Excess deaths associated with major depression alone were estimated at more than 2.2 million in 2010. This figure is significantly higher than other attempts to quantify these deaths (Walker, McGee, and Druss 2015), and indicates a potentially higher degree of mortality associated with MNS disorders than that captured by GBD 2010 YLLs.

Since these estimates of excess deaths include deaths from causal and non-causal origins, however, they must

be interpreted carefully. Table 1.1 summarizes cause-specific and excess deaths attributable to each MNS disorder. Comparative risk analyses have also highlighted mental and substance use disorders as significant risk factors of premature death from a range of other health outcomes (Lim and others 2012). For example, an estimated 60 percent of suicide deaths can be re-attributed to mental and substance use disorders, elevating them from the fifth to third leading cause of burden of disease (Ferrari and others 2014). These findings strongly suggest the importance of continued assessment of the role MNS disorders play in premature death and as risk factors for other health outcomes.

The estimates of disease burden do not fully take into account the significant social and economic consequences of MNS disorders, not only for affected individuals and households, but also for communities and economies. Notable examples of such impacts include the effects of maternal mental disorders on the well-being of children, contributing to the intergenerational transmission of ill-health and poverty; the effects of

Table 1.1 Cause-Specific and Excess Deaths Associated with Mental, Neurological, and Substance Use Disorders, Global Burden of Disease Study, 2010

Disorder	Cause-specific deaths (uncertainty range)	Excess deaths (uncertainty range)	Contributors to excess deaths
Alzheimer's disease and other dementias	486,000 (308,000–590,000)	2,114,000 (1,304,000–2,882,000)	Lifestyle factors including smoking, hypercholesterolemia, high blood pressure, low forced vital capacity; comorbid physical conditions including cardiovascular disease; infectious disease including pneumonia.
Epilepsy	178,000 (20,000–222,000)	296,000 (261,000–331,000)	Underlying conditions including neoplasms, cerebrovascular diseases, and cardiac disease; accident or injury resultant from status epilepticus including drowning and burns.
Migraine	0	0	N/A
Alcohol use disorders	111,000 (64,000–186,000)	1,954,000 (1,910,000–1,997,000)	Comorbid disease including cancer; mental, neurological, and substance use disorders; cardiovascular disease; liver and pancreas diseases; epilepsy, injuries; and infectious disease.
Opioid dependence	43,000 (27,000–68,000)	404,000 (304,000–499,000)	Acute toxic effects and overdose; accidental injuries, violence, and suicide; comorbid disease including cardiovascular disease, liver disease, mental disorders, and blood-borne bacterial and viral infections.
Cocaine dependence	500 (200–500)[c]	96,000 (60,000–130,000)	
Amphetamine dependence	500 (100–300)[c]	202,000 (155,000–250,000)	
Cannabis dependence	0	0	
Schizophrenia	20,000 (17,000–25,000)	699,000 (504,000–886,000)	Suicide and comorbid disease including cardiovascular disease and diabetes.
Major depressive disorder	0	2,224,000 (1,900,000–2,586,000)	Suicide and comorbid disease such as cardiovascular disease and infectious disease.
Anxiety disorders	0	0[a]	Comorbid disease such as cardiovascular disease and neoplasms; intentional and unintentional injuries.
Bipolar disorder	0	1,320,000 (1,147,000–1,495,000)	Comorbid disease such as cardiovascular disease; causes including intentional injuries/suicide.
Disruptive behavioral disorders	0	0[b]	Unintentional injuries including traffic accidents; lifestyle factors such as smoking, binge drinking, and obesity.
Autistic spectrum disorders	0	109,000 (96,000–122,000)	Accidents, respiratory diseases, and seizures; comorbid conditions, particularly epilepsy and intellectual disability.

Source: Whiteford and others 2015.

a. In GBD 2010, the anxiety disorders category represents "any" anxiety disorder. Although mortality data are available for individual anxiety disorders, estimates of mortality associated with "any" anxiety disorder required for GBD purposes are unavailable.

b. There are currently insufficient data to derive estimates of excess mortality for disruptive behavioral disorders.

c. In the GBD 2010 cause of death modeling, the mean value for cocaine and amphetamine use disorders falls outside of the 95% uncertainty interval. This was because the full distribution of 1,000 draws is asymmetric with a long tail, and a small number of high values in the uncertainty distribution pushes the mean above the 97.5 percentile of distribution.

substance use disorders on criminal behavior and incarceration; and the effects of a range of severe conditions on the economic productivity of affected persons and family members engaged in caregiving.

A recent study estimated that total economic output lost to MNS disorders globally was US$8.5 trillion in 2010, a sum expected to nearly double by 2030 if a concerted response is not mounted (Bloom and others 2011). A separate study estimated the economic costs attributable to alcohol use and alcohol use disorders to amount to the equivalent of between 1.3 and 3.3 percent of gross domestic product (GDP) in a range of high- and middle-income countries, with over two-thirds of the loss represented by productivity losses (Rehm and others 2009).

The global cost of dementia in 2010 was estimated to be US$604 billion, equivalent to 1 percent of global GDP (WHO 2012). In addition, a rising tide of social adversities is associated with MNS disorders (box 1.2). Moreover, large and growing proportions of the global population have been affected by conflict or displacement because of environmental degradation and climate change, which bodes for a grim forecast on the future burden of these conditions.

Finally, the disease burden estimates do not account for the significant hazards faced by persons with MNS disorders in relation to the systematic denial of basic human rights. These costs range from limited opportunities for education and employment, to torture and denial of freedom, sometimes within health care institutions (Patel, Kleinman, and Saraceno 2012).

WHAT WORKS? EFFECTIVE INTERVENTIONS FOR THE PREVENTION AND TREATMENT OF MNS DISORDERS

This section addresses the evidence on effective interventions for a subset of MNS disorders selected because of their contribution to the burden of disease and the availability of cost-effective and scalable interventions. The disorders are organized under five broad groups: adult mental disorders (chapter 4), neurological disorders (chapter 5), illicit drug use disorders (chapter 6), alcohol use disorders (chapter 7), and child mental and developmental disorders (chapter 8). Self-harm and suicide (chapter 9), which are commonly associated with MNS disorders, are also addressed.

The selected disorders have their onset across the life course: epilepsy, anxiety disorders, autism, and intellectual disability in childhood; migraine, depression, psychotic disorders (schizophrenia and bipolar disorders), illicit drug use, and alcohol use disorders in adolescence and young adulthood; and dementia late in life. The epidemiologies of these disorders share some important characteristics: with the exception of dementia, the vast majority of cases have their onset before age 30 years and most tend to run a chronic or relapsing course. In addition, several of the disorders are associated with other health concerns. For example, injecting drug use is associated with HIV/AIDS, alcohol use disorders are associated with road traffic injuries and liver cirrhosis, depression is associated with cardiovascular disease, and maternal depression is associated with child undernutrition and delayed cognitive development (Prince and others 2007).

The evidence on interventions presented in this section builds on the work published in *DCP2* and its findings (Chandra and others 2006; Hyman and others 2006; Rehm and others 2006). The evidence is derived from various sources: the mhGAP guidelines developed by the World Health Organization (WHO) for use in non-specialized health settings, which used the Grading of Recommendations Assessment, Development and Evaluation (GRADE) methodology to review the literature published up to 2009 (Dua and others 2011); other recent reviews, where appropriate, such as Strang and others (2012) for illicit drugs; interventions that require a specialist for delivery but that were not addressed by mhGAP or DCP2, assessed with GRADE; and a review of all reviews. The review of all reviews includes systematic reviews and any type of evaluation evidence from LMICs published since mhGAP and assessed with GRADE. The findings are summarized in table 1.2.

Effective Essential Interventions

A wide variety of effective medicines and psychological and social interventions is available to prevent and treat the range of MNS disorders covered in this volume. As shown in table 1.2, it is possible to identify for this group of conditions a set of *essential medicines* (such as antipsychotic, antidepressant, and anti-epileptic medications) and *essential psychosocial interventions* (such as cognitive behavioral therapy and parent skills training). Although there are very few curative interventions for these disorders, the severity and course of most of them can be greatly attenuated by psychosocial treatment or generic formulations of essential psychotropic medicines, including in combinations tailored to the needs of individuals. A small minority of patients with more severe, refractory, or emergency clinical presentations will require specialist interventions, such as inpatient care with expert nursing for acute psychosis, modified electroconvulsive therapy for severe depression, or surgery for epilepsy.

Table 1.2 Effective Interventions for the Prevention, Treatment, and Care of Mental, Neurological, and Substance Use Disorders

Type of disorder	Preventive interventions	Drug and physical interventions	Psychosocial interventions
MENTAL DISORDERS IN ADULTHOOD			
Schizophrenia (5.3% of total MNS DALYs) *Chronic or relapsing condition characterized by delusions, hallucinations, and disturbed behavior*		Antipsychotic medication***	• Family therapy/support** • Community-based rehabilitation* • Self-help and support groups*
Mood and anxiety disorders (41.9% of total MNS DALYs) *Group of conditions characterized by somatic, emotional, cognitive, and behavioral symptoms; bipolar disorder associated with episodes of elated and depressed mood*	CBT for persons with subthreshold symptoms**	Antidepressant, anxiolytic, mood stabilizer, and antipsychotic medication;*** ECT for severe refractory depression**	• CBT*** • Interpersonal therapy**
MENTAL AND DEVELOPMENTAL DISORDERS IN CHILDHOOD AND ADOLESCENCE			
Conduct disorder (2.2% of total MNS DALYs) *Pattern of antisocial behaviors that violate the basic rights of others or major age-appropriate societal norms*	Life skills education to build social and emotional well-being and competencies;** parenting skills training;** maternal mental health interventions*		• Parenting skills training*** • CBT*
Anxiety disorders (2.3% of total MNS DALYs) *Excessive or inappropriate fear, with associated behavioral disturbances that impair functioning*	Parenting skills training;** maternal mental health interventions**		• CBT***
Autism (1.6% of total MNS DALYs) *Severe impairment in reciprocal social interactions and communication skills, as well as the presence of restricted and stereotypical behaviors*			• Parental education and skills training* • Educational support*
ADHD (0.2% of total MNS DALYs) *Neurodevelopmental disorder characterized by inattention and disorganization, with or without hyperactivity-impulsivity, causing impairment of functioning*	Psychosocial stimulation of infants and young children*	Methylphenidate**	• Parenting skills training** • Cognitive behavioral therapy**

table continues next page

Table 1.2 Effective Interventions for the Prevention, Treatment, and Care of Mental, Neurological, and Substance Use Disorders (continued)

	Type of disorder	Preventive interventions	Drug and physical interventions	Psychosocial interventions
Intellectual disability (idiopathic) (0.4% of total MNS DALYs)	Significantly impaired cognitive functioning and deficits in two or more adaptive behaviors	Psychosocial stimulation of infants and young children;* perinatal interventions, for example screening for congenital hypothyroidism;** population-based interventions targeting intellectual disability risk factors (such as reducing maternal alcohol use)*		• Parental education and skills training* • Educational support*
NEUROLOGICAL DISORDERS				
Migraine (8.7% of total MNS DALYs)	Episodic attacks where headache and nausea are the most characteristic attack features; headache lasting for hours to 2–3 days, typically moderate or severe and likely to be unilateral, pulsating, and aggravated by routine physical activity	Prophylactic drug treatment with propranolol or amitriptyline***	Drug treatments, aspirin or one of several other nonsteroidal anti-inflammatory drugs***	• Behavioral and cognitive interventions*
Epilepsy (6.8% of total MNS DALYs)	A brain disorder traditionally defined as the occurrence of two unprovoked seizures occurring more than 24 hours apart with an enduring predisposition to generate further seizures	Population-based interventions targeting epilepsy risk factors (preventing head injuries, neurocysticercosis prevention)*	Standard anti-epileptic medications (phenobarbital, phenytoin, carbamazepine, valproic acid);*** epilepsy surgery**	
Dementia (4.4% of total MNS DALYs)	A neuropsychiatric syndrome characterized by a combination of progressive cognitive impairment, BPSD, and functional difficulties	Cardiovascular risk factors management (healthy diet, physical activity, tobacco use cessation)*	Cholinesterase inhibitors and memantine for cognitive functions; medications for management of BPSD*	• Caregiver education and support*** • Behavioral training and environmental modifications ** • Interventions to support caregivers of people with dementia*

Table 1.2 Effective Interventions for the Prevention, Treatment, and Care of Mental, Neurological, and Substance Use Disorders (continued)

	Type of disorder	Preventive interventions	Drug and physical interventions	Psychosocial interventions
SUBSTANCE USE DISORDERS				
Alcohol use disorders (6.9% of total MNS DALYs)	*Harmful use is a pattern of alcohol use that causes damage to physical or mental health* *Alcohol dependence is a cluster of physiological, behavioral, and cognitive phenomena in which the use of a substance takes on a much higher priority for a given individual than other behaviors that once had greater value*	• Excise taxes*** • Restriction on sales** • Minimum legal age** • Drunk driving countermeasures** • Advertising bans* • Restrictions on density* • Opening and closing hours and days of sale** • Family interventions*	• Naltrexone, acamprosate*	• Family support* • Motivational enhancement, brief advice, CBT** • Screening and brief interventions*** • Self-help groups*
Illicit drug use disorders (7.8% of total MNS DALYs)	*A pattern of regular use of illicit drugs characterized by significantly impaired control over use and physiological adaptation to regular consumption as indicated by tolerance and withdrawal*	• Psychosocial interventions with primary school children, such as the Good Behavior Game or Strengthening Families Program*	• Opioid substitution therapy (methadone, buprenorphine)***	• Self-help groups, psychological interventions, CBT*
SUICIDE AND SELF-HARM				
Suicide and self-harm (1.47% of GBD; 22.5 million YLLs or 62.1% of suicide YLLs are attributed to mental and substance use disorders in 2010)	*The act of deliberately killing oneself; suicide attempt refers to any nonfatal suicidal behavior and intentional self-inflicted poisoning, injury, or self-harm that may or may not have a fatal intent or outcome*	• Policies and legislation to reduce access to the means of suicide (such as pesticides)*** • Decriminalization of suicide* • Responsible media reporting of suicide*	• Effective drug interventions for underlying MNS disorders** • Emergency management of poisoning**	• Social support and psychological therapies for underlying MNS disorders, Planned follow-up and monitoring of suicide attempters*

Notes: ADHD = Attention Deficit Hyperactivity Disorder; BPSD = behavioral and psychological symptoms; CBT = cognitive behavioral therapy; DALY = disability-adjusted life year; ECT = electroconvulsive therapy; GBD = Global Burden of Diseases; MNS = mental, neurological, and substance use; YLLs = years of life lost.

*** = evidence of cost-effectiveness; ** = strong evidence of effectiveness but not cost-effectiveness;

*** = evidence of effectiveness and either no cost-effectiveness or no evidence of cost-effectiveness.

* = modest evidence of effectiveness and either no cost-effectiveness or no evidence of cost-effectiveness.

Certain preventive interventions that are primarily intended to target disorders covered in other DCP3 volumes, for example, to prevent cardiovascular diseases or neurocysticercosis, will also have benefits for disorders covered in this volume, such as dementia and epilepsy, respectively. Conversely, some interventions targeting MNS disorders are also associated with benefits to health outcomes for other disorders. Examples include injury prevention as a result of reduced alcohol or drug use or effective treatment of Attention Deficit Hyperactivity Disorder, reduced antisocial behaviors and associated social consequences as a result of treatment of conduct disorders in childhood, improved cardiovascular health as a result of recovery from depression, and enhanced early child development as a result of psychosocial stimulation in infancy. Even for those conditions for which there are currently no highly effective treatments for the primary disorder, such as autism and dementia, psychosocial interventions have been shown to be effective in addressing their adverse social consequences and supporting family caregivers.

Limited Access to Essential Interventions

Despite this evidence, many persons affected by MNS disorders do not have access to the interventions. In general, severe MNS disorders tend to have higher rates of contact coverage, while treatment gaps for less visible conditions, such as harmful drinking and depression and anxiety disorders, approach or exceed 90 percent in many populations. Similarly, the coverage rates tend to be much higher for medicines than for psychosocial interventions. Across all disorders, the rates of effective coverage are low. Supply-side and demand-side barriers play a role in explaining these low coverage rates. The lack of adoption of effective interventions is often influenced by concerns about financial resources. This issue is being addressed by a mounting evidence base demonstrating the effectiveness of the delivery of these interventions by nonspecialist health workers (van Ginneken and others 2013), as well as their costs and cost-effectiveness (chapter 12 in this volume, Levin and Chisholm 2015).

A related resource constraint concerns the low availability of appropriately trained mental health workers. Cultural attitudes and beliefs may also pose specific barriers. For example, the moral model of addiction sees it as largely a voluntary behavior in which people freely engage in substance use. By contrast, the medical model of addiction recognizes that a minority of users will lose control over their use and develop a mental or physical disorder—an addiction—that requires specific treatment if sufferers are to become abstinent. As another example, the symptoms associated with depression or anxiety disorders are commonly interpreted as being normative consequences of social adversity, and proven biomedical or psychological causal models are rare, leading to low demand for care and low visibility of the condition from the view of health policy makers and providers (Aggarwal and others 2014). It is clear that these competing views will affect the societal preference for and acceptability of investment in the wider adoption of effective interventions for MNS disorders. More generally, stigma, lack of awareness, and discrimination are major factors behind low levels of political commitment and the paucity of demand for care for persons with MNS disorders in many populations (Saraceno and others 2007).

HOW TO DELIVER EFFECTIVE INTERVENTIONS?

The implementation of evidence-based interventions for MNS disorders seldom occurs through the delivery of single, vertical interventions. More frequently, these interventions are delivered via platforms—the level of the health or welfare system at which interventions or packages can be most appropriately, effectively, and efficiently delivered. A specific delivery channel, such as a school or a primary health care center, can be viewed as the vehicle for delivery of a particular intervention on a specified platform. Identifying the set of interventions that fall within the realm of a particular delivery channel or platform is of interest and relevance to decision makers because it enables potential opportunities, synergies, and efficiencies to be identified. It also reflects how resources are often allocated in practice, for example, to schools or primary health care services, rather than to specific interventions or disorders. This section identifies three broad platforms: population, community, and health care.

There is a fair amount of good evidence from HICs for interventions across these platforms and along the continuum of primary, secondary, and tertiary prevention. However, the evidence base for LMICs is far less robust. Recommendations for best practice and good practice interventions for the platforms are shown in table 1.3. Best practice interventions were identified on the basis of evidence for their effectiveness and contextual acceptability and scalability in LMICs, plus evidence of their cost-effectiveness at least in HICs. Good practice interventions were identified on the basis of sufficient evidence of their effectiveness in HICs and/or promising evidence of their effectiveness in LMICs. The lack of evidence of cost-effectiveness in LMICs reflects the absence

Table 1.3 Intervention Priorities for Mental, Neurological, and Substance Use Disorders by Delivery Platform

| | | **Platforms for intervention delivery** | | | | |
| | | | | **Health care platforms** | | |
Target area	**Population platform**	**Community platform**	**Self-care**	**Primary health care**	**First-level hospital care**	**Specialized care**
All MNS disorders	Awareness campaigns to increase mental health literacy and address stigma and discrimination Legislation on protection of human rights of persons affected by MNS disorders	Training of gatekeepers (community workers, police, teachers) in early identification of priority disorders, provision of low-intensity psychosocial support, and referral pathways Self-help and support groups (for example, for alcohol use disorders, epilepsy, parents of children with developmental disorders, and survivors of suicide)				
Adult mental disorders	Child protection laws	Workplace stress reduction programs and awareness of alcohol and drug abuse	Physical activity Relaxation training Education about early symptoms and their management Web- and smartphone-based psychological therapy for depression and anxiety disorders	Screening and proactive case finding of psychosis, depression, and anxiety disorders **Diagnosis and management of depression (including maternal) and anxiety disorders*** **Continuing care of schizophrenia and bipolar disorder** Management of depression and anxiety disorders in people with HIV, with other NCDs*	Diagnosis and management of acute psychoses Management of severe maternal depression* Management of depression and anxiety disorders in people with HIV, and people with other NCDs*	ECT for severe or refractory depression Management of refractory psychosis with clozapine
Child mental and developmental disorders	Child protection laws	Parenting programs in infancy to promote early child development **Life skills training in schools to build social and emotional competencies** Parenting programs in early and middle childhood (ages 2-14 years) Early child enrichment/preschool education programs Identification of children with	Web- and smartphone-based psychological therapy for depression and anxiety disorders in adolescents	Screening for developmental disorders in children Maternal mental health interventions Parent skills training for developmental disorders **Psychological treatment for mood, anxiety, ADHD, and disruptive behavior disorders*** Improve the quality of antenatal and perinatal care to reduce risk factors	Diagnosis of childhood mental disorders such as autism and ADHD Stimulant medication for severe cases of ADHD Newborn screening for modifiable risk factors for intellectual disability	

Table 1.3 Intervention Priorities for Mental, Neurological, and Substance Use Disorders by Delivery Platform (continued)

Target area	Platforms for intervention delivery			Health care platforms		
	Population platform	Community platform	Self-care	Primary health care	First-level hospital care	Specialized care
Neurological disorders	Policy interventions to address the risk factors for cardio-vascular diseases, for example, tobacco control Improved control of neurocysticercosis		**Self-managed treatment of migraine** Self-identification/management of seizure triggers Self-management of risk factors for vascular disease (healthy diet, physical activity, tobacco use)	**Diagnosis and management of epilepsy and headaches** Screening for detection of dementia Interventions to support caregivers of patients with dementia Management of prolonged seizures or status epilepticus	Diagnosis of dementia and secondary causes of headache	Surgery for refractory epilepsy
Alcohol and illicit drug use disorders	**Regulate the availability and demand for alcohol (for example, increases in excise taxes on alcohol products, advertising bans)** Penalize risky behaviors associated with alcohol (enforcement of BAC limits)	Awareness campaigns to reduce maternal alcohol use during pregnancy	Self-monitoring of substance use	**Screening and brief interventions for alcohol use disorders** **Opioid substitution therapy (methadone and buprenorphine) for opioid dependence**	Management of severe dependence and withdrawal	Psychological treatments (CBT) for refractory cases*
Suicide and self-harm	**Control the sale and distribution of means of suicide (such as pesticides)** Decriminalize suicide	Safer storage of pesticides in the community and farming households	Web- and smartphone-based treatment for depression and self-harm	Primary health care packages for underlying MNS disorders (as described above)* Planned follow-up and monitoring of suicide attempters* Emergency management of poisoning	Treatment of comorbid mood and substance use disorder*	Specialist health care packages for underlying MNS disorders (as described above)

Note: Red type denotes urgent care; blue type denotes continuing care, black type denotes routine care. Recommendations in **bold** = best practice, recommendations in normal font = good practice.

ADHD = Attention Deficit Hyperactivity Disorder; BAC = blood alcohol concentration; CBT = cognitive behavioral therapy; ECT = electroconvulsive therapy; HIV = human immunodeficiency virus; MNS = mental, neurological, and substance use; NCDs = noncommunicable diseases.

*There is no fixed time period for the management of these complex conditions; for example, in the management of depression, some individuals need relatively short periods of engagement (for example, 6–12 months for a single episode) at the one end, while others may need maintenance care for several years (for example, when there is a relapsing course).

of evidence rather than the lack of cost-effectiveness for most interventions.

In addition to bridging the treatment gap for MNS disorders by improving access to evidence-based interventions, it is imperative to enhance the quality of service delivery, which together with need and utilization make up the concept of *effective coverage*. The quality of care should not be subservient to the quantity of available and accessible services, not least since robust quality improvement mechanisms ensure that limited resources are utilized appropriately. Good quality services also build people's confidence in care, thereby fueling the demand for and increased utilization of preventive and treatment interventions.

Population and Community Platforms

Chapter 10 in this volume (Petersen and others 2015) outlines the intervention packages for delivery through the population and community platforms. *Population* platform interventions typically apply to the entire population and mainly revolve around promoting mental health, preventing MNS disorders, and addressing demand-side barriers. Best practice packages include legislative and regulatory measures to restrict access to means of self-harm/suicide (notably pesticides) and reduce the availability of and demand for alcohol, including increased taxes and advertising bans. Good practice packages include interventions aimed at raising mental health literacy and reducing stigma and discrimination. The criminal justice system offers an important channel for the delivery of interventions for a range of MNS disorders, notably those associated with alcohol and illicit drug use, behavior disorders in adolescents, and psychoses.

Other preventive and promotion interventions do not require such a populationwide approach. These interventions are best delivered by targeting a group of people in the community that share a certain characteristic or are part of a particular setting, such as children in school. This platform is referred to as the *community*. Best practice packages at the community level include life skills training to build social and emotional competencies in children and adolescents (school-based programs and programs that target vulnerable children). Good practice packages at the community level are reported in table 1.3.

Health Care Platform

Chapter 11 in this volume (Shidhaye, Lund, and Chisholm 2015) outlines the packages pertaining to the *health care* platform through three specific delivery channels: self-management and care, primary health care (which includes outreach services in the community), and hospital care (which include MNS specialist services and other specialist services, such as HIV or maternal health care).

Examples of best or good practice packages for self-care include the self-management of conditions, such as migraines, and web-based psychological therapy for depression and anxiety disorders, increasingly enabled by internet- and smartphone-based delivery.

At the primary health care level, a range of case-finding, detection, and diagnostic measures, as well as the psychological and pharmacological management of such conditions, can be effectively performed. The conditions include depression (including maternal depression), anxiety disorders, migraines, and alcohol and illicit drug use disorders, as well as continuing care for severe disorders such as epilepsy or psychosis.

The recommended delivery model is collaborative stepped care, in which patient care is coordinated by a primary care–based nonspecialist case manager who carries out a range of tasks including screening, provision of psychosocial interventions, and proactive monitoring, while working in close liaison with, and acting as a link between the patient, primary care physician, and specialist services. A robust evidence base supports the delivery of psychosocial interventions by appropriately trained and supervised nonspecialist health workers (van Ginneken and others 2013) and the collaborative stepped care model of delivery (Patel and others 2013).

At the hospital level, first-level hospitals, typically district hospitals, offer a range of medical care services focused on providing integrated care for MNS disorders, by implementing the same packages as recommended for the primary care channel. In particular, first-level hospitals offer those services where MNS disorders frequently co-occur, such as maternal health, other noncommunicable diseases, and HIV/AIDS (Kaaya and others 2013; Ngo and others 2013; Rahman and others 2013). Specialist health care may be offered in first-level hospitals or separate specialist hospitals, such as psychiatric hospitals or de-addiction centers. Specialist health care delivery channels focus on the diagnosis and management of complex, refractory, and severe cases (for example for psychosis, bipolar disorder, or refractory epilepsy); childhood behavioral disorders; dementia; severe alcohol or illicit drug dependence and withdrawal; and severe depression.

A small minority of individuals with MNS disorders will require ongoing care in community-based residential facilities because of their disability and lack of alternative sources of care and support. The role of community outreach teams that can provide variable levels of intensity of care appropriate for individuals' needs is also crucial as they provide support to enable these individuals to function in an independent way, in the community, alongside close liaison with general primary care services and other social and criminal justice services.

Humanitarian Aid and Emergency Response

In humanitarian contexts and emergency affected populations, such as those arising from conflicts or natural disasters, the humanitarian aid and emergency response channel is yet another channel for delivering much needed mental health care. These populations are at an increased risk of MNS disorders that can overwhelm the local capacity to respond, particularly if the existing infrastructure or health system was already weak or may have been rendered dysfunctional as a result of the emergency situation. There is a heightened need to identify and allocate resources for providing mental health care and psychosocial support in these settings, for those with disorders induced by the emergency and for those with preexisting disorders. International humanitarian aid and emergency response at the national level can be a channel for rapidly enabling or supporting the availability of and access to basic or specialist care. In several countries, such emergencies have actually provided opportunities for systemic change or service reform in public mental health (WHO 2013b; see also box 1.4).

Box 1.4

Country Case Studies on Scaling Up Interventions for Mental, Neurological, and Substance Use Disorders

The 686 Project: China (Hong 2012)

The Central Government Support for the Local Management and Treatment of Severe Mental Illnesses Project was initiated in China in 2004 with the first financial allotment of ¥ 6.86 million (US$829,000 in 2004 dollars). Subsequently it was referred to as the 686 Project. Modeled on the World Health Organization's (WHO's) recommended method for integrating hospital-based and community-based mental health services, this program provides care for a range of severe mental disorders through the delivery of a community-based package by multidisciplinary teams.

The interventions are functionality oriented and provide free outpatient treatment through insurance coverage (New Rural Cooperative Medical Care system) along with subsidized inpatient treatment for poor patients. The program covered 30 percent of the population of China by the end of 2011. Evaluation of the program showed improved outcomes for the more than 280,000 registered patients, as the proportion of patients with severe mental illnesses who did not suffer a relapse for five years or longer increased from a baseline of 67 percent to 90 percent, along with large reductions in the rates of "creating disturbances" and "causing serious accidents."

Government investment in the program amounted to ¥ 280 million in 2011. The program's key innovations were the increase in the availability of human resources, including the involvement of non-mental-health professionals and their intensive capacity building, which increased the number of psychiatrists in the country by one-third.

The National Depression Detection and Treatment Program: Chile (MHIN)

The National Depression Detection and Treatment Program in Chile is a national mental health program that integrates detection and treatment of depression in primary care. The program is based on scaling up an evidence-based collaborative stepped care intervention in which most patients diagnosed with depression are provided medications and psychotherapy at primary care clinics, while only severe cases are referred to specialists. Launched in 2001, the program operates through a network of 500 primary care centers, and presently covers 50 percent of Chile's population.

box continues next page

Box 1.4 (continued)

The program has added many psychologists in primary care, amounting to an increase of 344 percent between 2003 and 2008. Enrollment of patients in the program has grown steadily, with around 100,000 to 125,000 patients starting treatment each year from 2004 to 2006 and close to 170,000 patients starting treatment in 2007. Nationwide implementation of the program has led to greater utilization of health services by women and the less educated, contributing to reduced health inequalities. The program's success can be attributed to the use of an evidence-based design that was made available to policy makers, teamwork, proactive leadership, strategic alliances across sectors, sustained investment and ring-fencing new and essential financial resources, program institutionalization, and sustained development of human resources that can implement the program.

Building Back Better: Burundi (WHO 2013a)

Civil war in the last decade of the 20th century and first decade of this century resulted in widespread massacres and forced migrations and internal displacement of around one million individuals in Burundi. To address this humanitarian crisis, Healthnet Transcultural Psychosocial Organization (TPO) started providing mental health services in Burundi during 2000 when the then Ministry of Public Health had no mental health policy, plan, or unit, and virtually all the psychiatric services were provided by one psychiatric hospital. Healthnet TPO first conducted a needs assessment and then built a network of psychosocial and mental health services in communities in the national capital, Bujumbura, and in seven of the country's 17 provinces. A new health worker cadre, the psychosocial worker, played a pivotal role in delivery of these services.

Considerable progress has been made in the past decade. The government now supplies essential psychiatric medications through its national drug distribution center, and outpatient mental health clinics are established in several provincial hospitals. From 2000 to 2008, more than 27,000 people were helped by newly established mental health and psychosocial services. Between 2006 and 2008, the mental health clinics in the provincial hospitals registered almost 10,000 people, who received more than 60,000 consultations. The majority (65 percent) were people with epilepsy.

In 2011, funding from the Dutch government enabled HealthNet TPO and the Burundian government to initiate a five-year project aimed at strengthening health systems. One of the project's components is the integration of mental health care into primary care using WHO Mental Health Gap Action Programme guidelines. The government has established a national commission for mental health and appropriate steps are being taken to support the provision of mental health care in general hospitals and follow-up within the community.

Suicide Prevention through Pesticide Regulation: Sri Lanka (Gunnell and others 2007)

In Sri Lanka, as well as in other Asian countries, pesticide self-poisoning is one of the most commonly used methods of suicide. Suicide rates in Sri Lanka increased eight-fold from 1950 to 1995, and the country had the highest rate of suicide worldwide (approximately 47 per 100,000 population) during this period. A series of policy and legislative actions around this time reduced the suicide rate by half by 2005.

Gunnell and others (2007) carried out an ecological analysis of trends in suicide and risk factors for suicide in Sri Lanka during 1975–2005. The analysis suggests that the marked decline in Sri Lanka's suicide rate in the mid-1990s coincided with the culmination of a series of legislative activities that systematically banned the most highly toxic pesticides that had been responsible for the majority of pesticide deaths in the preceding two decades. The Registrar of Pesticides banned methyl parathion and parathion in 1984 and over the following years gradually phased out all the remaining Class I (the most toxic) organophosphate pesticides, culminating in July 1995 with bans on the remaining Class I pesticides monocrotophos and methamidophos. By December 1998, endosulfan (a Class II pesticide) was also banned as farmers had substituted Class I pesticides with endosulfan.

By 2005, suicide rates halved to around 25 per 100,000 population. This case study underlines the fact that in countries where pesticides are commonly used in acts of self-poisoning, regulatory controls on the sale of the most toxic pesticides may help to reduce the number of suicides.

HOW MUCH WILL IT COST? MOVING TOWARD UNIVERSAL HEALTH COVERAGE FOR MNS DISORDERS

For successful and sustainable scale-up of effective interventions and innovative service delivery strategies, such as task-sharing and collaborative care, decision makers require not only evidence of an intervention's health impact, but also the costs and cost-effectiveness. Even when cost-effectiveness evidence is available, there remains the question of whether or how an intervention might confer wider economic and social benefits on households or society, such as restored productivity, reduced medical impoverishment, or greater equality.

This volume reviews existing cost-effectiveness evidence and new analyses of the distributional and financial protection effects of interventions (box 1.5).

Intervention Costs and Cost-Effectiveness

There is a small but growing economic evidence base to inform decision making in LMICs, mainly on the treatment of specific disorders. Analysis undertaken at the global level by WHO, updated to 2012 values for DCP3, reveals a marked variation in the cost per DALY averted, not only between different regions of the world, but also between different disorders and interventions (Chisholm and Saxena 2012; Hyman and others 2006).

Box 1.5

Economic Evaluation of the Treatment and Prevention of Mental, Neurological, and Substance Use Disorders

Economic evaluations aim to inform decision making by quantifying the trade-offs between the resource inputs needed for alternative investments and the resulting outcomes. Four approaches to economic evaluation in health are particularly prominent:

1. Assessment of how much of a specific health outcome (for example, depressive episodes or epileptic seizures averted) can be attained for a particular level of resource input.
2. Assessment of how much of an aggregate measure of health (for example, averted deaths, disability, or quality-adjusted life years) can be attained from a particular level of resource inputs applied to alternative interventions. This approach of cost-effectiveness analysis enables comparison of the attractiveness of interventions addressing many different health outcomes (such as tuberculosis or HIV treatment versus prevention of harmful alcohol use or treatment of psychosis).
3. Assessment of how much health and financial risk protection can be attained for a particular level of public sector finance of a particular intervention. This approach (extended cost-effectiveness analysis) enables assessment not only of efficiency in improving the health of a population, but also of efficiency in achieving the other major goal of a health system (that is, protection of the population from financial risk).

4. Assessment of the economic benefits, measured in monetary terms, from investment in a health intervention and weighing that benefit against its cost (benefit-cost analysis). This analysis enables comparison of the attractiveness of health investments compared with those in other sectors.

Cost-effectiveness analyses predominate among economic evaluations in the care and prevention of mental, neurological, and substance use (MNS) disorders. These types of analysis are reviewed in the disorder-specific chapters of the volume and, in a more synthesized format, in chapter 12 (Levin and Chisholm 2015). This review shows that the economic evidence base for mental health policy and planning continues to strengthen. Thus, the overgeneralized claim that treatment of MNS disorders is not a cost-effective use of scarce health care resources can be increasingly debunked.

Extended cost-effectiveness analyses remain a fairly new evaluation approach developed for *Disease Control Priorities*, 3rd edition (*DCP3*). In this volume, Chisholm and others (chapter 13) apply extended cost-effectiveness analysis to a range of MNS disorder interventions in Ethiopia and India. The chapter shows that moving toward universal coverage via scaled-up provision of publicly financed services leads to significant financial protection effects as well as health gains in the population.

Brief interventions for harmful alcohol use and treatment of epilepsy with first-line anti-epileptic medicines fall toward the lower (more favorable) end, while community-based treatment of schizophrenia and bipolar disorder with first-generation medications and psychosocial care fall toward the upper end. Figure 1.2 shows the range for the most cost-effective intervention identified for each of these four conditions (for details, see chapter 12 in this volume, Levin and Chisholm 2015).

Anderson, Chisholm, and Fuhr (2009) analyze the cost-effectiveness of alcohol demand reduction measures. They estimate that one DALY could be averted for as little as US$200–US$400 through increases in excise taxes on alcoholic beverages, and for US$200–US$1,200 through comprehensive advertising bans or reduced availability of retail outlets. Other than that study, there is hardly any published evidence on the cost-effectiveness of population-based or community-level strategies in or for LMICs. For example, there remains a startling paucity of robust economic studies with which to inform planners and policy makers in LMICs about scaled-up efforts to prevent self-harm and suicide, or to enhance the mental and social development of children through parent skills training.

The combined cost of implementing alcohol control measures is estimated to range between US$0.10 and US$0.30 per capita (Anderson, Chisholm, and Fuhr 2009; WHO 2011). A new cost analysis carried out for this volume estimates that a school-based, life skills program would cost between US$0.05 and US$0.25 per capita (Levin and Chisholm 2015). The annual cost of delivering a defined package of cost-effective interventions for schizophrenia, depression, epilepsy, and alcohol use disorders in two WHO subregions (one in Sub-Saharan Africa, the other in South Asia) has been estimated to be US$3–US$4 per capita (Chisholm and Saxena 2012); in HICs and upper-middle-income countries, the cost of such a package is expected to be at least double this amount (chapter 12 in this volume, Levin and Chisholm 2015).

Financial Risk Protection: Extended Cost-Effectiveness Analysis

By considering important goals or attributes of health systems other than health improvement itself, such as equity and financial risk protection, this volume has taken some initial steps toward addressing and analyzing the concept of universal health coverage for MNS disorders (Chisholm and others 2015). These disorders are chronic and disabling, often go undetected, and are regularly omitted from essential packages of care or insurance schemes. Therefore, these health conditions pose a direct threat to households' well-being and economic viability, as a result of private out-of-pocket (OOP) expenditures on health services and goods, as well as diminished production or income opportunities.

Through the application of a newly developed approach to economic evaluation called extended cost-effectiveness analysis (Verguet, Laxminarayan, and Jamison 2015; see also box 1.5), an effort has been made to identify how scaled-up, community-based public services might contribute to greater equality of access and less OOP spending in two distinct settings, India and Ethiopia. Both countries have recently articulated ambitious plans to enhance mental health service quality and coverage, as well as extend financial protection or health insurance for their citizens. Across these two geographical settings, it is evident that publicly financing the scale-up of mental health service leads to a more equitable allocation of public health resources across income groups, with the lowest-income groups benefiting most in financial protection.

For example, an extended cost-effectiveness analysis was done for schizophrenia treatment in India. The analysis shows that public financing of the 70 percent of total treatment costs incurred by households would remove US$140,000 of OOP spending per one million population at current treatment coverage rates. Public financing of a concerted effort to provide an enhanced level of service coverage (80 percent) for all segments of the Indian population would result in a more equitable allocation of resources (as shown in figure 1.3, panel a). This effort would have a clear pro-poor effect (figure 1.3, panel b): 30 percent of the total estimated value of insurance (estimated at US$24,582 for a population of one million persons) is bestowed on the poorest quintile of the population, compared with 10 percent for the richest quintile.

In Ethiopia, where current treatment coverage for psychosis and other mental disorders is very low (10 percent or less), the averted OOP spending arising from a switch to public finance of treatment costs would also be low. Only when a substantial increase in service coverage is modeled does the true scale of the private expenditures that would pertain in the absence of publicly financed care become apparent.

It is therefore vital for increased financial protection of persons with MNS disorders to go hand in hand with scaled-up coverage of an essential package of care. Improved service access without financial protection for persons with MNS disorders will lead to inequitable rates of service uptake and outcomes, while improved financial protection without appropriate service scale-up will bring little public health gain at all. In short, a concerted, multidimensional effort is needed if the move toward universal health coverage for MNS disorders is to occur.

Figure 1.2 Cost-Effectiveness of Selected Interventions for Addressing Mental, Neurological and Substance Use Disorders in Low-income and Middle-income Countries (2012 US$ per DALY averted)

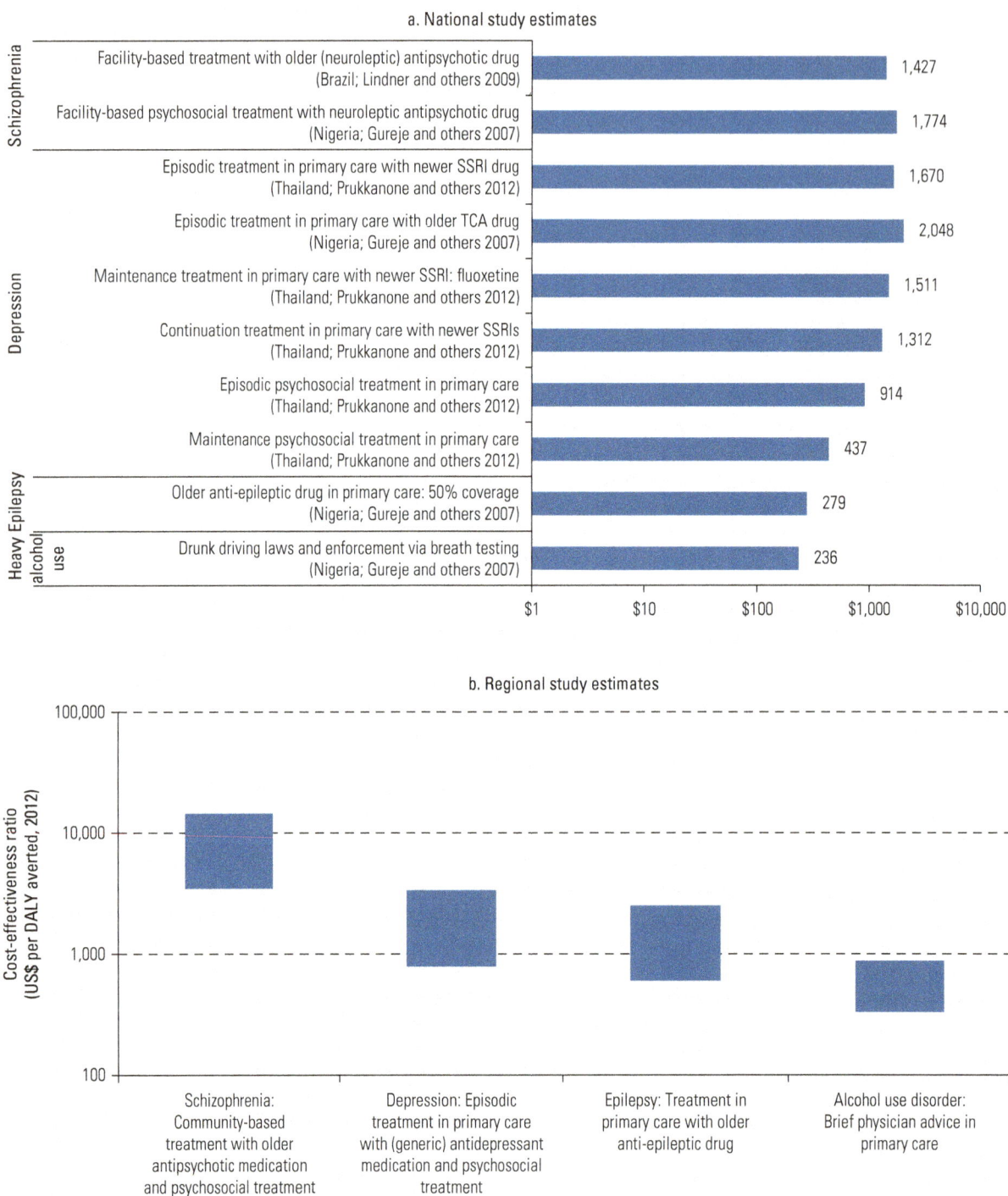

a. National study estimates

Category	Intervention	Value
Schizophrenia	Facility-based treatment with older (neuroleptic) antipsychotic drug (Brazil; Lindner and others 2009)	1,427
Schizophrenia	Facility-based psychosocial treatment with neuroleptic antipsychotic drug (Nigeria; Gureje and others 2007)	1,774
Depression	Episodic treatment in primary care with newer SSRI drug (Thailand; Prukkanone and others 2012)	1,670
Depression	Episodic treatment in primary care with older TCA drug (Nigeria; Gureje and others 2007)	2,048
Depression	Maintenance treatment in primary care with newer SSRI: fluoxetine (Thailand; Prukkanone and others 2012)	1,511
Depression	Continuation treatment in primary care with newer SSRIs (Thailand; Prukkanone and others 2012)	1,312
Depression	Episodic psychosocial treatment in primary care (Thailand; Prukkanone and others 2012)	914
Depression	Maintenance psychosocial treatment in primary care (Thailand; Prukkanone and others 2012)	437
Epilepsy	Older anti-epileptic drug in primary care: 50% coverage (Nigeria; Gureje and others 2007)	279
Heavy alcohol use	Drunk driving laws and enforcement via breath testing (Nigeria; Gureje and others 2007)	236

Axis: $1 $10 $100 $1,000 $10,000

b. Regional study estimates

Cost-effectiveness ratio (US$ per DALY averted, 2012)

Axis: 100,000 / 10,000 / 1,000 / 100

- Schizophrenia: Community-based treatment with older antipsychotic medication and psychosocial treatment
- Depression: Episodic treatment in primary care with (generic) antidepressant medication and psychosocial treatment
- Epilepsy: Treatment in primary care with older anti-epileptic drug
- Alcohol use disorder: Brief physician advice in primary care

Source: Hyman and others 2006; Chisholm and Saxena 2012; Levin and Chisholm 2015.
Note: In panel a, all reported cost-effectiveness estimates have been converted to 2012 US$. In panel b, previously published findings have been converted to 2012 US$ values, based on International Monetary Fund inflation estimates for World Bank reporting regions. Bars show the range in cost-effectiveness for six low- and middle-income world regions: Sub-Saharan Africa, Latin America and the Caribbean, Middle East and North Africa, Europe and Central Asia, South Asia, and East Asia and Pacific. DALY = disability-adjusted life year; SSRI = selective serotonin reuptake inhibitor; TCA = tricyclic antidepressants.

Figure 1.3 Distribution of Public Spending and Insurance Value of Enhanced Public Finance for Schizophrenia Treatment in India, by Income Quintile

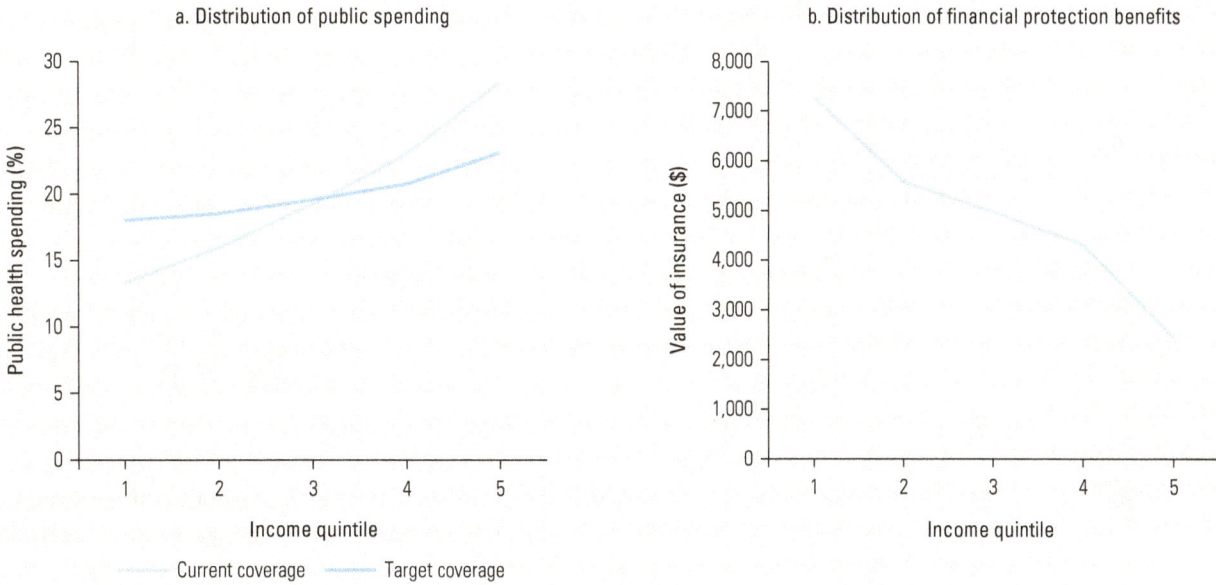

a. Distribution of public spending

b. Distribution of financial protection benefits

Current coverage Target coverage

Source: Chisholm and others 2015 (chapter 13 in this volume).
Note: Results are based on a population of one million people, divided into equal income quintiles of 200,000 persons (quintile 1 has the lowest income and quintile 5 the highest). Monetary values are expressed in 2012 US$. Target coverage for schizophrenia treatment for all income groups is set at 80 percent. Current coverage ranges from 30 percent in the poorest income group 50 percent in the richest. Panel A shows the distribution of public health spending across income groups before and after the introduction of universal public finance. Panel B shows the distribution of financial protection benefits across income groups resulting from a policy of universal public finance; the value of insurance is per income quintile (each with 200,000 persons).

HOW TO SCALE UP? HEALTH SYSTEM BARRIERS AND OPPORTUNITIES

Despite the need for renewed attention and scaled-up investment, there is relatively little action on addressing MNS disorders in most LMICs. There are several reasons for this lack of action, perhaps the most important one being the overall lack of policy commitment to MNS disorders, as is evident from the fact that less than 1 percent of the health budget is allocated to mental health in most LMICs (Saxena and others 2007). Similarly, despite the evidence-based calls to action for scaling up services for almost a decade (Lancet Global Mental Health Group 2007), less than 1 percent of development assistance for health is devoted to mental health (Gilbert and others 2015).

Political Will

Key contributors to the lack of political will and consequently low levels of resource allocation include the low demand for mental health care interventions, which is in part caused by low levels of mental health literacy and high levels of stigma attached to MNS

disorders. In addition, the following are lacking: technically sound leadership in designing and implementing evidence-based programs; adequate absorptive capacity in the existing health care system; competing policy priorities and vested interests; and effective agency and advocacy by affected people. And there is a persisting belief in the importance of hospital-based specialized models of care, which continue to absorb disproportionate amounts of the already meager budgetary allocations for this sector (Saraceno and others 2007).

Knowledge Gaps

There is a lack of evidence from LMICs, especially on the cost-effectiveness of many interventions and the integration of care for MNS disorders in routine health and social care platforms. This lack continues to represent a constraint to investment for many stakeholders, and is partly a result of low levels of political commitment to this dimension of health through disproportionately less funding for research. The critical knowledge gaps are related to implementation science, that is, research to bridge the gap between what we know works and how to implement it at scale (Collins and others 2011).

Research that seeks to address the significant knowledge gaps on the causes of MNS disorders and the discovery of novel interventions is also urgently needed. An empirical approach to analysis of the impact of macroeconomic and structural factors on the burden of MNS disorders, such as global conventions on the regulation of illicit drugs and climate change, is warranted to guide evidence-based policy making in the wider context. However, these knowledge gaps cannot explain why even known cost-effective interventions have not been adopted.

A complicating factor is the limitations of the evidence synthesized in this chapter. In particular, there are significant gaps in the evidence in support of some interventions in LMICs and limited effectiveness of the best available interventions for some disorders. To address these barriers, the scaling-up of interventions for MNS disorders requires an approach that embraces public health principles, systems thinking, and a whole-of-government perspective. Reassuringly, several countries are now demonstrating how a combination of these ingredients can lead to significant increases in the coverage of evidence-based interventions (box 1.4).

Strategies for Strengthening the Health System

Key strategies for strengthening the health system include the following:

- Mainstreaming a rights-based perspective throughout the health system and ensuring health policies, plans, and laws are updated to be consistent with international human rights standards and conventions
- Implementing multicomponent initiatives to address stigma, enhance mental health literacy and demand for care, and mobilize people with the conditions to support one another and be effective advocates
- Engaging other key sectors concerned with MNS disorders to improve services, notably the social care, non-governmental organizations, private sector, criminal justice, education, and indigenous medical sectors, as they all have complementary roles.
- Providing inpatient care through units in general or district hospitals rather than standalone psychiatric hospitals
- Implementing large-scale or national rollouts of training and supervision programs for nonspecialist human resource cadres that can perform the roles of case managers for delivery of collaborative care in primary care and other health care platforms to improve treatment coverage
- Ensuring the supply of essential medicines at relevant platforms

- Investing in research across the translational continuum to improve knowledge on more effective interventions and more effective delivery systems, including innovative financing options such as raising and diverting income from taxes on unhealthy products (such as alcohol and tobacco)
- Emphasizing the use of low-cost generic medicines throughout the health care systems, and reallocating expenditure on ineffective or low-value interventions, such as overprescription of benzodiazepines and vitamins in primary care.
- Finally, it will be important to embed health indicators for MNS disorders within national health information and surveillance systems so that progress and achievements can be monitored and evaluated (WHO 2015).

The WHO Comprehensive Mental Health Action Plan (Saxena, Funk, and Chisholm 2013) offers a clear road map for countries at any stage of the journey to scale up. Some regions (such as the Eastern Mediterranean) have adapted this new policy instrument to initiate consultations with international experts and regional policy makers and develop frameworks for action (box 1.6) across all four domains of the plan, along with priority interventions and indicators for evaluation of progress (Gater, Saeed, and Rahman 2015).

TIME TO ACT NOW

MNS disorders account for a substantial proportion of the global disease burden. This burden has increased dramatically since 1990 and is likely to continue to rise with the epidemiological transition from infectious diseases to noncommunicable diseases, the demographic transition in LMICs, and the increase in the prevalence of several social determinants associated with these conditions.

Despite the challenges in quantifying causal mortality in these disorders, new analyses presented in this volume suggest that the mortality-associated disease burden is very large and was previously underestimated. This volume also summarizes evidence to document effective treatment and prevention interventions that are feasible to implement across diverse socioeconomic and cultural settings for a range of priority MNS disorders. A critically relevant aspect of these disorders is their propensity to strike early in life, which is a key factor behind their large contribution to the global burden of disease.

Populationwide platforms are primarily suited for policy-level interventions for promoting mental health, preventing MNS disorders, improving mental health literacy, and protecting the human rights of persons affected by these disorders. The community platform provides opportunities for leveraging non-health

Box 1.6

Proposed Regional Framework to Scale Up Action on Mental Health in the WHO Eastern Mediterranean Region

Domain	Strategic interventions	Proposed indicators
Leadership and governance	• Establish/update a multisector national policy/ strategic action plan for mental health in line with international and regional human rights instruments. • Establish a structure, as appropriate for the national context, to facilitate and monitor implementation of the multisector national policy/strategic action plan. • Review legislation related to mental health in line with international human rights covenants and instruments. • Include defined priority mental health conditions in the basic health delivery package of the government and social and private insurance reimbursement schemes. • Increase and prioritize budgetary allocations to address the agreed upon service targets and priorities, including providing transitional or bridge funding.	• Country has an operational multisectoral national mental health policy or plan in line with international and regional human rights instruments. • Country has an updated mental health law in line with international and regional human rights instruments. • Inclusion of specified priority mental health conditions in the basic health care packages for public and private insurance and reimbursement schemes.
Reorientation and scaling-up of mental health services	• Establish mental health services in general hospitals for outpatient and short-stay inpatient care. • Integrate delivery of evidence-based interventions for priority mental health conditions in primary health care and other priority health programs. • Enable people with mental health conditions and their families through self-help and community-based interventions. • Downsize the existing long-stay mental hospitals (in parallel with investment increases in integrated inpatient and general hospitals and supported residential care in the community).[a] • Embed mental health and psychosocial support in national emergency preparedness and recovery plans. • Strengthen the capacity of health professionals for recognition and management of priority mental health conditions during emergencies. • Implement evidence-informed interventions for psychosocial assistance to vulnerable groups.	• Proportion of general hospitals that have mental health units including inpatient and outpatient units. • Proportion of persons with mental health conditions utilizing health services (disaggregated by age, sex, diagnosis, and setting). • Proportion of PHC facilities having regular availability of essential psychotropic medicines. • Proportion of PHC facilities with at least one staff trained to deliver nonpharmacological interventions. • Proportion of mental health facilities monitored annually to ensure use of quality and rights standards for the protection of human rights of persons with mental health conditions. • Mental health and psychosocial support provision is integrated in the national emergency preparedness plans. • Proportion of health care workers trained in recognition and management of priority mental health conditions during emergencies.

box continues next page

Box 1.6 (continued)

Domain	Strategic interventions	Proposed indicators
Promotion and prevention	• Integrate recognition and management of maternal depression and parenting skills training in maternal and child health programs. • Integrate life skills education with a whole-school approach. • Reduce access to means of suicide. • Employ evidence-based methods to improve mental health literacy and reduce stigma.	• Proportion of community workers trained in early recognition and management of maternal depression and providing early childhood care and development and parenting skills to mothers and families. • Proportion of schools implementing the whole-school approach to promote life skills.
Information, evidence, and research	• Integrate the core indicators within the national health information systems. • Enhance the national capacity to undertake prioritized research. • Engage stakeholders in research planning, implementation, and dissemination.	• Routine data and reports at the national level available on core set of mental health indicators. • Annual reporting of national data on numbers of deaths by suicide.

Source: Gater, Saeed, and Rahman 2015.
Note: PHC = primary health care; WHO = World Health Organization.
a. Modified by authors.

resources for prevention and promotion interventions targeting particular groups of people or particular settings. The health care interventions primarily comprise generic medicines, brief psychological treatments, and social interventions. Interventions for diverse disorders can be packaged together to deploy low-cost and widely available human resources in primary health care and non-health care platforms, with appropriate support and supervision provided by mental health care professionals. In settings with a higher level of resources, as is the case in many middle-income countries, specialist platforms offer incremental value in addressing the needs of the relatively small proportion of persons with complex, severe, or refractory clinical presentations.

Apart from being effective and feasible and providing benefits that improve the lifelong trajectories of individuals, many of these interventions are also inexpensive to implement and represent a cost-effective use of resources for health. Furthermore, a policy of moving toward universal public finance for MNS disorders can be expected to lead to a far more equitable allocation of public health resources across income groups. With universal public finance, the lowest-income groups would benefit most from the value of insurance (used here as a measure of financial protection).

Country case studies show that the most important drivers of change are the political will and commitment of countries and development agencies to allocate the necessary resources and provide technical leadership. As also emphasized in the WHO Mental Health Action Plan, this will and commitment are essential to address the avoidable toll of suffering caused by MNS disorders, not least among the poorest people and least resourced countries in the world.

This volume presents strong clinical and economic evidence to back this investment. Ultimately there must also be a moral case for scaling up care for the hundreds of millions of people whose health care needs have been systematically neglected and whose basic human rights have been routinely denied (Patel, Saraceno, and Kleinman 2006). The time to act on this evidence is therefore now.

NOTE

Disclaimer: Dan Chisholm and Tarun Dua are staff members of the World Health Organization. The authors alone are responsible for the views expressed in this publication and they do not necessarily represent the decisions, policy, or views of the World Health Organization.

World Bank Income Classifications as of July 2014 are as follows, based on estimates of gross national income (GNI) per capita for 2013:

• Low-income countries (LICs) = US$1,045 or less
• Middle-income countries (MICs) are subdivided:
  a) Lower-middle-income = US$1,045 to US$4,125
  b) Upper-middle-income (UMICs) = US$4,126 to US$12,735
• High-income countries (HICs) = US$12,736 or more.

REFERENCES

Aggarwal, N. K., M. Balaji, S. Kumar, R. Mohanraj, A. Rahman, and others. 2014. "Using Consumer Perspectives to Inform the Cultural Adaptation of Psychological Treatments for Depression: A Mixed Methods Study from South Asia." *Journal of Affective Disorders* 163: 88–101.

Anderson, P., D. Chisholm, and D. Fuhr. 2009. "Effectiveness and Cost-Effectiveness of Policies and Programmes to Reduce the Harm Caused by Alcohol." *The Lancet* 373: 2234–46.

Bloom, D. E., E. T. Cafiero, E. Jane-Llopis, S. Abrahams-Gessel, L. R. Bloom, and others. 2011. *The Global Economic Burden of Noncommunicable Diseases*. Geneva: World Economic Forum.

Chandra, V., R. Pandav, R. Laxminarayan, C. Tanner, B. Manyam, and others. 2006. "Neurological Disorders." In *Disease Control Priorities in Developing Countries*, 2nd ed., edited by D. T. Jamison, J. G. Breman, A. R. Measham, G. Alleyene, M. Claeson, and D. B. Evans, P. Jha, A. Mills, and P. Musgrove. Washington, DC: World Bank and Oxford University Press.

Chang, C. K., R. D. Hayes, G. Perera, M. T. Broadbent, A. C. Fernandes, and others. 2011. "Life Expectancy at Birth for People with Serious Mental Illness and Other Major Disorders from a Secondary Mental Health Care Case Register in London." *PLoS One* 6 (5): e19590. doi:10.1371/journal.pone.0019590.

Charlson, F. J., A. J. Baxter, T. Dua, L. Degenhardt, H. A. Whiteford, and T. Vos. 2015. "Excess Mortality from Mental, Neurological and Substance Use Disorders in the Global Burden of Disease Study 2010." In *Disease Control Priorities* (third edition): Volume 4, *Mental, Neurological, and Substance Use Disorders*, edited by V. Patel, D. Chisholm, T. Dua, R. Laxminarayan, and M. E. Medina-Mora. Washington, DC: World Bank.

Chisholm, D., and S. Saxena. 2012. "Cost Effectiveness of Strategies to Combat Neuropsychiatric Conditions in Sub-Saharan Africa and South East Asia: Mathematical Modelling Study." *BMJ* 344:e609. doi:10.1136/bmj.e609.

Chisholm, D., K. A. Raykar, N. Meggido, I. Nigam, A. Nigam, K. B. Strand, A. Colson, A. Fekadu, and S. Verguet. 2015. "Universal Health Coverage for Mental, Neurological, and Substance Use Disorders: An Extended Cost-Effectiveness Analysis." In *Disease Control Priorities* (third edition): Volume 4, *Mental, Neurological, and Substance Use Disorders*, edited by V. Patel, D. Chisholm, T. Dua, R. Laxminarayan, and M. E. Medina-Mora. Washington, DC: World Bank.

Collins, P. Y., V. Patel, S. S. Joestl, D. March, T. R. Insel, and others. 2011. "Grand Challenges in Global Mental Health." *Nature* 475 (7354): 27–30. doi:10.1038/475027a.

Dua, T., C. Barbui, N. Clark, A. Fleischmann, V. Poznyak, and others. 2011. "Evidence-Based Guidelines for Mental, Neurological, and Substance Use Disorders in Low- and Middle-Income Countries: Summary of WHO Recommendations." *PLoS Med* 8 (11): e1001122. doi:10.1371/journal.pmed.1001122.

Ferrari, A. J., R. E. Norman, G. Freedman, A. J. Baxter, J. E. Pirkis, and others. 2014. "The Burden Attributable to Mental and Substance Use Disorders As Risk Factors for Suicide: Findings from the Global Burden of Disease Study 2010." *PLoS One* 9 (4):e91936. doi:10.1371/journal.pone.0091936.

Gater, R., K. Saeed, and A. Rahman, A. 2015. "From Plan to Framework: The Process Followed in the Development of the Regional Framework for Scaling Up Action on Mental Health towards the Implementation of the Comprehensive Mental Health Action Plan 2013-2020 in the Eastern Mediterranean Region." *Eastern Mediterranean Health Journal* 21 (7): 464–66.

Gilbert, B., V. Patel, P. Farmer, and C. Lu. 2015. "Assessing Development Assistance for Mental Health in Developing Countries: 2007-2013. " *PLoS Medicine* 12 (6): e1001834.

Global Burden of Disease Study 2013 Collaborators. 2015. "Global, Regional, and National Incidence, Prevalence, and Years Lived with Disability for 301 Acute and Chronic Diseases and Injuries in 188 Countries, 1990–2013: A Systematic Analysis for the Global Burden of Disease Study 2013." *The Lancet* 386: 743–800. http://www.thelancet.com/journals/lancet/article/PIIS0140-6736%2815%2960692-4/abstract.

Gunnell, D., R. Fernando, M. Hewagama, W. D. Priyangika, F. Konradsen, and others. 2007. "The Impact of Pesticide Regulations on Suicide in Sri Lanka." *International Journal of Epidemiology* 36 (6): 1235–42. doi:dym164 [pii]10.1093/ije/dym164.

Gureje, O., D. Chisholm, L. Kola, V. Lasebikan, and S. Saxena. 2007. "Cost-Effectiveness of an Essential Mental Health Intervention Package in Nigeria." *World Psychiatry* 6 (1): 42–48.

Hong, M. A. 2012. "Integration of Hospital and Community Services—The '686 Project'—Is a Crucial Component in the Reform of China's Mental Health Services." *Shanghai Archives of Psychiatry* 24 (3): 172–74. doi:10.3969/j.issn.1002-0829.2012.03.007.

Hyman, S., D. Chisholm, R. Kessler, V. Patel, and H. Whiteford. 2006. "Mental Disorders." In *Disease Control Priorities in Developing Countries*, 2nd ed., edited by D. T. Jamison, J. G. Breman, A. R. Measham, G. Alleyne, M. Claeson, and D. B. Evans, P. Jha, A. Mills and P. Musgrove. Washington, DC: World Bank and Oxford University Press.

Jamison, D. T., J. G. Breman, A. R. Measham, G. Alleyne, M. Claeson, D. B. Evans, P. Jha, A. Mills, and P. Musgrove, eds. 2006. *Disease Control Priorities in Developing Countries*, 2nd edition. Washington, DC: World Bank and Oxford University Press.

Jamison, D. T., W. H. Mosley, A. R. Measham, and J. L. Bobadilla, eds. 1993. *Disease Control Priorities in Developing Countries*. New York: Oxford University Press.

Kaaya, S. F., E. Eustache, I. Lapidos-Salaiz, S. Musisi, C. Psaros, and others. 2013. "Grand Challenges: Improving HIV Treatment Outcomes by Integrating Interventions for Co-morbid Mental Illness." *PLoS Med* 10: e1001447.

Lancet Global Mental Health Group. 2007. "Scale Up Services for Mental Disorders: A Call for Action." *The Lancet* 370: 1241–52.

Lawrence, D., K. J. Hancock, and S. Kisely. 2013. "The Gap in Life Expectancy from Preventable Physical Illness in Psychiatric Patients in Western Australia: Retrospective Analysis of Population Based Registers." *BMJ* 346: f2539. doi:10.1136/bmj.f2539.

Levin, C., and D. Chisholm. 2015. "Cost and Cost-Effectiveness of Interventions, Policies, and Platforms for the Prevention and Treatment of Mental, Neurological, and Substance Use Disorders." In *Disease Control Priorities* (third edition): Volume 4, *Mental, Neurological, and Substance Use Disorders*, edited by V. Patel, D. Chisholm, T. Dua, R. Laxminarayan, and M. E. Medina-Mora. Washington, DC: World Bank.

Lim, S. S., T. Vos, A. D. Flaxman, G. Danaei, K. Shibuya, and others. 2012. "A Comparative Risk Assessment of Burden of Disease and Injury Attributable to 67 Risk Factors and Risk Factor Clusters in 21 Regions, 1990-2010: A Systematic Analysis for the Global Burden of Disease Study 2010." *The Lancet* 380 (9859): 2224–60. doi:10.1016/s0140-6736(12)61766-8.

Lindner, L. M., A. C. Marasciulo, M. R. Farias, and G. E. M. Grohs. 2009. "Economic Evaluation of Antipsychotic Drugs for Schizophrenia Treatment within the Brazilian Healthcare System." *Revista de saúde pública* 43: 62–69.

Lund, C., M. De Silva, S. Plagerson, S. Cooper, D. Chisholm, and others. 2011. "Poverty and Mental Disorders: Breaking the Cycle in Low-Income and Middle-Income Countries." *The Lancet* 378 (9801): 1502–14.

MHIN (Mental Health Innovation Network). "Program for Screening, Diagnosis and Comprehensive Treatment of Depression." MHIN. http://mhinnovation.net/innovations/program-screening-diagnosis-and-comprehensive-treatment-depression#.VVYpd46qqkp.

Ngo, V. K., A. Rubinstein, V. Ganju, P. Kanellis, N. Loza, and others. 2013. "Grand Challenges: Integrating Mental Health Care into the Non-Communicable Disease Agenda." *PLoS Med* 10: e1001443.

Patel, V., G. S. Belkin, A. Chockalingam, J. Cooper, S. Saxena, and others. 2013. "Integrating Mental Health Services into Priority Health Care Platforms: Addressing a Grand Challenge in Global Mental Health." *PLoS Med* 10: e1001448.

Patel, V., A. Kleinman, and B. Saraceno. 2012. "Protecting the Human Rights of People with Mental Disorders: A Call to Action for Global Mental Health." In *Mental Health & Human Rights*, edited by M. Dudley, D. Silove, and F. Gale. Oxford: Oxford University Press.

Patel, V., C. Lund, S. Heatherill, S. Plagerson, J. Corrigal, and others. 2009. "Social Determinants of Mental Disorders." In *Priority Public Health Conditions: From Learning to Action on Social Determinants of Health*, edited by E. Blas and A. Sivasankara Kurup. Geneva: World Health Organization.

Patel, V., B. Saraceno, and A. Kleinman. 2006. "Beyond Evidence: The Moral Case for International Mental Health." *American Journal of Psychiatry* 163 (8): 1312–15.

Petersen, I., S. Evans-Lacko, M. Semrau, M. Barry, D. Chisholm, P. Gronholm, C. O. Egbe, and G. Thornicrost. 2015. "Population Platforms." In *Disease Control Priorities*

(third edition): Volume 4, *Mental, Neurological, and Substance Use Disorders*, edited by V. Patel, D. Chisholm, T. Dua, R. Laxminarayan, and M. E. Medina-Mora. Washington, DC: World Bank.

Prince, M., V. Patel, S. Saxena, M. Maj, J. Maselko, and others. 2007. "No Health without Mental Health." *The Lancet* 370 (9590): 859–77.

Prukkanone, B., T. Vos, M. Bertram, and S. Lim. 2012. "Cost-Effectiveness Analysis for Antidepressants and Cognitive Behavioral Therapy for Major Depression in Thailand." *Value in Health* 15 (1): S3–8.

Rahman, A., P. J. Surkan, C. E. Cayetano, P. Rwagatare, and K. E. Dickson. "Grand Challenges: Integrating Maternal Mental Health into Maternal and Child Health programmes." *PLoS Med* 2013; 10: e1001442.

Rehm, J., D. Chisholm, R. Room, and A. D. Lopez. 2006. "Alcohol." In *Disease Control Priorities in Developing Countries*, 2nd ed., edited by D. T. Jamison, J. G. Breman, A. R. Measham, G. Alleyene, M. Claeson, and D. B. Evans, P. Jha, A. Mills, and P. Musgrove. Washington, DC: World Bank and Oxford University Press.

Rehm, J., C. Mathers, S. Popova, M. Thavorncharoensap, Y. Teerawattananon, and others. 2009. "Global Burden of Disease and Injury and Economic Cost Attributable to Alcohol Use and Alcohol-Use Disorders." *The Lancet* 373 (9682): 2223–33.

Saraceno, B., M. van Ommeren, R. Batniji, A. Cohen, O. Gureje, and others. 2007. "Barriers to Improvement of Mental Health Services in Low-Income and Middle-Income Countries." *The Lancet* 370 (9593): 1164–74.

Saxena, S., M. Funk, and D. Chisholm. 2013. "World Health Assembly Adopts Comprehensive Mental Health Action Plan 2013—2020." *The Lancet* 381 (9882): 1970–71. doi:10.1016/S0140-6736(13)61139-3.

Saxena, S., G. Thornicroft, M. Knapp, and H. Whiteford. 2007. "Resources for Mental Health: Scarcity, Inequity, and Inefficiency." *The Lancet* 370 (9590): 878–89.

Shidhaye, R., C. Lund, and D. Chisholm. 2015. "Health Care Delivery Platforms." In *Disease Control Priorities* (third edition): Volume 4, *Mental, Neurological, and Substance Use Disorders*, edited by V. Patel, D. Chisholm, T. Dua, R. Laxminarayan, and M. E. Medina-Mora. Washington, DC: World Bank.

Strang, J., T. Babor, J. Caulkins, B. Fischer, D. Foxcroft, and others. 2012. "Drug Policy and the Public Good: Evidence for Effective Interventions." *The Lancet* 379 (9810): 71–83. doi:10.1016/s0140-6736(11)61674-7.

United Nations. 2015. *Global Sustainable Development Report, 2015 Ediion*. New York: United Nations.

van Ginneken, N., P. Tharyan, S. Lewin, G. N. Rao, S. Meera, and others. 2013. "Non-Specialist Health Worker Interventions for the Care of Mental, Neurological and Substance-Abuse Disorders in Low- and Middle-Income Countries." *Cochrane Database Systematic Reviews* 11: CD009149. doi:10.1002/14651858.CD009149.pub2.

Verguet, S., R. Laxminarayan, and D. T. Jamison. 2015. "Universal Public Finance of Tuberculosis Treatment in

India: An Extended Cost-Effectiveness Analysis." *Health Economics* 24 (3): 318–32. doi:10.1002/hec.3019.

Walker, E. R., R. E. McGee, and B. G. Druss. 2015. "Mortality in Mental Disorders and Global Disease Burden Implications: A Systematic Review and Meta-analysis." *JAMA Psychiatry* 72 (4): 334–41. doi:10.1001/jamapsychiatry.2014.2502.

Whiteford, H. A., L. Degenhardt, J. Rehm, A. J. Baxter, A. J. Ferrari, and others. 2013. "Global Burden of Disease Attributable to Mental and Substance Use Disorders: Findings from the Global Burden of Disease Study 2010." *The Lancet* 382 (9904): 1575–86. doi:10.1016/S0140-6736(13)61611-6.

Whiteford, H. A., A. J. Ferrari, L. Degenhardt, V. Feigin, and T. Vos. 2015. "The Global Burden of Mental, Neurological and Substance Use Disorders: An Analysis from the Global Burden of Disease Study 2010." *PLoS One* 10 (2): e0116820. doi:10.1371/journal.pone.0116820.

———. 2015. "The Global Burden of Mental, Neurological and Substance Use Disorders: An Analysis from the Global Burden of Disease Study 2010." In *Disease Control Priorities* (third edition): Volume 4, *Mental, Neurological, and Substance Use Disorders,* edited by V. Patel, D. Chisholm, T. Dua, R. Laxminarayan, and M. E. Medina-Mora. Washington, DC: World Bank.

WHO (World Health Organization). 2008. *Mental Health Gap Action Programme (mhGAP): Scaling Up Care for Mental, Neurological and Substance Abuse Disorders.* Geneva: WHO.

———. 2011. *Scaling Up Action Against NCDs: How Much Will It Cost?* Geneva: WHO.

———. 2012. *Dementia: A Public Health Priority.* Geneva: WHO.

———. 2013a. *Building Back Better: Sustainable Mental Health Care after Emergencies.* Geneva: WHO.

———. 2013b. *WHO Humanitarian Response Compendium of Health Priorities and WHO Projects in Consolidated Appeals and Response Plans.* Geneva: WHO.

———. 2014. *Global Health Estimates.* http://www.who.int/healthinfo/global_burden_disease/estimates/en/index2.html.

———. 2015. *Mental Health Atlas 2014.* Geneva: WHO.

Chapter 2

Global Burden of Mental, Neurological, and Substance Use Disorders: An Analysis from the Global Burden of Disease Study 2010

Harvey A. Whiteford, Alize J. Ferrari, Louisa Degenhardt, Valery Feigin, and Theo Vos

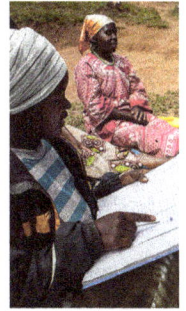

INTRODUCTION

A substantial proportion of the world's health problems in high-income countries (HICs) and low- and middle-income countries (LMICs) arises from mental, neurological, and substance use disorders (Murray, Vos, and others 2012; WHO 2008). Treatment rates for these disorders are low, particularly in LMICs, where treatment gaps of more than 90 percent have been documented (Wang, Aguilar-Gaxiola, and others 2007). Even in HICs, where rates of treatment are comparatively higher, treatment for mental, neurological, and substance use disorders tends to be provided many years after the onset of the disorder (Wang, Aguilar-Gaxiola, and others 2007; Wang, Angermeyer, and others 2007).

Global Burden of Mental, Neurological, and Substance Use Disorders

Historically, major health policy decisions have been informed by mortality statistics. Although our understanding of diseases causing premature mortality has expanded, the lack of emphasis on morbidity has undervalued the global impact of prevalent and disabling disorders with lower mortality, such as mental, neurological, and

substance use disorders. Until recently, there was a poor understanding of the comparative global epidemiology of mental, neurological, and substance use disorders and slower progress compared with other diseases in identifying the most cost-effective interventions. To improve the health outcomes of people with mental, neurological, and substance use disorders in HICs and LMICs, it is important to understand not only the number and distribution of affected people among countries, but also the way the disorders affect their health compared with other diseases. There are many summary measures available to measure population health (Alonso, Chatterji, and He 2013; Sassi 2006). In this chapter, we focus on the approach in the Global Burden of Disease Study 2010 (GBD 2010) to measure disease burden—the most comprehensive measure of population health to date, which combines in one metric the disability and mortality associated with a given disease (Murray, Vos, and others 2012).

The first Global Burden of Disease Study, which published data on disease burden in 1990 (GBD 1990) (Murray and Lopez 1996), reported that the category of mental, neurological, and substance use disorders—a grouping that included depression, selected anxiety disorders, bipolar disorder, schizophrenia, epilepsy, dementia, Parkinson's disease, multiple sclerosis,

Corresponding author: Harvey A. Whiteford, Queensland Centre for Mental Health Research, University of Queensland, the Park Centre for Mental Health, Wacol, QLD 4076, Australia; h.whiteford@uq.edu.au.

and alcohol and drug use disorders—accounted for 10.5 percent of the world's disease burden, as measured by disability-adjusted life years (DALYs). The DALY is a health metric that captures the nonfatal component of the disease burden as years lived with disability (YLDs), and the fatal component as years of life lost (YLLs) to premature mortality (Murray and Lopez 1996). GBD 1990 showed that five of the top 10 causes of disability—making up more than 25 percent of global YLDs for 1990—belonged to the category of mental, neurological, and substance use disorders (Murray and Lopez 1996). In its update of burden estimates for 2000–05, the World Health Organization (WHO) assigned 31.7 percent of all YLDs to mental, neurological, and substance use conditions; the five main contributors of this burden were depression (11.8 percent), alcohol use disorders (3.3 percent), schizophrenia (2.8 percent), bipolar disorder (2.4 percent), and dementia (1.6 percent) (WHO 2008).

Global Burden of Disease Study 2010

In this chapter we present findings from GBD 2010. The GBD 2010 estimated the burden for 291 diseases and injuries and 67 risk factors and was the first comprehensive re-analysis of the burden since GBD 1990 (Lim and others 2012; Lozano and others 2012; Murray, Vos, and others 2012; Salomon and others 2012; Vos and others 2012; Wang and others 2012). GBD 2010 estimated burden for three main cause groups:

- Communicable diseases: infectious or transmissible diseases
- Noncommunicable diseases: noninfectious or non transmissible diseases
- Injuries (accidental or intentional).

The study included a complete epidemiological reassessment of these communicable and noncommunicable diseases and injuries across 187 countries; 21 world regions; males and females; estimated burden for 1990, 2005, and 2010; and 20 age groups. Rather than rely on a selective sample of data points as previous GBD studies had, burden estimates were based on a systematic review of the literature to obtain all available epidemiological data. The estimates were also derived through the use of new statistical methods to model the epidemiological data, quantify disability, adjust for comorbidity between diseases, and propagate uncertainty to final burden estimates (Murray, Vos, and others 2012; Vos and others 2012).

GBD 2010 highlighted a shift in burden from communicable to noncommunicable diseases and from YLLs to YLDs (Murray, Vos, and others 2012; Vos and others 2012). Although communicable diseases remain a health

priority in many LMICs, increasing life expectancies due to better reproductive health, childhood nutrition, and control of communicable diseases meant that more people in 2010 were living to ages where mental, neurological, and substance use disorders were most prevalent (Whiteford, Degenhardt, and others 2013).

In GBD 2010, the burden of mental and substance use disorders was estimated separately from that of neurological disorders, such as dementia, Parkinson's disease, and epilepsy. This approach enabled us to investigate more comprehensively the differences in the epidemiology and burden between these groups of disorders compared with previous GBD studies. Mental and substance use disorders were among the leading causes of disease burden in 2010. They were responsible for 7.4 percent of global DALYs and 22.9 percent of global YLDs, making them the fifth-leading cause of DALYs and the leading cause of YLDs (Whiteford, Degenhardt, and others 2013). Neurological disorders explained 3.0 percent of global DALYs and 5.6 percent of global YLDs (Murray, Vos, and others 2012; Vos and others 2012).

The overarching findings of the study for all 291 diseases and injuries have been presented (Lim and others 2012; Lozano and others 2012; Murray, Ezzati, and others 2012; Murray, Vos, and others 2012; Salomon and others 2012; Vos and others 2012), as have the GBD 2010 results for mental and substance use disorders (Degenhardt, Whiteford, and others 2013; Whiteford, Degenhardt, and others 2013). This chapter presents GBD 2010 burden estimates of mental, neurological, and substance use disorders as a group. Specifically, we quantify the global disease burden attributable to mental, neurological, and substance use disorders and explore variations in burden by disorder type, age, gender, year, and region. This approach provides background and context for chapter 3 in this volume (Charlson and others 2015), which responds to the lack of deaths and fatal burden estimated by GBD 2010 for mental, neurological, and substance use disorders. Most important, this chapter for the first time presents GBD 2010 burden of disease estimates at the aggregated level of mental, neurological, and substance use disorders. Analysis of burden estimates at this aggregated level is important from the clinical and population health perspectives, given that the organization of services in many LMICs does not separate neurological disorders from mental disorders, something seen as a progression of Western medical subspecialization.

METHODOLOGY

Annex 2A summarizes the mental, neurological, and substance use disorders investigated in GBD 2010 and describes how the YLDs, YLLs, and DALYs for each disorder were estimated. More detailed information about the input data and methods can be accessed elsewhere (Baxter and others 2013; Baxter and others 2014a; Baxter and others 2014b; Degenhardt and others 2011; Degenhardt, Baxter, and others 2014; Degenhardt, Charlson, and others 2014; Degenhardt, Ferrari, and others 2013; Degenhardt, Whiteford, and others 2013; Erskine and others 2014; Ferrari, Baxter, and Whiteford 2010; Ferrari and others 2013a; Ferrari and others 2013b; Saha and others 2005; Whiteford, Degenhardt, and others 2013; Whiteford, Ferrari, and others 2013).

To allow for comparability in measurement, the definitions of dementia and mental and substance use disorders used for GBD 2010 were restricted to diagnostic classifications provided in the *Diagnostic and Statistical Manual of Mental Disorders* (APA 2000) and the *International Classification of Diseases* (ICD-10) (WHO 1992). The epilepsy definition was based on ICD-10 (WHO 1992). For each disorder, YLDs and YLLs were summed to estimate DALYs. For disorders where there were insufficient data to estimate YLLs, YLDs were equated with DALYs. Uncertainty was estimated at all stages of the analysis through microsimulation methods and propagated to the final burden estimates. YLDs, YLLs, and DALYs in this chapter are presented for 1990 and 2010 at the following levels:

- Global
- Disaggregated by disorder type, age, gender, and year
- Disaggregated by the seven superregion groups in GBD 2010: East Asia and Pacific, Eastern Europe and Central Asia, high-income regions (North America, Australasia, Western Europe, high-income Asia Pacific, and southern Latin America), Latin America and the Caribbean, the Middle East and North Africa, South Asia, and Sub-Saharan Africa
- Disaggregated by developed and developing regions.

The terms *developed* and *developing* regions are used here rather than HICs and LMICs for consistency with the presentation of the GBD 2010 estimates. The classification of countries into regions and regions into superregions was based on geographical proximity and epidemiological likeness in cause of death patterns (Murray, Vos, and others 2012; Vos and others 2012). Whiteford, Degenhardt, and others (2013) provide a list of all countries in each region and superregions. Where age-standardized DALY rates are presented, these were estimated using direct standardization to the global standard population that WHO proposed in 2001 (http://www.who.int/healthinfo/paper31.pdf).

BURDEN OF MENTAL, NEUROLOGICAL, AND SUBSTANCE USE DISORDERS

Mental, neurological, and substance use disorders accounted for 258 million DALYs in 2010, which was equivalent to 10.4 percent of total all-cause DALYs. Within mental, neurological, and substance use disorders, mental disorders accounted for the highest proportion of DALYs (56.7 percent), followed by neurological disorders (28.6 percent) and substance use disorders (14.7 percent). For all three groups of disorders, DALYs occurred across the lifespan (figure 2.1); however, there was a peak in early adulthood (between ages 20 and 30 years) for mental and substance use disorders compared with neurological disorders, where DALYs were highest in the elderly.

Absolute DALYs for mental, neurological, and substance use disorders increased by 41 percent between 1990 and 2010, from 182 million to 258 million DALYs. With the exception of substance use disorders, where age-standardized DALY rates for opioid, cocaine, and amphetamine dependence increased over time, the increase in absolute DALYs for the other disorders was largely caused by changes in population growth and aging. Table 2.1 summarizes the age-standardized DALY rates for 1990 and 2010.

Table 2.2 summarizes the DALYs assigned to each mental, neurological, and substance use disorder in 2010. These disorders as a group ranked as the third-leading cause of DALYs (explaining 10.4 percent of DALYs), after cardiovascular and circulatory diseases (explaining 11.9 percent of DALYs), and diarrhea, lower

Figure 2.1 DALYs Attributable to Mental, Neurological, and Substance Use Disorders, by Age, 2010

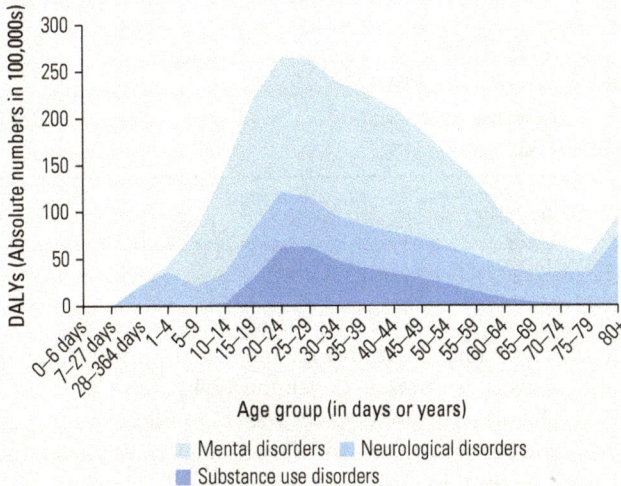

Source: http://vizhub.healthdata.org/gbd-compare.
Note: DALYs = disability-adjusted life years.

Table 2.1 Age-Standardized DALY Rates Attributable to Mental, Neurological, and Substance Use Disorders, 1990 and 2010

Disorder	Age-standardized DALY rates (per 100,000)			
	Male		Female	
	1990	2010	1990	2010
Mental disorders				
Major depressive disorder	694.8	689.9	1,171.7	1,161.2
Dysthymia	135.3	135.8	189.7	190.0
Bipolar disorder	172.0	172.1	204.6	204.8
Schizophrenia	230.7	223.0	187.8	180.6
Anxiety disorders	274.3	273.0	508.9	510.3
Eating disorders	4.4	3.9	47.6	59.5
Autism	85.1	85.8	29.5	29.6
Asperger's syndrome	85.2	85.0	20.3	20.3
Attention-deficit hyperactivity disorder	10.8	10.6	3.1	3.1
Conduct disorder	111.9	113.3	47.0	47.6
Idiopathic intellectual disability	25.3	17.7	18.2	11.9
Other mental and behavioral disorders	25.5	23.3	21.5	20.8
Neurological disorders				
Alzheimer's disease and other dementias	125.7	155.5	153.7	178.6
Parkinson's disease	32.7	36.6	23.2	23.3
Epilepsy	261.6	269.3	226.0	232.9
Multiple sclerosis	16.3	12.3	23.7	19.8
Migraine	233.1	236.6	405.9	415.8
Tension-type headache	24.1	24.0	28.3	28.3
Other neurological disorders	228.0	259.9	200.0	266.7
Substance use disorders				
Alcohol use disorders[a]	431.0	409.9	117.2	106.0
Opioid dependence	139.0	184.4	63.8	78.4
Cocaine dependence	22.5	22.0	10.3	9.7
Amphetamine dependence	45.4	47.3	26.9	27.6
Cannabis dependence	38.8	36.7	22.3	21.3
Other drug use disorders	83.7	97.0	44.6	47.9

Source: http://vizhub.healthdata.org/gbd-compare/.
Note: DALY = disability-adjusted life year.
a. Alcohol use disorders include alcohol dependence and fetal alcohol syndrome.

respiratory infections, meningitis, and other common infectious diseases (explaining 11.4 percent of DALYs). Major depressive disorder was responsible for the highest proportion of mental, neurological, and substance use disorder DALYs (24.5 percent); attention-deficit hyperactivity disorder was responsible for the lowest (0.2 percent).

Overall, in 2010, 124 million mental, neurological, and substance use DALYs occurred among males and 134 million among females. Figure 2.2 shows DALY rates for each mental, neurological, and substance use disorder by gender. Females accounted for more DALYs for most of the mental and neurological disorders, except for mental disorders occurring in childhood, schizophrenia,

Table 2.2 DALYs Attributable to Mental, Neurological, and Substance Use Disorders, 2010

Disorder	Absolute DALYs (to the nearest 100,000)	Proportion of total (all-cause) DALYs (%)	Proportion of mental, neurological, and substance use disorder DALYs (%)
Mental disorders			
Major depressive disorder	63,200,000	2.5	24.5
Dysthymia	11,100,000	0.4	4.3
Bipolar disorder	12,900,000	0.5	5.0
Schizophrenia	13,600,000	0.5	5.3
Anxiety disorders	26,800,000	1.1	10.4
Eating disorders	2,200,000	0.1	0.9
Autism	4,000,000	0.2	1.6
Asperger's syndrome	3,700,000	0.1	1.4
Attention-deficit hyperactivity disorder	500,000	0.02	0.2
Conduct disorder	5,800,000	0.2	2.2
Idiopathic intellectual disability	1,000,000	0.04	0.4
Other mental disorders	1,500,000	0.1	0.6
Subtotal	146,300,000	5.9	56.7
Neurological disorders			
Alzheimer's disease and other dementias	11,400,000	0.5	4.4
Parkinson's disease	1,900,000	0.1	0.7
Epilepsy	17,400,000	0.7	6.8
Multiple sclerosis	1,100,000	0.04	0.4
Migraine	22,400,000	0.9	8.7
Tension-type headache	1,800,000	0.1	0.7
Other neurological disorders	17,900,000	0.7	6.9
Subtotal	73,900,000	3.0	28.6
Substance use disorders			
Alcohol use disorders[a]	17,700,000	0.7	6.9
Opioid dependence	9,200,000	0.4	3.6
Cocaine dependence	1,100,000	0.04	0.4
Amphetamine dependence	2,600,000	0.1	1.0
Cannabis dependence	2,100,000	0.1	0.8
Other drug use disorders	5,100,000	0.2	2.0
Subtotal	37,800,000	1.5	14.7

Source: http://vizhub.healthdata.org/gbd-compare/.

Note: DALYs = disability-adjusted life years. DALYs were aggregated across all country, gender, and age groups for 2010.

a. Alcohol use disorders include alcohol dependence and fetal alcohol syndrome.

Parkinson's disease, and epilepsy, where males accounted for more DALYs. Males also accounted for more DALYs than females in all substance use disorders.

Figure 2.3 shows the burden attributable to mental, neurological, and substance use disorders as a group in 2010 by the GBD 2010 superregion groupings and by developed and developing world regions. Overall, the burden of these disorders as age-standardized rates was approximately 1.6 times higher in developed regions (explaining 15.5 percent of total DALYs) compared

Figure 2.2 Age-Standardized DALY Rates Attributable to Individual Mental, Neurological, and Substance Use Disorders, by Gender, 2010

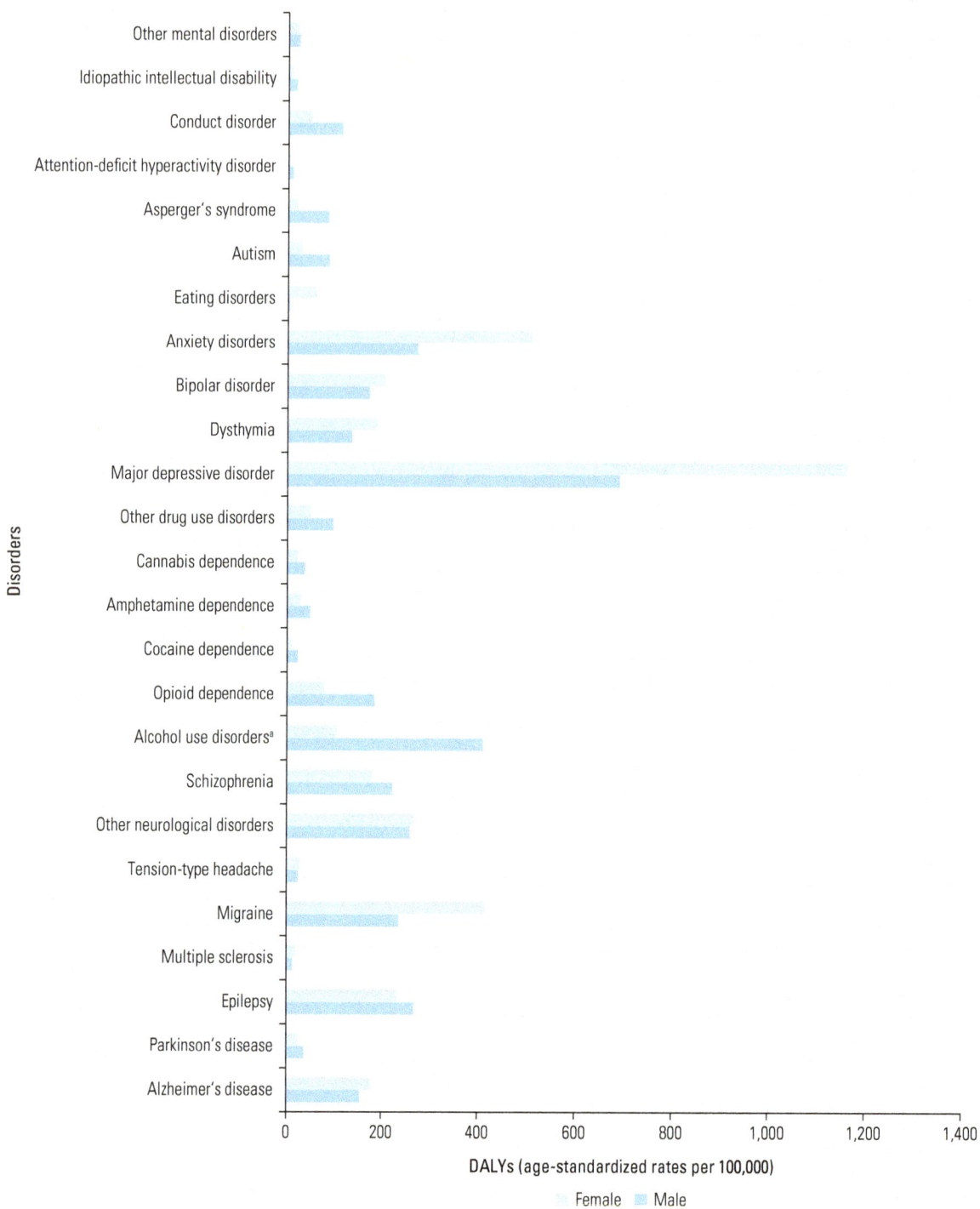

Source: http://vizhub.healthdata.org/gbd-compare/.
Note: DALY = disability-adjusted life year.
a. Alcohol use disorders include alcohol dependence and fetal alcohol syndrome.

with developing regions (explaining 9.4 percent of total DALYs). When disaggregated by GBD superregions, the burden of mental, neurological, and substance use disorders was highest in Eastern Europe and Central Asia and lowest in East Asia and Pacific. Mental disorders maintained the highest proportion of DALYs in all superregions; the greatest variation in DALYs occurred within substance use disorders, where DALYs were almost three times higher in Eastern Europe and Central Asia, compared with Sub-Saharan Africa, where DALYs were lowest.

Figure 2.4 illustrates the decomposition of global burden by YLDs and YLLs for the overall categories of communicable diseases, noncommunicable diseases, and injuries. Noncommunicable diseases explained a large proportion of YLDs and YLLs in 2010. Within this group, mental, neurological, and substance use disorders were responsible for 28.5 percent of all YLDs, making them the leading cause of YLDs worldwide.

In comparison, mental, neurological, and substance use disorders contributed to only 2.3 percent of YLLs. Deaths and YLLs could be assigned to a mental, neurological, or substance use disorder only when the disorder was considered as a direct cause of death in the ICD-10 cause-of-death directory. Using this approach, the majority of excess deaths in individuals with a mental disorder, in particular, were coded to the direct physical cause of death (for example, suicide deaths were coded

Figure 2.3 Age-Standardized DALY Rates Attributable to Mental, Neurological, and Substance Use Disorders, by Region, 2010

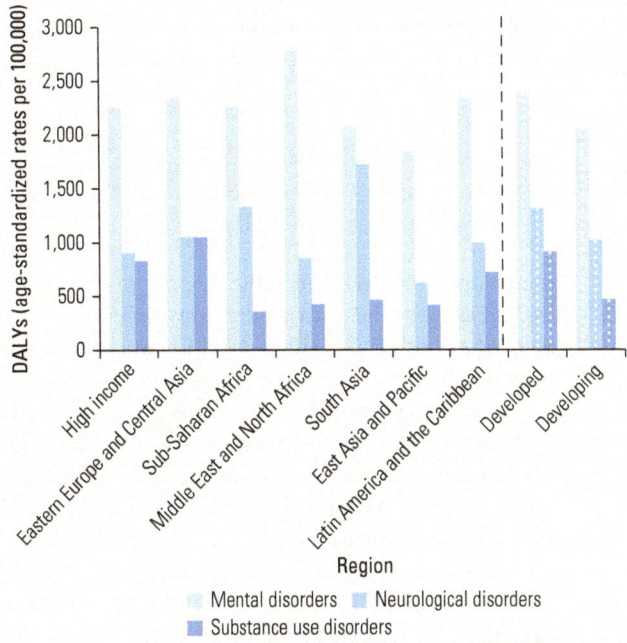

Source: http://vizhub.healthdata.org/gbd-compare/.
Note: DALY = disability-adjusted life year. DALYs were disaggregated by GBD 2010's seven superregion groups—East Asia and Pacific, Eastern Europe and Central Asia, high-income regions (North America, Australasia, Western Europe, high-income Asia Pacific, and southern Latin America), Latin America and the Caribbean, the Middle East and North Africa, South Asia, and Sub-Saharan Africa—and by developed and developing regions.

Figure 2.4 Proportion of Global YLDs and YLLs Attributable to Mental, Neurological, and Substance Use Disorders, 2010

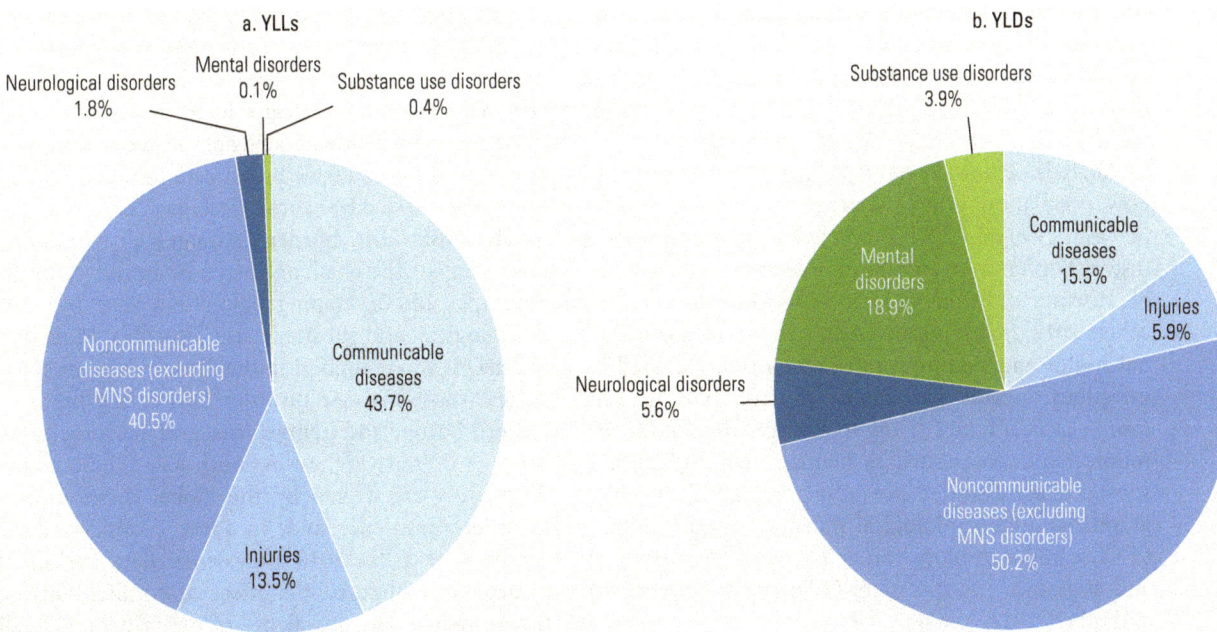

Source: http://vizhub.healthdata.org/gbd-compare/.
Note: MNS = mental, neurological, and substance use; YLLs = years of life lost; YLDs = years lived with disability.

under injuries as self-harm) rather than to the disorder. An analysis of excess mortality in individuals with mental, neurological, and substance use disorders and the implications for burden of disease estimates is presented in chapter 3 in this volume (Charlson and others 2015).

IMPLICATIONS OF THE GBD 2010 FINDINGS FOR MENTAL, NEUROLOGICAL, AND SUBSTANCE USE DISORDERS

Mental, neurological, and substance use disorders are a leading cause of the disease burden worldwide, substantially contributing to health loss in individuals of all ages, from developed and developing regions.

In GBD 2010, the differences in DALYs between mental, neurological, and substance use disorders were guided by differences in the prevalence, death, and disability weights associated with each disorder. The input data that were used to estimate burden are presented in greater detail elsewhere (Baxter and others 2015; Baxter and others 2014a; Baxter and others 2014b; Degenhardt, Baxter, and others 2014; Degenhardt, Charlson, and others 2014; Degenhardt, Ferrari, and others 2013; Erskine and others 2013; Ferrari and others 2013a; Ferrari and others 2013b; Saha and others 2005). Mental disorders, such as anxiety and depressive disorders, were associated with high levels of prevalence and disability. In comparison, schizophrenia was associated with low prevalence but high levels of disability; an acute state of schizophrenia obtained the highest disability weight in GBD 2010. The same was true for opioid dependence, which, although it had lower prevalence in comparison with other substance use disorders like cannabis dependence, was associated with high disability and death. Migraine, in contrast, was associated with high levels of prevalence but low disability.

Analysis of burden estimates across time illustrated how population growth and a changing age profile between 1990 and 2010 produced a shift in the global disease burden from communicable to noncommunicable diseases and from YLLs to YLDs (Murray, Vos, and others 2012). With improvements in infant and maternal health and declining rates of mortality caused by infectious diseases, particularly in developing regions, more people are now living to the age where noncommunicable diseases such as mental, neurological, and substance use disorders are most prevalent. This demographic and epidemiological transition is contributing to a rise in the absolute burden of mental, neurological, and substance use disorders (Whiteford, Degenhardt, and others 2013).

Although not adopted in GBD 2010, the use of age weighting in many economic analyses and in earlier GBD studies (Murray and Acharya 1997) recognizes and attempts to incorporate the social preference for avoiding health loss in young adults. In spite of the absence of age weighting in the GBD 2010 estimates, the peak impact of mental, neurological, and substance use disorders in early adulthood remained and demonstrated the ubiquitous effect of these disorders at a time of life when individuals are starting to make significant social and economic contributions to their families and societies. The peak in the total burden of mental, neurological, and substance use disorders was found in young adults. However, unlike many chronic diseases, there is a significant burden in children, lending further evidence to the importance of early intervention strategies for mental, neurological, and substance use disorders.

The presentation of burden estimates by age in GBD 2010 facilitates the selection and tailoring of intervention strategies for mental, neurological, and substance use disorders. For instance, it allows us to identify the ages at which interventions would be most beneficial. Historically, mental, neurological, and substance use disorders occurring in childhood have not been well represented in burden of disease analyses. GBD 2010 was the first study to estimate the burden associated with childhood mental disorders like autism, Asperger's disorder, attention-deficit hyperactivity disorder, and conduct disorder. For countries such as those in Sub-Saharan Africa, where children constitute 40 percent of the population (UN 2011), these findings highlight the need for prevention and treatment services targeted to children and adolescents. The availability of such services is often more sporadic than that of adult services. In addition, the high burden of neurological disorders in elderly persons emphasizes the need for the development and implementation of more effective prevention strategies for these disorders, especially given the worldwide aging of the population, as well as the need for equitable health care resource allocation for people affected by neurological disorders.

The GBD 2010 burden estimates also underlined the extent of the challenge faced by health systems in developed and developing regions as a result of mental, neurological, and substance use disorders. Mental disorder DALYs are highest in the Middle East and North Africa, substance use disorder DALYs are highest in Eastern Europe and Central Asia, and neurological disorder DALYs are highest in South Asia. These regional differences are driven by the global distribution of disorder prevalence and, in some instances, deaths. Analysis of GBD 2010 prevalence data for mental disorders highlighted the effect of conflict status on the estimates. The prevalence of major depressive disorder and anxiety disorders was highest in countries with a history of conflict or war, many of which are in the Middle East and North Africa (Baxter and others 2014b; Ferrari and others 2013a).

The prevalence of opioid and cannabis dependence was highest in Australasia and Western Europe (Degenhardt, Charlson, and others 2014; Degenhardt, Ferrari, and others 2013). Cocaine dependence was highest in the North America, high-income, and southern Latin America. Although there was less regional variation in the prevalence of amphetamine dependence, the rates were highest in Southeast Asia and Australasia (Degenhardt, Baxter, and others 2014). The largest contributor of deaths and YLLs for drug use disorders was opioid dependence, with particularly high proportions of deaths caused by opioid dependence occurring in the North America high-income region, Eastern Europe, and southern Sub-Saharan Africa.

In many Eastern European and Sub-Saharan African countries, access to interventions found to be effective in reducing the risk of mortality from opioid dependence—such as opioid substitution therapy, needle and syringe programs, and HIV treatment for those who are HIV-positive—is limited. Access to these interventions in the North America High-income region varies subnationally, with insufficient data to determine access rates at the national level (Degenhardt, Charlson, and others 2014). Prevalence and deaths attributable to Alzheimer's disease were highest in North America, high-income Western Europe, and Australasia. In contrast, prevalence and deaths attributable to epilepsy were highest in Sub-Saharan Africa. The geographic differences in the burden of such neurological disorders should be used to inform research priorities and evidence-based, region-specific service delivery and health care planning. Effective interventions have been identified for mental, neurological, and substance use disorders and are described in the following chapters.

YLDs explained a larger proportion of the burden due to mental, neurological, and substance use disorders compared with YLLs. To estimate YLLs, GBD 2010 followed the ICD-10 cause-of-death categories, whereby deaths can only be assigned to a given condition when it is considered a direct cause of death. This approach can only account for some of the excess deaths attributable to mental, neurological, and substance use disorders, given that deaths will also be coded to the direct physical cause of death. For instance, ischemic heart disease or suicide deaths occurring as a result of major depressive disorder will be coded to cardiovascular disease or injuries rather than to major depressive disorder.

The additional burden attributable to mental, neurological, and substance use disorders as a risk factor for other health outcomes can be investigated through comparative risk assessment analysis, which compares the current health status with a theoretical minimum risk exposure, in this case, the counterfactual status of the absence of mental, neurological, and substance use disorders in the population. The use of this method to estimate the additional burden due to mental and substance use disorders as risk factors for suicide showed that these disorders could account for approximately 60 percent of suicide YLLs in GBD 2010; this would have increased the overall burden of mental and substance use disorders in 2010 from 7.4 percent to 8.3 percent of global DALYs (Ferrari and others 2014). Chapter 3 in this volume (Charlson and others 2015) explores this issue further and presents an analysis of excess mortality in individuals with mental, neurological, and substance use disorders and the implications of this for burden of disease estimates.

LIMITATIONS OF GBD 2010 AND DIRECTIONS FOR FUTURE RESEARCH

Although it represents the most comprehensive assessment of the burden due to mental, neurological, and substance use disorders to date, not all elements of the burden were captured in GBD 2010. By focusing on health loss, the burden in GBD 2010 does not extend to welfare loss; hence, it does not capture all the consequences of mental, neurological, and substance use disorders for families or societies. For a more complete picture of the burden imposed by mental, neurological, and substance use disorders, future research should focus on quantifying the associated welfare losses.

Disability weights in GBD 2010 were derived by surveying the general population (rather than by clinicians, as in previous GBD studies), with the aim of better capturing the societal view of health loss. Nevertheless, adequately encompassing the complexity of health states that represent mental, neurological, and substance use disorders within the survey was challenging; the extent to which the GBD 2010 disability weights entirely reflected the associated health loss is an important area for further research.

Furthermore, the established definitions of mental, neurological, and substance use disorders used in the study may not be sensitive to non-Western presentations of these disorders, which may have led to an underestimation of burden in developing regions. Although these disorders exist in all countries, cultures influence their development and presentation. The predominantly Western-based definitions of mental, neurological, and substance use disorders can be in conflict with cultural contexts (Jorm 2006), leading to challenges in assembling data on global epidemiology. For example, some languages do not have the words to describe concepts such as "sadness" or "depression" consistent with how they are described in Western countries. Explanations for the onset and progression of mental, neurological, and substance use disorders may be explained through mechanisms such the presence of spirits or curses, rather than as medical disorders (Jorm 2006).

Epidemiological surveys in many LMICs tend to capture somatic manifestations of disorders such as depression and anxiety, which may not be as relevant to other countries and cultures (Cheng 2001; Whiteford, Ferrari, and others 2013; Yang and Link 2009). In their survey of mental disorders in China, Phillips and others (2009) concluded that some cases of minor depression were likely misdiagnosed cases of major depressive disorder, given that standard diagnostic criteria were not sensitive to cross-cultural presentations of this disorder. A task for upcoming GBD analyses will be to explore the extent to which certain disorders are misdiagnosed as other mental or physical disorders in developing countries and the consequence on burden.

Finally, regular updating of burden of disease estimates, using the most up-to-date epidemiological data and burden estimation methodology is important. After GBD 2010 was published, the Institute for Health Metrics and Evaluation at the University of Washington endeavored to make available yearly updates of burden of disease estimates. The Global Burden of Disease Study 2013 (GBD 2013) published in 2015 was the first of these updates (GBD 2013 DALYs Hale Collaborators 2015). Although high-level findings were largely consistent between GBD 2010 and GBD 2013, continued updating of estimates presented in this chapter is required.

CONCLUSIONS

According to the findings in GBD 2010, mental, neurological, and substance use disorders contribute to a significant proportion of the global burden of disease and will continue to do so as the shift in burden from communicable to noncommunicable diseases continues. Health systems worldwide can respond to these findings by implementing proven, cost-effective interventions; where these are limited, it will be important to support the research necessary to develop better prevention and treatment options.

Although GBD 2010 represents the most comprehensive assessment of the burden due to mental, neurological, and substance use disorders to date, some limitations need to be acknowledged. For instance, the definition of burden in GBD 2010 does not extend to welfare loss; accordingly, it does not capture all the consequences of mental, neurological, and substance use disorders on

societies. Definitions of mental, neurological, and substance use disorders and the subsequent quantification of disability may not be fully representative of non-Western presentations of these disorders. Further research into the cross-cultural presentations of these disorders is required for a more comprehensive analysis of burden.

ANNEX

The annex to this chapter is as follows. It is available at http://www.dcp-3.org/mentalhealth.

- Annex 2A. Global Burden of Mental, Neurological, and Substance Use Disorders: An Analysis from the Global Burden of Disease Study 2010

NOTE

This chapter was previously published in an article by H. A. Whiteford, A. J. Ferrari, L. Degenhardt, V. Feigin, and T. Vos, entitled "The Global Burden of Mental, Neurological, and Substance Use Disorders: An Analysis for the Global Burden of Disease Study 2010." *PLoS ONE*, 2015: 10 (2): e0116820. doi:10.1371/journal.pone.0116820. http://www.ncbi.nlm.nih.gov/pmc/articles/PMC4320057/pdf/pone.0116820.pdf.

REFERENCES

Alonso, J., S. Chatterji, and Y. He, eds. 2013. *The Burdens of Mental Disorders: Global Perspectives from the WHO World Mental Health Surveys.* Cambridge, U.K.: Cambridge University Press.

APA (American Psychiatric Association). 2000. *Diagnostic and Statistical Manual of Mental Disorders (DSM-IV-TR).* 4th ed. Text Revision ed. Washington, DC: APA.

Baxter, A. J., T. S. Brugha, H. E. Erskine, R. W. Scheurer, T. Vos, and others. 2015. "The Epidemiology and Global Burden of Autism Spectrum Disorders." *Psychological Medicine* 45 (3): 601–13. doi:21.1017/S003329171400172X.

Baxter, A. J., G. Patton, L. Degenhardt, K. M. Scott, and H. A. Whiteford. 2013. "Global Epidemiology of Mental Disorders: What Are We Missing?" *PLoS One* 8 (6): e65514.

Baxter, A. J., T. Vos, K. M. Scott, A. J. Ferrari, and H. A. Whiteford. 2014a. "The Global Burden of Anxiety Disorders in 2010." *Psychological Medicine* 44 (11): 2363–74.

Baxter, A. J., T. Vos, K. M. Scott, R. E. Norman, A. D. Flaxman, and others. 2014b. "The Regional Distribution of Anxiety Disorders: Implications for the Global Burden of Disease Study, 2010." *International Journal of Methods in Psychiatric Research* 23 (4): 422–38. doi:10.1002/mpr.1444.

Charlson, F. J., A. J. Baxter, T. Dua, L. Degenhardt, H. A. Whiteford, and T. Vos. 2015. "Excess Mortality from Mental, Neurological, and Substance Use Disorders in the Global Burden of Disease Study 2010." In *Disease*

Control Priorities (third edition): Volume 4, *Mental, Neurological, and Substance Use Disorders*, edited by V. Patel, D. Chisholm, T. Dua, R. Laxminarayan, and M. E. Medina-Mora. Washington, DC: World Bank.

Cheng, A. T. 2001. "Case Definition and Culture: Are People All the Same?" *British Journal of Psychiatry* 179: 1–3.

Degenhardt, L., A. J. Baxter, Y. Y. Lee, W. Hall, G. E. Sara, and others. 2014. "The Global Epidemiology and Burden of Psychostimulant Dependence: Findings from the Global Burden of Disease Study 2010." *Drug and Alcohol Dependence* 137: 37–47.

Degenhardt, L., C. Bucello, B. Calabria, P. Nelson, A. Roberts, and others. 2011. "What Data Are Available on the Extent of Illicit Drug Use and Dependence Globally? Results of Four Systematic Reviews." *Drug and Alcohol Dependence* 117 (2–3): 85–101.

Degenhardt, L., F. Charlson, B. Mathers, W. D. Hall, A. D. Flaxman, and others. 2014. "The Global Epidemiology and Burden of Opioid Dependence: Results from the Global Burden of Disease 2010 Study." *Addiction* 109 (8): 1320–33.

Degenhardt, L., A. J. Ferrari, B. Calabria, W. D. Hall, R. E. Norman, and others. 2013. "The Global Epidemiology and Contribution of Cannabis Use and Dependence to the Global Burden of Disease: Results from the GBD 2010 Study." *PLoS One* 8 (10): e76635.

Degenhardt, L., H. A. Whiteford, A. J. Ferrari, A. J. Baxter, F. J. Charlson, and others. 2013. "The Global Burden of Disease Attributable to Illicit Drug Use: Results from the GBD 2010 Study." *The Lancet* 382 (9904): 1564–74.

Erskine, H. E., A. J. Ferrari, P. Nelson, G. V. Polanczyk, A. D. Flaxman, and others. 2013. "Research Review: Epidemiological Modelling of Attention-Deficit/Hyperactivity Disorder and Conduct Disorder for the Global Burden of Disease Study 2010." *Journal of Child Psychology and Psychiatry* 54 (12): 1263–74.

Erskine, H. E., A. J. Ferrari, G. V. Polanczyk, T. E. Moffitt, C. J. L. Murray, and others. 2014. "The Global Burden of Conduct Disorder and Attention-Deficit/Hyperactivity Disorder in 2010." *Journal of Child Psychology and Psychiatry, and Allied Disciplines* 55 (4): 328–36.

Ferrari, A. J., A. J. Baxter, and H. A. Whiteford. 2010. "A Systematic Review of the Global Distribution and Availability of Prevalence Data for Bipolar Disorder." *Journal of Affective Disorders* 34 (1–3): 1–13.

Ferrari, A. J., F. J. Charlson, R. Norman, A. D. Flaxman, S. B. Patten, and others. 2013. "The Epidemiological Modelling of Major Depressive Disorder: Application for the Global Burden of Disease Study 2010." *PLoS One* 8 (7): e69637.

Ferrari, A. J., F. J. Charlson, R. E. Norman, S. B. Patten, C. J. L. Murray, and others. 2013. "Burden of Depressive Disorders by Country, Sex, Age, and Year: Findings from the Global Burden of Disease Study 2010." *PLoS Medicine* 10 (11): e1001547.

Ferrari, A. J., R. E. Norman, G. Freedman, A. J. Baxter, J. E. Pirkis, and others. 2014. "The Burden Attributable to Mental and Substance Use Disorders as Risk Factors for

Suicide: Findings from the Global Burden of Disease Study 2010." *PLoS One* 9 (4): e91936.

GBD 2013 DALYs Hale Collaborators. 2015. "Global, Regional, and National Disability-Adjusted Life Years (DALYs) for 306 Diseases and Injuries and Healthy Life Expectancy (HALE) for 188 countries, 1990–2013: Quantifying the Epidemiological Transition." *The Lancet* Epub August 26. doi: http://dx.doi.org/10.1016/S0140-6736(15)61340-X.

Jorm, A. F. 2006. "National Surveys of Mental Disorders: Are They Researching Scientific Facts or Constructing Useful Myths?"*Australian and New Zealand Journal of Psychiatry* 40: 830–34.

Lim, S. S., T. Vos, A. D. Flaxman, G. Danaei, K. Shibuya, and others. 2012. "A Comparative Risk Assessment of Burden of Disease and Injury Attributable to 67 Risk Factors and Risk Factor Clusters in 21 Regions, 1990–2010: A Systematic Analysis for the Global Burden of Disease Study 2010." *The Lancet* 380: 2224–60.

Lozano, R., M. Naghavi, K. Foreman, S. Lim, K. Shibuya, and others. 2012. "Global and Regional Mortality from 235 Causes of Death for 20 Age Groups in 1990 and 2010: A Systematic Analysis for the Global Burden of Disease Study 2010." *The Lancet* 380 (9859): 2095–128.

Murray, C. J. L., and A. K. Acharya. 1997. "Understanding DALYs." *Journal of Health Economics* 16: 703–30.

Murray, C. J. L., M. Ezzati, A. Flaxman, S. Lim, R. Lozano, and others. 2012. "GBD 2010: Design, Definitions, and Metrics." *The Lancet* 380 (9859): 2063–66.

Murray, C. J. L., and A. D. Lopez, eds. 1996. *The Global Burden of Disease: A Comprehensive Assessment of Mortality and Disability from Diseases, Injuries, and Risk Factors in 1990 and Projected to 2020.* Cambridge, MA: Harvard University Press.

Murray, C. J. L., T. Vos, R. Lozano, M. Naghavi, A. D. Flaxman, and others. 2012. "Disability-Adjusted Life Years (DALYs) for 291 Diseases and Injuries in 21 Regions, 1990–2010: A Systematic Analysis for the Global Burden of Disease Study 2010." *The Lancet* 380 (9859): 2197–223.

Phillips, M. R., J. Zhang, Q. Shi, Z. Song, Z. Ding, and others. 2009. "Prevalence, Treatment, and Associated Disability of Mental Disorders in Four Provinces in China during 2001–05: An Epidemiological Survey." *The Lancet* 373 (9680): 2041–53.

Saha, S., D. Chant, J. Welham, and J. McGrath. 2005. "A Systematic Review of the Prevalence of Schizophrenia." *PLoS Medicine* 2 (5): e141.

Salomon, J. A., H. Wang, M. K. Freeman, T. Vos, A. D. Flaxman, and others. 2012. "Healthy Life Expectancy for 187 Countries, 1990–2010: A Systematic Analysis for the Global Burden of Disease Study 2010." *The Lancet* 380 (9859): 2144–62.

Sassi, F. 2006. "Calculating QALYs, Comparing QALY and DALY Calculations." *Health Policy and Planning* 21 (5): 402–08.

UN (United Nations). 2011. *World Population Prospects: The 2010 Revision.* New York: UN.

Vos, T., A. D. Flaxman, M. Naghavi, R. Lozano, C. Michaud, and others. 2012. "Years Lived with Disability (YLDs) for 1,160 Sequelae of 289 Diseases and Injuries 1990–2010:

A Systematic Analysis for the Global Burden of Disease Study 2010." *The Lancet* 380 (9859): 2163–96.

Wang, H., L. Dwyer-Lindgren, K. T. Lofgren, J. K. Rajaratnam, J. R. Marcus, and others. 2012. "Age-Specific and Sex-Specific Mortality in 187 Countries, 1970–2010: A Systematic Analysis for the Global Burden of Disease Study 2010." *The Lancet* 380: 2071–94.

Wang, P. S., S. Aguilar-Gaxiola, J. Alonso, M. C. Angermeyer, G. Borges, and others. 2007. "Use of Mental Health Services for Anxiety, Mood, and Substance Disorders in 17 Countries in the WHO World Mental Health Surveys." *The Lancet* 370 (9590): 841–50.

Wang, P. S., M. Angermeyer, G. Borges, R. Bruffaerts, W. Tat Chiu, and others. 2007. "Delay and Failure in Treatment Seeking after First Onset of Mental Disorders in the World Health Organization's World Mental Health Survey Initiative." *World Psychiatry* 6 (3): 177–85.

Whiteford, H. A., L. Degenhardt, J. Rehm, A. J. Baxter, A. J. Ferrari, and others. 2013. "The Global Burden of Mental and Substance Use Disorders, 2010." *The Lancet* 382 (9904): 1575–86.

Whiteford, H. A., A. J. Ferrari, A. J. Baxter, F. J. Charlson, and L. Degenhardt. 2013. "How Did We Arrive at Burden of Disease Estimates for Mental and Illicit Drug Use Disorders in the Global Burden of Disease Study 2010?" *Current Opinion in Psychiatry* 26 (4): 376–83.

WHO (World Health Organization). 1992. *The ICD-10 Classification of Diseases: Clinical Descriptions and Diagnostic Guidelines.* Geneva: WHO.

———. 2008. *The Global Burden of Disease: 2004 Update.* Geneva: WHO.

Yang, L. H., and B. G. Link. 2009. "Comparing Diagnostic Methods for Mental Disorders in China." *The Lancet* 373 (9680): 2002–04.

Chapter **3**

Excess Mortality from Mental, Neurological, and Substance Use Disorders in the Global Burden of Disease Study 2010

Fiona J. Charlson, Amanda J. Baxter, Tarun Dua,
Louisa Degenhardt, Harvey A. Whiteford, and Theo Vos

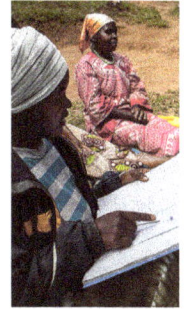

INTRODUCTION

Findings from the Global Burden of Disease Study 2010 (GBD 2010) have reinforced the understanding of the significant impact that mental, neurological, and substance use disorders have on population health (Murray and others 2012; Whiteford and others 2013). One key finding was the health transition from communicable to noncommunicable diseases across all regions. This transition was particularly evident in low- and middle-income countries (LMICs) (Murray and others 2012), where the proportion of burden attributable to noncommunicable disease increased from 36 percent in 1990 to 49 percent in 2010, compared with an increase from 80 percent to 83 percent in high-income countries (HICs) (IHME 2013).

GBD 2010 estimates that the majority of disease burden caused by mental, neurological, and substance use disorders is from nonfatal health loss; only 15 percent of the total burden is from mortality in years of life lost (YLLs) (IHME 2013). This finding may erroneously lead to the interpretation that premature death in people with mental, neurological, and substance use disorders is inconsequential. A recent review has shown higher mortality risks than the general population for a range of mental disorders, with a standardized mortality ratio (SMR) as high as 14.7 for opioid use

disorders (Chesney, Goodwin, and Fazel 2014). Excess mortality in people with epilepsy is reported to be two- to three-fold higher than that of the general population, with an increased risk up to six-fold higher in LMICs (Diop and others 2005). A significant proportion of these deaths is preventable (Diop and others 2005; Jette and Trevathan 2014).

There are multiple causes for lower life expectancy in people with mental disorders (Chang and others 2011; Crump and others 2013; Lawrence, Hancock, and Kisely 2013). Self-harm is an important cause of death, but the majority of premature deaths are caused by chronic physical disease, particularly ischemic heart disease (IHD), stroke, type II diabetes, respiratory diseases, and cancer (Crump and others 2013; Lawrence, Hancock, and Kisely 2013). Dementia is an independent risk factor for premature death; and patients with physical impairment, inactivity, and medical comorbidities are at increased risk (Park and others 2014).

In many HICs, the life expectancy gap between those with mental disorders and the general population is widening. The general population enjoys a longer life, while the lifespan for those with mental, neurological, and substance use disorders remains significantly lower and unchanged (Lawrence, Hancock, and Kisely 2013). Information on the extent and causes of premature mortality in people with mental, neurological, and substance

Corresponding author: Fiona J. Charlson, University of Queensland, School of Public Health, Herston, Queensland, Australia; fiona_charlson@qcmhr.uq.edu.au.

use disorders in LMICs is sparse, but these groups are understood to experience reduced life expectancy, although causes of death may vary across regions.

This chapter explores the cause-specific and excess mortality of individual mental, neurological, and substance use disorders estimated by GBD 2010 and discusses the results. We present the additional burden that can be attributed to these disorders, using GBD results for comparative risk assessments (CRAs) assessing mental, neurological, and substance use disorders as risk factors for other health outcomes. We focus on the following mental, neurological, and substance use disorders:

- Mental disorders, including schizophrenia, major depressive disorder, anxiety disorders, bipolar disorder, autistic disorder, and disruptive behavioral disorders (attention-deficit hyperactivity disorder [ADHD] and conduct disorder [CD])
- Substance use disorders, including alcohol use disorders (alcohol dependence and fetal alcohol syndrome) and opioid, cocaine, cannabis, and amphetamine dependence
- Neurological disorders, including dementia, epilepsy, and migraine.

For the purposes of GBD 2010, countries were grouped into 21 regions and 7 super-regions based on geographic proximity and levels of child and adult mortality (IHME 2014; Murray and others 2012). Regions were further grouped into developed and developing categories using the GBD 2010 method. Details of countries in each region and super-region can be found on the Institute for Health Metrics and Evaluation (IHME) website (IHME 2014).

The mortality associated with a disease can be quantified using two different, yet complementary, methods employed as part of the GBD analyses. First, cause-specific mortality draws on vital registration systems and verbal autopsy studies that identify deaths attributed to a single underlying cause using the International Classification of Diseases (ICD) death coding system. Second, GBD creates natural history models of disease, drawing on a range of epidemiological inputs, which ultimately provide epidemiological estimates for parameters including excess mortality—that is, the all-cause mortality rate in a population with the disorder above the all-cause mortality rate observed in a population without the disorder. By definition, the estimates of excess deaths include cause-specific deaths.

Although arbitrary, the ICD conventions are a necessary attempt to deal with the multi-causal nature of mortality and avoid the double-counting of deaths. Despite the system's clear strengths, cause-specific mortality estimated via the ICD obscures the contribution of other underlying causes of death—for example, suicide as a direct result of major depressive disorder—and likely underestimates the true number of deaths attributable to a particular disorder. However, the estimation of excess mortality using natural history models often includes deaths from causal and noncausal origins and likely overestimates the true number of deaths attributable to a particular disorder. The challenge is to parse out causal contributions to mortality, beyond those already identified as cause-specific, from the effects of confounders.

The quantification of the burden attributable to risk factors requires approaches such as CRA, which is now an integral part of the GBD studies. The fundamental approach is to calculate the proportion of deaths or disease burden caused by specific risk factors—for example, lung cancer caused by tobacco smoking—while holding all other independent factors constant. A counterfactual approach is used to compare the burden associated to an outcome with the amount expected in a hypothetical situation of ideal risk factor exposure, for example, zero prevalence. This provides a consistent method for estimating the changes in population health when decreasing or increasing the level of exposure to risk factors (Lim and others 2012).

METHODOLOGY

Years of Life Lost and Cause of Death

The GBD uses YLLs to quantify the fatal burden due to a given disease or injury (Lozano and others 2012). YLLs are computed by multiplying the number of deaths attributable to a particular disease at each age by a standard life expectancy at that age. The standard life expectancy represents the normative goal for survival; for GBD 2010, it was computed based on the lowest recorded death rates in any age group in countries with populations greater than five million (Salomon and others 2012).

Cause-specific death estimates in GBD 2010 were produced from available cause-of-death data for 187 countries from 1980 to 2010. Data sources included vital registration, verbal autopsy, mortality surveillance, censuses, surveys, hospitals, police records, and mortuaries (Lozano and others 2012). Because cause-of-death data are often not available or are subject to substantial problems of comparability, a method of modeling cause-of-death estimates and trends was developed. Cause of Death Ensemble Modeling (CODEm) was used for all mental, neurological, and substance use disorders (Foreman and others 2012). CODEm uses four families of statistical models testing a large set of different models using different permutations of covariates. Model ensembles were developed from these component models, and model performance was assessed with rigorous out-of-sample testing of prediction error and the coverage of 95 percent uncertainty intervals. Details relating to CODEm and the method for how these models were used in calculating YLLs are described in detail elsewhere (Foreman and others 2012; Lozano and others 2012).

Ultimately, YLLs for GBD 2010 were computed from cause-specific mortality estimates for only 7 of the 15 mental, neurological, and substance use disorders investigated in this chapter (Lozano and others 2012):

- Dementia
- Epilepsy
- Schizophrenia
- Alcohol use disorders (including alcohol dependence and fetal alcohol syndrome)
- Opioid dependence
- Amphetamine dependence
- Cocaine dependence.

The justification for this selection lies in the rules of the ICD, which specify that the recorded cause of death should be the primary or direct cause of death, resulting in several important disorders being absent from the ICD cause-of-death list (Lim and others 2012; WHO 1993). For example, a person dying from endocarditis caused by injecting drug use is likely to have the cause of death coded to endocarditis rather than the substance use disorder.

Excess Mortality from Natural History Models

The GBD 2010 methods for developing a natural history model of disease using DisMod-MR are discussed in chapter 2 in this volume (Whiteford and others 2015) and in detail elsewhere (Ferrari and others 2013; Murray and others 2012). DisMod-MR is a Bayesian meta-regression tool that estimates a generalized negative binomial model for all epidemiological data (Murray and others 2012). The primary role of this modeling is to derive internally consistent models of prevalence that are used to produce burden of disease estimates—years lived with disability (YLDs) and disability-adjusted life years (DALYs). The models also provide estimates of other epidemiological parameters, utilizing the relationship described in figure 3.1 (Murray and others 2012). Excess mortality estimates for mental, neurological, and substance use disorders were made available through this process.

Cause-specific mortality estimated using ICD coding rules does not consider the contribution of underlying causes of death. However, estimates of excess deaths produced by DisMod-MR include deaths from causal and noncausal origins and therefore overestimate the true number of deaths attributable to a particular disorder. In this chapter, although we compare GBD 2010 estimates from both of these data sources and discuss the discrepancies between the two, caution should be exercised in interpreting the excess mortality data attributable to mental, neurological, and substance use disorders.

Figure 3.1 Generic Disease Model

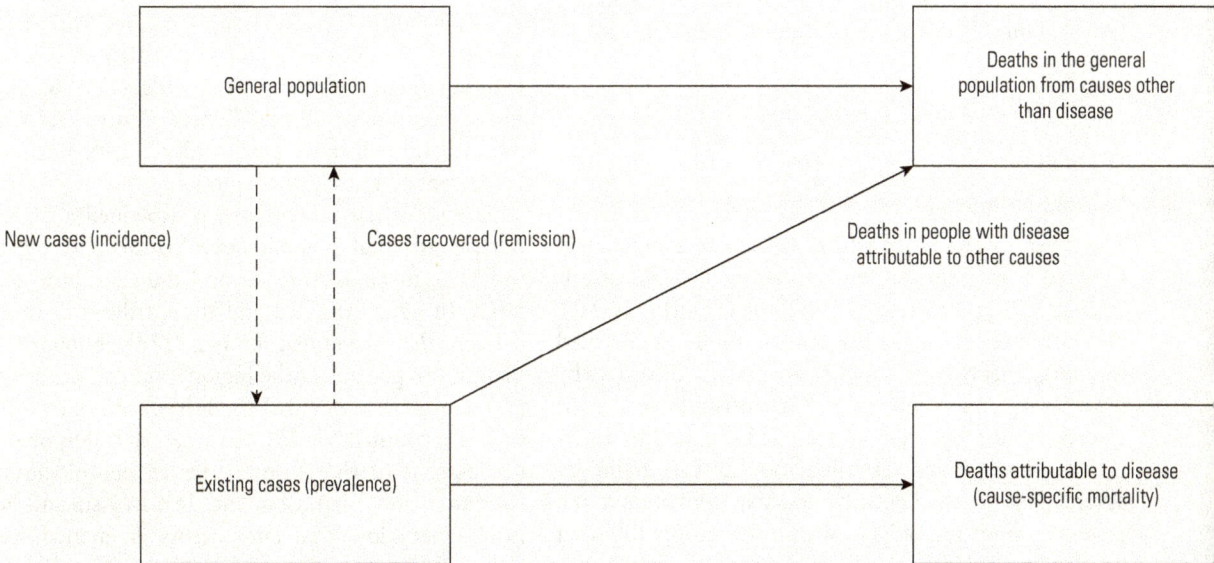

Source: Adapted from Barendregt and others 2003, figure 1.

Counterfactual Burden and Comparative Risk Assessment

Using counterfactual analysis, the effect of a risk factor can be quantified by comparing the burden associated with an outcome with the amount expected in a hypothetical situation of ideal risk factor exposure. Prince and others (2007) have summarized the evidence where causal relationships between mental and substance use disorders and other health outcomes have been proposed. In GBD 2010, reviews were conducted to assess the strength of evidence for mental, neurological, and substance use disorders as independent risk factors for other health outcomes (Charlson and others 2011; Degenhardt and Hall 2012; Degenhardt, Hall, and others 2009; Rehm, Baliunas, and others 2010). Risk factor studies were identified through systematic searches of published and unpublished data, and information on effect sizes and study characteristics was extracted and collated (Charlson and others 2013; Degenhardt, Whiteford, and others 2013; Ferrari and others 2014).

Data were metasynthesized to calculate relative risks (RR) for mental and alcohol use disorders (the exposures) as risk factors for other health outcomes. These included mental and substance use disorders collectively as risk factors for suicide, alcohol use as a risk factor for a range of health outcomes, and injecting drug use as a risk factor for blood-borne viruses. The RR was applied to prevalence distributions of the specific exposures by gender and age group for each region to derive population attributable fractions (PAFs). The additional burden (YLLs and YLDs) attributable to mental, neurological, and substance use disorders is the product of the PAFs and the burden for the health outcome as estimated in GBD 2010. More detail on the calculation of PAFs in GBD 2010 is provided by Lim and others (2012).

MORTALITY AND MENTAL, NEUROLOGICAL, AND SUBSTANCE USE DISORDERS

Causal Mortality and Years of Life Lost

The seven disorders for which YLLs were estimated in GBD 2010 were directly responsible for 840,000 deaths in 2010, or approximately 20 million YLLs (figure 3.2). Online annex 3A further summarizes the YLLs allocated to mental, neurological, and substance use disorders by disorder, age, and gender. The YLLs attributable to each disorder as a proportion of total YLLs caused by mental, neurological, and substance use disorders highlight several key points. Globally, epilepsy contributed the greatest proportion of YLLs within this group, followed by dementia. Although the impact of substance use disorders, specifically alcohol and opioid dependence,

is evident, the comparatively smaller contribution of several mental disorders is a finding that requires further explanation.

Examination of age-standardized YLL rates indicates large variations across the seven GBD 2010 geographical super-regions, primarily because of differences in patterns of alcohol use disorders, drug dependence, and mental and neurological disorder prevalence. Several regions have significant deviations from the global average YLL rates (figure 3.3).

In figure 3.3, amphetamine and cocaine dependence have been aggregated under psychostimulant dependence. Details of which countries are in each super-region can be found on the IHME website (IHME 2014).

In 2010, YLL rates were highest in Sub-Saharan Africa (604 YLLs per 100,000 population) and Central/Eastern Europe and Central Asia (593 YLLs per 100,000); the causes of these high fatal burden estimates vary considerably (figure 3.3). In Sub-Saharan Africa, the YLL burden was driven by epilepsy, which accounted for 511 YLLs per 100,000 population. This rate is fourfold higher than the global average and approximately 85 percent of all YLLs attributed to mental, neurological, and substance use disorders in the region. Sub-Saharan Africa has comparatively lower YLL rates for substance use disorders; however, illicit drug dependence YLLs increased by 3.0 percent from 1990 to 2010, almost double the average global increase and the highest of all regions. The Middle East and North Africa follows with a 2.6 percent increase (Degenhardt, Whiteford, and others 2013).

The high fatal burden in Central/Eastern Europe and Central Asia was largely caused by deaths attributed to alcohol use disorders. These disorders accounted for 331 YLLs per 100,000 population, compared with a global average of 57 YLLs per 100,000 population. High mortality caused by illicit drug use disorders also contributed to the YLL rate in Central/Eastern Europe and Central Asia, with all substance use disorders together explaining 73 percent of YLLs in the region.

Substance use disorders also explained a high proportion of total mental, neurological, and substance use YLLs in Latin America and the Caribbean and in HICs. In Latin America and the Caribbean, substance use disorders accounted for 142 YLLs per 100,000 population (54 percent of the region's mental, neurological, and substance use YLLs). In HICs, substance use disorders accounted for 151 YLLs per 100,000 population (49 percent of the region's mental, neurological, and substance use YLLs). Countries in East Asia and Pacific exhibit very low YLL rates across all mental, neurological, and substance use disorders, with little change observed between 1990 and 2010.

Globally, neurological disorders accounted for 58 percent of all mental, neurological, and substance use disorder YLLs in men, and 81 percent in women. Substance use disorders explained 39 percent of YLLs in men and 16 percent in women. The contribution of schizophrenia to total mental, neurological, and substance use disorder YLLs was similar for both genders, at 3 percent each.

Differences in YLL patterns between the genders were influenced in part by the differing contribution to YLLs of substance use disorders compared with neurological disorders across regions. Where substance use disorders dominated YLLs, their higher prevalence in men drove up the overall YLL rates in men, compared with women. Interestingly, the gender differential was not stable across regions: in Central/Eastern Europe and Central Asia, there was a smaller gender difference in the proportion of YLLs caused by alcohol use disorders (61 percent of mental, neurological, and alcohol use disorder YLLs in men and 40 percent in women). A much larger gender differential exists in Latin America and the Caribbean, where 57 percent of YLLs were caused by alcohol use disorders in men and 15 percent in women. The gender differential for YLLs caused by alcohol use disorders was comparatively smaller in HICs: 28 percent of YLLs in men and 13 percent of YLLs in women, compared with the global mean of 27 percent and 9 percent, for men and women, respectively.

In those regions where neurological disorders contribute the greater proportion of YLLs, the gender differential was considerably smaller, as shown in figure 3.4. In Sub-Saharan Africa, for example, where epilepsy deaths were very high, there was less of a gender difference: epilepsy explained 84 percent of mental, neurological, and substance use disorder YLLs in men, compared with 86 percent in women. In South Asia, epilepsy contributed 60 percent of YLLs in men and 65 percent in women.

Excess Mortality from a Natural History Model

The GBD cause-of-death modeling translates to a relatively small YLL burden attributable to mental, neurological, and substance use disorders; however, to conclude that mental disorders are not associated with premature death would be misleading. The mental disorders for which cause-specific deaths and YLLs were estimated in GBD 2010 were schizophrenia and anorexia nervosa (the latter is not considered in this chapter). Several other mental disorders, such as major depressive disorder and bipolar disorder, exhibit significant and documented excess mortality (Baxter, Page, and Whiteford 2011; Roshanaei-Moghaddam and Katon 2009) (table 3.1).

Figure 3.2 Age-Standardized YLL Rates by Disorder, as a Proportion of Global YLL Rates for Mental, Neurological, and Substance Use Disorders, per 100,000 Population, 2010

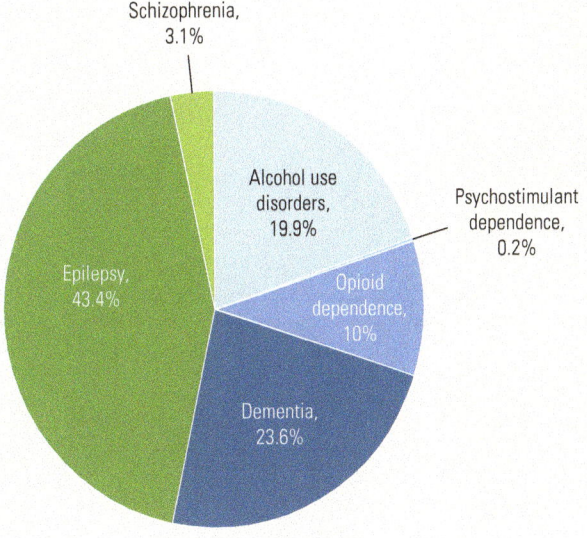

Source: IHME 2013.
Note: For the purposes of this graph, amphetamine and cocaine dependence have been aggregated under psychostimulant dependence. The individual disorder proportions are amphetamine dependence (0.1 percent) and cocaine dependence (0.1 percent). YLLs = years of life lost.

Figure 3.3 Age-Standardized YLL Rates for Mental, Neurological, and Substance Use Disorders, by GBD 2010 Super-Region and Disorder, per 100,000 Population, 2010

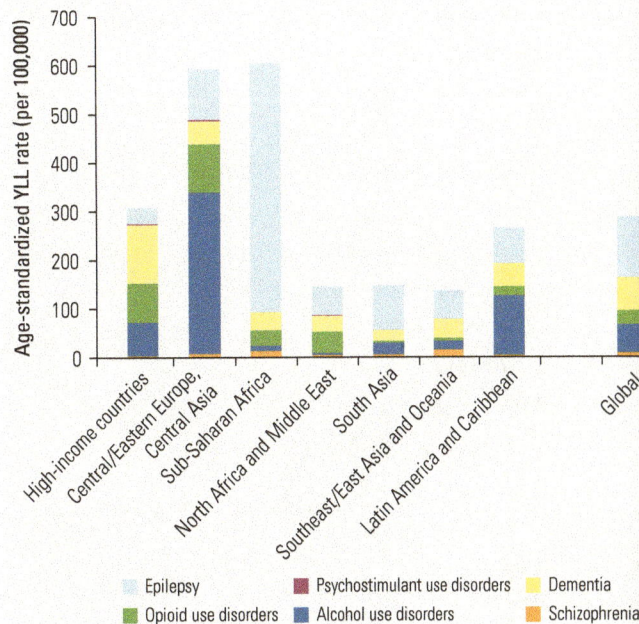

Source: IHME 2013.
Note: GBD = Global Burden of Disease; YLL = year of life lost.

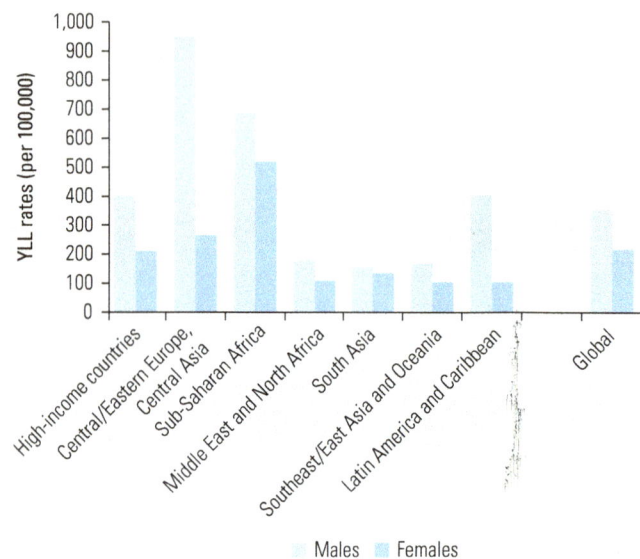

Figure 3.4 Age-Standardized YLL Rates for Mental, Neurological, and Substance Use Disorders, by GBD 2010 Super-Region and Gender, per 100,000 Population, 2010

Source: IHME 2013.
Note: GBD = Global Burden of Disease; YLL = year of life lost.

These were not included in the estimated cause-specific deaths and YLLs, because the method for cause-of-death estimation, where death counts are used to calculate YLLs, can only be attributed to the primary ICD cause of death.

Examination of excess mortality derived from natural history models of disease allows for a better appreciation of the contribution of underlying diseases to poor health outcomes. There were five disorders for which sufficient evidence of excess all-cause mortality could not be found in the literature—anxiety disorders, ADHD, CD, cannabis dependence, and migraine—and no estimations of excess mortality were made.

Mental Disorders

Figure 3.5 shows the estimated number of cause-specific and excess deaths for each of the five mental disorders, with estimated excess mortality by age and uncertainty bounds. Inspection of excess deaths suggests that schizophrenia, major depressive disorder, bipolar disorder, and autistic disorder are all associated with significant premature mortality not reflected in YLL calculations. This work should be interpreted with caution, given that not

Table 3.1 Presence of Cause-Specific Mortality and Excess Mortality Attributed to Mental, Neurological, and Substance Use Disorders in GBD 2010

Disorders	Cause-specific mortality attributed to disorders in GBD 2010	Excess mortality attributed to disorders in GBD 2010
Mental disorders		
Major depressive disorder	No	Yes
Anxiety disorders	No	No
Schizophrenia	Yes	Yes
Bipolar disorders	No	Yes
Disruptive behavioral disorders: ADHD and CD	No	No
Autistic disorder	No	Yes
Substance use disorders		
Alcohol use disorders[a]	Yes	Yes
Opioid dependence	Yes	Yes
Cannabis dependence	No	No
Amphetamine dependence	Yes	Yes
Cocaine dependence	Yes	Yes
Neurological disorders		
Epilepsy	Yes	Yes
Migraine	No	No
Dementia	Yes	Yes

Note: ADHD = attention-deficit hyperactivity disorder; CD = conduct disorder; GBD = Global Burden of Disease study.
a. Cause-specific deaths for alcohol use disorders include those from alcohol dependence and fetal alcohol syndrome; differentially, excess deaths represent those from alcohol dependence only.

Figure 3.5 Cause-Specific and Excess Deaths Attributed to Mental Disorders, by Age, with 95 percent Uncertainty, 2010

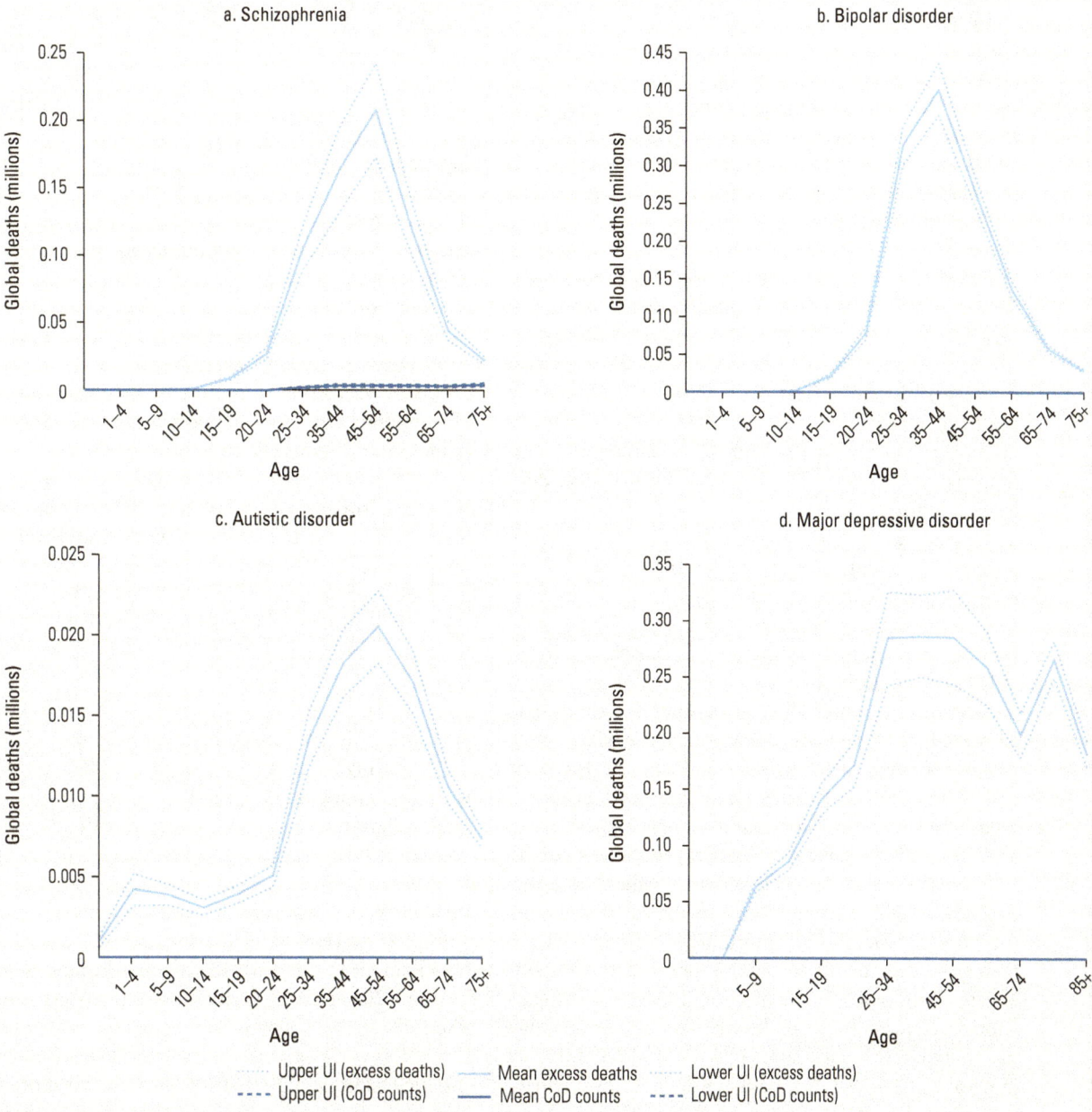

a. Schizophrenia

b. Bipolar disorder

c. Autistic disorder

d. Major depressive disorder

Upper UI (excess deaths) ···· Mean excess deaths —— Lower UI (excess deaths) ····
Upper UI (CoD counts) ‐‐‐‐ Mean CoD counts —— Lower UI (CoD counts) ‐‐‐‐

Source: IHME 2013.

Note: CoD = cause-specific deaths; UI = uncertainty interval. Disruptive behavioral disorders (attention-deficit hyperactivity disorder and conduct disorder) and anxiety are not shown, as cause-specific and excess mortality were not estimated.

all the excess deaths estimated by DisMod-MR will be causally attributable to the disorder. A complex interplay of risk factors will typically contribute to the high rates of all-cause mortality in people with mental disorders.

Mental disorders can directly impact the risk of chronic disease through underlying biochemical mechanisms (Stapelberg and others 2011). For example, major

depression is linked to higher rates of coronary heart disease (Charlson and others 2011). Lifestyle risk factors and the use of medications in the treatment of some mental disorders contribute to higher morbidity and mortality rates through increased risk of obesity and metabolic dysfunction. Smoking rates are significantly higher in people with mental disorders (Lasser and others 2000); this group experiences disproportionate tobacco-related harm.

Despite their increased exposure to chronic disease risk factors, people with mental disorders have inequitable access to health care, with less opportunity for metabolic risk factor screening (Crump and others 2013) and early cancer detection (Kisely, Campbell, and Wang 2009) and lower rates of common prescriptions and procedures (Kisely and others 2007; Laursen and others 2009), even in HICs.

Schizophrenia. People with schizophrenia have well-documented premature mortality (Laursen 2011), but very few YLLs in GBD 2010. Although schizophrenia is one of the few mental disorders with cause-specific deaths permissible by ICD, the number of cause-specific deaths globally (approximately 20,000) is noticeably lower compared with the number of all-cause deaths (approximately 700,000) ascribed by the disorder's natural history.

Research from HICs suggests that men with schizophrenia die about 15 years earlier than men without schizophrenia; women with schizophrenia die, on average, 12 years earlier than women without schizophrenia (Crump and others 2013; Lawrence, Hancock, and Kisely 2013). The majority of these deaths is due to chronic disease; cardiovascular disease accounts for more than 33 percent of all premature deaths in those with schizophrenia (Crump and others 2013; Lawrence, Hancock, and Kisely 2013). Suicide, homicide, and accidents account for less than 15 percent of excess deaths (Crump and others 2013; Lawrence, Hancock, and Kisely 2013).

The side effects of antipsychotic medications, particularly weight gain and impaired glucose tolerance, increase the risk of excess mortality in people regularly taking these medications. Despite concerns over the side effects of antipsychotic medication, the lack of antipsychotic treatment has been linked with higher all-cause mortality rates (hazard ratio [HR] 1.45; 95% confidence interval [CI], 1.20-1.76), with the highest risks attributed to suicide (HR 2.07; 95% CI, 0.73-5.87) and cancer (HR 1.94; 95% CI, 1.13-3.32) (Crump and others 2013). Research shows that although cancer-related death rates are higher in this group, people with schizophrenia are at lower risk of developing cancer (Grinshpoon and others 2005). High mortality rates therefore likely reflect inadequate and unequal access to health care and lower rates of diagnostic screening. Multiple medications and discontinuation of medication also appear to increase the risk of all-cause death (Haukka and others 2008; Joukamaa and others 2006).

Research suggests that the majority of excess mortality in people with schizophrenia could be directly attributable to their condition: a strong and consistent relationship between schizophrenia and higher death rates has been shown; the onset of schizophrenia generally precedes the physical health condition causally associated with their death; and plausible biological pathways exist through the side effects of medication and unhealthy behaviors directly related to the condition (Laursen, Nordentoft, and Mortensen 2014). Although poverty may be a confounding factor, with schizophrenia more prevalent in low socioeconomic populations that tend to experience poorer health outcomes, evidence indicates that people with schizophrenia move to these populations because of the impact of their disorder, such as difficulty in securing education and employment because of cognitive and social problems (Lambert, Velakoulis, and Pantelis 2003). Accordingly, schizophrenia can be the mediating factor for poorer socioeconomic and health outcomes.

Bipolar Disorder. Approximately 1.3 million excess deaths were estimated in the natural history model of bipolar disorder. However, in contrast to schizophrenia, no cause-specific deaths are attributed to the disorder. The natural history of the disease suggests that bipolar disorder is associated with more excess deaths globally than schizophrenia. Research from the United Kingdom suggests that the excess mortality rates in schizophrenia and bipolar disorder are comparable (Chang and others 2011); the higher number of deaths is likely explained by the higher population prevalence of bipolar disorders (58.9 million cases in 2010, compared with 23.8 million cases for schizophrenia) (Whiteford and others 2013). An estimated 80 percent of premature deaths in people with bipolar disorder is caused by physical disease, almost 50 percent of which is cardiovascular disease (Westman and others 2013). Unnatural causes account for nearly 20 percent of premature deaths (Westman and others 2013).

Autistic Disorder. GBD 2010 estimated that more than 100,000 excess deaths were caused by autistic disorder. There is clear evidence of premature mortality in the natural history of autistic disorder, despite lack of disorder-specific deaths registered using ICD codes. People with developmental disorders are at twice the risk of premature death compared with the general population (Mouridsen and others 2008). There are several causes of elevated death rates in autistic disorder, including accidents, respiratory diseases, and seizures (Mouridsen and others 2008; Shavelle, Strauss, and Pickett 2001). Autism spectrum disorders are highly comorbid, with a range of potentially life-limiting physical conditions, including epilepsy and chromosomal disorders such as fragile X syndrome (Gillberg and Billstedt 2000), which suggest shared underlying pathophysiology. Without an identified temporal sequence in onset of these comorbid disorders and a plausible biological pathway, it is likely that the causal relationship between autistic disorder and elevated mortality may be due more to the presence of comorbid conditions rather than autistic disorder itself (Bilder and others 2013; Lee and others 2008).

Major Depressive Disorder. No deaths were coded to major depressive disorder in GBD 2010, because the disorder was absent from the list of ICD cause-of-death codes. Natural history models of major depressive disorder suggest that more than 2.2 million excess deaths occurred in this group. In GBD 2010, no YLLs and no excess all-cause mortality were found for dysthymic disorder, consistent with previous findings (Baxter, Page, and Whiteford 2011).

As is the case for other disorders, YLL calculations based on cause-of-death estimates for major depressive disorder highlight the gap between those deaths that can be causally attributed to a disorder and excess deaths, some of which will not be directly attributable to the disorder. More than two million excess deaths produced by DisMod-MR in 2010 is high, and likely to be an overestimate of directly attributable deaths when considered in a strict cause-and-effect framework, but this finding highlights the importance of deciphering the complex interplay of factors linking major depressive disorder with other health outcomes.

Anxiety Disorders. The information on excess mortality in anxiety disorders is inconsistent. Some anxiety disorders, especially severe presentations of post-traumatic stress disorder, have been associated with increased deaths caused by IHD, neoplasms, and intentional and unintentional injuries (Ahmadi and others 2011; Lawrence, Hancock, and Kisely 2013). There is insufficient information, however, to determine whether premature mortality is significantly raised across the entire spectrum of anxiety disorders (Baxter and others 2014). In GBD 2010, no YLLs or excess mortality were associated with the natural history of disease applied to the broad category of anxiety disorders.

Disruptive Behavioral Disorders. Disruptive behavioral disorders are associated with poor health outcomes across the lifespan. Research shows that children with ADHD or CD are two to three times more likely to experience unintentional injuries requiring medical attention than children without behavioral disorders (Lee and others 2008; Rowe, Maughan, and Goodman 2004). The most commonly reported injuries included

burns, poisoning, and fractures (Rowe, Maughan, and Goodman 2004). Adolescents and young adults with inattention disorders are more likely to be involved in traffic accidents (Jerome, Segal, and Habinski 2006). Adults who were identified with behavioral disorders in childhood are at higher risk of cigarette smoking, binge drinking, and obesity (von Stumm and others 2011).

Despite the strong evidence of an association between childhood behavioral disorders and poorer health outcomes, insufficient data are available to model the natural history of disease; accordingly, no estimates quantify excess mortality in this group at the population level. However, it is likely that a significant proportion of excess mortality is causally attributable to these conditions. There is not only an implicit temporal relationship between onset of ADHD (that is, several symptoms must be present prior to age 12) and dangerous driving, but also a plausible biological mechanism in the relationship, specifically, the characteristic pattern of inattention and impulsivity of ADHD that leads to dangerous driving.

Substance Use Disorders

Figure 3.6 shows the estimated number of cause-specific and excess deaths for each substance use disorder, with estimated excess mortality by age and uncertainty bounds.

Alcohol Use Disorders. The number of cause-specific deaths attributed to alcohol use disorders in 2010 (111,000) was substantially lower than the number of excess deaths (1.95 million) calculated using natural history models.

Light to moderate alcohol consumption has been associated with lower rates of some diseases, such as diabetes mellitus and coronary heart disease. However, heavy consumption has been associated with increased rates of chronic diseases, including cancer; mental, neurological, and substance use disorders; cardiovascular disease; and liver and pancreas diseases (Rehm, Baliunas, and others 2010):

- Evidence suggests that alcohol may be a carcinogen in humans, with particularly strong causal links established between alcoholic beverage consumption and oral cavity, pharynx, larynx, esophagus, liver, colorectal, and female breast cancers (Rehm, Baliunas, and others 2010).
- A consistent relationship has been found between heavy alcohol consumption and epilepsy (Rehm, Baliunas, and others 2010).
- Alcohol has been implicated in the development of depression and personality disorders, although the

Cause-Specific and Excess Deaths Attributed to Substance Use Disorders, by Age, with Uncertainty, 2010

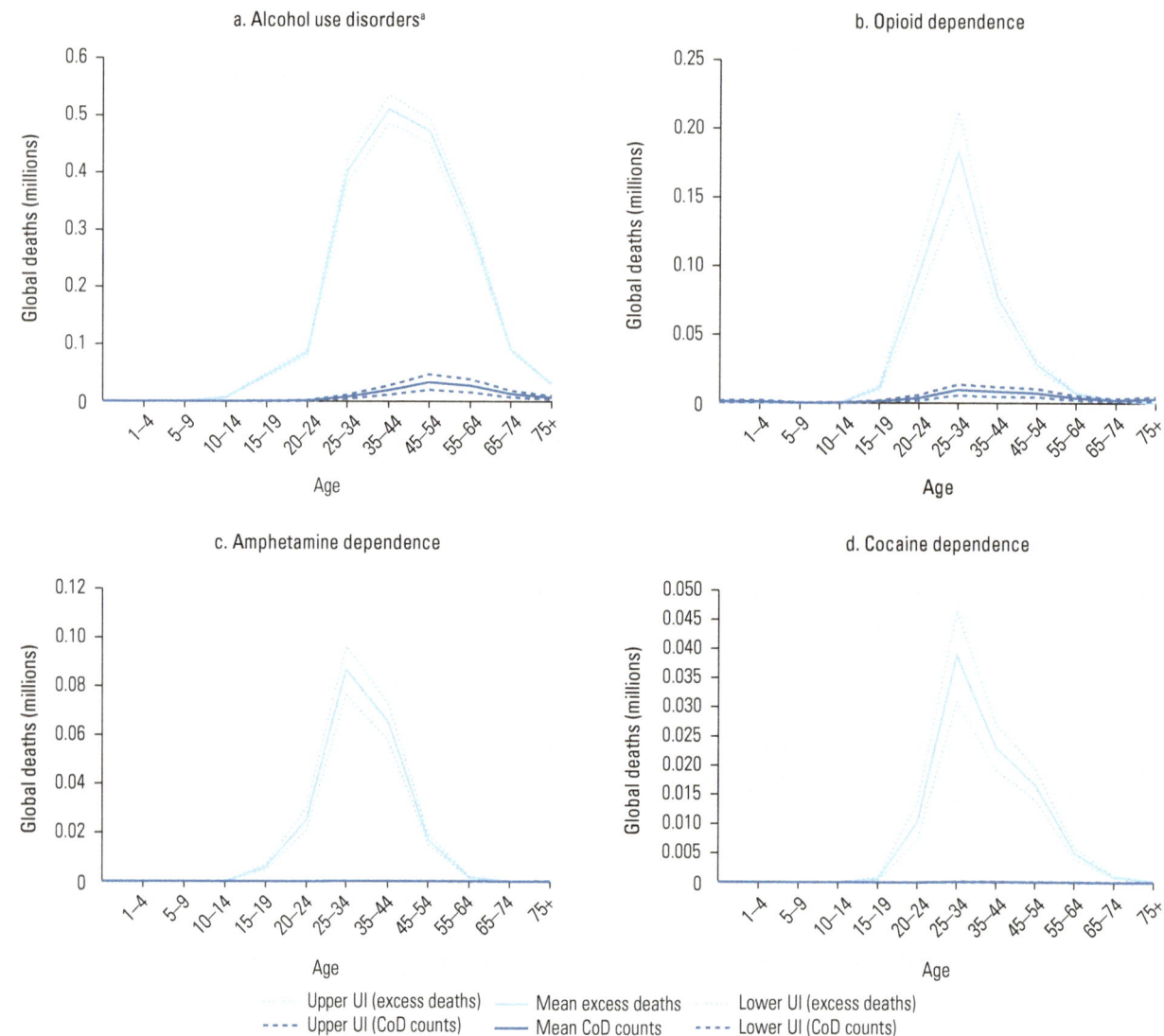

direction of causality and the effects of confounding factors remain uncertain (Rao, Daley, and Hammen 2000; Rohde and others 2001).

- The relationship between alcohol consumption and liver cirrhosis is well recognized, but alcohol use disorders appear to be more strongly related to cirrhosis mortality versus morbidity, as it negatively affects the course of existing liver disease (Rehm, Baliunas, and others 2010).
- Heavy alcohol use is related to higher rates of infectious diseases, such as tuberculosis, and unintentional and intentional injuries, with strong evidence for a dose-response relationship (Rehm, Baliunas, and others 2010).
- The risk of death through injuries and self-harm is elevated, accounting for approximately 30 million YLLs globally.

The elevated risks in those with alcohol use disorders appear to be mediated by the quantity of alcohol consumed and the drinking pattern (Rehm, Baliunas, and others 2010).

Illicit Drug Use Disorders. Between 95,800 (in cocaine dependence) and 404,000 (in opioid dependence) excess deaths occurred in dependent illicit drug users in 2010, compared with 78,000 deaths in which illicit drug use was identified as the explicit cause. The majority of these cause-specific deaths—43,000—are attributable to opioid dependence (Degenhardt, Whiteford, and others 2013).

Excess and premature deaths in illicit drug users occur in several ways, including the acute toxic effects of illicit drug use that may lead to overdose, specifically, the cause-specific deaths captured by the ICD coding system. In addition, substantial numbers of deaths are likely to be caused by the more indirect effects of intoxication that result in accidental injuries and violence, cardiovascular disease, liver disease, and a range of mental disorders. Suicide is an important outcome, particularly for opioid users, where an SMR of approximately 14 has been reported in two separate reviews (Chesney, Goodwin, and Fazel 2014; Degenhardt and others 2011). The injection of drugs carries a high risk of blood-borne bacterial and viral infections, notably, human immunodeficiency virus and acquired immune deficiency syndrome (HIV/AIDS), hepatitis B, and hepatitis C (Mathers and others 2010; Nelson and others 2011).

Neurological Disorders
Cause-specific death estimates are more substantial for neurological disorders (figure 3.7), resulting in a smaller gap between cause-specific and excess deaths. This finding may reflect the increasing recognition of neurological disorders as the primary cause of death.

Epilepsy. Epilepsy was modeled as an envelope condition in GBD 2010; idiopathic epilepsy and epilepsy were secondary to a range of causes, including meningitis, neonatal tetanus, iodine deficiency, and a variety of birth complications modeled as one disorder. Cause-of-death modeling estimated nearly 200,000 deaths caused by epilepsy in 2010; natural history models show approximately 300,000 excess deaths. The high number of deaths in young children is clear in figure 3.7.

Mortality in people with epilepsy is generally two- to three-fold higher than mortality in the general community (Preux and Druet-Cabanac 2005; Trinka and others 2013). The relative mortality in those with epilepsy in LMICs is significantly higher than in HICs (Carpio and others 2005; Diop and others 2005), particularly in poorer, rural populations (Carpio and others 2005). Mortality data from HICs show that most deaths are caused by underlying conditions, such as neoplasms, cerebrovascular diseases, and cardiac disease (Spencer 2014); a greater proportion of deaths in LMICs appears to be related to epilepsy (Carpio and others 2005; Diop and others 2005) or to accident or injury (Carpio and others 2005; Kamgno, Pion, and Boussinesq 2003;

Figure 3.7 Numbers of Cause-Specific and Excess Deaths Attributed to Neurological Disorders, by Age, with Uncertainty, 2010

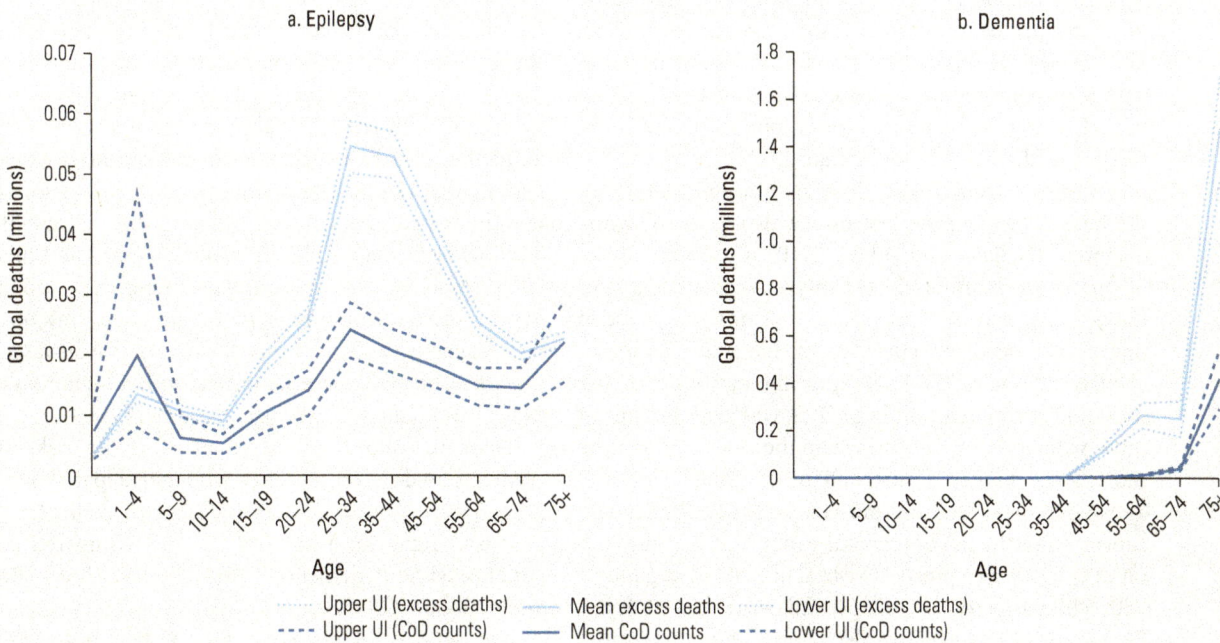

Source: IHME 2013.
Note: CoD = cause-specific deaths; UI = uncertainty interval. Migraine is not shown, as there was no cause-specific or excess mortality.

Mu and others 2011). These differences could be due partly to methodological differences or to genuine differences caused by the etiology of the disease and environmental risk factors.

The proportion of deaths attributable to epilepsy differs by region. In GBD 2010, Sub-Saharan Africa had the highest death rates caused by epilepsy (Murray and others 2012). Importantly, studies have shown that a large proportion of these deaths—those attributable to falls, drowning, burns, and status epilepticus—is preventable (Diop and others 2005; Jette and Trevathan 2014). In a large cohort of people with active convulsive epilepsy in rural Kenya, 38 percent of epilepsy-related deaths were caused by status epilepticus. Mortality in this cohort was more than six-fold greater than expected and associated with nonadherence to (or unavailability of) anti-epileptic drugs, cognitive impairment, and age (Ngugi and others 2014).

Kamgno, Pion, and Boussinesq (2003) found similarly high mortality rates in Cameroon, associated with poor access to or compliance with medical treatment. In a study of 164 patients with epilepsy followed for 30 years in Tanzania and treated with phenobarbital, 67.1 percent of the patients died, a mortality rate twice that of the rural Tanzanian population. The causes of death were related to epilepsy in more than 50 percent of the patients and included status epilepticus, drowning, and burns (Jilek-Aall and Rwiza 1992).

In other LMICs outside Sub-Saharan Africa, the preventable causes of death in epilepsy patients are also a significant factor. Drowning is the most common cause of premature death in rural China (proportional mortality ratio = 82.4 percent). This finding is attributed in part to geographic and occupational risk hazards that include living and working around ponds, paddy fields, cesspits, and wells (Mu and others 2011).

Epilepsy is associated with premature mortality, with the highest SMR in the first one to two years following diagnosis (Neligan and others 2010). Common causes of premature mortality in epilepsy include acute symptomatic disorders, such as brain tumor or stroke; sudden unexpected death in epilepsy; suicides; and accidents (Hitiris and others 2007). The epidemiology of premature mortality is very relevant in LMICs, where 85 percent of those with epilepsy live and where the risk of premature mortality is highest (Diop and others 2005; Jette and Trevathan 2014; Newton and Garcia 2012). Particularly concerning is the risk of premature mortality in childhood onset epilepsy. In a prospective trial in Finland of patients with childhood onset epilepsy followed for 40 years, 24 percent of the patients died. This rate is three times higher than the expected age- and gender-adjusted mortality in the general population (Sillanpää and Shinnar

2010); 55 percent of the deaths in the cohort were directly related to epilepsy, including sudden, unexplained death in 30 percent, definite or probable seizure in 15 percent, and accidental drowning in 10 percent.

Another important risk factor for premature mortality is comorbid mental illness. Most studies of mortality risk in this population have been conducted in HICs, and the extent of this risk factor in resource-limited settings is largely unknown. In a Swedish retrospective study, 75 percent of epilepsy patients dying from an external cause had comorbid psychiatric illness, most commonly depression and substance abuse (Fazel and others 2013). In a population-based study in the United Kingdom, mortality among epilepsy patients was associated with alcohol use and depression (Ridsdale and others 2011). In a meta-analysis of studies on suicide in epilepsy patients, Pompili and others (2005) found that the incidence of suicide was significantly higher among epilepsy patients than the general population. This striking mortality risk in epilepsy patients with mental disorders requires further study and intervention in LMICs, where the burden of epilepsy is highest.

Dementia. Our natural history model attributed more than two million excess deaths worldwide to dementia in 2010, compared with 500,000 cause-specific deaths derived from ICD records. Figure 3.7 shows that the majority of deaths caused by dementia, as expected, occur in the elderly.

Excess mortality in dementia has been associated with functional disability leading to unhealthy lifestyle factors and comorbid physical conditions (Guehne, Riedel-Heller, and Angermeyer 2005; Llibre and others 2008). Midlife cardiovascular risk factors have been associated with later mortality in patients who develop dementia. In a Norwegian prospective study following patients for 35 years, dementia mortality was associated with increased total cholesterol levels, diabetes mellitus, and low body mass index in midlife (Strand and others 2013). A study in seven countries found that smoking, hypercholesterolemia, high blood pressure, low forced vital capacity, and previous history of cardiovascular disease at baseline were associated with a higher risk of death from dementia (Alonso and others 2009).

Dementia shows an increased mortality risk. In a study of male civil servants who participated in the Israel Heart Disease study, patients with dementia had a hazard ratio for mortality of 2.27 compared with patients without dementia (95% CI, 1.92–2.68) (Beeri and Goldbourt 2001).

The severity of disease is one of the most significant predictors of premature death in individuals with dementia after controlling for other factors, with an HR for moderate cases of 2.0 (95% CI, 0.1-4.1) compared with mild cases, and an HR of 3.8 (95% CI, 2.7-3.4) for severe cases compared with mild cases (Gühne and others 2006). In a cohort of 15,209 patients in the Swedish Dementia Registry, lower scores on the mini-mental status examination, male gender, higher number of medications, institutionalization, and age were associated with increased death risk after dementia diagnosis (Garcia-Ptacek and others 2014).

Infections, particularly pneumonia, frequently lead to death in people with dementia (Mitchell and others 2009). Urinary tract infections caused by incontinence, as well as bedsores and deep venous clots caused by immobility, can lead to systemic bloodstream infections and death. Psychological agitation and aggression are frequent symptoms in patients with dementia, and antipsychotics are frequently prescribed, although significant increased mortality risk odds ratio (OR 1.7) is associated with typical and atypical antipsychotics. This practice has resulted in a formal black box warning by the United States Food and Drug Administration (U.S. FDA 2008). An independent, systematic review of 15 randomized control trials (RCTs) of atypical antipsychotics confirmed the significant increased risk (OR 1.54) for all antipsychotics (Schneider, Dagerman, and Insel 2005). The dementia antipsychotic withdrawal trial (DART-AD) trial reported increased mortality in patients who were prescribed agents in the long term and likely related to oversedation, dehydration, and prolongation of QT interval corrected for heart rate on electrocardiogram (Ballard and others 2009).

A clear causal relationship exists between dementia and premature death; however, other environmental factors can precede both outcomes and independently increase the risk of dementia and excess mortality. For example, education and literacy may confer a degree of protection against dementia and excess mortality (Prince and others 2012). Thus, these factors, which are already high on the agenda for LMICs, may be considered independent, modifiable risk factors in reduced life expectancy, explaining a portion of the excess mortality currently associated with dementia.

Deaths across the Lifespan

Cause-specific deaths from mental, neurological, and substance use disorders increase steadily across the lifespan, with the exception of a peak at ages one to four years caused by epilepsy-related deaths. The greatest number of deaths occurs in the oldest group (ages 75 years and older). This finding is explained almost entirely by dementia, including Alzheimer's disease, although it may, at least in part, be caused by the broad age-grouping at this age (table 3.2). If dementia deaths are excluded, the number of deaths attributable to mental, neurological, and substance use disorders is highest between ages 35 and 54 years; most are caused by epilepsy and alcohol use disorders.

Table 3.2 shows that the cause-specific deaths and excess deaths directly coded to mental, neurological, and substance use disorders are relatively similar up to age four years. After this age point, excess deaths rise sharply in relation to cause-specific deaths. As with cause-specific deaths, the greatest number of excess deaths occurs at ages 75 years and older due to dementia. If dementia deaths are excluded, excess deaths would peak between 25 and 54 years of age; the majority is attributable to alcohol use disorders.

Counter-Factual Burden and Comparative Risk Assessment

In GBD 2010, literature investigating mental, neurological, and substance use disorders as risk factors for other health outcomes was reviewed. Because of data limitations, only a few risk factor–outcome pairings could be established and assessed in the study's CRA analysis (Baxter and others 2011; Lim and others 2012). These risk factors are summarized in table 3.3. There were insufficient data to assess neurological disorders as risk factors in GBD 2010. From the data that were available for selected mental and substance use disorders, we can begin to appreciate the impact these disorders have on other health outcomes in the GBD cause list.

Online annex 3A summarizes the YLLs allocated to mental, neurological, and substance use disorders as direct causes of death; these were estimated using previously reported cause-specific death estimates. In addition to these cause-specific YLLs, mental and substance use disorders are responsible for 22.5 million YLLs caused by deaths from suicide; major depression is responsible for 3.5 million YLLs caused by deaths from IHD; injecting drug use is responsible for 7.2 million YLLs caused by deaths from blood-borne viruses and liver disease; and alcohol use is responsible for 78.7 million YLLs from death caused by various additional outcomes. Regular cannabis use as a risk factor for schizophrenia accounted for an estimated 7,000 DALYs globally, all of which were YLDs given that there was no evidence to suggest an elevated risk of mortality in cannabis users (Charlson and others 2013; Degenhardt, Ferrari, and others 2013; Ferrari and others 2014; Lim and others 2012).

Figure 3.8 shows the additional YLLs attributable to mental, neurological, and substance use disorders as risk factors for other health outcomes by region; these are

Table 3.2 Number of Cause-Specific and Excess Deaths, by Age, 2010

Cause-specific deaths	0–1 years	1–4 years	5–9 years	10–14 years	15–19 years	20–24 years	25–34 years	35–44 years	45–54 years	55–64 years	65–74 years	75+ years	Total
Alzheimer's disease and other dementias	-	-	869	605	578	642	1,259	2,302	4,575	12,559	41,622	420,710	485,721
Epilepsy	7,388	19,819	6,255	5,351	10,562	14,101	24,107	20,605	18,038	14,826	14,522	22,054	177,627
Schizophrenia	-	-	-	-	-	-	2,003	3,610	3,429	3,440	3,035	4,246	19,763
Alcohol use disorders	-	-	-	-	464	1,311	7,937	20,044	33,613	27,446	13,295	7,024	111,134
Opioid dependence	1,231	1,217	288	260	1,350	3,745	9,736	8,446	7,432	3,846	2,319	3,171	43,040
Cocaine dependence	13	12	3	3	16	47	120	107	96	53	33	44	549
Amphetamine dependence	13	11	3	3	14	40	102	88	75	44	30	41	465

Excess deaths	0–1 years	1–4 years	5–9 years	10–14 years	15–19 years	20–24 years	25–34 years	35–44 years	45–54 years	55–64 years	65–74 years	75+ years	Total
Alzheimer's disease and other dementias	-	-	-	-	-	-	-	1,160	114,334	267,613	251,719	1,478,957	2,113,783
Epilepsy	3,513	13,486	10,680	9,050	18,957	25,784	54,590	52,928	38,961	25,330	20,276	22,647	296,201
Schizophrenia	-	-	-	816	8,758	26,990	106,121	163,634	208,056	118,828	43,846	21,945	698,993
Alcohol use disorders	-	-	-	6,868	46,164	85,768	403,572	510,864	472,712	304,907	91,601	31,046	1,953,502
Opioid dependence	-	-	-	-	11,268	94,748	183,102	77,352	28,489	7,350	1,498	319	404,125
Cocaine dependence	-	-	-	-	638	10,334	38,838	23,083	16,682	5,023	984	237	95,818
Amphetamine dependence	-	-	-	-	5,856	25,306	86,702	65,420	17,058	1,765	101	11	202,219
Major depressive disorder	-	239	63,015	86,160	141,417	171,916	284,988	286,056	285,313	258,639	198,975	447,142	2,223,840
Bipolar disorder	-	-	-	1,337	21,063	78,773	327,425	401,817	266,179	136,888	58,706	28,204	1,320,391
Autistic disorder	963	4,220	3,883	3,087	3,918	5,102	13,468	18,276	20,536	17,133	10,675	7,384	108,645

Source: Lozano and others 2012.
Note: Larger than expected numbers in the 75+ age group may be an artefact of the age groupings. - = nil.

Table 3.3 Mental, Neurological, and Substance Use Disorders Included as Risk Factors in the GBD 2010 Comparative Risk Assessments and Attributable YLLs for Health Outcomes, 2010

Risk	Outcome	Millions of YLLs (95% uncertainty)
Alcohol use	Alcohol use disorders, tuberculosis, lower respiratory infections, multiple cancers, cardiovascular and circulatory diseases, cirrhosis of the liver, pancreatitis, epilepsy, diabetes mellitus, injuries, and interpersonal violence	78.7 (70.9–86.8)
Injecting drug use	HIV/AIDS, hepatitis B and C, liver cancer, and cirrhosis of the liver secondary to hepatitis	7.2 (5.6–9.7)
Mental and substance use disorders	Suicide	22.5 (14.8–29.8)
Major depression	Ischemic heart disease	3.6 (1.8–5.4)
Regular cannabis use[a]	Schizophrenia	0

Sources: Estimates based on Charlson and others 2013; Degenhardt, Ferrari, and others 2013; Ferrari and others 2014; Lim and others 2012.
Note: DALYs = disability-adjusted life years; HIV/AIDS = human immunodeficiency virus and acquired immune deficiency syndrome; YLD = years lived with disability; YLL = years of life lost.
a. Regular cannabis use as a risk factor for schizophrenia accounted for an estimated 7,000 DALYs globally, all of which were YLDs.

over and above cause-specific YLLs directly attributable to these disorders. Variation in absolute YLLs among regions is explained not only by population size, but also the distribution of the risk factors and outcomes in each region. For example, YLLs attributable to alcohol use as a risk factor are greatest in Central Europe, Eastern Europe, and Central Asia—rather than South Asia, which has the largest population size—because of high rates of alcohol use disorders in this region. In contrast, the lower contribution of attributable YLLs in Sub-Saharan Africa likely reflects the lower rates of alcohol use disorders in this region. Had there been sufficient data to estimate YLLs caused by neurological disorders as risk factors for other health outcomes, estimates of attributable YLLs may have been higher in Sub-Saharan Africa, where cause-specific deaths from neurological disorders are highest.

The attributable YLLs presented provide more comprehensive insight into the magnitude of the burden of mental, neurological, and substance use disorders. For example, the addition of attributable suicide YLLs would have changed total YLLs caused by mental and substance use disorders combined from 0.5 percent (allocated to them as a direct cause) to 1.8 percent of global YLLs, elevating them from the fifth to the third leading disease category of global burden (DALYs) in 2010 (Charlson and others 2013; Degenhardt, Ferrari, and others 2013; Ferrari and others 2014; Lim and others 2012). Attributable YLLs estimated for each risk factor–outcome pairing are not mutually exclusive of contributions of other risk factors; consequently, they cannot be aggregated to estimate the overall YLLs attributable

Figure 3.8 Absolute YLLs Attributable to Mental, Neurological, and Substance Use Disorders as Risk Factors for Other Health Outcomes, 2010

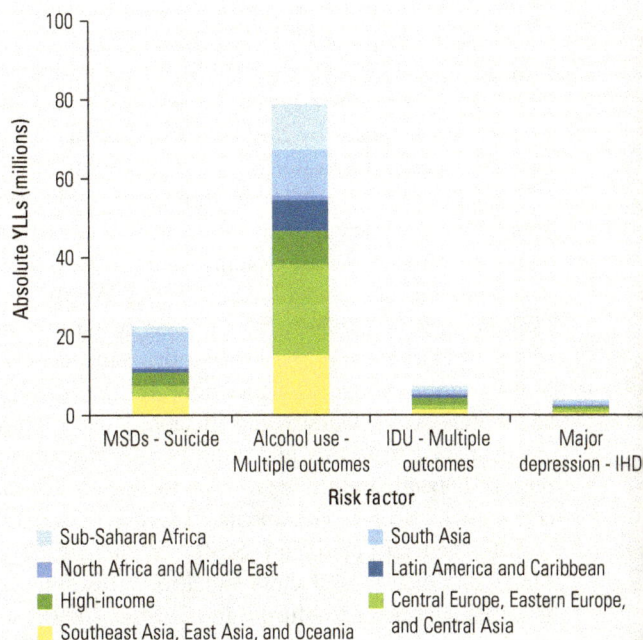

Source: IHME 2013.
Note: Risk factor–outcome pairings are defined in table 3.3. IDU = injecting drug use; IHD = ischemic heart disease; MSDs = mental and substance use disorders; YLLs = years of life lost to premature mortality.

to all mental, neurological, and substance use disorders combined. Nevertheless, presenting attributable YLLs is another example of the deaths and YLLs caused by these disorders, over and above the direct cause-specific deaths and YLLs allocated to each disorder in GBD 2010. It is clear that the mortality-associated disease is significant.

DISCUSSION AND IMPLICATIONS

Mental Disorders

The GBD findings of elevated rates of excess mortality across most mental and substance use disorders are supported by the findings of a recent meta-analytic review (Walker, McGee, and Druss 2015). Moreover, recent studies suggest that the majority of excess deaths are caused by preventable diseases, with a smaller proportion attributed to unnatural or unknown causes (Fekadu and others 2015; Lawrence, Hancock, and Kisely 2013). The question remains as to what proportion of these deaths can be directly attributed to mental disorders and how much to subsequent confounding factors.

Despite the existence of complex relationships between mental disorders and premature mortality, some relationships, such as that between mental disorders and suicide, are well-established (Li and others 2011). Mental disorders have also been linked to higher rates of death caused by cardiovascular disease, stroke, diabetes mellitus, respiratory diseases, and some cancers (Crump and others 2013; Hoyer, Mortensen, and Olesen 2000). The relationship between mental disorders and a specific physical disease, leading to premature death, is also complex. People with major depression are more likely to develop cardiovascular disease (Charlson and others 2011). Psychotropic medications can negatively impact cardiovascular and metabolic health (De Hert and others 2012). Obesity and metabolic disturbances are primary risk factors for cardiovascular disease and type II diabetes, and these are two- to three-fold more common in people with mental disorders, compared with the general population (Scott and Happell 2011). Major modifiable risk factors for chronic disease, such as smoking (Lawrence, Mitrou, and Zubrick 2009), poor diet, physical inactivity (Kilbourne and others 2007; Shatenstein, Kergoat, and Reid 2007), and substance abuse (Scott and Happell 2011), are overrepresented in people with mental disorders. These risk factors may be the consequences of symptoms of mental, neurological, and substance use disorders; medication effects; and poor emotional regulation (Scott and others 2013).

Mental disorders are associated with poorer clinical management of comorbid conditions. People with severe and persistent mental disorders may be less likely to receive a timely diagnosis of physical illness because of diagnostic overshadowing, that is, physical complaints may be overlooked and attributed to psychological and psychiatric factors (Bailey, Thorpe, and Smith 2013). A review by Happell, Scott, and Platania-Phung (2012) found a reduced likelihood for people with mental disorders to receive screening for breast, cervical, and colorectal cancer or immunizations for influenza and pneumonia, compared with the rest of the population. Even in countries with well-established health care systems, people with mental disorders receive lower-than-average prescriptions for medication treating cardiovascular disease (Kisely, Campbell, and Wang 2009; Mitchell and Lord 2010) and are less likely to receive coronary artery bypass grafting, cardiac catheterization, or cerebrovascular arteriography (Kisely, Campbell, and Wang 2009; Mitchell and Lawrence 2011).

Strategies for reducing mortality associated with mental and substance use disorders primarily target preventing onset, reducing case fatality, and preventing the development of fatal sequela. Growing evidence indicates that excess mortality in people with these disorders can be reduced through established evidence-based treatments and improved screening and treatment for chronic disease.

Psychiatric treatments, specifically pharmacotherapies, may have some protective effect against excess mortality (Weinmann, Read, and Aderhold 2009), although evidence suggests that this depends on the use of medications according to best practice guidelines (Cullen and others 2013). However, some antidepressants and second-generation antipsychotics may actually pose an elevated risk mediated by metabolic side effects (Newcomer 2005; Rummel-Kluge and others 2010; Smith and others 2008).

Collaborative care by community-based health teams has the potential to reduce overall mortality, as well as suicide deaths (Dieterich and others 2010; Malone and others 2007). The use of collaborative care models to improve physical health in people with mental, neurological, and substance use disorders is growing in HICs; these models have demonstrated a range of positive health outcomes, including reduced cardiovascular risk profiles (Druss and others 2010). The effectiveness of these strategies in preventing premature mortality in LMICs has yet to be tested, but this may be a cost-effective approach to treatment in settings in which trained mental health clinicians are scarce.

Known chronic disease risk factors, such as smoking and obesity, are potentially modifiable. Lifestyle interventions comprising a psycho-educational or behavioral approach can achieve modest but significant improvements, such as reduced smoking (Kisely and Campbell 2008; van Hasselt and others 2013), increased physical activity, and improved eating habits (Verhaeghe and others 2011), resulting in reduced body mass index and improved metabolic profiles (Gierisch and others 2013).

Screening, prevention of metabolic risk factors, and proactive provision of basic health care services are essential to improve life expectancy in people with comorbid mental and physical health issues. Strategies for early cancer detection need to be prioritized, and models of care need to be developed to ensure that people with these disorders receive the same level of physical health care and treatment as the rest of the population.

Several guidelines address the management of mental, neurological, and substance use disorders. The World Health Organization (WHO), for example, has developed specific strategies in its Mental Health Gap Action Programme, which aim to scale up services in LMICs (http://www.who.int/mental_health/mhgap/en/). The WHO has also developed guidelines for other related health priorities, such as suicide, which draws attention to the pivotal role that mental health care plays in suicide prevention (http://www.who.int/mental_health /prevention/suicide/suicideprevent/en/index.html).

Strategies to address self-harm remain critical, as evidence shows that a proportion of suicide deaths can be averted through public health measures. Policies that address restriction of access to common methods of suicide are effective in reducing suicide risk (WHO 2012). Strong evidence indicates that improved prevention and treatment of major depression and alcohol and substance abuse can reduce suicide rates.

The continuing life expectancy gap in persons with mental disorders is a clear example of discrimination and lack of parity between this portion of the population and the community in general (Thornicroft 2013). Differential access to usual care for this group leads to poorer outcomes in terms of health loss and mortality (Liao and others 2013) and incurs high costs in health care provision (Centre for Mental Health 2010). Accordingly, identification of physical health issues and equitable access to health care are essential to improve long-term health outcomes and reduce excess mortality among people with mental disorders (Bass and others 2012).

Substance Use Disorders

Opioid dependence and injecting drug use are significant contributors to the global burden of mental, neurological, and substance use disorders. Much of this burden could be averted by scaling up needle and syringe programs, opioid substitution treatment (OST), and HIV antiretroviral therapy (Degenhardt and others 2010; Turner and others 2011). Increasing evidence indicates that needle and syringe programs can reduce the burden of HIV/AIDS (Degenhardt and others 2010) and hepatitis C virus (HCV) (Turner and others 2011). The HCV burden can also be decreased by effectively treating chronic HCV (Turner and others 2011). The release of more effective and less toxic HCV drugs is expected to result in dramatic improvement in what have been extremely low rates of treatment uptake by people who inject drugs (Swan 2011).

More effective strategies to reduce the burden of disease attributable to opioid dependence include maintenance OST and HIV antiretroviral therapy (Degenhardt and others 2010; Turner and others 2011). The two most commonly used medications, methadone and buprenorphine, are on the *List of Essential Medicines* (WHO 2005) as core medications for the treatment of opioid dependence (Mattick and others 2008, 2009). OST reduces mortality among opioid dependent people (Brugal and others 2005; Caplehorn and Drummer 1999; Darke, Degenhardt, and Mattick 2006; Davoli and others 1994; Degenhardt, Randall, and others 2009; Gibson and others 2008), with time spent in treatment halving mortality compared with that of time spent not in treatment (Degenhardt and others 2011). A large evaluation study in multiple countries, including LMICs, demonstrated that OST is effective in reducing opioid use and injecting risk behaviors and improving physical and mental well-being (Lawrinson and others 2008).

There is scope for reducing the risk of overdose among people who continue to use opioids, particularly in countries with high injecting drug use rates but a low emphasis on harm reduction measures, such as the Russian Federation and the United States. Increasing evidence indicates that the provision of the opioid antagonist naloxone to users enables peers to intervene effectively if overdoses occur (Galea and others 2006; Sporer and Kral 2007). Additional strategies may include educating users about the risks of overdose and conducting motivational interviews with users who have recently overdosed (Sporer 2003). Safe injecting rooms have been proposed as an additional strategy to reduce overdose, although their population reach is likely to be more limited (Hall and Kimber 2005).

Psychosocial interventions, including self-help programs and cognitive behavioral therapy, can be effective (Baker, Lee, and Jenner 2005; Knapp and others 2007). There is no evidence to date that pharmacotherapies, such as mood stabilizers, antidepressants, or antipsychotics, are effective for the treatment of stimulant dependence (Srisurapanont, Jarusuraisin, and Kittirattanapaiboon 2001). The RCTs of prescribed psychostimulants in cocaine dependence have not found that they lead to greater abstinence or retention in care (Castells and others 2010).

In some regions, notably Asia, there is also widespread delivery of non-evidence-based responses to psychostimulant dependence (Degenhardt and others 2010, 2014). Illicit drug users may be detained in closed settings, typically operated by military, government security, or police for what is claimed to be treatment, most often for psychostimulant use (IHRD 2009; Pearson 2009; UNODC Regional Centre for East Asia and the Pacific 2006; WHO 2009). Detainees are often forced to comply with the interventions; evidence-based, effective drug treatment and HIV prevention are rarely delivered (General Department for Social Evils Prevention, Constella Group, and DFID 2008; IHRD 2009; UNODC Regional Centre for East Asia and the Pacific 2006; WHO 2009). External evaluations have concluded that there may be adverse impacts on drug use and HIV risk (Pearson 2009), in addition to human rights violations (Human Rights Watch 2004; IHRD 2009; Pearson 2009; Rehm, Csete, and others 2010; WHO 2009).

Although cannabis dependence had no YLLs, two million YLDs were attributed to the disorder. Behavioral interventions are effective in the treatment of cannabis dependence (Denis and others 2013; Knapp and others 2007); cognitive behavioral therapy and contingency management show the greatest promise. Public health campaigns may be necessary to advise young people of the risks of developing dependence on cannabis, because many users fail to appreciate this risk. More research is needed, however, into how to scale up these behavioral approaches to reduce the population prevalence of these disorders (Knapp and others 2007).

Neurological Disorders

As the incidence of neurological disorders, including epilepsy and dementia, grows in many resource-limited settings, strategies to decrease mortality rates in these regions in particular must be addressed. Improvements in access to medical treatment, patient and clinician education, and a focus on preventable causes of death can substantially decrease mortality rates.

In resource-constrained settings, the mortality risk in epilepsy patients is up to six times higher than in HICs and largely due to preventable causes (Kamgno, Pion, and Boussinesq 2003; Ngugi and others 2014). The epilepsy treatment gap is more than 75 percent in low-income countries, and more than 50 percent in many LMICs and upper-middle-income countries (Jette and Trevathan 2014). Legislation to ensure the availability of affordable and efficacious anti-seizure medications, clinician education in prescribing anti-epileptic medications, and patient education on the importance of medical adherence is critical to alleviate the epilepsy treatment gap. Cost-effective epilepsy treatments are available, and accurate diagnosis can be made without costly technical equipment. Targeting epilepsy risk factors, including more common structural and metabolic causes of epilepsy, can decrease mortality risk. Education and information on safe lifestyle habits in epilepsy patients will benefit populations in LMICs, as will education initiatives targeted to employers and teachers to dispel the myths associated with epilepsy.

The mortality risk of dementia in many LMICs is poorly known. Studies on the mortality rates due to dementia and the incidence of preventable risk factors in these regions are critical to develop strategies to alleviate mortality in this fragile patient population. Mortality in dementia patients is commonly caused by preventable medical conditions. Caregiver education and support services regarding proper care of patients with cognitive decline will likely decrease infection rates and mortality. Government financial support for health care services and caregiver support would benefit this population. Strategies to enhance nutrition, as well as monitoring and treatment of vascular risk factors, are important measures. Raising awareness of the mortality risk among the public, caregivers, and health workers can lead to increased demand for services.

CONCLUSIONS AND LIMITATIONS

Quantifying mortality presents several challenges. The cause-of-death data are affected by multiple factors, including certification skills among physicians, diagnostic and other data available for completing the death certificate, cultural variations in choosing and prioritizing the cause of death, and institutional parameters governing mortality reporting (Lozano and others 2012). In LMICs, where many deaths are not medically certified, different data sources and diagnostic approaches are used to derive cause-of-death estimates (Lozano and others 2012). Overall, improving and expanding sources of national mortality estimates is imperative.

Mortality directly related to mental, neurological, and substance use disorders is particularly difficult to capture in cause-of-death data because of the complex web of causality that links these disorders with other physical disorders. It is important to identify and quantify the excess premature mortality in people with these disorders by elucidating the pathway between the disorders and fatal sequelae. The estimates of excess mortality presented in this chapter include deaths from causal and noncausal origins and therefore cannot be interpreted as the number of deaths directly attributable to a particular disorder. In addition, DisMod-MR natural history models do not adjust for co-occurrence between disorders. Thus, it is important to note that excess deaths and YLLs (as is the case for estimates from risk factor analyses) cannot be aggregated across disorders.

Although valuable, the CRA undertaken as part of GBD 2010 also provides an incomplete picture. Given the lack of available data, we are not able to estimate and reassign all deaths attributable to mental, neurological, and substance use disorders. Assuming multiple risk factors are independent of each other is also a limitation. A more accurate quantification of the joint effects of multiple risk factors, that is, what explains the difference between excess and cause-specific deaths, is an important area for future research.

Our analysis of the excess and attributable deaths caused by mental, neurological, and substance use disorders demonstrates the elevated risk of mortality associated with these disorders, over and above what is captured in GBD 2010's estimation of cause-specific YLLs. Prevention of excess mortality in people with these disorders should be considered a high priority in the reform of health systems. A key step in the identification and treatment of comorbid health issues is to ensure equitable access to health care, thereby improving long-term health outcomes and reducing premature mortality among people with these disorders.

ANNEX 3A

The annex to this chapter is as follows. It is available at www.dcp-3.org/mentalhealth.

- Annex 3A. Cause-Specific Years of Life Lost as a Percentage of All-Cause Years of Life Lost, 2010

NOTE

A version of this chapter appeared in an article by F. J. Charlson, A. J. Baxter, T. Dua, L. Degenhardt, H. Whiteford, and T. Vos, titled "Excess Mortality from Mental, Neurological, and Substance Use Disorders in the Global Burden of Disease Study 2010." *Epidemiology and Psychiatric Sciences*, 2015: 24 (2): 121–40. doi:10.1017/S2045796014000687. <http://journals.cambridge.org/action/displayJournal?jid=EPS>. © Cambridge University Press 2015. Licensed under Creative Commons Attribution (CC BY). <http://creativecommons.org/licenses>.

World Bank Income Classifications as of July 2014 are as follows, based on estimates of gross national income (GNI) per capita for 2013:

- Low-income countries (LICs) = US$1,045 or less
- Middle-income countries (MICs) are subdivided:
  a) lower-middle-income = US$1,046 to US$4,125
  b) upper-middle-income (UMICs) = US$4,126 to US$12,745
- High-income countries (HICs) = US$12,746 or more.

REFERENCES

Ahmadi, N., F. Hajsadeghi, H. B. Mirshkarlo, M. Budoff, R. Yehuda, and R. Ebrahimi. 2011. "Post-Traumatic Stress Disorder, Coronary Atherosclerosis, and Mortality." *American Journal of Cardiology* 108 (1): 29–33.

Alonso, A., D. R. Jacobs, A. Menotti, A. Nissinen, A. Dontas, A. Kafatos, and others. 2009. "Cardiovascular Risk Factors and Dementia Mortality: 40 Years of Follow-up in the Seven Countries Study." *Journal of the Neurological Sciences* 280 (1): 79–83.

Bailey, S., L. Thorpe, and G. Smith. 2013. *Whole-Person Care: From Rhetoric to Reality. Achieving Parity between Mental and Physical Health*. London: Royal College of Psychiatrists.

Baker, A., N. Lee, and L. Jenner, eds. 2005. *Models of Intervention and Care for Psychostimulant Users*. Canberra: Australian Government Department of Health and Ageing.

Ballard, C., M. L. Hanney, M. Theodoulou, S. Douglas, R. McShane, K. Kossakowski, and others. 2009. "The Dementia Antipsychotic Withdrawal Trial (DART-AD): Long-Term Follow-up of a Randomised Placebo-Controlled Trial." *The Lancet Neurology* 8 (2): 151–57.

Barendregt, J. J., G. J. van Oortmarssen, T. Vos, and C. J. L. Murray. 2003. "A Generic Model for the Assessment of Disease Epidemiology: The Computational Basis of Dismod II." *Population Health Metrics* 1 (1): 4.

Bass, J. K., T. H. Bornemann, M. Burkey, S. Chehil, L. Chen, and others. 2012. "A United Nations General Assembly Special Session for Mental, Neurological, and Substance Use Disorders: The Time Has Come." *PLoS Medicine* 9 (1). doi:10.1371/journal.pmed.1001159.

Baxter, A. J., F. J. Charlson, A. J. Somerville, and H. A. Whiteford. 2011. "Mental Disorders as Risk Factors: Assessing the Evidence for the Global Burden of Disease Study." *BMC Medicine* 9 (1): 134.

Baxter, A. J., A. Page, and H. A. Whiteford. 2011. "Factors Influencing Risk of Premature Mortality in Community Cases of Depression: A Meta-Analytic Review." *Epidemiology Research International* (Article ID 832945). doi:10.1155/2011/832945.

Baxter, A. J., T. Vos, K. M. Scott, R. E. Norman, A. Flaxman, and others. 2014. "The Regional Distribution of Anxiety Disorders: Implications for the Global Burden of Disease Study, 2010." *International Journal of Methods in Psychiatric Research* 23 (4): 422–38. doi:10.1002/mpr.1444.

Beeri, M. S., and U. Goldbourt. 2001. "Late-Life Dementia Predicts Mortality beyond Established Midlife Risk Factors." *American Journal of Geriatric Psychiatry* 19 (1): 79–87.

Bilder, D., E. L. Botts, K. R. Smith, R. Pimentel, M. Farley, and others. 2013. "Excess Mortality and Causes of Death in Autism Spectrum Disorders: A Follow Up of the 1980s Utah/UCLA Autism Epidemiologic Study." *Journal of Autism and Developmental Disorders* 43 (5): 1196–204. doi:10.1007/s10803-012-1664-z.

Brugal, M. T., A. Domingo-Salvany, R. Puig, G. Barrio, P. Garcia de Olalla, and L. de la Fuente. 2005. "Evaluating the Impact of Methadone Maintenance Programmes on Mortality Due to Overdose and AIDS in a Cohort of Heroin Users in Spain." *Addiction* 100: 981–89.

Caplehorn, J. R. M., and O. H. Drummer. 1999. "Mortality Associated with New South Wales Methadone Programs in 1994: Lives Lost and Saved." *Medical Journal of Australia* 170: 104–09.

Carpio, A., N. E. Bharucha, P. Jallon, E. Beghi, R. Campostrini, and others. 2005. "Mortality of Epilepsy in Developing Countries." *Epilepsia* 46 (Suppl. 11): 28–32. doi:10.1111/j.1528-1167.2005.00404.x.

Castells, X., M. Casas, C. Perez-Mana, C. Roncero, and D. Capella. 2010. "Efficacy of Psychostimulant Drugs for Cocaine Dependence." *Cochrane Database of Systematic Reviews* (2). doi:10.1002/14651858.CD007380.pub3.

Centre for Mental Health. 2010. "The Economic and Social Costs of Mental Health Problems in 2009/10." Centre for Mental Health. http://www.centreformentalhealth.org.uk/pdfs/Economic_and_social_costs_2010.pdf.

Chang, C.-K., R. D. Hayes, G. Perera, M. T. M. Broadbent, A. C. Fernandes, and others. 2011. "Life Expectancy at Birth for People with Serious Mental Illness and Other Major Disorders from a Secondary Mental Health Care Case Register in London." *PLoS One* 6 (5). doi:10.1371/journal.pone.0019590.

Charlson, F. J., A. E. Moran, G. Freedman, R. E. Norman, N. J. C. Stapelberg, and others. 2013. "The Contribution of Major Depression to the Global Burden of Ischaemic Heart Disease: A Comparative Risk Assessment." *BMC Medicine* 11 (250). doi:10.1186/1741-7015-11-250.

Charlson, F. J., N. Stapelberg, A. J. Baxter, and H. Whiteford. 2011. "Should Global Burden of Disease Estimates Include Depression as a Risk Factor for Coronary Heart Disease?" *BMC Medicine* 9 (1): 47.

Chesney, E., G. E. Goodwin, and S. Fazel. 2014. "Risks of All-Cause and Suicide Mortality in Mental Disorders: A Meta-Review." *World Psychiatry* 13 (2): 153–60. doi:10.1002/wps.20128.

Crump, C., M. A. Winkleby, K. Sundquist, and J. Sundquist. 2013. "Comorbidities and Mortality in Persons with Schizophrenia: A Swedish National Cohort Study." *American Journal of Psychiatry* 170 (3): 324–33. doi:10.1176/appi.ajp.2012.12050599.

Cullen, B. A., E. E. McGinty, Y. Zhang, S. C. Dosreis, D. M. Steinwachs, and others. 2013. "Guideline-Concordant Antipsychotic Use and Mortality in Schizophrenia." *Schizophrenia Bulletin* 39 (5): 1159–68. doi:10.1093/schbul/sbs097.

Darke, S., L. Degenhardt, and R. P. Mattick, eds. 2006. *Mortality amongst Illicit Drug Users.* Cambridge, UK: Cambridge University Press.

Davoli, M., F. Forastiere, D. D. Abeni, E. Rapiti, and C. A. Perucci. 1994. "Longitudinal and Cross-Sectional Mortality Studies in Injecting Drug Users." *Journal of Epidemiology and Community Health* 48 (1): 101–02.

De Hert, M., J. Detraux, R. van Winkel, W. Yu, and C. U. Correll. 2012. "Metabolic and Cardiovascular Adverse Effects Associated with Antipsychotic Drugs." *Nature Reviews Endocrinology* 8: 114–26. doi:10.1038/nrendo.2011.156.

Degenhardt, L., C. Bucello, B. Mathers, C. Briegleb, H. Ali, M. Hickman, and J. McLaren. 2011. "Mortality among Regular or Dependent Users of Heroin and Other Opioids: A Systematic Review and Meta-Analysis of Cohort Studies." *Addiction* 106 (1): 32–51.

Degenhardt, L., A. J. Ferrari, B. Calabria, W. D. Hall, R. E. Norman, and others. 2013. "The Global Epidemiology and Contribution of Cannabis Use and Dependence to the Global Burden of Disease: Results from the GBD 2010 Study." *PLoS One* 8 (10): e76635. doi:10.1371/journal.pone.0076635.

Degenhardt, L., and W. Hall. 2012. "Extent of Illicit Drug Use and Dependence, and Their Contribution to the Global Burden of Disease." *The Lancet* 379 (9810): 55–70. doi:http://dx.doi.org/10.1016/S0140-6736(11)61138-0.

Degenhardt, L., W. D. Hall, M. Lynskey, J. McGrath, J. McLaren, and others. 2009. "Should Burden of Disease Estimates Include Cannabis Use as a Risk Factor for Psychosis?" *PLoS Medicine* 6 (9): e1000133.

Degenhardt, L., B. Mathers, P. Vickerman, T. Rhodes, C. Latkin, and others. 2010. "Prevention of HIV Infection for People Who Inject Drugs: Why Individual, Structural, and Combination Approaches Are Needed." *The Lancet* 376: 285–301.

Degenhardt, L., B. M. Mathers, A. L. Wirtz, D. Wolfee, A. Kamarulzamanf, and others. 2014. "What Has Been Achieved in HIV Prevention, Treatment and Care for People Who Inject Drugs, 2010–2012? A Review of the Six Highest Burden Countries." *International Journal of Drug Policy* 25 (1): 53–60. doi:10.1016/j.drugpo.2013.08.004.

Degenhardt, L., D. Randall, W. Hall, M. Law, T. Butler, and others. 2009. "Mortality among Clients of a State-Wide Opioid Pharmacotherapy Programme Over 20 Years: Risk Factors and Lives Saved." *Drug and Alcohol Dependence* 105 (1–2): 9–15.

Degenhardt, L., H. A. Whiteford, A. J. Ferrari, A. J. Baxter, F. J. Charlson, and others. 2013. "Global Burden of Disease Attributable to Illicit Drug Use and Dependence: Findings from the Global Burden of Disease Study 2010." *The Lancet* 382 (9904): 1564–74.

Denis, C., E. Lavie, M. Fatseas, and M. Auriacombe. 2013. "Psychotherapeutic Interventions for Cannabis Abuse and/or Dependence in Outpatient Settings." *Cochrane Database of Systematic Reviews.* doi:10.1002/14651858.CD005336.pub3.

Dieterich, M., C. B. Irving, B. Park, and M. Marshall. 2010. "Intensive Case Management for Severe Mental Illness." *Cochrane Database of Systematic Reviews* (10). doi:10.1002/14651858.CD007906.pub2.

Diop, A. G., D. C. Hesdorffer, G. Logroscino, and W. A. Hauser. 2005. "Epilepsy and Mortality in Africa: A Review of the Literature." *Epilepsia* 46: 33–35. doi:10.1111/j.0013-9580.2005.t01-1-53904.x-i1.

Druss, B. G., S. A. von Esenwein, M. T. Compton, K. J. Rask, L. Zhao, and others. 2010. "A Randomized Trial of Medical Care Management for Community Mental Health Settings: The Primary Care Access, Referral, and Evaluation (PCARE) Study." *American Journal of Psychiatry* 167 (2): 151–59. doi:10.1176/appi.ajp.2009.09050691.

Fazel, S., A. Wolf, N. Långström, C. R. Newton, and P. Lichtenstein. 2013. "Premature Mortality in Epilepsy and the Role of Psychiatric Comorbidity: A Total Population Study." *The Lancet* 382 (9905): 1646–54.

Fekadu, A., G. Medhin, D. Kebede, A. Alem, A. J. Cleare, and others. 2015. "Excess Mortality in Severe Mental Illness: 10-Year Population-Based Cohort Study in Rural Ethiopia." *British Journal of Psychiatry* 206 (4): 289–96.

Ferrari, A. J., F. J. Charlson, R. E. Norman, S. B. Patten, G. Freedman, and others. 2013. "Burden of Depressive Disorders by Country, Sex, Age, and Year: Findings from the Global Burden of Disease Study 2010." *PLoS Medicine* 10 (11): e1001547. doi:10.1371/journal.pmed.1001547.

Ferrari, A. J., R. E. Norman, G. Freedman, A. J. Baxter, J. E. Pirkis, and others. 2014. "The Burden Attributable to Mental and Substance Use Disorders as Risk Factors for Suicide: Findings from the Global Burden of Disease Study 2010." *PLoS One* 9 (4): e91936. doi:10.1371/journal.pone.0091936.

Foreman, K. J., R. Lozano, A. D. Lopez, and C. J. Murray. 2012. "Modeling Causes of Death: An Integrated Approach Using CODEm." *Population Health Metrics* 10 (1).

Galea, S., N. Worthington, T. M. Piper, V. V. Nandi, M. Curtis, and others. 2006. "Provision of Naloxone to Injection Drug Users as an Overdose Prevention Strategy: Early Evidence from a Pilot Study in New York City." *Addictive Behaviors* 31 (5): 907–12.

Garcia-Ptacek, S., B. Farahmand, I. Kåreholt, D. Religa, M. L. Cuadrado, and M. Eriksdotter. 2014. "Mortality Risk after Dementia Diagnosis by Dementia Type and Underlying Factors: A Cohort of 15,209 Patients Based on the Swedish Dementia Registry." *Dementia* 37: 38.

General Department for Social Evils Prevention, Constella Group, and DFID (Department of International Development). 2008. *Economic and Public Health Analysis of Institutional and Community Responses to Injecting Drug Use and HIV/AIDS in Vietnam.* Draft report of the findings from Data Collection and Cost Analysis in Four Rehabilitation Centres: Duc Hanh (HCMC), Ba Ria-Vung Tau, Khanh Hoa and Tay Ninh, Hanoi.

Gibson, A., L. Degenhardt, R. P. Mattick, R. Ali, J. White, and S. O'Brien. 2008. "Exposure to Opioid Maintenance Treatment Reduces Long-Term Mortality." *Addiction* 103 (3): 462–68.

Gierisch, J. M., J. A. Nieuwsma, D. W. Bradford, C. M. Wilder, M. C. Mann-Wrobel, and others. 2013. "Interventions to Improve Cardiovascular Risk Factors in People with Serious Mental Illness." Comparative Effectiveness Review 105, prepared by the Duke Evidence-Based Practice Center, Agency for Healthcare Research and Quality, Rockville, MD.

Gillberg, C., and E. Billstedt. 2000. "Autism and Asperger Syndrome: Coexistence with Other Clinical Disorders." *Acta Psychiatrica Scandinavia* 102: 321–30.

Grinshpoon, A., M. Barchana, A. Ponizovsky, I. Lipshitz, D. Nahon, and others. 2005. "Cancer in Schizophrenia: Is the Risk Higher or Lower?" *Schizophrenia Research* 73 (2-3): 333–41.

Guehne, U., S. Riedel-Heller, and M. C. Angermeyer. 2005. "Mortality in Dementia: A Systematic Review." *Neuroepidemiology* 25: 153–62. doi:10.1159/000086680.

Gühne, U., H. Matschinger, M. C. Angermeyer, and S. G. Riedel-Heller. 2006. "Incident Dementia Cases and Mortality: Results of the Leipzig Longitudinal Study of the Aged (LEILA75+)." *Dementia and Geriatric Cognitive Disorders* 22: 185–93.

Hall, W., and J. Kimber. 2005. "Being Realistic about Benefits of Supervised Injecting Facilities." *The Lancet* 366 (9482): 271–72.

Happell, B., D. Scott, and C. Platania-Phung. 2012. "Provision of Preventive Services for Cancer and Infectious Diseases among Individuals with Serious Mental Illness." *Archives of Psychiatric Nursing* 26 (3): 192–201. doi:http://dx.doi.org/10.1016/j.apnu.2011.09.002.

Haukka, J., J. Tiihonen, T. Härkänen, and J. Lönnqvist. 2008. "Association between Medication and Risk of Suicide, Attempted Suicide and Death in Nationwide Cohort of Suicidal Patients with Schizophrenia." *Pharmacoepidemiology and Drug Safety* 17 (7): 686–96. doi:10.1002/pds.1579.

Hitiris, N., R. Mohanraj, J. Norrie, and M. J. Brodie. 2007. "Mortality in Epilepsy." *Epilepsy and Behavior* 10 (3): 363–76.

Hoyer, E. H., P. Bo Mortensen, and A. V. Olesen. 2000. "Mortality and Causes of Death in a Total National Sample of Patients with Affective Disorders Admitted for the First Time between 1973 and 1993." *British Journal of Psychiatry* 176: 76–82.

Human Rights Watch. 2004. *Not Enough Graves: The War on Drugs, HIV/AIDS, and Violations of Human Rights.* New York: Human Rights Watch.

IHME (Institute of Health Metrics and Evaluation). 2013. "GBD Compare." University of Washington. http://viz.healthmetricsandevaluation.org/gbd-compare/.

———. 2014. "What Countries Are in Each Region?" University of Washington. http://www.healthdata.org/gbd/faq#What countries are in each region?

IHRD (International Harm Reduction Development Program). 2009. "Human Rights Abuses in the Name of Drug Treatment: Reports from the Field." In *Public Health Fact Sheet*, Open Society Institute, Public Health Program, New York, NY.

Jerome, L., A. Segal, and L. Habinski. 2006. "What We Know about ADHD and Driving Risk: A Literature Review, Meta-Analysis and Critique." *Journal of the Canadian Academy of Child and Adolescent Psychiatry* 15 (3): 105–25.

Jette, N., and E. Trevathan. 2014. "Saving Lives by Treating Epilepsy in Developing Countries." *Neurology* 82 (7): 552–53.

Jilek-Aall, L., and H. T. Rwiza. 1992. "Prognosis of Epilepsy in a Rural African Community: A 30-Year Follow-Up of 164 Patients in an Outpatient Clinic in Rural Tanzania." *Epilepsia* 33 (4): 645–50.

Joukamaa, M., M. Heliovaara, P. Knekt, A. Aromaa, R. Raitasalo, and V. Lehtinen. 2006. "Schizophrenia, Neuroleptic Medication and Mortality." *British Journal of Psychiatry* 188 (2): 122–27. doi:10.1192/bjp.188.2.122.

Kamgno, J., S. D. S. Pion, and M. Boussinesq. 2003. "Demographic Impact of Epilepsy in Africa: Results of a 10-Year Cohort Study in a Rural Area of Cameroon." *Epilepsia* 44 (7): 956–63. doi:10.1046/j.1528-1157.2003.59302.x.

Kilbourne, A. M., D. L. Rofey, J. F. McCarthy, E. P. Post, D. Welsh, and others. 2007. "Nutrition and Exercise Behavior among Patients with Bipolar Disorder 1." *Bipolar Disorders* 9 (5): 443–52. doi:10.1111/j.1399-5618.2007.00386.x.

Kisely, S., and L. A. Campbell. 2008. "Use of Smoking Cessation Therapies in Individuals with Psychiatric Illness: An Update for Prescribers." *CNS Drugs* 22 (4): 263–73.

Kisely, S., L. A. Campbell, and Y. Wang. 2009. "Treatment of ISCHAEMIC Heart Disease and Stroke in Individuals with Psychosis under Universal Healthcare." *The British Journal of Psychiatry* 195 (6): 545–50. doi:10.1192/bjp.bp.109.067082.

Kisely, S., M. Smith, D. Lawrence, M. Cox, L. A. Campbell, and others. 2007. "Inequitable Access for Mentally Ill Patients to Some Medically Necessary Procedures." *Canadian Medical Association Journal* 176 (6): 779–84. doi:10.1503/cmaj.060482.

Knapp, P. W., B. Soares, M. Farrell, and M. Silva de Lima. 2007. "Psychosocial Interventions for Cocaine and Psychostimulant Amphetamines Related Disorders." *Cochrane Database of Systematic Reviews* 3. doi:10.1002/14651858.CD003023.pub2.

Lambert, T. J. R., D. Velakoulis, and C. Pantelis. 2003. "Medical Comorbidity in Schizophrenia. Supplement: Comprehensive Care for People with Schizophrenia Living in the Community." *Medical Journal of Australia* 178 (9): 67–70.

Lasser, K., J. Boyd, S. Woolhandler, D. U. Himmelstein, D. McCormick, and others. 2000. "Smoking and Mental Illness: A Population-Based Prevalence Study." *Journal of the American Medical Association* 284 (20): 2606–10. doi:10.1001/jama.284.20.2606.

Laursen, T. M. 2011. "Life Expectancy among Persons with Schizophrenia or Bipolar Affective Disorder." *Schizophrenia Research* 131 (1–3): 101–04. doi:10.1016/j.schres.2011.06.008.

Laursen, T., T. Munk-Olsen, E. Agerbo, C. Gasse, and P. Mortensen. 2009. "Somatic Hospital Contacts, Invasive Cardiac Procedures, and Mortality from Heart Disease in Patients with Severe Mental Disorder." *Archives of General Psychiatry* 66 (7): 713–20. doi:10.1001/archgenpsychiatry.2009.61.

Laursen, T. M., M. Nordentoft, and P. B. Mortensen. 2014. "Excess Early Mortality in Schizophrenia." *Annual Review of Clinical Psychology* 10: 425–28. doi:10.1146/annurev-clinpsy-032813-153657.

Lawrence, D., K. J. Hancock, and S. Kisely. 2013. "The Gap in Life Expectancy from Preventable Physical Illness in Psychiatric Patients in Western Australia: Retrospective Analysis of Population Based Registers." *British Medical Journal* (346): f2539. doi:10.1136/bmj.f2539.

Lawrence, D., F. Mitrou, and S. Zubrick. 2009. "Smoking and Mental Illness: Results from Population Surveys in Australia and the United States." *BMC Public Health* 9 (1): 285.

Lawrinson, P., R. Ali, A. Buavirat, S. Chiamwongpaet, S. Dvoryak, and others. 2008. "Key Findings from the WHO Collaborative Study on Substitution Therapy for Opioid Dependence and HIV/AIDS." *Addiction* 103 (9): 1484–92.

Lee, L.-C., R. A. Harrington, J. J. Chang, and S. L. Connors. 2008. "Increased Risk of Injury in Children with Developmental Disabilities." *Research in Developmental Disabilities* 29: 247–55.

Li, Z., A. Page, G. Martin, and R. Taylor. 2011. "Attributable Risk of Psychiatric and Socio-Economic Factors for Suicide from Individual-Level, Population-Based Studies: A Systematic Review." *Social Science & Medicine* 72 (4): 608–16. doi:10.1016/j.socscimed.2010.11.008.

Liao, C. C., W. W. Shen, C. C. Chang, H. Chang, and T. L. Chen. 2013. "Surgical Adverse Outcomes in Patients with Schizophrenia: A Population-Based Study." *Annals of Surgery* 257 (3): 433–38.

Lim, S. S., T. Vos, A. D. Flaxman, G. Danaei, K. Shibuya, and others. 2012. "A Comparative Risk Assessment of Burden of Disease and Injury Attributable to 67 Risk Factors and Risk Factor Clusters in 21 Regions, 1990–2010: A Systematic Analysis for the Global Burden of Disease Study 2010." *The Lancet* 380 (9859): 2224–60.

Llibre R., J., A. Valhuerdi, I. I. Sanchez, C. Reyna, and M. A. Guerra. 2008. "The Prevalence, Correlates and Impact of Dementia in Cuba: A 10/66 Group Population-Based Survey." *Neuroepidemiology* 31: 243–51.

Lozano, R., M. Naghavi, K. Foreman, S. Lim, K. Shibuya, and others. 2012. "Global and Regional Mortality from 235 Causes of Death for 20 Age Groups in 1990 and 2010: A Systematic Analysis for the Global Burden of Disease Study 2010." *The Lancet* 380 (9859): 2095–128.

Malone, D., S. Marriott, G. Newton-Howes, S. Simmonds, and P. Tyrer. 2007. "Community Mental Health Teams (CMHTs) for People with Severe Mental Illnesses and Disordered Personality." *Cochrane Database of Systematic Reviews* 3. doi:10.1002/14651858.CD000270.pub2.

Mathers, B. M., L. Degenhardt, H. Ali, L. Wiessing, M. Hickman, and others. 2010. "HIV Prevention, Treatment, and Care Services for People Who Inject Drugs: A Systematic Review of Global, Regional, and National Coverage." *The Lancet* 375 (9719): 1014–28.

Mattick, R. P., C. Breen, J. Kimber, and M. Davoli. 2009. "Methadone Maintenance Therapy Versus No Opioid Replacement Therapy for Opioid Dependence." *Cochrane Database of Systematic Reviews* 2009 (3). doi:10.1002/14651858.CD002209.pub2.

Mattick, R. P., J. Kimber, C. Breen, and M. Davoli. 2008. "Buprenorphine Maintenance Versus Placebo or Methadone Maintenance for Opioid Dependence." *Cochrane Database of Systematic Reviews* 2008 (2). doi:10.1002/14651858 .CD002207.pub4.

Mitchell, A. J., and D. Lawrence. 2011. "Revascularisation and Mortality Rates Following Acute Coronary Syndromes in People with Severe Mental Illness: Comparative Meta-Analysis." *British Journal of Psychiatry* 198: 434–41. doi:10.1192/bjp.bp.109.076950.

Mitchell, A. J., and O. Lord. 2010. "Do Deficits in Cardiac Care Influence High Mortality Rates in Schizophrenia? A Systematic Review and Pooled Analysis." *Journal of Psychopharmacology* 24: 69–80.

Mitchell, S. L., J. M. Teno, D. K. Kiely, M. L. Shaffer, R. N. Jones, and others. 2009. "The Clinical Course of Advanced Dementia." *New England Journal of Medicine* 361 (16): 1529–38. doi:10.1056/NEJMoa0902234.

Mouridsen, S. E., H. Bronnum-Hansen, B. Rich, and T. Isager. 2008. "Mortality and Causes of Death in Autism Spectrum Disorders: An Update." *Autism* 12 (4): 403–14.

Mu, J., L. Liu, Q. Zhang, Y. Si, J. Hu, and others. 2011. "Causes of Death among People with Convulsive Epilepsy in Rural West China: A Prospective Study." *Neurology* 77 (2): 132–37. doi:10.1212/WNL.0b013e318223c784.

Murray, C. J. L., T. Vos, R. Lozano, M. Naghavi, A. D. Flaxman, and others. 2012. "Disability-Adjusted Life Years (DALYs) for 291 Diseases and Injuries in 21 Regions, 1990–2010: A Systematic Analysis for the Global Burden of Disease Study 2010." *The Lancet* 380 (9859): 2197–223.

Neligan, A., G. S. Bell, S. D. Shorvon, and J. W. Sander. 2010. "Temporal Trends in the Mortality of People with Epilepsy: A Review." *Epilepsia* 51 (11): 2241–46. doi:10.1111/j.1528-1167.2010.02711.x.

Nelson, P. K., B. M. Mathers, B. Cowie, H. Hagan, D. Des Jarlais, and others. 2011. "Global Epidemiology of Hepatitis B and Hepatitis C in People Who Inject Drugs: Results of Systematic Reviews." *The Lancet* 378 (9791): 571–83.

Newcomer, J. W. 2005. "Second-Generation (Atypical) Antipsychotics and Metabolic Effects." *CNS Drugs* 19 (1): 1–93. doi:10.2165/00023210-200519001-00001.

Newton, C. R., and H. H. Garcia. 2012. "Epilepsy in Poor Regions of the World." *The Lancet* 380 (9848): 1193–201. doi:10.1016/S0140-6736(12)61381-6.

Ngugi, A. K., C. Bottomley, G. Fegan, E. Chengo, R. Odhiambo, and others. 2014. "Premature Mortality in Active Convulsive Epilepsy in Rural Kenya: Causes and Associated Factors." *Neurology* 82 (7): 582–89. doi:10.1212 /WNL.0000000000000123.

Park, J.E., J.-Y. Lee, G.-H. Suh, B.-S. Kim, and M. J. Cho. 2014. "Mortality Rates and Predictors in Community-Dwelling Elderly Individuals with Cognitive Impairment: An Eight-Year Follow-up after Initial Assessment." *International Psychogeriatrics* 26 (08): 1295–304.

Pearson, R. 2009. *Compulsory Drug Treatment in Thailand: Observations on the Narcotic Addict Rehabilitation Act B.E. 2545 (2002)*. Toronto: Canadian HIV/AIDS Legal Network.

Pompili, P., P. Girardi, A. Ruberto, and R. Tatarelli. 2005. "Suicide in the Epilepsies: A Meta-Analytic Investigation of 29 Cohorts. *Epilepsy and Behaviour* 7 (2): 305–10.

Preux, P.-M., and M. Druet-Cabanac. 2005. "Epidemiology and Aetiology of Epilepsy in Sub-Saharan Africa." *The Lancet Neurology* 4 (1): 21–31. doi:http://dx.doi.org/10.1016 /S1474-4422(04)00963-9.

Prince, M., D. Acosta, C. P. Ferri, M. Guerra, Y. Huang, and others. 2012. "Dementia Incidence and Mortality in Middle-Income Countries, and Associations with Indicators of Cognitive Reserve: A 10/66 Dementia Research Group Population-Based Cohort Study." *The Lancet* 380 (9836): 50–58.

Prince, M., V. Patel, S. Saxena, M. Maj, J. Maselko, M. R. Phillips, and A. Rahman. 2007. "No Health without Mental Health." *The Lancet* 370 (9590): 859–77.

Rao, U. M. A., S. E. Daley, and C. Hammen. 2000. "Relationship between Depression and Substance Use Disorders in Adolescent Women during the Transition to Adulthood." *Journal of the American Academy of Child & Adolescent Psychiatry* 39 (2): 215–22. doi:http://dx.doi .org/10.1097/00004583-200002000-00022.

Rehm, J., D. Baliunas, G. L. G. Borges, K. Graham, H. Irving, and others. 2010. "The Relation between Different Dimensions of Alcohol Consumption and Burden of Disease: An Overview." *Addiction* 105 (5): 817–43. doi:10.1111/j.1360-0443.2010.02899.x.

Rehm, J., J. Csete, J. J. Amon, S. Baral, and C. Beyrer. 2010. "People Who Use Drugs, HIV, and Human Rights." *The Lancet* 376 (9739): 475–85.

Ridsdale, L., J. Charlton, M. Ashworth, M. P. Richardson, and M. C. Gulliford. 2011. "Epilepsy Mortality and Risk Factors for Death in Epilepsy: A Population-Based Study." *British Journal of General Practice* 61 (586): e271–e278.

Rohde, P., P. M. Lewinsohn, C. W. Kahler, J. R. Seeley, and R. A. Brown. 2001. "Natural Course of Alcohol Use Disorders from Adolescence to Young Adulthood." *Journal of the American Academy of Child & Adolescent Psychiatry* 40 (1): 83–90. doi:http://dx.doi.org/10.1097/00004583 -200101000-00020.

Roshanaei-Moghaddam, B., and W. Katon. 2009. "Premature Mortality from General Medical Illnesses among Persons with Bipolar Disorder: A Review." *Psychiatric Services* 60 (2): 147–56. doi:10.1176/appi.ps.60.2.147.

Rowe, R., B. Maughan, and R. Goodman. 2004. "Childhood Psychiatric Disorder and Unintentional Injury: Findings from a National Cohort Study." *Journal of Pediatric Psychology* 29 (2): 119–30.

Rummel-Kluge, C., K. Komossa, S. Schwarz, H. Hunger, F. Schmid, and others. 2010. "Head-to-Head Comparisons of Metabolic Side Effects of Second Generation

Antipsychotics in the Treatment of Schizophrenia: A Systematic Review and Meta-Analysis." *Schizophrenia Research* 123 (2–3): 225–33. doi:http://dx.doi.org/10.1016/j.schres.2010.07.012.

Salomon, J. A., H. Wang, M. K. Freeman, T. Vos, A. D. Flaxman, and others. 2012. "Healthy Life Expectancy for 187 Countries, 1990–2010: A Systematic Analysis for the Global Burden Disease Study 2010." *The Lancet* 380 (9859): 2144–62.

Schneider, L.S., K. S. Dagerman, and P. Insel. 2005. "Risk of Death with Atypical Antipsychotic Drug Treatment for Dementia: Meta-Analysis of Randomized Placebo-Controlled Trials." *Jama* 294 (15): 1934–43.

Scott, D., and B. Happell. 2011. "The High Prevalence of Poor Physical Health and Unhealthy Lifestyle Behaviours in Individuals with Severe Mental Illness." *Issues in Mental Health Nursing* 32: 589–97.

Scott, K. M., B. Wu, K. Saunders, C. Benjet, Y. He, and others. 2013. "Early-Onset Mental Disorders and Their Links to Chronic Physical Conditions in Adulthood." In *The Burdens of Mental Disorders. Global Perspectives from the WHO World Mental Health Surveys*, 87–96, edited by J. Alonso, S. Chatterji, and Y. He. New York: Cambridge University Press.

Shatenstein, B., M.-J. Kergoat, and I. Reid. 2007. "Poor Nutrient Intakes During 1-Year Follow-Up with Community Dwelling Older Adults with Early-Stage Alzheimer Dementia Compared to Cognitively Intact Matched Controls." *Journal of the American Dietetic Association* 107 (12): 2091–99. doi:http://dx.doi.org/10.1016/j.jada.2007.09.008.

Shavelle, R. M., D. J. Strauss, and J. Pickett. 2001. "Causes of Death in Autism." *Journal of Autism and Developmental Disorders* 31 (6): 569–76.

Sillanpää, M., and S. Shinnar. 2010. "Long-Term Mortality in Childhood-Onset Epilepsy." *New England Journal of Medicine* 363 (26): 2522–29.

Smith, M., D. Hopkins, R. C. Peveler, R. I. G. Holt, M. Woodward, and others. 2008. "First- v. Second-Generation Antipsychotics and Risk for Diabetes in Schizophrenia: Systematic Review and Meta-Analysis." *British Journal of Psychiatry* 192 (6): 406–11. doi:10.1192/bjp.bp.107.037184.

Spencer, D. 2014. "Understanding the Sources of Excess Mortality in Epilepsy." *Epilepsy Currents* 14 (1): 31–32. doi:10.5698/1535-7597-14.1.31.

Sporer, K. A. 2003. "Strategies for Preventing Heroin Overdose." *British Medical Journal* 326 (7386).

Sporer, K. A., and A. H. Kral. 2007. "Prescription Naloxone: A Novel Approach to Heroin Overdose Prevention." *Annals of Emergency Medicine* 49 (2): 172–77.

Srisurapanont, M., N. Jarusuraisin, and P. Kittirattanapaiboon. 2001. "Treatment for Amphetamine Dependence and Abuse." *Cochrane Database of Systematic Reviews* (4). doi:10.1002/14651858.CD003022.pub2.

Stapelberg, N. J. C., D. L. Neumann, D. H. K. Shum, H. McConnell, and I. Hailton-Craig. 2011. "A Topographical Map of the Causal Network of Mechanisms Underlying the Relationship between Major Depressive Disorder and Coronary Heart Disease." *Australian and New Zealand Journal of Psychiatry* 45: 351–69.

Strand, B. H., E. M. Langballe, V. Hjellvik, M. Handal, O. Næss, G. P. Knudsen, and others. 2013. "Midlife Vascular Risk Factors and Their Association with Dementia Deaths: Results from a Norwegian Prospective Study Followed Up for 35 Years." *Journal of Neurological Sciences* 324 (1-2): 124–30.

Swan, T. 2011. *Hepatitis C Treatment Pipeline Report*. New York, NY: Treatment Action Group.

Thornicroft, G. 2013. "Premature Death among People with Mental Illness: At Best a Failure to Act on Evidence; at Worst a Form of Lethal Discrimination." *British Medical Journal* 346. doi:10.1136/bmj.f2969.

Trinka, E., G. Bauer, W. Oberaigner, J. P. Ndayisaba, K. Seppi, and others. 2013. "Cause-Specific Mortality among Patients with Epilepsy: Results from a 30-Year Cohort Study." *Epilepsia* 54 (3): 495–501. doi:10.1111/epi.12014.

Turner, K. M. E., S. Hutchinson, P. Vickerman, V. Hope, N. Craine, and others. 2011. "The Impact of Needle and Syringe Provision and Opiate Substitution Therapy on the Incidence of Hepatitis C Virus in Injecting Drug Users: Pooling of UK Evidence." *Addiction* 106 (11): 1978–88.

UNODC (United Nations Office on Drugs and Crime) Regional Centre for East Asia and the Pacific. 2006. *HIV/AIDS and Custodial Settings in South East Asia: An Exploratory Review into the Issues of HIV/AIDS and Custodial Settings in Cambodia, China, Lao PDR, Myanmar, Thailand and Viet Nam*. Bangkok: UNODC.

U.S. FDA (U.S. Food and Drug Administration). 2008. "Information for Healthcare Professionals: Conventional Antipsychotics." http://www.fda.gov/Drugs/DrugSafety/PostmarketDrugSafetyInformationforPatientsandProviders/ucm124830.htm.

van Hasselt, F. M., P. F. Krabbe, D. G. van Ittersum, M. J. Postma, and A. J. Loonen. 2013. "Evaluating Interventions to Improve Somatic Health in Severe Mental Illness: A Systematic Review." *Acta Psychiatrica Scandinavica* 128: 251–60. doi:10.1111/acps.12096.

Verhaeghe, N., J. De Maeseneer, L. Maes, C. Van Heeringen, and L. Annemans. 2011. "Effectiveness and Cost-Effectiveness of Lifestyle Interventions on Physical Activity and Eating Habits in Persons with Severe Mental Disorders: A Systematic Review." *International Journal of Behavioral Nutrition and Physical Activity* 8: 28.

von Stumm, S., I. J. Deary, M. Kivimäki, M. Jokela, H. Clark, and others. 2011. "Childhood Behavior Problems and Health at Midlife: 35-Year Follow-Up of a Scottish Birth Cohort." *Journal of Child Psychology and Psychiatry* 52 (9): 992–1001. doi:10.1111/j.1469-7610.2011.02373.x.

Walker, E., R. E. McGee, and B. G. Druss. 2015. "Mortality in Mental Disorders and Global Disease Burden Implications: A Systematic Review and Meta-Analysis." *JAMA Psychiatry* 72 (4): 334–41. doi:10.1001/jamapsychiatry.2014.2502.

Weinmann, S., J. Read, and V. Aderhold. 2009. "Influence of Antipsychotics on Mortality in Schizophrenia: Systematic Review." *Schizophrenia Research* 113 (1): 1–11. doi:http://dx.doi.org/10.1016/j.schres.2009.05.018.

Westman, J., J. Hallgren, K. Wahlbeck, D. Erlinge, L. ALfredsson, and others. 2013. "Cardiovascular Mortality in Bipolar Disorder: A Population-Based Cohort Study in Sweden." *BMJ Open* 3. doi:10.1136/bmjopen-2012-002373.

Whiteford, H. A., L. Degenhardt, J. Rehm, A. J. Baxter, A. J. Ferrari, and others. 2013. "Global Burden of Disease Attributable to Mental and Substance Use Disorders: Findings from the Global Burden of Disease Study 2010." *The Lancet* 382 (9904): 1575–86.

Whiteford, H. A., A. J. Ferrari, L. Degenhardt, V. Feigin, and T. Vos. 2015. "The Global Burden of Mental, Neurological and Substance Use Disorders: An Analysis from the Global Burden of Disease Study 2010." In *Disease Control Priorities* (third edition): Volume 4, *Mental, Neurological, and Substance Use Disorders*, edited by V. Patel, D. Chisholm, T. Dua, R. Laxminarayan, and M. E. Medina-Mora. Washington, DC: World Bank.

WHO (World Health Organization). 1993. *The ICD-10 Classification of Mental and Behavioral Disorders: Diagnostic Criteria for Research*. Geneva: WHO.

———. 2005. *WHO Model List of Essential Medicines*. Geneva: WHO.

———. 2009. *Assessment of Compulsory Treatment of People Who Use Drugs in Cambodia, China, Malaysia and Viet Nam: An Application of Selected Human Rights Principles*. Manila: WHO.

———. 2012. *Public Health Action for the Prevention of Suicide: A Framework*. Geneva: WHO.

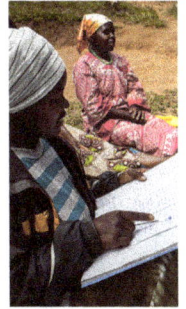

Chapter **4**

Adult Mental Disorders

Steven Hyman, Rachana Parikh,
Pamela Y. Collins, and Vikram Patel

INTRODUCTION

Burden of Disease

Mental disorders are a diverse group of conditions that primarily impair cognition, emotion, and behavioral control; occur early in life; and have a high aggregate prevalence in all countries where epidemiology has been investigated (Demyttenaere and others 2004; Kessler, Berglund, and others 2005; WHO 1992). The combination of high prevalence, early onset, clinical course that is either chronic or remitting and relapsing, and impairment of critical brain functions makes mental disorders a major contributor to the global disease burden discussed in chapter 2 in this volume (Whiteford and others 2015). The greatest fraction of the burden results from years lived with disability (YLDs), particularly for ages 15–49 years—a critical life interval for completing education, starting a family, and increasing productivity at work (figure 4.1) (WHO 2014b). The global cost of mental health conditions is projected to be as high as US$6 trillion by 2030, of which 35 percent would be contributed by low- and middle-income countries (LMICs) (Bloom and others 2011).

Although mental disorders directly account for fewer than half of one percent of all deaths, they contribute significantly to premature mortality through multiple medical causes (discussed in chapter 3 in this volume, Charlson and others 2015) and are a major risk factor for suicide (WHO 2014c; chapter 9 in this volume, Vijayakumar and others 2015). An estimated 8 million deaths annually due to medical conditions are attributable to mental disorders (Walker, McGee, and Druss 2015).

Mental disorders are associated with social stigma in many countries and cultures (Weiss and others 2001). The slow emergence of scientific explanations for the etiologies of mental disorders and the mistaken belief that symptoms reflect either a lack of will power or some moral failure facilitate negative attitudes and discrimination. Patients with psychotic symptoms can seem frightening, but persons with mental illnesses are far more likely to commit suicide than homicide and to be victims of crimes than perpetrators (*The Lancet* 2013; Walsh and others 2003). Shame and fear are substantial obstacles to help-seeking, diagnosis, and treatment. Individuals with mental disorders are often imprisoned, without access to adequate care, for minor legal transgressions that result directly from their illnesses. In many mental hospitals and other settings, people with these disorders may not be accorded basic human rights. Stigmatization has contributed to disparities in availability and access to care and medications and insurance coverage, as well as research funding, compared with other chronic illnesses (Wang, Aguilar-Gaxiola, and others 2007).

This chapter updates data on the disease burden, as well as interventions to treat the four leading contributors to adult mental illness globally—schizophrenia, bipolar disorder, depressive disorders, and anxiety disorders. These were selected because of their high contribution to the global disease burden, accounting

Corresponding author: Steven Hyman, Stanley Center for Psychiatric Research, Broad Institute of the Massachusetts Institute of Technology and Harvard University; and Department of Stem Cell and Regenerative Biology, Harvard University, Cambridge, Massachusetts, United States of America, seh@harvard.edu.

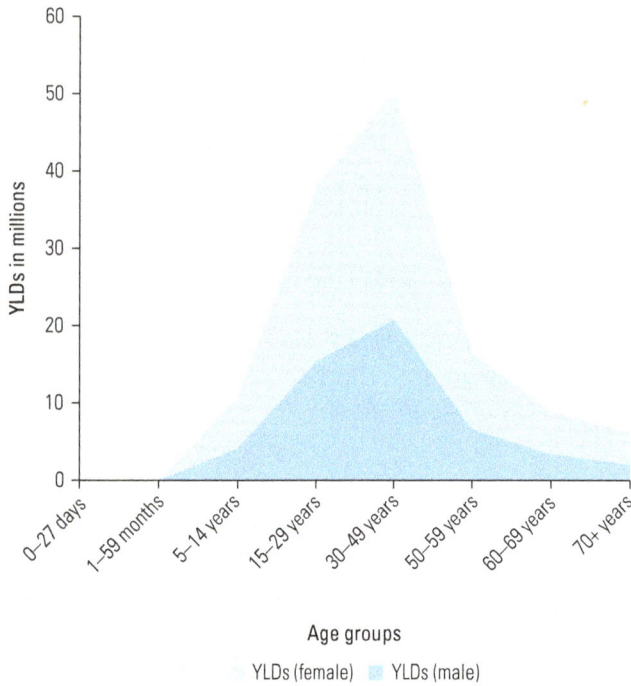

Figure 4.1 Years Lived with Disability Caused by Unipolar Depression, Anxiety Disorders, Bipolar Disorder, and Schizophrenia Globally

Source: WHO 2014b.
Note: YLDs = years lived with disability.

for 66 percent of disability-adjusted life years (DALYs) lost and 69 percent of YLDs due to mental and behavioral disorders, as well as based on the availability of data for cost-effectiveness analyses. We begin with a brief summary of the etiology of these disorders, followed by a more detailed description of the burden and epidemiology of each group of disorders and the evidence on treatment. Throughout this chapter, although we attempt to emphasize data from LMICs, most of the data are from high-income countries (HICs).

Risk Factors

The etiologies of mental disorders involve interactions among genetic, developmental, social, and environmental risk factors. Mental disorders are polygenic, meaning that hundreds of risk variants in DNA sequence exist across global populations, much like type 2 diabetes mellitus and hypertension. An individual's risk results from the aggregation of some disease-associated alleles (alternative forms of a gene at a given locus) in combination with environmental factors. Strong evidence suggests that multiple psychiatric disorders share a significant fraction of genetic risk factors (Lee and others 2013).

Among the disorders discussed in this chapter, schizophrenia and bipolar disorder are the most highly influenced by genes, with estimated heritabilities of 65 to 80 percent (Sullivan, Daly, and O'Donovan 2012). Genotyping of nearly 40,000 individuals with schizophrenia and a larger number of healthy comparison subjects has revealed 108 genomewide significant loci that contribute to risk, with different combinations of risk alleles acting in different individuals (Ripke and others 2014). Genes exert less influence, and environmental risk factors more, in depressive and anxiety disorders (Sullivan, Daly, and O'Donovan 2012).

The relative risk of developing psychopathology involves interactions with genetic and developmental risk factors (Digangi and others 2013). Adverse circumstances in childhood have been associated with risk; histories of early childhood abuse, violence, poverty, and experiences of significant loss correlate with risk of multiple mood and anxiety disorders (Heim and others 2010; Patel and Kleinman 2003). Through complex pathways, people with chronic physical illnesses like diabetes, chronic obstructive pulmonary disease, cardiovascular disease, arthritis, and cancer have a greater likelihood of developing mental disorders, particularly depression (Moussavi and others 2007). Similarly, individuals who have sustained traumatic brain injuries have a greater likelihood of developing mental disorders (Jorge and others 2004). Environmental triggers are best documented in post-traumatic stress disorder (PTSD), but even here individuals vary enormously in the threshold of stress severity associated with PTSD. Replicated environmental risk factors for schizophrenia include urban birth, migrant status, season of birth, and possibly viral infections during pregnancy (Sorensen and others 2014). These environmental risk factors are proxies for causal mechanisms that remain to be identified and that interact with genetic risk factors to produce illness (McGrath and Scott 2006).

Gender is associated with the risk of many mental disorders; men have higher rates of schizophrenia, and women have higher rates of depressive and anxiety disorders (Patel and others 2006). The reasons for these differences are likely related to genetic and social factors that may expose a particular gender to a higher burden of risk factors. Bipolar disorder affects men and women equally.

MOOD AND ANXIETY DISORDERS

Mood disorders differ from normal variation in emotional state by their persistence across time and situations—each episode lasting weeks or even months—and accompanying physiological and cognitive symptoms. Mood disorders are divided into unipolar depressive disorders and bipolar disorder, in which manic episodes also occur. The unipolar-bipolar distinction is well supported by studies of families, genetics, and treatment response.

During an episode of a mood disorder, a person may be predominantly sad or emotionally withdrawn (depressive disorders), elated (mania), or irritable (mania or depression). The emotions are relatively inflexible; for example, a person with a depressive disorder cannot respond appropriately to happy or rewarding stimuli. The physiological disturbances typical of mood disorders include abnormalities in sleep, appetite, libido, and energy. Cognitive abnormalities associated with mood disorders include impairment in attention and memory, as well as mood-dependent changes in the content of thought.

Severe depression and mania may be characterized by psychotic symptoms. Due to frequent occurrence of psychotic symptoms during the manic phase of bipolar disorder, it can also be considered a type of psychotic disorder. In many LMICs, concurrent somatic symptoms are commonly reported with mood and anxiety disorders and may be the chief complaint. For example, patients suffering from depression might not complain of emotional symptoms but of fatigue or multiple aches and pains. Many reasons have been suggested for this phenomenon, including the stigma associated with mental disorders and patients' expectation that physical symptoms have more salience in medical consultations.

Depressive Disorder

Clinical Features and Course

Clinically significant depression is distinguished from normal sadness or grief by its severity, persistence across time and situations, duration, and associated physiological and behavioral symptoms. The cardinal symptoms include a period of persistent sadness or other negative affective states, such as loss of interest in previously pleasurable pursuits, or anhedonia (inability to experience pleasure). Physiological symptoms occur across cultures, including sleep disturbance, most often insomnia (with early morning awakening), but occasionally excessive sleeping; appetite disturbance (usually loss of appetite and weight loss), but occasionally excessive eating; and decreased energy, fatigue, multiple aches, and pains.

The cognitive symptoms may include thoughts of worthlessness and guilt, suicidal thoughts, difficulty concentrating, slow thinking, ruminations, and poor memory. Some individuals with depression exhibit slowed motor movements (psychomotor retardation), while others may be agitated. Psychotic symptoms occur in a minority of cases, most often congruent with the depressed mood. Thus, a person might hear relentlessly critical voices.

Epidemiology and Burden of Disease

Depression is an episodic disorder that generally begins early in life (median age of onset is in the mid- to late 20s), although new onsets can be observed across the lifespan. Childhood onset is being increasingly recognized, although not all childhood precursors of adult depression take the form of a clearly diagnosable depressive disorder. A pattern of remissions and relapses is typical, with recurrence risk greater among those with early-onset disease (Lewinsohn and others 2000). Many individuals do not recover fully from acute episodes and suffer a persistent depressive disorder that exerts negative effects on public health worldwide (Gureje 2011) and is a risk factor for suicide.

Depression is often comorbid with other mental disorders (Kessler, Chiu, and others 2005); roughly half of the people who have a history of depression also have an anxiety disorder in their lifetime. Depression is frequently comorbid with obesity and general medical disorders, such as type 2 diabetes mellitus, coronary artery disease, and chronic pain disorders.

The 12-month prevalence of depressive disorder, dysthymia, or bipolar disorder among the 17 countries that participated in the World Health Organization's (WHO) World Mental Health (WMH) surveys ranged between 1.1 percent in Nigeria and 9.7 percent in the United States, with an interquartile range (IQR)—which covers the 25th to 75th percentiles—of 3.4 to 6.8 percent and substantial cross-country variations (Kessler and others 2008).[1] These wide differences in prevalence may represent both methodological differences (notably difficulties in self-reporting conditions that are stigmatized across cultures) and true differences due to the interplay among the genetic, developmental, and environmental factors that might differ across countries.

Depression also leads to substantial impairments in productive and social roles (Wang, Simon, and Kessler 2003) and is the single largest contributor to the nonfatal burden globally (WHO 2014b). Depression is a leading risk factor for suicide—a risk that is exacerbated if concurrent with substance use disorders or psychotic symptoms (Isometsa 2014).

People with depression frequently delay seeking professional treatment—particularly those with early-onset cases (Olfson and others 1998)—and frequently receive undertreatment. The WMH surveys found that the proportion of persons with mood disorders receiving any treatment in the first year of onset of the disorder ranged from 6 percent in China and Nigeria to 52.1 percent in the Netherlands, with an IQR of 16.0–42.7 percent. Overall, the use of mental health services is lower in LMICs and largely corresponds to countries' overall spending on health. A higher proportion of people receives care from general medical services (except in some countries, including Colombia, Israel, and Mexico), indicating the need to focus on interventions through general health care platforms (Wang, Aguilar-Gaxiola, and others 2007).

Anxiety Disorders

Clinical Features and Course
Anxiety disorders represent symptomatically diverse, albeit related, forms of dysregulation of fear responses in the brain, likely excessive activation of subcortical fear circuitry with inadequate regulation by the prefrontal cortex. In anxiety disorders, even innocuous stimuli induce a significant and often prolonged response including tension, vigilance, activation of the sympathetic nervous system, subjective fear, and, in some circumstances, panic.

Although anxiety per se is likely to feature in the clinical presentation of most patients, somatic complaints such as chest pain, palpitations, respiratory difficulty, or headaches are common. These symptoms may be more commonly reported in LMICs.

Panic Disorder. The central feature of panic disorder is an unexpected panic attack: a discrete period of intense fear accompanied by physiological symptoms, such as a racing heart, shortness of breath, sweating, or dizziness, with an intense fear of losing control or dying. Panic disorder is diagnosed when the attacks are recurrent and give rise to anticipatory anxiety about additional attacks. People with panic disorder may progressively restrict their lives and ultimately stop leaving their homes altogether to avoid situations like crowds, traveling, bridges, or elevators, in which panic attacks occur.

Generalized Anxiety Disorder. Generalized anxiety disorder is characterized by chronic, unrealistic and excessive worry, accompanied by anxiety-related symptoms such as sympathetic nervous system arousal, excessive vigilance, and motor tension.

Post-Traumatic Stress Disorder. PTSD follows significant trauma and is characterized by emotional numbness, punctuated by intrusive reliving of the traumatic episode triggered by cues that act as reminders of the trauma; disturbed sleep (including nightmares); and hyperarousal, such as exaggerated startle responses.

Social Anxiety Disorder. *Social anxiety disorder (social phobia)* is characterized by a persistent fear of social situations or performance situations that expose a person to potential scrutiny by others. It may be difficult to separate social anxiety disorder from extremes of normal temperament, such as shyness. Nonetheless, social anxiety disorder can be quite disabling.

Simple Phobias. *Simple phobias* are extreme fear in the presence of discrete stimuli or cues such as heights or spiders.

Obsessive-Compulsive Disorder. Obsessive-compulsive disorder (OCD) was historically considered an anxiety disorder, but is now recognized to reflect dysfunction of a different brain circuit, striatal-thalamic-cortical loops (Pauls and others 2014). While OCD symptoms engender severe anxiety, the core symptoms are intrusive, unwanted thoughts followed by actions and rituals meant to neutralize them. For example, the thought that a doorknob is contaminated may lead to excessive handwashing. When severe, OCD rituals can consume much time in the day and can be distressing and disabling. Childhood onsets are common and are more likely to be familial than later onsets.

Epidemiology and Burden of Disease
Anxiety disorders are the most common mental disorders in most of the countries that participated in the WMH surveys. The 12-month prevalence of anxiety disorders ranges between 3.0 percent (China) and 19.0 percent (the United States), with an IQR of 6.5–12.2 percent (Kessler and others 2008). Despite wide variation in overall prevalence, specific phobia and social phobia are generally the most prevalent lifetime anxiety disorders, with a weighted mean prevalence of 6.4 percent and 4.6 percent, respectively. Panic disorder and OCD are generally the least prevalent, with weighted means of 1.7 percent and 1.3 percent, respectively.

Anxiety disorders have consistently been found in epidemiological surveys to be highly comorbid, both among themselves (multiple anxiety disorders) and in combination with mood disorders. Most people with a history of one anxiety disorder typically have a second anxiety disorder. More than half of the people with a history of either an anxiety or mood disorder typically have both types of disorders. Retrospective reports from community surveys consistently show that anxiety disorders have early average ages of onset, a median of approximately age 15 years, based on cross-national patterns (de Graaf and others 2003; Kessler, Chiu, and others 2005).

There is considerable delay in seeking care for anxiety disorders. Data from the WMH surveys report that, among the countries studied, the proportion of persons with anxiety disorders receiving treatment within the first year of the onset of the disorder ranged from 0.8 percent in Nigeria to 36.4 percent in Israel among the countries studied, with an IQR of 3.6–19.8 percent. The median delay in seeking care varied significantly between countries, ranging from three years in Israel to as many as 30 years in Mexico (Wang, Angermeyer, and others 2007).

Anxiety disorders have consistently been found in epidemiological surveys to be associated with substantial impairments in productive roles (such as work absenteeism, work performance, unemployment, and underemployment) and social roles (such as social isolation, interpersonal tensions, and marital disruption).

Bipolar Disorder

Clinical Features and Course
Bipolar disorder is defined by the presence of mania as well as depression, but the relative frequency and duration of the two poles vary widely. Moreover, mixtures of symptoms are quite common. Patients with bipolar disorder have recurrent episodes of illness—manias and depression—and may recover to baseline functioning between episodes. However, many patients have residual symptoms, most often depressive symptoms, which may cause significant impairment (Angst and Sellaro 2000). Individuals who have had at least one manic episode are considered to have bipolar disorder, even if they have not yet experienced a depressive episode. Some classification systems distinguish bipolar I disorder, in which patients meet the full criteria for manic episodes, from bipolar II disorder, in which patients experience only mild manic episodes.

Mania is typically characterized by euphoria or irritability, a marked increase in energy, and a decreased need for sleep. Individuals with mania often exhibit impulsive and disinhibited behaviors. There may be excessive involvement in goal-directed behaviors characterized by poor judgment. Self-esteem is typically inflated, frequently reaching delusional proportions. Speech is typically rapid and difficult to interrupt. Individuals with mania may exhibit cognitive symptoms; patients cannot stick to a topic and may jump rapidly from idea to idea, making comprehension of their train of thought difficult. Psychotic symptoms are common during manic episodes. The depressive episodes of people with bipolar disorder are symptomatically indistinguishable from those of people who have unipolar depression, but those with bipolar disorder tend to be less responsive to treatment. Mixed states may occur, with symptoms of both mania and depression.

The rate of cycling between mania and depression varies widely among individuals. One common pattern of illness is for episodes initially to be separated by a relatively long period, perhaps a year, and then to become more frequent with age. A minority of patients with bipolar disorder has four or more cycles per year (Coryell and others 2003). These individuals tend to be more disabled and less responsive to treatment. Once cycles are established, acute relapses may occur without an identifiable precipitant, with the exception of sleep deprivation (Leibenluft and others 1996), making a regular daily sleep schedule and avoidance of shift work important in disease management.

Epidemiology and Burden of Disease
Bipolar disorder has an equal gender ratio. Retrospective reports from community epidemiological surveys consistently show that bipolar disorder has an early age of onset in the late teens through mid-20s. Onset in childhood has been recognized (Geller and Luby 1997), but childhood diagnoses remain controversial; the revision in the recent *Diagnostic and Statistical Manual of Mental Disorders, 5th ed. (DSM-5)* offers disruptive mood dysregulation disorder as an alternative explanation of severe childhood mood disturbance with temper tantrums (APA 2013).

Epidemiological surveys have consistently found bipolar disorder to be highly comorbid with other psychiatric disorders, especially anxiety and substance use disorders (ten Have and others 2002). The extent of comorbidity is much greater than for unipolar depressive disorders or anxiety disorders. Some individuals with classical symptoms of bipolar disorder also exhibit chronic psychotic symptoms superimposed on their mood syndrome—and are then diagnosed with schizoaffective disorder. Their prognosis tends to be less favorable than for the classical bipolar patient, although somewhat better than for individuals with schizophrenia. Schizoaffective disorder may also be diagnosed when chronic psychotic symptoms are superimposed on unipolar depression. The latter have outcomes similar to patients with schizophrenia (Tsuang and Coryell 1993).

A recent systematic review of 29 epidemiological studies covering 20 countries reported 6- and 12-month point prevalence estimates of bipolar disorder of 0.74 and 0.84 percent, respectively, with no significant differences correlated with gender or economic status (Ferrari, Baxter, and Whiteford 2011). Notably, good evidence exists that bipolar disorder has a wide subthreshold spectrum that includes people who are often seriously impaired even though they do not meet full *DSM* or International Classification of Diseases criteria for bipolar I or II disorders (Perugi and Akiskal 2002). This spectrum might include as much as 5 percent of the general population. The ratio of recent-to-lifetime prevalence of bipolar disorder in community surveys is quite high (0.71), indicating that bipolar disorder is persistent.

Bipolar disorder is associated with substantial impairments in productive and social roles (Das Gupta and Guest 2002), and there are consistent delays in initially seeking professional treatment (Olfson and others 1998), particularly among early-onset cases, and substantial undertreatment of current cases. Each of these characteristics—chronic, recurrent course; significant impairments to functioning; and modest treatment rates—contributes to the significant disease burden approaching that for schizophrenia.

PSYCHOTIC DISORDERS: SCHIZOPHRENIA

Clinical Features and Course

Schizophrenia is a severe neuropsychiatric syndrome associated with significant lifelong disability as well as premature mortality from suicide and other causes. Schizophrenia exhibits three main symptom domains:

- *Psychotic, or positive, symptoms* include hallucinations and delusions that are generally experienced as having a basis in reality outside the person's psyche.
- *Negative, or deficit, symptoms* include loss of motivation, blunted affect, and impoverishment of thought and language.
- *Cognitive symptoms* include significant impairments in attention, working memory, declarative memory, verbal fluency, and multiple aspects of social cognition. In addition, many individuals with schizophrenia suffer from mood disturbances, usually depression.

Negative and cognitive symptoms, currently untreatable, are highly disabling, in great measure because of a loss of ability to control thought, emotion, and behavior (Lesh and others 2011). Indeed, individuals with schizophrenia remain disabled even when their positive symptoms are well controlled.

Schizophrenia typically begins in the mid-teen years with a prodrome (also described as a psychosis risk state) characterized by significant declines across multiple cognitive domains, social isolation, odd and eccentric thinking, and later by attenuated psychotic symptoms (Fusar-Poli and others 2013). Longitudinal structural magnetic resonance imaging studies suggest that the prodrome is associated with excessive cortical thinning, especially in prefrontal and temporal cortices (Vidal and others 2006). Abnormal synaptic loss (pruning) beginning in the prodrome is thought to cause significant loss of neural processes and synapses, consistent with the significant observed cognitive impairment (Lesh and others 2011).

The diagnosis of schizophrenia is generally made with a first onset of florid psychotic symptoms. First episodes of schizophrenia generally respond well to antipsychotic drugs, but the response attenuates over time. Ultimately, most patients have residual psychotic symptoms and acute psychotic relapses despite treatment.

The course of schizophrenia, beyond the first psychotic episode, is typically one of relapses of severe psychotic symptoms, followed by partial remission. The time between relapses is extended by maintenance treatment with antipsychotic drugs at lower doses than are needed to treat acute episodes. Cognitive and occupational functioning tend to decline over the first years of the illness and then to plateau at a level well below what would have been expected for the individual (Lesh and others 2011). Nonetheless, residual impairment has substantial cross-cultural variation that is hypothesized to reflect greater maintenance of social integration in societies where outcomes are better.

Based on emerging genetic findings as well as observation of symptom diversity, severity, and treatment response, it is clear that schizophrenia is highly heterogeneous (Ripke and others 2014; Sullivan, Daly, and O'Donovan 2012). Schizophrenia is now seen as a spectrum of disorders that includes both related nonaffective psychoses and likely some affective psychoses, such as schizoaffective disorder, although the *DSM-5* does not yet recognize this breadth (APA 2013).

Epidemiology and Burden of Disease

Schizophrenia affects between 0.5 and 1.0 percent of the population worldwide, with a male-female ratio of 1.4 to 1.0 (McGrath and others 2004). Seven or eight persons per 1,000 are likely to be affected by schizophrenia in their lifetime. Point prevalence is estimated to be 4.6 per 1,000 persons (Saha and others 2005). The incidence rates vary greatly by gender, urban status, and migrant status. A systematic review of 158 studies found a median incidence rate of 15.2 per 100,000 persons, with a 10 and 90 percent quantiles range of 7.7–43.0. The incidence rate was found to be influenced by gender, with a higher incidence in men (median male-female ratio of 1.4 to 1.0, with a 10 and 90 percent quantiles range of 0.9–2.4). And there was a higher incidence in migrants than native-born individuals (median migrant–native-born incidence rate ratio of 4.6, with a 10 and 90 percent quantiles range of 1.0–12.8) (McGrath and others 2004).

Although schizophrenia is a relatively uncommon disorder, aggregate estimates of disease burden are high because the condition is associated with early onset, long duration, and severe disability. Schizophrenia leads to loss of approximately 1,994 DALYs per one million population (WHO 2014a).

INTERVENTIONS FOR MOOD, ANXIETY, AND PSYCHOTIC DISORDERS

This section updates the evidence contained in *Disease Control Priorities in Developing Countries*, 2nd ed., based on a systematic search of systematic reviews. Where no reviews were found, randomized controlled trials testing the effectiveness of interventions for mood, anxiety, and psychotic disorders were included.

Population Platform Interventions

Mental Health Awareness Campaigns

Awareness campaigns through mass media can be instrumental in reducing prejudice (Clement and others 2013) and improving the use of services (Grilli, Ramsay, and Minozzi 2002). A community-based awareness program in Nigeria was helpful in making mental disorders a priority on the local political agenda (Eaton and Agomoh 2008).

Awareness campaigns must attempt to dispel myths and fight discrimination against people affected by mental disorders while educating and increasing awareness of mental disorders. Interventions based on education and improvement of social contact with persons with mental disorders appear to be the most effective to increase knowledge, reduce stigma, change behavior, and decrease the "desire for social distance" (Evans-Lacko and others 2012; Yamaguchi and others 2013). However, campaigns focused on increasing public understanding of the biological correlates alone may not lead to better social acceptance of people with mental disorders (Schomerus and others 2012). Experience from the mass media interventions in the United Kingdom suggests that it may be helpful to include messages on how to help (Evans-Lacko and others 2010).

Mental Health Legislation

Fewer than half of LMICs have enacted legislation focused on mental health (WHO 2011). Where they exist, mental health laws focus on human rights protection, involuntary admission and treatment, guardianship, freedom from discrimination, and inspection of institutions. The WHO's Assessment Instrument for Mental Health Systems (WHO-AIMS) survey in 2009 observed that about 42 percent of all participating low-income countries and 30 percent of the lower-middle-income countries had legislation to protect people with mental disorders against discrimination in employment, compared with 80 percent of upper-middle-income countries (WHO 2009).

By means of action or inaction, legislation can itself contribute to human rights abuses. In the WHO-AIMS survey, LMICs reported higher frequency of involuntary admissions to mental hospitals and other inpatient units, as well as higher incidences of human rights abuses in hospitals and many fewer provisions for inspections of health facilities (WHO 2009).

Community Platform Interventions

Community-based interventions primarily seek to promote health and prevent illness in settings such as workplaces and schools, as well as within families and other community networks.

Workplaces

Workplace attributes related to organizational culture, employment status, exposure to workplace trauma, and job dissatisfaction can contribute to psychosocial risk factors for mood disorders. Although largely drawn from studies in HICs, work-related stress management through physical exercise and cognitive and behavioral approaches such as problem-solving techniques, meditation, and relaxation training can help prevent and improve symptoms of anxiety and depression among employees (Martin, Sanderson, and Cocker 2009; Penalba, McGuire, and Leite 2008). For employees with diagnosed depression, collaboration among all parties dealing with the management of affected employees is important. Provision of integrated care and access to worksite stress reduction programs, with assured confidentiality for the employee, can reduce symptoms of depression (Furlan and others 2012).

Schools

Schools are a good platform for increasing community awareness about mental health. Evidence from a randomized controlled trial in rural Pakistan demonstrated that increasing mental health awareness among school children also increased awareness among parents and neighbors (Rahman and others 1998).

Preventive interventions, such as structured physical activity, delivered in schools can reduce students' anxiety and improve self-esteem (Bonhauser and others 2005).

Similarly, programs that advance positive thinking have been effective in preventing depression in school children (Yu and Seligman 2002). As in workplace stress reduction programs, psychological and educational counseling can decrease anxiety among students (Sharif and Armitage 2004).

Family

Family interventions through support groups or formal family therapies promote understanding of mental disorders among family members and support positive family environments by reducing overinvolvement and excessive criticism of affected members within families. The ultimate goal is to reduce relapse and hospitalization events in patients and reduce the stress felt by family members living with the patient.

Family interventions—including brief interventions over a limited number of sessions—are effective for schizophrenia (Okpokoro, Adams, and Sampson 2014; Pharaoh and others 2010) and bipolar disorder (Justo, Soares, and Calil 2007). Although there is a relative paucity of high-quality studies on family interventions, it is reasonable to utilize family interventions in the management of psychotic disorders, particularly in LMICs where most people with psychosis stay with families who are also the primary caregivers. Existing interventions can be used with relevant adaptation of the therapies according to the local social and cultural context.

Health Care Platform Interventions

Treatments for Mood and Psychotic Disorders

Self-Care and Management. Self-care enables people living with mental disorders to take the first step in effective prevention and management of their conditions. Systematic reviews suggest that regular exercise promotes physical and mental well-being in individuals with depression (Cooney and others 2013) and psychoses (Gorczynski and Faulkner 2010). Similarly, relaxation techniques (Jorm, Morgan, and Hetrick 2008) and music therapy (Maratos and others 2008) effectively reduce depressive symptoms. The use of media-delivered psychotherapy interventions is effective for self-care in persons with anxiety disorders (Mayo-Wilson and Montgomery 2013). For people with psychotic disorders, education forms a component of self-care: knowing early warning symptoms and signs of bipolar disorder and schizophrenia and their management has been found to improve functioning and delay recurrence, reducing the need for hospitalization (Morriss and others 2007).

Pharmacotherapy and Psychotherapy. Many psychotherapies based on cognitive mechanisms underlying the symptoms of mood and anxiety disorders have been developed and subjected to well-designed clinical trials that have demonstrated their efficacy for depressive and anxiety disorders (Beck and Haigh 2014). Cognitive remediation therapies for schizophrenia are in the early stages of development, but appear promising.

Table 4.1 reviews the evidence for pharmacotherapy and psychotherapy for mood, anxiety, and psychotic disorders. Although the evidence that strongly supports the efficacy of a range of pharmacological and psychotherapeutic interventions is from HICs, the interventions have been validated in a wide range of cultures, ethnicities, and levels of economic development. However, contextual adaptation of psychosocial interventions should occur routinely. Integration with social welfare departments in LMICs could also be helpful in addressing the burden of life stressors in these settings.

This substantial body of knowledge is relevant for guiding treatment in nonspecialist health care platforms in LMICs and has formed the basis of the recent WHO Mental Health Gap Action Programme (mhGAP) guidelines (WHO 2010). Unfortunately, this information is far too rarely applied in practice (Hyman 2014; Simon and others 2004) despite implementation research in LMICs that has sought to bridge the gap between what we know and what we do. These packages of care are described in the next section.

Specialist Care. Electroconvulsive therapy (ECT) is a well-established, effective, and relatively low-cost therapy for adults with severe or treatment-resistant depression, older people with depression (Martinez-Amoros and others 2012), and acute mania when a patient cannot tolerate medications. ECT must be administered in a clinical setting with the help of qualified personnel to deliver the treatment as well as anesthesia and muscle relaxants. Once symptoms have improved (generally six to eight treatments delivered no more frequently than every other day), the person may receive antidepressant medications. In treatment refractory cases, ECT is also used as a maintenance therapy for depression.

Combined with antipsychotic medications, ECT may also be an option for people with schizophrenia, particularly when rapid global improvement and reduction of symptoms is desired as well as in cases with no response to medications, although it has only short-term benefits (Tharyan and Adams 2005).

Among the newer treatment modalities, transcranial magnetic stimulation, which involves the use of a magnet to stimulate selected areas of the brain, may be effective for refractory depression, but the evidence remains inconclusive. Moreover, it is expensive and limited in scalability because of the need for the appropriate technology.

Table 4.1 Review of Evidence for Pharmacologic and Psychological Treatment of Mood, Anxiety, and Psychotic Disorders

Disorder	First-line treatment	Second-line treatments or adjunct treatment
Mood disorders		

Depressive disorder	• Antidepressants:
	  • Tricyclic antidepressants and selective serotonin reuptake inhibitors (Silva de Lima and Hotopf 2003; von Wolff and others 2013)[a]
	• Psychotherapy:
	  • Brief psychological interventions (Cuijpers and others 2009)[b]
	  • Problem-solving therapy (Cuijpers, van Straten, and Warmerdam 2007; Huibers and others 2007)[b]
	  • Cognitive behavioral therapy (Orgeta and others 2014; Wilson, Mottram, and Vassilas 2008)[a]
	  • Behavioral therapies (Shinohara and others 2013)[a]
	  • Psychodynamic therapies (Abbass and others 2014)[a]
	  • Interpersonal psychotherapy (de Mello and others 2005)[a]
		• For postpartum depression:
		  • Psychological and social interventions (Dennis and Hodnett 2007)[a]
		  • SSRIs, but safety concerns for breastfeeding neonates are not known (Molyneaux and others 2014)[a]
		• For psychotic depression: Combination of an antipsychotic and an antidepressant (Wijkstra and others 2013)[a]
		• For refractory depression:
		  • Combined CBT and antidepressant (Wiles and others 2013)[c]
		  • Electroconvulsive therapy (Martinez-Amoros and others 2012; UK ECT Review Group 2003)[a]
		  • Transcranial magnetic stimulation (Gaynes and others 2014)[a]

Notes	• Antidepressants are also effective for depression in people with physical illnesses (Rayner and others 2010).[a] • Antidepressants can be effectively prescribed in primary care settiings (Arroll and others 2009).[a] • Problem-solving therapy can be delivered by general practitioners (Huibers and others 2007).[a] • Group interpersonal therapy is effective in community-based, low-resource settings (Bass and others 2006).[c] • Older tricyclic antidepressants are similar in efficacy to newer drugs, but have greater side effects (Mottram, Wilson, and Strobl 2006).[a] • Continuation of treatment with drugs for 9–12 months following response to medication reduces the risk of relapse (Kaymaz and others 2008;[b] Wilkinson and Izmeth 2012[a]). • Evidence to suggest the superiority of one type of psychological intervention over another is limited (Cuijpers and others 2008;[b] Moradveisi and others 2013[c]).	
Bipolar disorder	• Combination of second-generation antipsychotics and mood stabilizers for acute mania (Scherk, Pajonk, and Leucht 2007)[a] • Lithium, valproate, lamotrigine, and olanzapine for maintenance therapy to prevent relapse (Soares-Weiser and others 2007)[a]	• Psychotherapies like CBT, group psychoeducational therapy, and family therapy (Soares-Weiser and others 2007)[a]
Anxiety disorders		
Anxiety disorders	• Antidepressants (Kapczinski and others 2003)[a]	
Generalized anxiety disorder	• CBT-based psychotherapies (Hunot and others 2007)[a]	
Panic disorder	• Combined therapy (CBT and antidepressants) or CBT alone (Furukawa, Watanabe, and Churchill 2007)[a]	
Post-traumatic stress disorder	• No psychological intervention can be recommended routinely following traumatic events, and this may also have adverse effects on some individuals (Roberts and others 2009). • SSRI antidepressants (Stein, Ipser, and Seedat 2006)[a] • CBT (particularly trauma-focused CBT) (Roberts and others 2010)	• Non-trauma focused CBT and eye movement desensitization and reprocessing (Bisson and others 2013)[a]

table continues next page

Disorder	First-line treatment	Second-line treatments or adjunct treatment
Notes	• There is no conclusive evidence of greater effectiveness of combined pharmacotherapy and psychotherapy over either of them alone for PTSD (Hetrick and others 2010).[a]	
Schizophrenia	• First-generation antipsychotics, such as haloperidol and fluphenazine, for positive symptoms (Tardy, Huhn, Engel, and Leucht 2014; Tardy, Huhn, Kissling, and Leucht 2014)[a] • Combination of antipsychotics and antidepressants is effective for negative symptoms (Rummel, Kissling, and Leucht 2006).[a] • Second-generation antipsychotics (amisulpride, clozapine, olanzapine, and risperidone). These are superior to first-generation antipsychotics in efficacy and have different side-effect profiles (Leucht and others 2009).[a]	• CBT as adjunctive treatment for positive symptoms (Zimmermann and others 2005)[b] • Cognitive remediation therapies, in early stages of the disorder (Fisher and others 2013)[d] • Psychoeducation reduces relapse, readmission, and length of hospital stay while encouraging medication compliance (Xia, Merinder, and Belgamwar 2011).[a] • Psychosocial interventions for reducing the need for antipsychotic medications (Richter and others 2012)[a] • Clozapine for refractory schizophrenia but needs monitoring for side effects (Essali and others 2009)[a]
Notes	• Continued antipsychotic medication following a clinical response helps prevent relapse (Leucht and others 2012; Sampson and others 2013).[a] • Acetylcholinesterase inhibitors are effective to overcome anticholinergic side effects of antipsychotic drugs (Leucht and others 2012).[a] • Evidence for clear and convincing advantage for CBT over other therapies is limited (Jones and others 2012).[a]	

Note: CBT = cognitive behavioral therapy; PTSD = post-traumatic stress disorder; SSRI = selective serotonin reuptake inhibitor.
[a] Systematic review.
[b] Meta-analysis.
[c] Randomized controlled trials in low- and middle-income countries.
[d] Review.

Persons with severe mental illnesses occasionally require short periods of hospitalization and/or longer-term supported housing because of the severity of their disorders and associated behaviors or abandonment by family. Systematic reviews have suggested that acute day hospitals can be as effective as inpatient care (Marshall and others 2011) and that day hospitals may prevent the need for inpatient care (Shek and others 2009).

Occupational Therapy. Occupational therapy interventions aim to support and improve skills for daily living through life skills training, cognitive rehabilitation, supportive employment and education, and social and interpersonal skills training. Occupational therapy is effective in rehabilitating persons with depression by increasing productivity, reducing work-related stress, and helping in recovery (Hees and others 2013; Schene and others 2007). Supported employment is effective in improving a number of vocational outcomes in persons

with severe mental illnesses (Kinoshita and others 2013). Systematic reviews have shown that life skills and social skills training have moderate to strong effectiveness to promote integration of persons with severe mental illnesses in communities where they live; and interventions with a greater client-centered approach have a larger impact (Gibson and others 2011).

Packages of Care
Promotion and Prevention. Indicated or targeted prevention of mental disorders is effective in the early and subclinical stages. A meta-analysis of 32 studies (largely from Europe and the United States) concluded that preventive interventions could lower the incidence of depression by 21 percent through psychological interventions such as cognitive behavioral therapy (CBT), interpersonal therapy, individual counseling, and group sessions (van Zoonen and others 2014). Psychological treatment of subclinical

depression was shown to have some effect in preventing the onset of major depression after six months (Cuijpers and others 2014).

For people with early psychosis, early intervention services (including CBT and family interventions) appear to have clinically important benefits over standard care, but the longer-term benefits of this approach remain unclear (Bird and others 2010; Marshall and Rathbone 2011). Specifically designated early intervention teams are in place in many HICs, but LMICs have few programs and no formal evaluations.

Case Detection and Diagnosis. The WHO advocates symptom-based algorithms for the detection of mental disorders by nonspecialized health care providers in general medical service settings (WHO 2008, 2010). Cultural influence on the clinical presentation of mental disorders should be accounted for in case detection and screening programs. For example, the inclusion of unexplained somatic symptoms in screening for anxiety and depression might improve case detection in LMICs. Training and screening for detection of mood and anxiety disorders in primary care settings are being implemented globally; however, screening must be accompanied by health system changes to ensure clinical benefits for patients by allowing sustained access to evidence-based treatments (Gilbody, House, and Sheldon 2005; Kauye, Jenkins, and Rahman 2014; Patel and others 2009).

When appropriately trained, health workers can identify probable cases of rare disorders such as schizophrenia, although community case-finding should be confirmed with diagnostic interviews (de Jesus and others 2009).

Collaborative and Stepped Care. Collaborative care is an approach to the care of chronic illnesses that has been successfully implemented for management of mental disorders in primary care. These models emphasize self-care and care management, blended with other pharmacotherapeutic, psychotherapeutic and specialist care interventions, and community supports. Specifically, the model adopts a patient-centric approach and includes active collaboration with mental health professionals, so that patients with severe disorders receive specialist intervention.

Collaborative care for depression and anxiety disorders is associated with significant improvement in clinical outcomes and leads to improvement in adherence, patient satisfaction, and mental health quality of life (Archer and others 2012; Patel and others 2009). Collaborative care can also be effective for severe mental illnesses (Reilly and others 2013), as demonstrated in a randomized controlled trial in India (Chatterjee and others 2014).

Key principles of the collaborative model include proactive case detection; a structured management plan; patient education; systematic monitoring and follow-up; and close collaboration among the patient, a case manager, primary care providers, and specialists. Successful implementation of such a model, however, depends on trained primary care staff, clear protocols and guidelines, and specialist supervision and support in the implementation of the guidelines (Patel and others 2013). Notably, the case manager's role is critical: this person acts as the link between the patient or the patient's family, the primary care physician, and the specialist, and undertakes proactive case detection, monitors progress, and provides psychosocial interventions and adherence support (if medication is prescribed). The case manager could also be an appropriately trained and supervised lay counselor or community health worker. Compelling evidence from LMICs suggests that community health workers, nonspecialized health workers, and paraprofessionals, based in primary care or community settings, can detect cases (Patel and others 2008) and effectively deliver psychosocial interventions for depressive disorder, postpartum depression, and PTSD (den Boer and others 2005; van Ginneken and others 2013).

Community Outreach for Severe Mental Disorders. The WHO's mhGAP intervention guidelines for providing mental health care in nonspecialized settings in LMICs explicitly include revival of social networks and participation in community activities as a part of treatment and care for patients with depression, anxiety, and psychosis (WHO 2010).

Community mental health teams that include outreach workers can effectively manage severe mental illnesses with greater acceptance and fewer hospital admissions and suicides (Malone and others 2007). A systematic review of trials from HICs suggests that intensive case management, based on an assertive community care model that involves providing community-based care for people with severe mental illnesses, focusing on the health and social care needs of the patients by a team of trained health workers, leads to a reduced need for hospitalization, increased retention in care, and improved social functioning (Dieterich and others 2010). Randomized controlled trials in the United Kingdom also show that crisis interventions delivered by a trained team can provide acceptable care to people with severe mental illnesses during the crisis phase, improve short-term mental health outcomes, reduce repeat admissions, and provide greater satisfaction for patients and families (Murphy and others 2012).

Longitudinal studies from India have observed that community-based rehabilitation for people with psychotic disorders have a beneficial impact on disability (Chatterjee and others 2009). Recently published results from a clinical trial in India also suggest that community-based care along with facility-based care is more effective than facility-based care alone for reducing disability and symptoms due to psychoses (Chatterjee and others 2014). Close participation of families, community members, and local health providers, in concert with continuous treatment, form the foundation of community-based care and rehabilitation. Activities to facilitate economic and social rehabilitation (Chatterjee and others 2003)—such as supported housing for people with severe mental illnesses (Chilvers, Macdonald, and Hayes 2006) and vocational rehabilitation (Crowther and others 2001)—are effective in promoting rehabilitation of people with severe mental disorders.

Information and Communication Packages. Information and communications technology (ICT) is emerging as a promising tool for providing care for people with mental disorders. The diverse technologies under this umbrella, along with the considerable presence of mobile phones and Internet access in most LMICs, make outreach and delivery of personalized interventions feasible. These technologies can also be effectively used to deliver interventions for self-care. Telemedicine is effective in reaching out to rural and remote areas (Pyne and others 2010), and can be provided effectively for the management of anxiety, depression, and psychotic disorders (Thara, John, and Rao 2008). Telephones and other Internet-based applications can be used to deliver health messages and prompts and peer support interventions, as well as evidence-based psychotherapies such as cognitive behavior therapy (Andersson and Cuijpers 2009).

COST-EFFECTIVENESS OF INTERVENTIONS

The preceding review reveals a diverse array of intervention approaches and models that can be utilized at different levels of the health (and welfare) system for the prevention and management of adult mental disorders, and includes an increasing body of evidence from and for settings in LMICs. However, the availability of cost-effectiveness information to complement this large and growing evidence base on effectiveness remains comparatively sparse. There is currently no cost-effectiveness evidence from LMICs relating to mental health awareness campaigns, family interventions, or use of ICT for early detection or treatment.

However, a few clinical trials have been conducted in LMICs that included an economic evaluation. These demonstrated not only the feasibility, but also the informational value of such analyses (Araya and others 2006; Buttorff and others 2012; Patel and Kleinman 2003). Explaining that a depression-free day could be gained for the price of a bus ticket, for example, was a helpful argument in the roll-out of depression care in Chile (Araya and others 2006). In India, the MANAS (MANashanti Sudhar Shodh, or project to promote mental health) trial showed that a task-shifting intervention for common mental disorders was not only cost-effective, but also cost-saving when time costs were taken into consideration (Buttorff and others 2012).

Partly because of the lack of available primary data, several cost-effectiveness modeling studies have been conducted, at the national and international levels. These studies, which rely on secondary data to generate estimates of expected cost and health gain, are reviewed in chapter 12 in this volume (Levin and Chisholm 2015). Overall, the studies indicate that, depending on the particular context and content of the interventions, cost-effectiveness ranges between US\$100 and US\$2,000 per healthy life year gained. Chapter 13 in this volume (Chisholm and others 2015) applies an extended cost-effectiveness analysis approach to several adult mental disorders (psychosis, bipolar disorder, and depression) to assess the distribution of costs and health gains across different income groups in the population, as well as the financial protection effects of scaled-up care and treatment. The analysis indicates that universal public finance can lead to a far more equitable allocation of public health resources, with lower-income groups benefitting most from enhanced financial protection (Chisholm and others 2015).

CONCLUSIONS AND RECOMMENDATIONS

Mood disorders, anxiety disorders, and psychotic disorders are a diverse group of adult mental disorders that are highly disabling and are caused by a complex interaction of genetic, developmental, and environmental risk factors. These disorders are highly stigmatized in most countries and cultures and often lead to shame and fear of rejection and discrimination.

The good news is that awareness campaigns, particularly those involving engagement with people with mental disorders, can improve general knowledge about these disorders. Appropriate legislation also can address the discrimination and human rights abuses that result from social stigma. On the whole, however, these interventions remain inadequately disseminated and implemented.

Since the mid-20th century, many medications have been discovered and psychotherapies have been validated for the treatment of mental disorders. In the context of the disorders addressed in this chapter, notable examples of pharmacotherapies are antidepressants, antipsychotics, and mood stabilizers. Notable examples of psychotherapies are brief treatments based on cognitive, behavioral, and interpersonal approaches. Collaborative care models with appropriately trained and supervised nonspecialist frontline workers can effectively deliver evidence-based packages, often constituting a combination of drug or psychological treatments as needed, with the active participation of the patient and family. These pharmacotherapies and psychotherapies have been validated across a wide range of cultures, ethnicities, and stages of economic development. There is clear evidence that these can be delivered successfully in resource-poor settings.

Families are traditionally closely involved in the care of persons with mental disorders in LMICs and should be considered important partners in treatment and rehabilitation. Occupational therapy and community-based rehabilitation are extremely important for providing those suffering from mental disorders with opportunities to live engaged, productive lives.

Even so, the treatment gap for mental disorders remains significant around the world. It is particularly large in LMICs, whose weaker health systems and fewer resources—financial and human—for mental health services limit the options for care. Although there are several potential innovations to reduce the costs and improve access to care, for example through task-sharing and use of ICT (Patel and Saxena 2014), the most urgent need of all is increased financial investment and political will to integrate mental health at all levels of the health care system in LMICs.

NOTES

World Bank Income Classifications as of July 2014 are as follows, based on estimates of gross national income (GNI) per capita for 2013:

- Low-income countries (LICs) = US$1,045 or less
- Middle-income countries (MICs) are subdivided:
  a) lower-middle-income = US$1,046 to US$4,125
  b) upper-middle-income (UMICs) = US$4,126 to US$12,745
- High-income countries (HICs) = US$12,746 or more.

1. The 17 countries participating in the WMH surveys are Belgium, China, Colombia, France, Germany, Israel, Italy, Japan, Lebanon, Mexico, the Netherlands, New Zealand, Nigeria, South Africa, Spain, Ukraine, and the United States.

REFERENCES

Abbass, A. A., S. R. Kisely, J. M. Town, F. Leichsenring, E. Driessen, and others. 2014. "Short-Term Psychodynamic Psychotherapies for Common Mental Disorders." *Cochrane Database of Systematic Reviews* 7: CD004687. doi:10.1002/14651858.CD004687.pub4.

Andersson, G., and P. Cuijpers. 2009. "Internet-Based and Other Computerized Psychological Treatments for Adult Depression: A Meta-Analysis." *Cognitive Behavioral Therapy* 38 (4): 196–205. doi:10.1080/16506070903318960.

Angst, J., and R. Sellaro. 2000. "Historical Perspectives and Natural History of Bipolar Disorder." *Biological Psychiatry* 48 (6): 445–57.

APA (American Psychiatric Association). 2013. *Diagnostic and Statistical Manual of Mental Disorders* (fifth edition). Washington, DC: APA.

Araya, R., T. Flynn, G. Rojas, R. Fritsch, and G. Simon. 2006. "Cost-Effectiveness of a Primary Care Treatment Program for Depression in Low-Income Women in Santiago, Chile." *American Journal of Psychiatry* 163 (8): 1379–87. doi:10.1176/appi.ajp.163.8.1379.

Archer, J., P. Bower, S. Gilbody, K. Lovell, D. Richards, and others. 2012. "Collaborative Care for Depression and Anxiety Problems." *Cochrane Database of Systematic Reviews* 10 (100909747): CD006525.

Arroll, B., C. R. Elley, T. Fishman, F. A. Goodyear-Smith, T. Kenealy, and others. 2009. "Antidepressants versus Placebo for Depression in Primary Care." *Cochrane Database of Systematic Reviews* (3): CD007954.

Bass, J., R. Neugebauer, K. F. Clougherty, H. Verdeli, P. Wickramaratne, and others. 2006. "Group Interpersonal Psychotherapy for Depression in Rural Uganda: 6-Month Outcomes: Randomised Controlled Trial." *The British Journal of Psychiatry* 188: 567–73. doi:10.1192/bjp.188.6.567.

Beck, A. T., and E. A. Haigh. 2014. "Advances in Cognitive Theory and Therapy: The Generic Cognitive Model." *Annual Review of Clinical Psychology* 10: 1–24. doi:10.1146/annurev-clinpsy-032813-153734.

Bird, V., P. Premkumar, T. Kendall, C. Whittington, J. Mitchell, and others. 2010. "Early Intervention Services, Cognitive–Behavioural Therapy and Family Intervention in Early Psychosis: Systematic Review." *The British Journal of Psychiatry* 197 (5): 350–56.

Bisson, J. I., N. P. Roberts, M. Andrew, R. Cooper, and C. Lewis. 2013. "Psychological Therapies for Chronic Post-Traumatic Stress Disorder (PTSD) in Adults." *Cochrane Database of Systematic Reviews* 12 (100909747): CD003388.

Bloom, D. E., E. T. Cafiero, E. Jané-Llopis, S. Abrahams-Gessel, L. R. Bloom, and others. 2011. *The Global Economic Burden of Noncommunicable Diseases*. Geneva: World Economic Forum.

Bonhauser, M., G. Fernandez, K. Puschel, F. Yanez, J. Montero, and others. 2005. "Improving Physical Fitness and Emotional Well-Being in Adolescents of Low Socioeconomic Status in Chile: Results of a School-Based Controlled Trial."

Health Promotion International 20 (2): 113–22. doi:10.1093/heapro/dah603.

Buttorff, C., R. S. Hock, H. A. Weiss, S. Naik, R. Araya, and others. 2012. "Economic Evaluation of a Task-Shifting Intervention for Common Mental Disorders in India." *Bulletin of the World Health Organization* 90 (11): 813–21.

Charlson, F. J., A. J. Baxter, T. Dua, L. Degenhardt, H. A. Whiteford, and T. Vos. 2015. "Excess Mortality from Mental, Neurological, and Substance Use Disorders in the Global Burden of Disease Study 2010." In *Disease Control Priorities* (third edition): Volume 4, *Mental, Neurological, and Substance Use Disorders*, edited by V. Patel, D. Chisholm, T. Dua, R. Laxminarayan, and M. E. Medina-Mora. Washington, DC: World Bank.

Chatterjee, S., S. Naik, S. John, H. Dabholkar, M. Balaji, and others. 2014. "Effectiveness of a Community-Based Intervention for People with Schizophrenia and Their Caregivers in India (COPSI): A Randomised Controlled Trial." *The Lancet* 383 (9926): 1385–94. doi:10.1016/s0140-6736(13)62629-x.

Chatterjee, S., V. Patel, A. Chatterjee, and H. A. Weiss. 2003. "Evaluation of a Community-Based Rehabilitation Model for Chronic Schizophrenia in Rural India." *The British Journal of Psychiatry* 182: 57–62.

Chatterjee, S., A. Pillai, S. Jain, A. Cohen, and V. Patel. 2009. "Outcomes of People with Psychotic Disorders in a Community-Based Rehabilitation Programme in Rural India." *The British Journal of Psychiatry* 195 (5): 433–39. doi:10.1192/bjp.bp.108.057596.

Chilvers, R., G. M. Macdonald, and A. A. Hayes. 2006. "Supported Housing for People with Severe Mental Disorders." *Cochrane Database of Systematic Reviews* (4): Cd000453. doi:10.1002/14651858.CD000453.pub2.

Chisholm, D., K. A. Johansson, N. Raykar, I. Megiddo, A. Nigam, K. Bjerkreim Strand, A. Colson, A. Fekadu, and S. Verguet. 2015. "Moving toward Universal Health Coverage for Mental, Neurological, and Substance Use Disorders: An Extended Cost-Effectiveness Analysis." In *Disease Control Priorities* (third edition): Volume 4, *Mental, Neurological, and Substance Use Disorders*, edited by V. Patel, D. Chisholm, T. Dua, R. Laxminarayan, and M. E. Medina-Mora. Washington, DC: World Bank.

Clement, S., F. Lassman, E. Barley, S. Evans-Lacko, P. Williams, and others. 2013. "Mass Media Interventions for Reducing Mental Health-Related Stigma." *Cochrane Database of Systematic Reviews* 7: Cd009453. doi:10.1002/14651858.CD009453.pub2.

Cooney, G. M., K. Dwan, C. A. Greig, D. A. Lawlor, J. Rimer, and others. 2013. "Exercise for Depression." *Cochrane Database of Systematic Reviews* 9: Cd004366. doi:10.1002/14651858.CD004366.pub6.

Coryell, W., D. Solomon, C. Turvey, M. Keller, A. C. Leon, and others. 2003. "The Long-Term Course of Rapid-Cycling Bipolar Disorder." *Archives of General Psychiatry* 60 (9): 914–20. doi:10.1001/archpsyc.60.9.914.

Crowther, R., M. Marshall, G. Bond, and P. Huxley. 2001. "Vocational Rehabilitation for People with Severe Mental Illness." *Cochrane Database of Systematic Reviews* (2): Cd003080. doi:10.1002/14651858.cd003080.

Cuijpers, P., S. L. Koole, A. van Dijke, M. Roca, J. Li, and others. 2014. "Psychotherapy for Subclinical Depression: Meta-Analysis." *The British Journal of Psychiatry* 205 (4): 268–74. doi:10.1192/bjp.bp.113.138784.

Cuijpers, P., A. van Straten, G. Andersson, and P. van Oppen. 2008. "Psychotherapy for Depression in Adults: A Meta-Analysis of Comparative Outcome Studies." *Journal of Consulting and Clinical Psychology* 76 (6): 909–22. doi:10.1037/a0013075.supp (Supplemental).

Cuijpers, P., A. van Straten, A. van Schaik, and G. Andersson. 2009. "Psychological Treatment of Depression in Primary Care: A Meta-Analysis." *The British Journal of General Practice: The Journal of the Royal College of General Practitioners* 59 (559): e51–60.

Cuijpers, P., A. van Straten, and L. Warmerdam. 2007. "Problem Solving Therapies for Depression: A Meta-Analysis." *European Psychiatry: The Journal of the Association of European Psychiatrists* 22 (1): 9–15.

Das Gupta, R., and J. F. Guest. 2002. "Annual Cost of Bipolar Disorder to UK Society." *The British Journal of Psychiatry* 180: 227–33.

de Graaf, R., R. V. Bijl, J. Spijker, A. T. Beekman, and W. A. Vollebergh. 2003. "Temporal Sequencing of Lifetime Mood Disorders in Relation to Comorbid Anxiety and Substance Use Disorders—Findings from the Netherlands Mental Health Survey and Incidence Study." *Social Psychiatry and Psychiatric Epidemiology* 38 (1): 1–11. doi:10.1007/s00127-003-0597-4.

de Jesus, M. J., D. Razzouk, R. Thara, J. Eaton, and G. Thornicroft. 2009. "Packages of Care for Schizophrenia in Low- and Middle-Income Countries." *PLoS Medicine* 6 (10): e1000165. doi:10.1371/journal.pmed.1000165.

de Mello, M. F., J. de Jesus Mari, J. Bacaltchuk, H. Verdeli, and R. Neugebauer. 2005. "A Systematic Review of Research Findings on the Efficacy of Interpersonal Therapy for Depressive Disorders." *European Archives of Psychiatry and Clinical Neuroscience* 255 (2): 75–82. doi:10.1007/s00406-004-0542-x.

Demyttenaere, K., R. Bruffaerts, J. Posada-Villa, I. Gasquet, V. Kovess, and others. 2004. "Prevalence, Severity, and Unmet Need for Treatment of Mental Disorders in the World Health Organization World Mental Health Surveys." *Journal of the American Medical Association* 291 (21): 2581–90.

den Boer, P. C., D. Wiersma, S. Russo, and R. J. van den Bosch. 2005. "Paraprofessionals for Anxiety and Depressive Disorders." *Cochrane Database of Systematic Reviews* (2): Cd004688. doi:10.1002/14651858.CD004688.pub2.

Dennis, C. L., and E. Hodnett. 2007. "Psychosocial and Psychological Interventions for Treating Postpartum Depression." *Cochrane Database of Systematic Reviews* (4): Cd006116. doi:10.1002/14651858.CD006116.pub2.

Dieterich, M., C. B. Irving, B. Park, and M. Marshall. 2010. "Intensive Case Management for Severe Mental Illness." *Cochrane Database of Systematic Reviews* (10): Cd007906. doi:10.1002/14651858.CD007906.pub2.

Digangi, J., G. Guffanti, K. A. McLaughlin, and K. C. Koenen. 2013. "Considering Trauma Exposure in the Context of Genetics Studies of Posttraumatic Stress Disorder: A Systematic Review." *Biology of Mood & Anxiety Disorders* 3 (1): 2. doi:10.1186/2045-5380-3-2.

Eaton, J., and A. O. Agomoh. 2008. "Developing Mental Health Services in Nigeria: The Impact of a Community-Based Mental Health Awareness Programme." *Social Psychiatry and Psychiatric Epidemiology* 43 (7): 552–58. doi:10.1007 /s00127-008-0321-5.

Essali, A., N. Al-Haj Haasan, C. Li, and J. Rathbone. 2009. "Clozapine versus Typical Neuroleptic Medication for Schizophrenia." *Cochrane Database of Systematic Reviews* (1): CD000059. doi:10.1002/14651858.CD000059 .pub2.

Evans-Lacko, S., J. London, S. Japhet, N. Rusch, C. Flach, and others. 2012. "Mass Social Contact Interventions and Their Effect on Mental Health Related Stigma and Intended Discrimination." *BMC Public Health* 12: 489. doi:10.1186/1471-2458-12-489.

Evans-Lacko, S., J. London, K. Little, C. Henderson, and G. Thornicroft. 2010. "Evaluation of a Brief Anti-Stigma Campaign in Cambridge: Do Short-Term Campaigns Work?" *BMC Public Health* 10: 339. doi:10.1186/1471-2458-10-339.

Ferrari, A. J., A. J. Baxter, and H. A. Whiteford. 2011. "A Systematic Review of the Global Distribution and Availability of Prevalence Data for Bipolar Disorder." *Journal of Affective Disorders* 134 (1–3): 1–13. doi:10.1016 /j.jad.2010.11.007.

Fisher M., R. Loewy, K. Hardy, D. Schlosser, and S. Vinogradov. 2013. "Cognitive Interventions Targeting Brain Plasticity in the Prodromal and Early Phases of Schizophrenia." *Annual Review of Clinical Psychology* 9: 435–63.

Furlan, A. D., W. H. Gnam, N. Carnide, E. Irvin, B. C. Amick, 3rd, and others. 2012. "Systematic Review of Intervention Practices for Depression in the Workplace." *Journal of Occupational Rehabilitation* 22 (3): 312–21. doi:10.1007 /s10926-011-9340-2.

Furukawa, T. A., N. Watanabe, and R. Churchill. 2007. "Combined Psychotherapy Plus Antidepressants for Panic Disorder with or without Agoraphobia." *Cochrane Database of Systematic Reviews* (1): Cd004364. doi:10.1002/14651858 .CD004364.pub2.

Fusar-Poli, P., S. Borgwardt, A. Bechdolf, J. Addington, A. Riecher-Rossler, and others. 2013. "The Psychosis High-Risk State: A Comprehensive State-of-the-Art Review." *JAMA Psychiatry* 70 (1): 107–20. doi:10.1001 /jamapsychiatry.2013.269.

Gaynes, B. N., S. W. Lloyd, L. Lux, G. Gartlehner, R. A. Hansen, and others. 2014. "Repetitive Transcranial Magnetic Stimulation for Treatment-Resistant Depression: A Systematic Review and Meta-Analysis." *Journal of Clinical Psychiatry* 75 (5): 477–89; quiz 489. doi:10.4088/JCP.13r08815.

Geller, B., and J. Luby. 1997. "Child and Adolescent Bipolar Disorder: A Review of the Past 10 Years." *Journal of the American Academy of Child and Adolescent Psychiatry* 36 (9): 1168–76. doi:10.1097/00004583-199709000-00008.

Gibson, R. W., M. D'Amico, L. Jaffe, and M. Arbesman. 2011. "Occupational Therapy Interventions for Recovery in the Areas of Community Integration and Normative Life Roles for Adults with Serious Mental Illness: A Systematic Review." *American Journal of Occupational Therapy* 65 (3): 247–56.

Gilbody, S., A. O. House, and T. A. Sheldon. 2005. "Screening and Case Finding Instruments for Depression." *Cochrane Database of Systematic Reviews* (4): Cd002792. doi:10.1002/14651858.CD002792.pub2.

Gorczynski, P., and G. Faulkner. 2010. "Exercise Therapy for Schizophrenia." *Cochrane Database of Systematic Reviews* (5): Cd004412. doi:10.1002/14651858.CD004412.pub2.

Grilli, R., C. Ramsay, and S. Minozzi. 2002. "Mass Media Interventions: Effects on Health Services Utilisation." *Cochrane Database of Systematic Reviews* (1): Cd000389. doi:10.1002/14651858.cd000389.

Gureje, O. 2011. "Dysthymia in a Cross-Cultural Perspective." *Current Opinion in Psychiatry* 24 (1): 67–71. doi:10.1097 /YCO.0b013e32834136a5.

Hees, H. L., G. de Vries, M. W. Koeter, and A. H. Schene. 2013. "Adjuvant Occupational Therapy Improves Long-Term Depression Recovery and Return-to-Work in Good Health in Sick-Listed Employees with Major Depression: Results of a Randomised Controlled Trial." *Occupational and Environmental Medicine* 70 (4): 252–60. doi:10.1136 /oemed-2012-100789.

Heim, C., M. Shugart, W. E. Craighead, and C. B. Nemeroff. 2010. "Neurobiological and Psychiatric Consequences of Child Abuse and Neglect." *Developmental Psychobiology* 52 (7): 671–90. doi:10.1002/dev.20494.

Hetrick, S. E., R. Purcell, B. Garner, and R. Parslow. 2010. "Combined Pharmacotherapy and Psychological Therapies for Post Traumatic Stress Disorder (PTSD)." *Cochrane Database of Systematic Reviews* (7): CD007316. doi:10.1002/14651858.CD007316.pub2.

Huibers, M. J., A. J. Beurskens, G. Bleijenberg, and C. P. van Schayck. 2007. "Psychosocial Interventions by General Practitioners." *Cochrane Database of Systematic Reviews* (3): Cd003494. doi:10.1002/14651858.CD003494.pub2.

Hunot, V., R. Churchill, M. Silva de Lima, and V. Teixeira. 2007. "Psychological Therapies for Generalised Anxiety Disorder." *Cochrane Database of Systematic Reviews* (1): CD001848. doi:10.1002/14651858.CD001848.pub4.

Hyman, S. E. 2014. "The Unconscionable Gap between What We Know and What We Do." *Science Translational Medicine* 6 (253): 253cm9. doi:10.1126/scitranslmed.3010312.

Isometsa, E. 2014. "Suicidal Behaviour in Mood Disorders—Who, When, and Why?" *Canadian Journal of Psychiatry* 59 (3): 120–30.

Jones, C., D. Hacker, I. Cormac, A. Meaden, and C. B. Irving. 2012. "Cognitive Behaviour Therapy versus Other Psychosocial Treatments for Schizophrenia." *Cochrane Database of Systematic Reviews* 4: CD008712. doi:10.1002/14651858.CD008712.pub2.

Jorge, R. E., R. G. Robinson, D. Moser, A. Tateno, B. Crespo-Facorro, and others. 2004. "Major Depression Following Traumatic Brain Injury." *Archives of General Psychiatry* 61 (1): 42–50. doi:10.1001/archpsyc.61.1.42.

Jorm, A. F., A. J. Morgan, and S. E. Hetrick. 2008. "Relaxation for Depression." *Cochrane Database of Systematic Reviews* (4): Cd007142. doi:10.1002/14651858.CD007142.pub2.

Justo, L. P., B. G. Soares, and H. M. Calil. 2007. "Family Interventions for Bipolar Disorder." *Cochrane Database of Systematic Reviews* 4: CD005167.

Kapczinski, F., M. S. Lima, J. S. Souza, and R. Schmitt. 2003. "Antidepressants for Generalized Anxiety Disorder." *Cochrane Database of Systematic Reviews* (2): Cd003592. doi:10.1002/14651858.cd003592.

Kauye, F., R. Jenkins, and A. Rahman. 2014. "Training Primary Health Care Workers in Mental Health and Its Impact on Diagnoses of Common Mental Disorders in Primary Care of a Developing Country, Malawi: A Cluster-Randomized Controlled Trial." *Psychological Medicine* 44 (3): 657–66. doi:10.1017/s0033291713001141.

Kaymaz, N., J. van Os, A. J. Loonen, and W. A. Nolen. 2008. "Evidence that Patients with Single versus Recurrent Depressive Episodes Are Differentially Sensitive to Treatment Discontinuation: A Meta-Analysis of Placebo-Controlled Randomized Trials." *Journal of Clinical Psychiatry* 69 (9): 1423–36.

Kessler, R. C., S. Aguilar-Gaxiola, J. Alonso, M. C. Angermeyer, J. C. Anthony, and others. 2008. "Prevalence and Severity of Mental Disorders in the World Mental Health Survey Initiative." In *The WHO World Mental Health Survey: Global Perspectives on the Epidemiology of Mental Disorders*, edited by R. C. Kessler and T. B. Ustun, 534–40. Cambridge, U.K.: Cambridge University Press.

Kessler, R. C., P. Berglund, O. Demler, R. Jin, K. R. Merikangas, and others. 2005. "Lifetime Prevalence and Age-of-Onset Distributions of DSM-IV Disorders in the National Comorbidity Survey Replication." *Archives of General Psychiatry* 62 (6): 593–602. doi:10.1001/archpsyc.62.6.593.

Kessler, R. C., W. T. Chiu, O. Demler, K. R. Merikangas, and E. E. Walters. 2005. "Prevalence, Severity, and Comorbidity of 12-Month DSM-IV Disorders in the National Comorbidity Survey Replication." *Archives of General Psychiatry* 62 (6): 617–27. doi:10.1001/archpsyc.62.6.617.

Kinoshita, Y., T. A. Furukawa, K. Kinoshita, M. Honyashiki, I. M. Omori, and others. 2013. "Supported Employment for Adults with Severe Mental Illness." *Cochrane Database of Systematic Reviews* 9: Cd008297. doi:10.1002/14651858.CD008297.pub2.

Lee, S. H., S. Ripke, B. M. Neale, S. V. Faraone, S. M. Purcell, and others. 2013. "Genetic Relationship between Five Psychiatric Disorders Estimated from Genome-Wide SNPs." *Nature Genetics* 45 (9): 984–94. doi:10.1038/ng.2711.

Leibenluft, E., P. S. Albert, N. E. Rosenthal, and T. A. Wehr. 1996. "Relationship between Sleep and Mood in Patients with Rapid-Cycling Bipolar Disorder." *Psychiatry Research* 63 (2–3): 161–68.

Lesh, T. A., T. A. Niendam, M. J. Minzenberg, and C. S. Carter. 2011. "Cognitive Control Deficits in Schizophrenia: Mechanisms and Meaning." *Neuropsychopharmacology* 36 (1): 316–38. doi:10.1038/npp.2010.156.

Leucht, S., C. Corves, D. Arbter, R. R. Engel, C. Li, and others. 2009. "Second-Generation versus First-Generation Antipsychotic Drugs for Schizophrenia: A Meta-Analysis." *The Lancet* 373 (9657): 31–41. doi:10.1016/s0140-6736(08)61764-x.

Leucht, S., M. Tardy, K. Komossa, S. Heres, W. Kissling, and others. 2012. "Maintenance Treatment with Antipsychotic Drugs for Schizophrenia." *Cochrane Database of Systematic Reviews* 5: Cd008016. doi:10.1002/14651858.CD008016.pub2.

Levin, C., and D. Chisholm. 2015. "Cost and Cost-Effectiveness of Interventions, Policies, and Platforms for the Prevention and Treatment of Mental, Neurological, and Substance Use Disorders." In *Disease Control Priorities* (third edition): Volume 4, *Mental, Neurological, and Substance Use Disorders*, edited by V. Patel, D. Chisholm, T. Dua, R. Laxminarayan, and M. E. Medina-Mora. Washington, DC: World Bank.

Lewinsohn, P. M., P. Rohde, J. R. Seeley, D. N. Klein, and I. H. Gotlib. 2000. "Natural Course of Adolescent Major Depressive Disorder in a Community Sample: Predictors of Recurrence in Young Adults." *American Journal of Psychiatry* 157 (10): 1584–91.

Malone, D., G. Newron-Howes, S. Simmonds, S. Marriot, and P. Tyrer. 2007. "Community Mental Health Teams (CMHTs) for People with Severe Mental Illnesses and Disordered Personality." *Cochrane Database of Systematic Reviews* (3): Cd000270. doi:10.1002/14651858.CD000270.pub2.

Maratos, A. S., C. Gold, X. Wang, and M. J. Crawford. 2008. "Music Therapy for Depression." *Cochrane Database of Systematic Reviews* (1): Cd004517. doi:10.1002/14651858.CD004517.pub2.

Marshall, M., R. Crowther, W. H. Sledge, J. Rathbone, and K. Soares-Weiser. 2011. "Day Hospital versus Admission for Acute Psychiatric Disorders." *Cochrane Database of Systematic Reviews* (12): Cd004026. doi:10.1002/14651858.CD004026.pub2.

Marshall, M., and J. Rathbone. 2011. "Early Intervention for Psychosis." *Schizophrenia Bulletin* 37 (6): 1111–14.

Martin, A., K. Sanderson, and F. Cocker. 2009. "Meta-Analysis of the Effects of Health Promotion Intervention in the Workplace on Depression and Anxiety Symptoms." *Scandinavian Journal of Work, Environment and Health* 35 (1): 7–18.

Martinez-Amoros, E., N. Cardoner, V. Galvez, and M. Urretavizcaya. 2012. "Effectiveness and Pattern of Use of Continuation and Maintenance Electroconvulsive Therapy." *Revista Psiquiatría y Salud Mental* 5 (4): 241–53. doi:10.1016/j.rpsm.2012.06.004.

Mayo-Wilson, E., and P. Montgomery. 2013. "Media-Delivered Cognitive Behavioural Therapy and Behavioural Therapy (Self-Help) for Anxiety Disorders in Adults." *Cochrane Database of Systematic Reviews* 9: Cd005330. doi:10.1002/14651858.CD005330.pub4.

McGrath, J., S. Saha, J. Welham, O. El Saadi, C. MacCauley, and others. 2004. "A Systematic Review of the Incidence of Schizophrenia: The Distribution of Rates and the Influence of Sex, Urbanicity, Migrant Status and Methodology." *BMC Medicine* 2: 13. doi:10.1186/1741-7015-2-13.

McGrath, J., and J. Scott. 2006. "Urban Birth and Risk of Schizophrenia: A Worrying Example of Epidemiology Where the Data Are Stronger Than the Hypotheses." *Epidemiologia e psichiatria sociale* 15 (4): 243–46.

Molyneaux, E., L. M. Howard, H. R. McGeown, A. M. Karia, and K. Trevillion. 2014. "Antidepressant Treatment for Postnatal Depression." *Cochrane Database of Systematic Reviews* (9): CD002018. doi:10.1002/14651858.CD002018 .pub2.

Moradveisi, L., M. J. Huibers, F. Renner, M. Arasteh, and A. Arntz. 2013. "Behavioural Activation v. Antidepressant Medication for Treating Depression in Iran: Randomised Trial." *The British Journal of Psychiatry* 202 (3): 204–11. doi:10.1192/bjp.bp.112.113696.

Morriss, R. K., M. A. Faizal, A. P. Jones, P. R. Williamson, C. Bolton, and others. 2007. "Interventions for Helping People Recognise Early Signs of Recurrence in Bipolar Disorder." *Cochrane Database of Systematic Reviews* (1): Cd004854. doi:10.1002/14651858.CD004854.pub2.

Mottram, P., K. Wilson, and J. Strobl. 2006. "Antidepressants for Depressed Elderly." *Cochrane Database of Systematic Reviews* (1): CD003491. doi:10.1002/14651858.CD003491 .pub2.

Moussavi, S., S. Chatterji, E. Verdes, A. Tandon, V. Patel, and others. 2007. "Depression, Chronic Diseases, and Decrements in Health: Results from the World Health Surveys." *The Lancet* 370 (9590): 851–58. doi:http://dx.doi .org/10.1016/S0140-6736(07)61415-9.

Murphy, S., C. B. Irving, C. E. Adams, and R. Driver. 2012. "Crisis Intervention for People with Severe Mental Illnesses." *Cochrane Database of Systematic Reviews* 5: Cd001087. doi:10.1002/14651858.CD001087.pub4.

Okpokoro, U., C. E. Adams, and S. Sampson. 2014. "Family Intervention (Brief) for Schizophrenia." *Cochrane Database of Systematic Reviews* 3: Cd009802. doi:10.1002/14651858 .CD009802.pub2.

Olfson, M., R. C. Kessler, P. A. Berglund, and E. Lin. 1998. "Psychiatric Disorder Onset and First Treatment Contact in the United States and Ontario." *American Journal of Psychiatry* 155 (10): 1415–22.

Orgeta, V., A. Qazi, A. E. Spector, and M. Orrell. 2014. "Psychological Treatments for Depression and Anxiety in Dementia and Mild Cognitive Impairment." *Cochrane Database of Systematic Reviews* 1: Cd009125. doi:10.1002/14651858.CD009125.pub2.

Patel, V., R. Araya, N. Chowdhary, M. King, B. Kirkwood, and others. 2008. "Detecting Common Mental Disorders in Primary Care in India: A Comparison of Five Screening Questionnaires." *Psychological Medicine* 38 (2): 221–28. doi:10.1017/s0033291707002334.

Patel, V., G. S. Belkin, A. Chockalingam, J. Cooper, S. Saxena, and others. 2013. "Grand Challenges: Integrating Mental Health Services into Priority Health Care Platforms." *PLoS Medicine* 10 (5): e1001448. doi:10.1371/journal .pmed.1001448.

Patel, V., B. R. Kirkwood, S. Pednekar, B. Pereira, P. Barros, and others. 2006. "Gender Disadvantage and Reproductive Health Risk Factors for Common Mental Disorders in Women: A Community Survey in India." *Archives of General Psychiatry* 63 (4): 404–13. doi:10.1001/archpsyc.63.4.404.

Patel, V., and A. Kleinman. 2003. "Poverty and Common Mental Disorders in Developing Countries." *Bulletin of the World Health Organization* 81 (8): 609–15.

Patel, V., and S. Saxena. 2014. "Transforming Lives, Enhancing Communities—Innovations in Global Mental Health." *New England Journal of Medicine* 370 (6): 498–501. doi:10.1056 /NEJMp1315214.

Patel, V., G. Simon, N. Chowdhary, S. Kaaya, and R. Araya. 2009. "Packages of Care for Depression in Low- and Middle-Income Countries." *PLoS Medicine* 6 (10): e1000159. doi:10.1371/journal.pmed.1000159.

Pauls, D. L., A. Abramovitch, S. L. Rauch, and D. A. Geller. 2014. "Obsessive-Compulsive Disorder: An Integrative Genetic and Neurobiological Perspective." *Nature Reviews Neuroscience* 15 (6): 410–24. doi:10.1038/nrn3746.

Penalba, V., H. McGuire, and J. R. Leite. 2008. "Psychosocial Interventions for Prevention of Psychological Disorders in Law Enforcement Officers." *Cochrane Database of Systematic Reviews* (3): Cd005601. doi:10.1002/14651858 .CD005601.pub2.

Perugi, G., and H. S. Akiskal. 2002. "The Soft Bipolar Spectrum Redefined: Focus on the Cyclothymic, Anxious-Sensitive, Impulse-Dyscontrol, and Binge-Eating Connection in Bipolar II and Related Conditions." *Psychiatric Clinics of North America* 25 (4): 713–37.

Pharoah, F., J. Mari, J. Rathbone, and W. Wong. 2010. "Family Intervention for Schizophrenia." *Cochrane Database of Systematic Reviews* (12): Cd000088. doi:10.1002/14651858 .CD000088.pub2.

Pyne, J. M., J. C. Fortney, S. P. Tripathi, M. L. Maciejewski, M. J. Edlund, and others. 2010. "Cost-Effectiveness Analysis of a Rural Telemedicine Collaborative Care Intervention for Depression." *Archives of General Psychiatry* 67 (8): 812–21. doi:10.1001/archgenpsychiatry.2010.82.

Rahman, A., M. H. Mubbashar, R. Gater, and D. Goldberg. 1998. "Randomised Trial of Impact of School Mental-Health Programme in Rural Rawalpindi, Pakistan." *The Lancet* 352 (9133): 1022–25.

Rayner, L., A. Price, A. Evans, K. Valsraj, I. J. Higginson, and others. 2010. "Antidepressants for Depression in Physically Ill People." *Cochrane Database of Systematic Reviews* (3): CD007503. doi:10.1002/14651858.CD007503.pub2.

Reilly, S., C. Planner, L. Gask, M. Hann, S. Knowles, and others. 2013. "Collaborative Care Approaches for People with Severe Mental Illness." *Cochrane Database of Systematic Reviews* (11): CD009531. doi:10.1002/14651858.CD009531 .pub2.

Richter, T., G. Meyer, R. Mohler, and S. Kopke. 2012. "Psychosocial Interventions for Reducing Antipsychotic Medication in Care Home Residents." *Cochrane Database of Systematic Reviews* 12: Cd008634. doi:10.1002/14651858 .CD008634.pub2.

Ripke, S., B. M. Neale, A. Corvin, J. T. Walters, K. H. Farh, and others. 2014. "Biological Insights from 108 Schizophrenia-Associated Genetic Loci." *Nature* 511 (7510): 421–72. doi:10.1038/nature13595.

Roberts, N. P., N. J. Kitchiner, J. Kenardy, and J. Bisson. 2009. "Multiple Session Early Psychological Interventions for the Prevention of Post-Traumatic Stress Disorder." *Cochrane Database of Systematic Reviews* (3): Cd006869. doi:10.1002/14651858.CD006869.pub2.

———. 2010. "Early Psychological Interventions to Treat Acute Traumatic Stress Symptoms." *Cochrane Database of Systematic Reviews* (3): Cd007944. doi:10.1002/14651858.CD007944.pub2.

Rummel, C., W. Kissling, and S. Leucht. 2006. "Antidepressants for the Negative Symptoms of Schizophrenia." *Cochrane Database of Systematic Reviews* (3): Cd005581. doi:10.1002/14651858.CD005581.pub2.

Saha, S., D. Chant, J. Welham, and J. McGrath. 2005. "A Systematic Review of the Prevalence of Schizophrenia." *PLoS Medicine* 2 (5): e141. doi:10.1371/journal.pmed.0020141.

Sampson, S., M. Mansour, N. Maayan, K. Soares-Weiser, and C. E. Adams. 2013. "Intermittent Drug Techniques for Schizophrenia." *Cochrane Database of Systematic Reviews* 7: Cd006196. doi:10.1002/14651858.CD006196.pub2.

Schene, A. H., M. W. Koeter, M. J. Kikkert, J. A. Swinkels, and P. McCrone. 2007. "Adjuvant Occupational Therapy for Work-Related Major Depression Works: Randomized Trial Including Economic Evaluation." *Psychological Medicine* 37 (3): 351–62. doi:10.1017/s0033291706009366.

Scherk, H., F. G. Pajonk, and S. Leucht. 2007. "Second-Generation Antipsychotic Agents in the Treatment of Acute Mania: A Systematic Review and Meta-Analysis of Randomized Controlled Trials." *Archives of General Psychiatry* 64 (4): 442–55.

Schomerus, G., C. Schwahn, A. Holzinger, P. W. Corrigan, H. J. Grabe, and others. 2012. "Evolution of Public Attitudes about Mental Illness: A Systematic Review and Meta-Analysis." *Acta Psychiatrica Scandinavica* 125 (6): 440–52. doi:10.1111/j.1600-0447.2012.01826.x.

Sharif, F., and P. Armitage. 2004. "The Effect of Psychological and Educational Counselling in Reducing Anxiety in Nursing Students." *Journal of Psychiatric and Mental Health Nursing* 11 (4): 386–92. doi:10.1111/j.1365-2850.2003.00720.x.

Shek, E., A. T. Stein, F. M. Shansis, M. Marshall, R. Crowther, and others. 2009. "Day Hospital versus Outpatient Care for People with Schizophrenia." *Cochrane Database of Systematic Reviews* (4): CD003240. doi:10.1002/14651858.CD003240.pub2.

Shinohara, K., M. Honyashiki, H. Imai, V. Hunot, D. M. Caldwell, and others. 2013. "Behavioural Therapies versus Other Psychological Therapies for Depression." *Cochrane Database of Systematic Reviews* 10 (100909747): CD008696. doi:10.1002/14651858.CD008696.pub2.

Silva de Lima, M., and M. Hotopf. 2003. "Pharmacotherapy for Dysthymia." *Cochrane Database of Systematic Reviews* CD004047. doi:10.1002/14651858.CD004047.

Simon, G. E., M. Fleck, R. Lucas, and D. M. Bushnell. 2004. "Prevalence and Predictors of Depression Treatment in an International Primary Care Study." *American Journal of Psychiatry* 161 (9): 1626–34. doi:10.1176/appi.ajp.161.9.1626.

Soares-Weiser, K., Y. Bravo Vergel, S. Beynon, G. Dunn, M. Barbieri, and others. 2007. "A Systematic Review and Economic Model of the Clinical Effectiveness and Cost-Effectiveness of Interventions for Preventing Relapse in People with Bipolar Disorder." *Health Technology Assessment* 11 (39): iii–iv, ix–206.

Sorensen, H. J., P. R. Nielsen, C. B. Pedersen, M. E. Benros, M. Nordentoft, and others. 2014. "Population Impact of Familial and Environmental Risk Factors for Schizophrenia: A Nationwide Study." *Schizophrenia Research* 153 (1–3): 214–19. doi:10.1016/j.schres.2014.01.008.

Stein, D. J., J. C. Ipser, and S. Seedat. 2006. "Pharmacotherapy for Post Traumatic Stress Disorder (PTSD)." *Cochrane Database of Systematic Reviews* (1): Cd002795. doi:10.1002/14651858.CD002795.pub2.

Sullivan, P. F., M. J. Daly, and M. O'Donovan. 2012. "Genetic Architectures of Psychiatric Disorders: The Emerging Picture and Its Implications." *Nature Reviews Genetics* 13 (8): 537–51. doi:10.1038/nrg3240.

Tardy, M., M. Huhn, R. R. Engel, and S. Leucht. 2014. "Fluphenazine versus Low-Potency First-Generation Antipsychotic Drugs for Schizophrenia." *Cochrane Database of Systematic Reviews* 8: Cd009230. doi:10.1002/14651858.CD009230.pub2.

Tardy, M., M. Huhn, W. Kissling, R. R. Engel, and S. Leucht. 2014. "Haloperidol versus Low-Potency First-Generation Antipsychotic Drugs for Schizophrenia." *Cochrane Database of Systematic Reviews* 7: Cd009268. doi:10.1002/14651858.CD009268.pub2.

ten Have, M., W. Vollebergh, R. Bijl, and W. A. Nolen. 2002. "Bipolar Disorder in the General Population in The Netherlands (Prevalence, Consequences and Care Utilisation): Results from The Netherlands Mental Health Survey and Incidence Study (NEMESIS)." *Journal of Affective Disorders* 68 (2–3): 203–13.

Thara, R., S. John, and K. Rao. 2008. "Telepsychiatry in Chennai, India: the SCARF Experience." *Behavioral Sciences and the Law* 26 (3): 315–22. doi:10.1002/bsl.816.

Tharyan, P., and C. E. Adams. 2005. "Electroconvulsive Therapy for Schizophrenia." *Cochrane Database of Systematic Reviews* (2): Cd000076. doi:10.1002/14651858.CD000076.pub2.

The Lancet. 2013. "Truth versus Myth on Mental Illness, Suicide, and Crime." *The Lancet* 382 (9901): 1309. doi:10.1016/s0140-6736(13)62125-x.

Tsuang, D., and W. Coryell. 1993. "An 8-Year Follow-Up of Patients with DSM-III-R Psychotic Depression, Schizoaffective Disorder, and Schizophrenia." *American Journal of Psychiatry* 150 (8): 1182–88.

UK ECT Review Group. 2003. "Efficacy and Safety of Electroconvulsive Therapy in Depressive Disorders: A Systematic Review and Meta-Analysis." *The Lancet* 361 (9360): 799–808. doi:10.1016/s0140-6736(03)12705-5.

van Ginneken, N., P. Tharyan, S. Lewin, G. N. Rao, S. M. Meera, and others. 2013. "Non-Specialist Health Worker Interventions for the Care of Mental, Neurological and Substance-Abuse Disorders in Low- and Middle-Income Countries." *Cochrane Database of Systematic Reviews* 11 (100909747): CD009149. doi:10.1002/14651858.CD009149.pub2.

van Zoonen, K., C. Buntrock, D. D. Ebert, F. Smit, C. F. Reynolds, 3rd, and others. 2014. "Preventing the Onset of Major Depressive Disorder: A Meta-Analytic Review of Psychological Interventions." *International Journal of Epidemiology* 43 (2): 318–29. doi:10.1093/ije/dyt175.

Vidal, C. N., J. L. Rapoport, K. M. Hayashi, J. A. Geaga, Y. Sui, and others. 2006. "Dynamically Spreading Frontal and Cingulate Deficits Mapped in Adolescents with Schizophrenia." *Archives of General Psychiatry* 63 (1): 25–34. doi:10.1001/archpsyc.63.1.25.

Vijayakumar, L., M. Phillips, M. M. Silverman, D. Gunnell, and V. Carli. 2015. "Suicide and Self-Harm Disorders." In *Disease Control Priorities* (third edition): Volume 4, *Mental, Neurological, and Substance Use Disorders*, edited by V. Patel, D. Chisholm, T. Dua, R. Laxminarayan, and M. E. Medina-Mora. Washington, DC: World Bank.

von Wolff, A., L. P. Holzel, A. Westphal, M. Harter, and L. Kriston. 2013. "Selective Serotonin Reuptake Inhibitors and Tricyclic Antidepressants in the Acute Treatment of Chronic Depression and Dysthymia: A Systematic Review and Meta-Analysis." *Journal of Affective Disorders* 144 (1–2): 7–15.

Walker, E. R., R. E. McGee, and B. G. Druss. 2015. "Mortality in Mental Disorders and Global Disease Burden Implications: A Systematic Review and Meta-Analysis." *JAMA Psychiatry* 72 (4): 334–41. doi:10.1001/jamapsychiatry.2014.2502.

Walsh, E., P. Moran, C. Scott, K. McKenzie, T. Burns, and others. 2003. "Prevalence of Violent Victimisation in Severe Mental Illness." *The British Journal of Psychiatry* 183: 233–38.

Wang, P. S., S. Aguilar-Gaxiola, J. Alonso, M. C. Angermeyer, G. Borges, and others. 2007. "Use of Mental Health Services for Anxiety, Mood, and Substance Disorders in 17 Countries in the WHO World Mental Health Surveys." *The Lancet* 370 (9590): 841–50. doi:10.1016/s0140-6736(07)61414-7.

Wang, P. S., M. C. Angermeyer, G. Borges, R. Bruffaerts, W. Tat Chiu, and others. 2007. "Delay and Failure in Treatment Seeking after First Onset of Mental Disorders in the World Health Organization's World Mental Health Survey Initiative." *World Psychiatry* 6 (3): 177–85.

Wang, P. S., G. Simon, and R. C. Kessler. 2003. "The Economic Burden of Depression and the Cost-Effectiveness of Treatment." *International Journal of Methods in Psychiatric Research* 12 (1): 22–33.

Weiss, M. G., S. Jadhav, R. Raguram, P. Vounatsou, and R. Littlewood. 2001. "Psychiatric Stigma across Cultures: Local Validation in Bangalore and London." *Anthropology and Medicine* 8 (1): 71–87.

Whiteford, H. A., A. J. Ferrari, L. Degenhardt, V. Feigin, and T. Vos. 2015. "Global Burden of Mental, Neurological, and Substance Use Disorders: An Analysis from the Global Burden of Disease Study 2010." In *Disease Control Priorities* (third edition): Volume 4, *Mental, Neurological, and Substance Use Disorders*, edited by V. Patel, D. Chisholm, T. Dua, R. Laxminarayan, and M. E. Medina-Mora. Washington, DC: World Bank.

WHO (World Health Organization). 1992. *The ICD-10 Classification of Mental and Behavioral Disorders: Clinical Descriptions and Diagnostic Guidelines.* Geneva: WHO.

——— 2008. *mhGAP: Mental Health Gap Action Programme: Scaling Up Care for Mental, Neurological and Substance Use Disorders.* Geneva: WHO.

———. 2009. *Mental Health Systems in Selected Low- and Middle-Income Countries: A WHO-AIMS Cross-National Analysis.* Geneva: WHO.

———. 2010. *mhGAP Intervention Guide for Mental, Neurological and Substance Use Disorders in Non-Specialized Health Settings: Mental Health Gap Action Programme (mhGAP).* Geneva: WHO.

———. 2011. *Mental Health Atlas 2011.* Geneva: WHO.

———. 2014a. "Global Health Estimates 2014 Summary Tables: DALY by Cause, Age and Sex, 2000–2012." WHO, Geneva. http://www.who.int/healthinfo/global_burden_disease/en/.

———. 2014b. "Global Health Estimates 2014 Summary Tables: YLD by Cause, Age and Sex, 2000–2012." WHO, Geneva. http://www.who.int/healthinfo/global_burden_disease/en/.

———. 2014c. *Preventing Suicide: A Global Imperative.* Geneva: WHO.

Wijkstra, J., J. Lijmer, H. Burger, J. Geddes, and W. A. Nolen. 2013. "Pharmacological Treatment for Psychotic Depression." *Cochrane Database of Systematic Reviews* 11: Cd004044. doi:10.1002/14651858.CD004044.pub3.

Wiles, N., L. Thomas, A. Abel, N. Ridgway, N. Turner, and others. 2013. "Cognitive Behavioural Therapy as an Adjunct to Pharmacotherapy for Primary Care Based Patients with Treatment Resistant Depression: Results of the CoBalT Randomised Controlled Trial." *The Lancet* 381 (9864): 375–84. doi:10.1016/s0140-6736(12)61552-9.

Wilkinson, P., and Z. Izmeth. 2012. "Continuation and Maintenance Treatments for Depression in Older People." *Cochrane Database of Systematic Reviews* (11): CD006727. doi:10.1002/14651858.CD006727.pub2.

Wilson, K., P. Mottram, and C. Vassilas. 2008. "Psychotherapeutic Treatments for Older Depressed People." *Cochrane Database of Systematic Reviews* (1): CD004853. doi:10.1002/14651858.CD004853.pub2.

Xia, J., L. B. Merinder, and M. R. Belgamwar. 2011. "Psychoeducation for Schizophrenia." *Cochrane Database of Systematic Reviews* (6): Cd002831. doi:10.1002/14651858.CD002831.pub2.

Yamaguchi, S., S. I. Wu, M. Biswas, M. Yate, Y. Aoki, and others. 2013. "Effects of Short-Term Interventions to Reduce Mental Health-Related Stigma in University or College Students: A Systematic Review." *Journal of*

Nervous and Mental Disease 201 (6): 490–503. doi:10.1097 /NMD.0b013e31829480df.

Yu, D. L., and M. E. P. Seligman. 2002. "Preventing Depressive Symptoms in Chinese Children." *Prevention and Treatment* 5 (1): 9a.

Zimmermann, G., J. Favrod, V. H. Trieu, and V. Pomini. 2005. "The Effect of Cognitive Behavioral Treatment on the Positive Symptoms of Schizophrenia Spectrum Disorders: A Meta-Analysis." *Schizophrenia Research* 77 (1): 1–9. doi:10.1016/j.schres.2005.02.018.

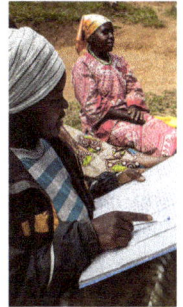

Chapter 5

Neurological Disorders

Kiran T. Thakur, Emiliano Albanese, Panteleimon
Giannakopoulos, Nathalie Jette, Mattias Linde,
Martin J. Prince, Timothy J. Steiner, and Tarun Dua

INTRODUCTION

Neurological disorders pose a large burden on world-wide health. The most recent estimates show that the neurological disorders included in the Global Burden of Disease (GBD) Study–Alzheimer's and other dementias, Parkinson's disease, multiple sclerosis, epilepsy, and headache disorders (migraine, tension-type headache [TTH], and medication-overuse headache [MOH])–represent 3 percent of the worldwide burden of disease. Although this is a seemingly small overall percentage, dementia, epilepsy, migraine, and stroke rank in the top 50 causes of disability-adjusted life years (DALYs) (Murray and others 2012).

Migraine and epilepsy represent one-third and one-fourth of this neurological burden, respectively (Murray and others 2012), and dementia and Parkinson's disease are among the top 15 conditions with the most substantial increase in burden in the past decade. In 2010, neurological disorders constituted 5.5 percent of years lived with disability (YLDs), or 42.9 million YLDs; migraine, epilepsy, and dementia were among the top 25 causes of YLDs. Migraine leads the list of neurological disorders, representing more than 50 percent of neurological YLDs or 2.9 percent of global YLDs; epilepsy represents 1.1 percent of global YLDs (Vos and others 2012).

The neurological burden of disease is expected to grow exponentially in low- and middle-income countries (LMICs) in the next decade (Murray and others 2012). Despite the significant impact of neurological disorders on patients and societies, knowledge of their epidemiology, including variation in disease frequency across place and time and understanding of associated risk factors and outcomes, remains limited, particularly in LMICs. Patients with neurological disorders often require significant social and economic support because of physical, cognitive, and psychosocial limitations (WHO 2006). Despite the high prevalence of disability, there is increasing recognition that services and resources are disproportionately scarce, especially in LMICs (WHO 2004). In addition, knowledge of the cost-effectiveness of interventions to improve neurological care in these settings remains limited.

This chapter addresses three neurological disorders: epilepsy, dementia, and headache disorders. The chapter reviews current knowledge of the epidemiology, risk factors, and cost-effective interventions for these conditions. The focus is on interventions that provide meaningful reduction in the burden to the global population, with particular emphasis on applicability to LMICs. Neurological disorders are an emerging challenge to health care systems globally, requiring further study, government and social engagement, and improvements in health care infrastructure.

This chapter uses the World Health Organization (WHO) regions—African, the Americas, Eastern Mediterranean, European, South-East Asia, and Western Pacific—to describe the global burden of the highlighted neurological disorders.

Corresponding author: Tarun Dua, MD, MPH Programme for Neurological Diseases and Neuroscience Evidence, Research and Action on Mental and Brain Disorders, Department of Mental Health and Substance Abuse, World Health Organization; duat@who.int.

EPILEPSY

Definitions

Epilepsy is a brain disorder traditionally defined as the occurrence of two unprovoked seizures occurring more than 24 hours apart with an enduring predisposition to generate further seizures (Fisher and others 2014). In 2014, the International League against Epilepsy provided an enhanced definition of epilepsy (box 5.1).

Epilepsy is considered to be resolved if a person has an age-dependent syndrome that is now beyond the expected age for this syndrome, or if the individual remained seizure free for the past 10 years and was off anti-epileptic drugs for at least the past five years (Fisher and others 2014). Those who continue to have seizures despite an adequate trial of a regimen of two tolerated and appropriately chosen anti-epileptic drugs (AEDs), whether in monotherapy or polytherapy, are considered to be drug resistant. Epilepsy can be classified in three categories:

- Structural or metabolic epilepsies, for example, epilepsy caused by a remote stroke
- Epilepsies of genetic or presumed genetic origin, for example, juvenile myoclonic epilepsy
- Epilepsies of unknown causes (Berg and others 2010).

Examples of more common causes of epilepsy include brain tumors, infectious diseases, brain injury, stroke, and hippocampal sclerosis. Less frequent causes include genetic causes, autoimmune causes, and malformations of cortical development (Bhalla and others 2011). Perinatal and infection-related etiologies often predominate in LMICs.

Box 5.1

Definition of Epilepsy

A person has epilepsy if he or she meets any of the following criteria (Fisher and others 2014):

- At least two unprovoked (or reflex) seizures occurring more than 24 hours apart
- One unprovoked (or reflex) seizure and a probability of further seizures similar to the general recurrence risk (at least 60 percent) after two unprovoked seizures, occurring over the next 10 years
- Diagnosis of an epilepsy syndrome.

Epidemiology and Burden of Disease

A worldwide systematic review of prevalence has not yet been published; in general, the prevalence in door-to-door studies has been reported to range from 2.2 per 1,000 to 41.0 per 1,000 persons, often with higher estimates in LMICs (Banerjee, Filippi, and Allen Hauser 2009; Benamer and Grosset 2009; Burneo, Tellez-Zenteno, and Wiebe 2005; Forsgren and others 2005; Mac and others 2007). The median incidence per 100,000 per year is higher in LMICs at 81.7 (interquartile range (IQR) 28.0-239.5) compared with HICs at 45.0 (IQR 30.3-66.7) (Ngugi and others 2011).

The higher estimates of prevalence or incidence rates reported in many LMICs are thought to be caused by the occurrence of endemic conditions, such as malaria or neurocysticercosis; the higher incidence of road traffic injuries; birth-related injuries; and variations in medical infrastructure, availability of preventative health programs, and accessible care. In HICs, the prevalence of epilepsy is stable until after age 50, when it increases; in contrast, the prevalence in LMICs tends to be stable in the third and fourth decade of life, drops in the fifth decade, and, in some studies, increases again after age 60 (Banerjee, Filippi, and Allen Hauser 2009).

Epilepsy is associated with premature mortality, with the highest standardized mortality ratio encountered in the first year or two after diagnosis (Neligan and others 2010). In general, the standardized mortality ratio for epilepsy is approximately 3 (Hitiris and others 2007). The epidemiology of premature mortality is particularly relevant in LMICs, where 85 percent of those with epilepsy live and where the risk of premature mortality is highest (Diop and others 2005; Jette and Trevathan 2014; Newton and Garcia 2012). Most concerning is the fact that a greater proportion of deaths in LMICs are potentially preventable, such as falls, drowning, burns, and status epilepticus (Diop and others 2005; Jette and Trevathan 2014). For example, 38 percent of all epilepsy-related deaths in a large cohort of people with convulsive epilepsy in rural Kenya were caused by status epilepticus (Ngugi and others 2014). Status epilepticus is defined as ongoing seizure activity lasting five minutes or more, or two or more seizures without recovery of consciousness in between (Lowenstein and others 2001). This is an important definition, as evidence suggests that seizures lasting more than five minutes are unlikely to self-terminate. Other common causes of premature mortality in those with epilepsy include acute symptomatic disorders (for example, brain tumor or stroke), sudden unexpected death in epilepsy, suicide, and accidents (Hitiris and others 2007).

Epilepsy ranks as the 36th leading cause of DALYs globally, according to the GBD 2010 report. Epilepsy ranks as high as the 14th leading cause of DALYs in western Sub-Saharan Africa. Epilepsy ranks as the 20th leading cause of YLDs globally, second only to migraine for brain disorders (Vos and others 2012). Importantly, models in the GBD 2010 report that calculate the global burden of epilepsy consider only the previously termed idiopathic/cryptogenic epilepsy and not epilepsy secondary to causes such as infections, stroke, or genetic syndromes, which may be responsible for more than 50 percent of the deaths in these regions (Murray and other 2012). Therefore, the data likely underrepresent the true burden of epilepsy, especially in LMICs.

Interventions

Population-Based Interventions

Targeting Epilepsy Risk Factors. Although genetic causes of epilepsy cannot be prevented, the more common structural or metabolic causes can be the target of primary prevention through public health policies. For example, helmet use for motorcyclists and laws against drinking and driving can reduce the risk of traumatic brain injury, a common risk factor. Improved perinatal care, particularly in rural areas, can reduce the incidence and subsequent prevalence of epilepsy. In one Tanzanian community-based, case-control study, adverse perinatal events were present in 14 percent of children with epilepsy but absent in all controls (Burton and others 2012). A population-based cross-sectional and case-control study in Ghana, Kenya, South Africa, Tanzania, and Uganda reported an association between abnormal antenatal period and active convulsive epilepsy (Ngugi and others 2013). Although abnormal delivery and home delivery did not reach statistical significance, there was a trend for these to be associated with active convulsive epilepsy.

Policies to control neurocysticercosis, a common risk factor in LMICs, would be an effective way to reduce epilepsy worldwide. An extensive eight-year public health and educational intervention program aimed at reducing symptomatic epilepsies (particularly those caused by perinatal insults and neurocysticercosis) was implemented in rural Salama, Honduras, starting in 1997 (Medina and others 2011). The program included education and media campaigns, animal husbandry training for pig farmers, construction of water projects and proper sewage disposal, deworming of school students, ongoing taeniasis surveillance, and other initiatives (Medina and others 2011). The proportion of epilepsy caused by neurocysticercosis was reduced from 36.9 percent in 1997 to 13.9 percent in 2005 (Medina and others 2011). The overall cost of this study was US$1.33 million, although an economic analysis was not conducted to determine if it was cost-effective.

A smaller-scale study examined the efficacy of teaching methods to prevent epilepsy caused by neurocysticercosis in western Kenya (Wohlgemut and others 2010). The authors found that knowledge improved significantly using this teaching method. Whether this program reduced the incidence of epilepsy caused by taenia solium was not examined, but the findings represent a positive step. The expert consultation report on foodborne infections, such as taeniasis/cysticercosis, proposes some approaches to ensure sustainable prevention and control of this often endemic agent. These approaches are listed in box 5.2; however, the report did not define the costs of implementing these approaches (WHO 2011).

Anti-Stigma Interventions. Civil rights violations, such as unequal access to health and life insurance or prejudicial weighting of health insurance provisions, are common. Discrimination in the workplace and restricted access to education are frequent. School teachers often have poor knowledge and negative attitudes toward children with seizure disorders (Akpan, Ikpeme, and Utuk 2013). Stigma is associated with social and economic consequences. Persons with epilepsy may not seek treatment or convey related health concerns to their care providers, further widening the treatment gap.

Improved knowledge about epilepsy is associated with positive attitudes and reduced stigma, but the

---

Box 5.2

Approaches to Ensure Sustainable Prevention and Control of Neurocysticercosis

- Preventive chemotherapy of human taeniasis through mass or targeted treatment of humans
- Mass treatment and vaccination of pigs
- Community education in health and pig husbandry
- Improved sanitation to end open defecation
- Improved meat inspection, control, and handling
- Better pig management.

The costs of implementing these approaches are not well defined.

Source: WHO 2009a.

sustainability and impact remain to be determined (Fiest and others 2014). A broad approach is needed to target stigma at the population level through legislation and advocacy. In addition, education and information provision to dispel myths and enhance seizure management among employers and teachers should empower those with epilepsy to seek treatment and encourage them to be more actively engaged in their communities. The cost-effectiveness of interventions to reduce stigma has not been formally assessed.

Legislation. One of the greatest contributors to the epilepsy treatment gap in LMICs is the lack of availability of anti-epileptic drugs. The second-generation medications are not available in the majority of countries, and even the older anti-epileptic drugs are only available sporadically. Investigators in Zambia who surveyed 111 pharmacies found that 49.1 percent did not carry anti-epileptic drugs. Pediatric syrups that are extensively used in HICs were universally unavailable (Chomba and others 2010). Regrettably, personal communications with epilepsy care providers in other LMICs suggested that this problem may be widespread (Chomba and others 2010).

Clearly, policies are warranted to guarantee the ongoing availability of affordable and efficacious anti-epileptic drugs to patients worldwide. Few countries have a separate budget for epilepsy services, and national funding support for epilepsy care is needed. Out-of-pocket expenses are the primary source of financing epilepsy care in 73 percent of low-income countries, including many countries in Africa, the Eastern Mediterranean, and South-East Asia, where the burden is highest (WHO 2011). Disability benefits do not exist in many regions, and patients are unable to receive monetary support.

Self-Management

Self-management is empowering patients to participate more actively in managing their care. Patients are likely to improve their understanding, adopt healthier lifestyles, and improve adherence to treatment (Fitzsimons and others 2012). Self-management can help those with epilepsy better identify and manage their seizure triggers, which can reduce frequency and decrease health services utilization and health care costs (Fitzsimons and others 2012). A few studies have examined the effectiveness of self-management education programs in adults and children and demonstrated some evidence of benefits; future research is needed to examine the cost-effectiveness of such programs in LMICs (Bradley and Lindsay 2008; Lindsay and Bradley 2010).

Pharmacological Interventions

The decision to initiate treatment with anti-epileptic drugs can be challenging. Analysis of the Multicentre trial for Early Epilepsy and Single Seizures suggests little benefit in initiating treatment for those who present with a single seizure, with no known neurological disorder, and normal electroencephalograms (EEGs) (Kim and others 2006). However, medical management should be considered in those who are at moderate to high risk, defined as more than two to three seizures at presentation, underlying neurological disorders, and abnormal EEGs (Kim and others 2006). More than 60 randomized control trials (RCTs), mostly in HICs, have examined the efficacy of anti-epileptic drugs, but there continues to be a lack of well-designed RCTs examining the efficacy of these medications for patients with generalized epilepsy syndromes and for children (Glauser and others 2013). Newer AEDs tend to be better tolerated, with fewer long-term side effects, but otherwise their superiority has not been proven.

Studies comparing the cost-effectiveness of anti-epileptic drugs in new onset epilepsy have not been conducted. A recent systematic review summarizes the evidence regarding their efficacy as initial monotherapy in those with epilepsy. Monotherapy with any of the standard anti-epileptic drugs (carbamazepine, phenobarbital, phenytoin, and valproic acid) should be offered to children and adults with convulsive epilepsy. Several lower-quality studies have demonstrated efficacy for phenobarbital in adults and children with partial onset seizures and generalized onset tonic-clonic seizures (Glauser and others 2013). Given the acquisition costs, phenobarbital should be offered as a first option if availability can be ensured. If available, carbamazepine should be offered to children and adults with partial onset seizures (WHO 2009b). Using the lowest possible dose should minimize side effects, improve seizure outcomes, and decrease the treatment gap. Valproic acid and ethosuximide have been shown to be most effective in the management of absence seizures, especially in children, although valproic acid is recommended, as it is on the list of essential medicines. Ethosuximide is available as a complementary medication. However, the medication should be avoided, when possible, in women of childbearing potential because of its higher association with major congenital malformations and poorer neurodevelopmental outcomes. Although newer therapeutic agents that are not metabolized by the liver are available, such as levetiracetam, the cost-effectiveness of such therapies has not been studied in LMICs.

Unfortunately, in LMICs, the availability and affordability of standard medications are poor and constitute barriers to treatment. One study found that the average availability of generic medications in the public sector is less than 50 percent for all medicines, except diazepam injection. The private sector availability of generic oral medications ranged from 42 percent for phenytoin to 70 percent for phenobarbital. Public sector patient prices for generic carbamazepine and phenytoin were 5 and 18 times higher than international reference prices, respectively; private sector patient prices were 11 and 25 times higher, respectively. For both medicines, originator brand prices were about 30 times higher. The highest prices were observed in the lowest-income countries (Cameron and others 2012). Ensuring a consistent supply at affordable prices should be a priority.

Approximately 60 percent of patients in Sub-Saharan Africa do not have access to AEDs, increasing the risk of seizures, accidents related to seizures, and status epilepticus, a significant cause of morbidity and mortality in patients with epilepsy (Ba-Diop and others 2014). Some of the best patient-related strategies to avoid status epilepticus include adherence to treatment and avoidance of other seizure triggers. On a population level, the best way to avoid the morbidity and mortality associated with status epilepticus is through health policy to increase the availability of and access to AEDs, and through health professional education such that health professionals are aware that time is brain. Aggressive treatment of status epilepticus should be implemented after five minutes, not after 30 minutes of ongoing seizures, in accordance with the current operational definition of status epilepticus (Lowenstein and others 2001).

Management of Infectious Etiologies of Epilepsy

Neurocysticercosis is a common cause of epilepsy in LMICs. Recent evidence-based guidelines are available to guide the treatment of parenchymal neurocysticercosis (Baird and others 2013). These guidelines suggest that therapy with albendazole, with or without corticosteroids, along with AEDs, is likely to be effective in improving outcomes (Baird and others 2013).

Evidence-based guidelines were published to guide the selection of anti-epileptic drugs for people with HIV/AIDS, because concomitant AED-antiretroviral administration may be indicated in up to 55 percent of people (Birbeck and others 2012). The guidelines state that it may be important to avoid enzyme-inducing AEDs in people on antiretroviral regimens that include protease inhibitors or nonnucleoside reverse transcriptase inhibitors, because pharmacokinetic interactions may result in virologic failure. If such regimens are required for seizure control, patients may be monitored through pharmacokinetic assessments to ensure the efficacy of the antiretroviral regimen (Birbeck and others 2012).

Surgical Management

The probability of achieving one-year seizure freedom after trying up to three anti-epileptic drugs occurs in the majority of cases (70 percent in those presenting with new onset epilepsy). However, drug resistance occurs in up to 40% of patients overall, particularly in those with focal epilepsy (Berg and others 2009; Kwan and Brodie 2000; Schiller and Najjar 2008; Semah and others 1998). In those who have failed three anti-epileptic drugs, attempting to treat with additional anti-epileptic drugs is unlikely to achieve sustained seizure freedom (Jette, Reid, and Wiebe 2014). Experts generally agree that those who are drug resistant and have failed two appropriate AED trials should be considered for a surgical evaluation (Jette, Reid, and Wiebe 2014; Kwan and others 2010; Wiebe and Jette 2012). Other patients who should be referred to a comprehensive epilepsy program for a surgical evaluation include children with complex syndromes, patients with stereotyped or lateralized seizures or focal findings, and children with a magnetic resonance imaging lesion amenable to surgical resection regardless of seizure frequency (Jette, Reid, and Wiebe 2014; Wiebe and Jette 2012). Strategies for surgical therapy of epilepsies in resource-poor settings have been proposed, and epilepsy surgery is increasingly performed in LMICs, with excellent outcomes (Asadi-Pooya and Sperling 2008).

Alternative Therapies

Proposed alternative therapies for epilepsy include dietary therapies, medical marijuana, and acupuncture; only dietary therapies have been subjected to randomized trials. The ketogenic diet can improve seizure outcome in those with drug-resistant epilepsy, but is difficult to tolerate, particularly in adults (Levy, Cooper, and Giri 2012). The Atkins diet was associated with improved seizure control in one observational study, but future studies are required to examine its benefit and the benefit of other dietary therapies, such as the modified Atkins diet and the low glycemic index diet (Levy, Cooper, and Giri 2012). Despite their increased use, dietary therapies are resource intensive, costly, and remain largely limited to HICs (Cross 2013). Cost-effective and simpler means of implementing these therapies in LMICs are needed. The efficacy of oral cannabinoids and acupuncture for the treatment of epilepsy remains uncertain (Cheuk and Wong 2014; Koppel and others 2014).

Interventions to Optimize Health Care Delivery

The treatment gap is defined as the number of people with active epilepsy who need appropriate anti-epileptic treatment but do not receive adequate medical therapy.

Regrettably, those living in LMICs, where the burden of epilepsy is extensive, are the most affected by the epilepsy treatment gap (Jette and Trevathan 2014). The treatment gap is more than 75 percent in low-income countries, more than 50 percent in many LMICs and upper-middle-income countries, and less than 10 percent in most HICs (figure 5.1) (Meyer and others 2010).

Proposed mechanisms for the epilepsy treatment gap can be divided into two broad categories: health care system and patient-related reasons (Cameron and others 2012; Kale 2002; Mbuba and others 2008). Health care system issues include lack of availability of anti-epileptic drugs, missed or delayed diagnosis, wrong treatment prescribed, treatment not offered to patients, and lack of resources and personnel (Cameron and others 2012; Kale 2002; Mbuba and others 2008). Epilepsy diagnosis is predominantly based on clinical history, and primary care physicians can be trained to provide basic treatment. Patient-related potential mechanisms for the treatment gap include cultural beliefs, stigma, fear of side effects, the hassle factor, and cost of treatment (Cameron and others 2012; Kale 2002; Mbuba and others 2008). All these reasons for the epilepsy treatment gap should be considered as potential targets for evaluation and action.

One study examined the availability, price, and affordability of anti-epileptic drugs in 46 countries (Cameron and others 2012). The study found that not only is the availability of these medications lower in LMICs, but their costs are highest where the treatment gap is the greatest (Cameron and others 2012). This study supports the view that availability and affordability of anti-epileptic drugs are likely major drivers in resource-poor countries. Box 5.3 provides a summary of the potential targets for evaluation and action to improve the epilepsy treatment gap.

Figure 5.1 Epilepsy Treatment Gap and Standard Errors Calculated from Lifetime Prevalence Estimates

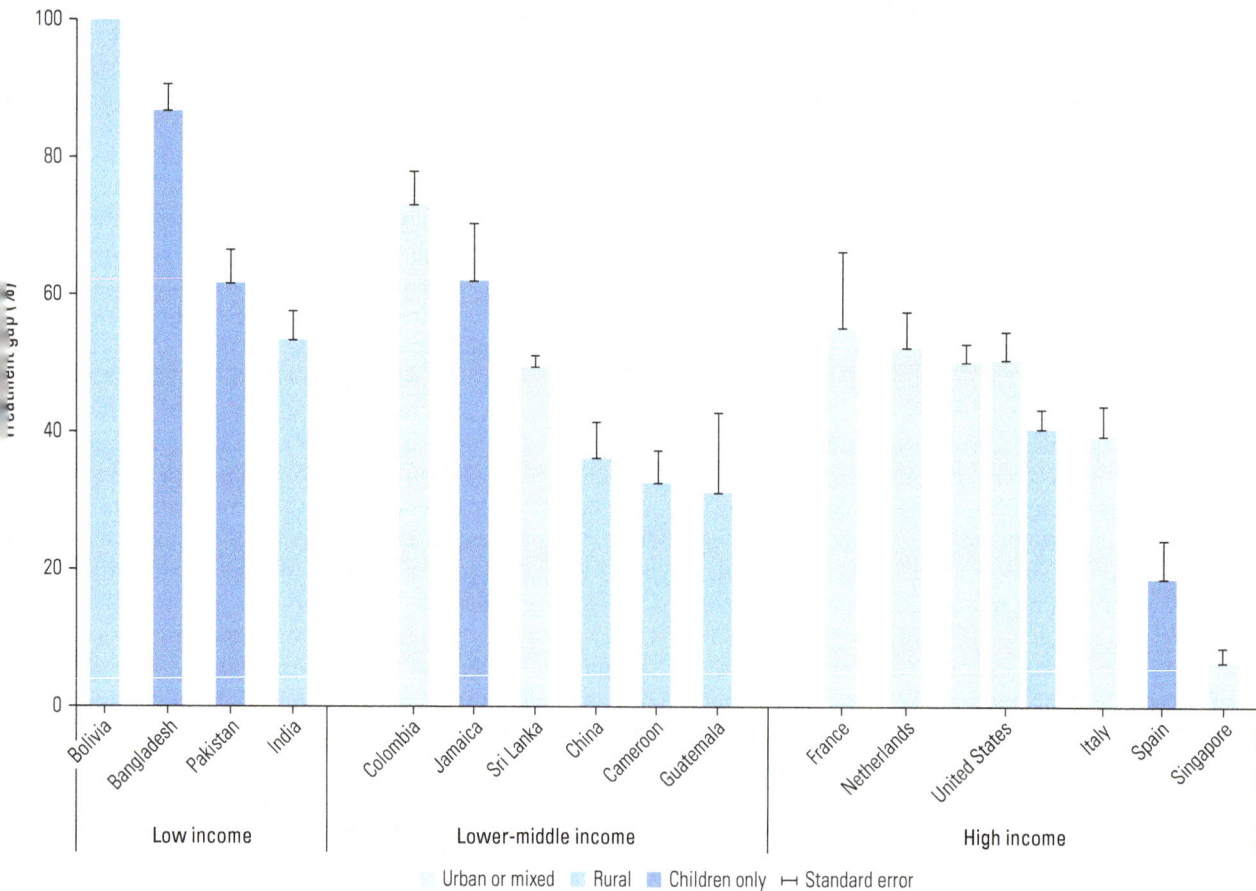

Source: Meyer and others 2010.

Two of the most impactful approaches to target the treatment gap are legislative and anti-stigma interventions. Unfortunately, their cost-effectiveness has not been evaluated.

Cost-Effectiveness of Interventions

The cost-effectiveness literature is focused on the pharmacological management of seizures, meaning that economic evidence concerning interventions at the population and community levels, such as stigma reduction strategies, are minimal. A recent study in India showed that covering costs for both first- and second-line therapy and other medical costs alleviates the financial burden from epilepsy and is cost-effective across wealth quintiles and in all Indian states (Megiddo and others 2016). WHO conducted a cost-effectiveness analysis of epilepsy treatment in nine developing regions of the world (Chisholm and WHO-CHOICE 2005). Both studies found that first-line medications, such as phenobarbital, represent a highly cost-effective use of resources for health (see also chapter 12 in this volume [Levin and Chisholm 2015]).

Surgery has been shown to be cost-effective in appropriately selected candidates in HICs, with health care costs declining significantly after successful surgery (Jette, Reid, and Wiebe 2014, Langfitt and others 2007). A summary of health economic analyses of epilepsy surgery found that, in general, the costs per quality-adjusted life year for epilepsy surgery are well within the "very cost-effective" range recommended by the WHO (Jette and Wiebe 2015; Langfitt 1997). In the United States, for example, the incremental cost-effectiveness ratio was US$27,200, considering direct and indirect costs, which is well below the country's gross domestic product per capita of US$40,000. Unfortunately, economic evaluations of epilepsy surgery in children, older adults, and from LMICs are generally lacking. In addition, most economic analyses focus on temporal lobe surgery.

Conclusions

The dire consequences of poorly treated epilepsy include significant morbidity and mortality caused by seizures and related injuries. The ongoing stigma associated with seizures remains a major challenge to clinical care in many regions, as well as the poor access to proper medications that can adequately treat this population. Ultimately, it is likely that the most effective target to address the treatment gap of epilepsy globally will be legislative changes and anti-stigma interventions. Among the required legislative efforts are those that advocate better provision of benefits for functionally disabled persons with epilepsy, especially in resource-poor countries where they are most needed.

DEMENTIA

Dementia poses a unique burden to those affected, their families, and societies. Substantial projected increases of patients with dementia in LMICs will pose additional economic and social burdens. Dementia is often erroneously considered an unavoidable part of aging or a condition for which nothing can be done; limited understanding and the persistence of stigma and discrimination limit help-seeking. Consequently, timely diagnosis is the exception rather than the norm; most people are not diagnosed and have limited access to adequate health or social care. Because pharmacotherapy and psychological and psychosocial interventions that can ameliorate symptoms and lessen the impact on family members and caregivers are often unavailable, the treatment gap remains very large, particularly in countries where cultural and infrastructure barriers persist.

Definitions

Dementia is a neuropsychiatric syndrome characterized by a combination of cognitive decline, progressive behavioral and psychological symptoms (BPSD), and functional disability (WHO 2012). Dementia is usually chronic and progressive; its insidious onset is typically characterized by objective deficits in one or more cognitive domains, such as memory, orientation, language, and executive function that are at the late stages accompanied by behavioral disturbances. Although age is the most significant risk factor, dementia is not a normal part of aging (Ganguli and others 2000; Kukull and others 2002; Launer and others 1999). The clinical onset of dementia is marked by the impact of cognitive decline in everyday activities, and diagnosis is often made by physical and neurological examination with supporting evidence from informant interviews.

Dementia is a syndrome that includes Alzheimer's disease; vascular dementia; frontotemporal dementia; Lewy body dementia; and reversible causes, for example, hypercalcemia, thyroid hormone abnormalities, vitamin B12 and folic acid deficiencies, HIV, subdural hematoma, and normal pressure hydrocephalus. Alzheimer's disease accounts for 50–60 percent of all late-life dementias, and vascular dementia accounts for up to 15–20 percent. Although brain pathological lesions differ across dementia subtypes, mixed forms of dementia are common, and vascular brain damage often co-occurs.

Epidemiology and Burden of Dementia

The most significant risk factor of dementia is increasing age; the incidence doubles with every five-year increment after age 65 (WHO 2015). The graying of societies in all global regions is expected to increase the number affected substantially. In 2015, approximately 47 million people had some form of dementia; 63 percent of those were in LMICs. This figure will nearly double to 76 million in 2030 and to 145 million by 2050. The majority (71 percent) of new cases will occur in LMICs (figure 5.2) (Prince and others 2015; WHO 2015). The steepest projected increases in numbers of people with dementia are expected in these settings because of rapid demographic changes. A new dementia case is diagnosed every four seconds in the world, leading to 7.7 million new cases per year; nearly 50 percent of new cases occur in Asia (WHO 2015).

In community-based samples, the prevalence of dementia varies from 38 to 400 per 100,000 inhabitants, with an increasing incidence over 55 years. Frontotemporal dementia (9.7 percent), alcohol-related dementia (9.4 percent), traumatic brain injury (3.8 percent), and Huntington's disease (3 percent) are more frequently present in early-onset dementia (EOD) compared with late-onset dementia (Picard and others 2011). Although dementia is more common in older age, some people develop symptoms at a younger age compatible with EOD, a poorly understood and frequently underdiagnosed condition.

Independent of the age at onset, most patients are cared for at home by close relatives. Need for one-on-one care starts early, becomes increasingly intense, and may change significantly throughout the natural history of the disease. Mood and behavioral changes, memory impairment for recent events, and spatiotemporal disorientation, as well as problem-solving deficits that characterize the early stage, may expose people with dementia

Figure 5.2 Projected Growth in Number of People with Dementia in All Income Groups, 2010–50

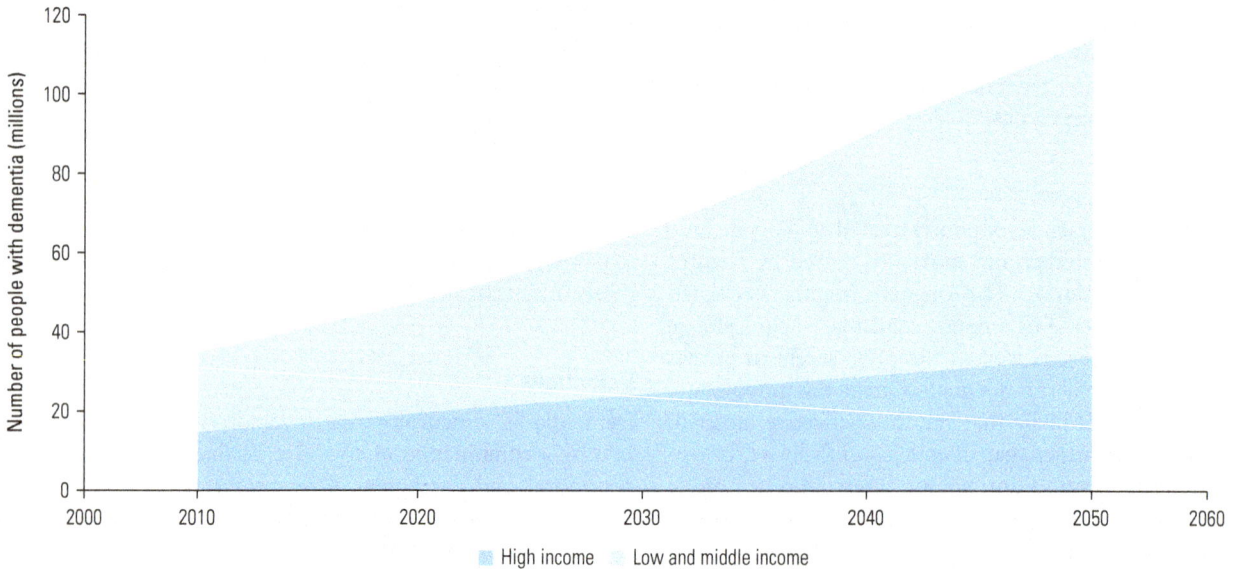

and their families to stressful situations well before the clinical diagnosis is made. Later, mood and behavioral disorders further increase the burden of the disease.

The later stages are characterized by diffuse involvement with psychological and behavioral symptoms, including repetitive behaviors, hallucinations, aggression, and wandering (Kales and others 2014). In contrast to cognitive deficits, these symptoms are strongly related to institutionalization (Richardson and others 2013). Caring for persons with dementia is associated with increasing physical and emotional stress. Studies show that caregivers often have feelings of isolation, anxiety, and depression that reduce the quality of life and may impact the quality of care they provide (Reitz, Brayne, and Mayeux 2011). The cumulative distress of caregivers constitutes a central component of the dementia burden (Donaldson and Burns 1999).

Global Burden of Dementia

Dementia has become a significant economic burden across the world (figure 5.3). The disease is the leading cause of dependence in older adults in all world regions; up to 50 percent of older adults who need care have dementia. According to the 2010 GBD report, the DALYs attributable to Alzheimer's disease and other dementias doubled in the past 20 years, and dementia is estimated as the major driver of DALYs in late life among all chronic diseases by virtue of its strong association with mortality and dependence. The dementia-attributable DALYs may increase further in LMICs, where life expectancy is increasing, and resources for the provision of health care for older adults are limited or unavailable.

In HICs, the level of care needed is the single strongest predictor of institutionalization of older adults. In LMICs, institutionalization is less likely; people with dementia tend to stay in their homes through the very advanced stages of the disease, cared for by informal caregivers, who are almost invariably close relatives and women.

The direct costs include health service use, health care, and institutionalization; the indirect costs include those associated with cutting back on work to provide care. Both pose significant financial burdens on individuals, families, and societies.

The global economic cost in 2013 was US$604 billion, approximately 1 percent of the global gross domestic product (WHO 2015). The direct and indirect costs are proportionally higher in HICs. Moreover, the distribution of costs across medical, societal, and informal care varies strikingly across regions and health system organizations. Hospital inpatient costs contributed 70 percent of the direct costs for prevalent dementia, mainly related to psychiatric care (Leibson and others 2015). The indirect costs of informal care likely go far beyond foregone income. There are potentially pernicious repercussions on families and social ties, caused by caring for persons with dementia, particularly in settings where there are false beliefs about the causes and course.

Figure 5.3 Distribution of the Total Societal Costs of Dementia Care, by World Bank Income Level

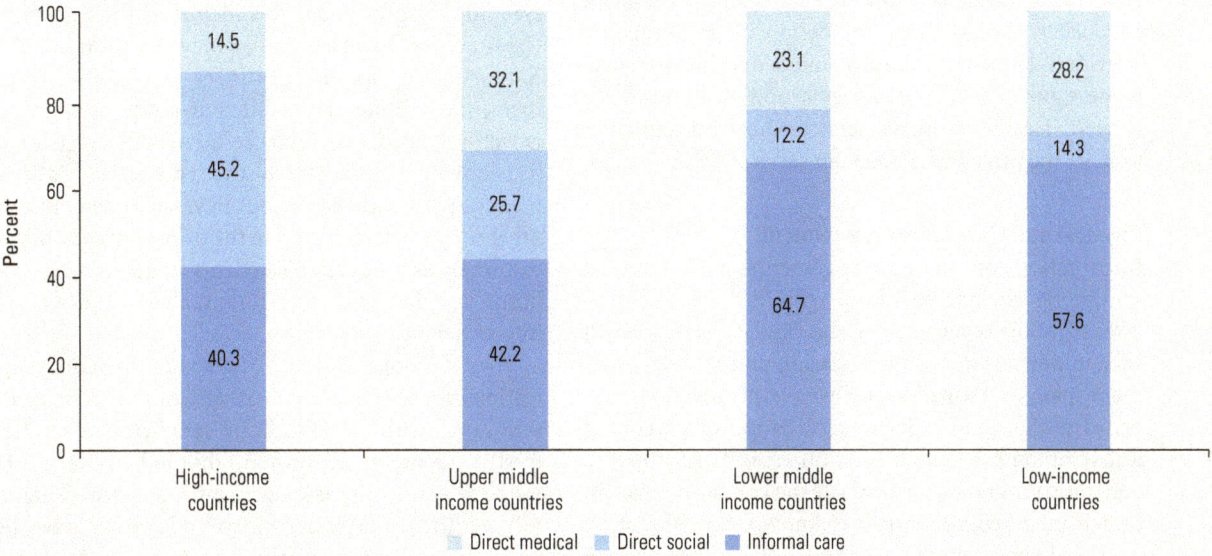

Interventions

Interventions need to address four key areas:

- Timely diagnosis
- Assessment and maintenance of physical health
- Cognition, activity, and well-being; assessment and treatment of BPSD
- Support for caregivers.

Detection and Diagnosis of Dementia

The evidence does not support dementia screening in the general population at present. Screening tools in primary health services may be used for those who report initial concerns about their cognitive function. Short versions of the Mini-Mental State Examination (Folstein, Folstein, and McHugh 1973) take as little as five minutes. However, unlike the Mini-Mental State Examination, which has been validated in several settings and languages, none of the short versions has been validated in LMICs, and their use is not recommended at present.

Diagnosis requires a clinical and informant interview and physical examination. Evidence from population-based studies, for example, the 10/66 culture-fair diagnostic algorithm (Prince and others 2003), suggests that diagnosis can be achieved using highly structured interviews and examinations conducted by trained community health workers. Adaptations for use in clinical practice are required, but the feasibility and cost-effectiveness of laboratory tests used in HICs to exclude treatable forms of dementia may limit their use in LMICs. Evidence from HICs indicates that the good practice of disclosure of the dementia diagnosis allows better planning and may limit distress; evidence from LMICs is lacking.

Appropriate adaptation to local culture, language, and beliefs should shape the design of programs and activities planned and implemented, and involve stakeholders, policy makers, the media, and local health care services. Health and social services should be enhanced to meet the projected increase in services.

Physical and Care Needs Assessment

Information on care arrangements and resources should be considered along with the evaluation of BPSD and the severity. A careful physical assessment is very important to monitor hearing and visual impairment, pain, constipation, urinary tract infections, and bedsores that may explain exacerbation of psychological symptoms. Whether physical assessment improves dementia prognosis, particularly the course of cognitive impairment, remains largely unknown. Nutritional status should be carefully monitored during the course of the disease. Weight loss is common and may start even before diagnosis. Loss of body weight may increase morbidity and mortality; yet, caregivers may be instructed on simple practices and techniques to overcome problems related to apathy and aversive feeding behaviors and may receive nutritional education to improve the caloric and nutritional content of meals. Finally, monitoring and effective treatment of vascular risk factors—including high blood pressure, hypercholesterolemia, smoking, obesity, and diabetes—should be encouraged to improve secondary prevention of cerebrovascular events. Moreover, there is extensive and persuasive evidence from mechanistic and well-designed prospective cohort studies that reducing the exposure to high blood pressure and hypertension in mid-life, and to diabetes in mid- and late life, as well as the reduction in tobacco use and increase in educational level of populations, can effectively reduce the dementia risk for populations (Prince and others 2014).

Pharmacological Interventions

Targets for pharmacological treatment include cognitive impairment; behavioral symptoms, such as agitation and aggression; and psychological symptoms, such as depression, anxiety, and psychosis. There is a large body of evidence for the efficacy of cholinesterase inhibitors (ChEIs), such as donepezil, rivastigmine, and galantamine, in the treatment of mild to moderate Alzheimer's disease (Institute for Quality and Efficiency in Healthcare 2014). The use of each of these medications is associated with modest and short-term comparable improvements in cognitive function, global clinical state, and activities of daily living. However, the evidence base for ChEIs in LMICs is limited. Moreover, the efficacy of this class of drugs in severe dementia is unclear, although behavioral symptom improvement was identified for galantamine (Institute for Quality and Efficiency in Healthcare 2014). A fourth drug for the treatment of cognitive impairment, memantine, has a different mode of action and is well tolerated, but evidence for its efficacy is limited to people with moderate to severe dementia. ChEIs and memantine are less efficacious in vascular dementia than other forms. Their efficacy in the treatment of behavioral disturbances is not established; manufacturer-sponsored licensing trials and post hoc analyses indicate small improvements.

Use of haloperidol and atypical antipsychotic medications for the treatment of agitation and behavioral symptoms with BPSD indicate small treatment effects, most evident for aggression, although these must be weighed against the associated mortality risk (Kales and others 2012). Atypical antipsychotic drugs have been widely prescribed for psychosis in dementia, but a meta-analysis of their efficacy indicated that only aripiprazole and risperidone had a statistically and clinically significant effect on psychiatric symptoms (Tan and others 2015). An important caveat to the use of these medications in dementia is the associated increased risk of death and cerebrovascular adverse events. The literature of antipsychotic treatment in older people with dementia reveals that although improvement in behavioral disturbance was minimal after 6–12 weeks, there was a significant increase in absolute mortality risk of approximately 1 percent (Banerjee, Filippi, and Allen Hauser 2009). As the literature suggests that prescribing antipsychotics in dementia continues beyond 6–12 weeks, the harm of continued antipsychotic treatment in dementia is likely to be substantial. Therefore, many recommend nonpharmacological treatments, such as psychological and training interventions, to reduce BPSD rather than antipsychotic management (Deudon and others 2009).

A meta-analysis of the efficacy of antidepressants in people with dementia was inconclusive (Leong 2014). Antidepressants have been proposed for the treatment of BPSD with encouraging results (Henry, Williamson, and Tampi 2011).

Nonpharmacological Interventions

A well-conducted RCT of cognitive stimulation (reality orientation, games, and discussions based on information processing rather than knowledge) conducted in the United Kingdom as a group intervention, and a small pilot trial from Brazil, suggest that cognitive benefits from this intervention are similar to those for ChEIs (Aguirre and others 2013). More specific cognitive training produced no benefits. Cognitive rehabilitation, an individualized therapy designed to enhance residual cognitive skills and the ability to cope with deficits, showed promise in uncontrolled case series in HICs. A meta-analysis of four trials of reminiscence therapy (the discussion of past activities, events, and experiences) provides evidence for short-term improvement in cognition, mood, and caregiver strain, but the quality of these trials was poor (Bahar-Fuchs, Clare, and Woods 2013; Woods and others 2005; Woods and others 2012).

Interventions for Caregivers

A large literature attests to the benefits of caregiver interventions. These include psycho-educational interventions, often including caregiver training; psychological therapies, such as cognitive behavioral therapy and counseling; caregiver support; and respite care. Many interventions combine several of these elements. The outcomes studied include caregiver strain, depression, and subjective well-being; behavior disturbance and mood in the care recipient; and institutionalization.

Most caregiver-focused interventions reduce strain and depression, with cognitive behavioral therapy having the largest impact on depression (Aboulafia-Brakha and others 2014; Martín-Carrasco and others 2009; Selwood and others 2007; Van Mierlo and others 2012). Caregiver training models have been developed for dementia care, including the Maximizing Independence at Home project (Tanner and others 2015). Psycho-educational interventions required the active participation of the caregiver to be effective. Caregiver support increased well-being but no other outcomes.

For respite care, methodologically flawed RCTs showed no benefit on any outcome (Grant and others 2003; Maayan, Soares-Weiser, and Lee 2014). However, nonrandomized studies suggest that respite care significantly reduces caregiver strain and psychological morbidity (Ornstein and others 2014). Interventions targeting the caregiver may also have small but significant beneficial effects on the behavior of the person with dementia. A systematic review of 10 RCTs indicated a 40 percent reduction in the pooled odds of institutionalization; the effective interventions were structured, intensive, and multicomponent, offering a choice of services and supports (Tam-Tham and others 2013). Two small trials of a brief caregiver education and training intervention, one from India and one from Russia, indicated much larger treatment effects on caregiver psychological morbidity and strain than typically seen for such interventions in HICs (Gavrilova and others 2009; Dias and others 2008).

Interventions to Optimize Health Care Delivery

Interventions to Increase Demand for Services. Raising awareness among the public, caregivers, and health workers can lead to increased demands for services. Intergenerational solidarity can be promoted through awareness-raising among children and young adults. In many LMICs, many people with dementia live in multigenerational households with young children, who are the most frequent caregivers and the most likely to initiate help-seeking. The provision of disability pensions and caregiver benefits in LMICs is likely to increase requests for diagnostic assessment. Importantly, however, efforts to increase awareness must be accompanied by health system and service reforms, so that help-seeking is met with a supply of better prepared, more responsive services.

Interventions to Improve the Capacity of Health Care Teams. Primary health care services in LMICs often fail older people because the services are clinic-based, often focused on simple curative interventions, and face high workloads. Given the frailty of many older people with dementia, there is a need for outreach to assess and manage patients in their own homes. Dementia care should be an essential component of any chronic disease care strategy. Training of nonspecialist health professionals should focus on case-finding and conveying the diagnosis to patients and caregivers together with information, needs assessment, and training and support. Training can be service-based, as well as through changes to medical and nursing schools, public health, and rural health curricula. Medical and community care services should be planned and coordinated to respond to the increasing need for support as the disease progresses.

Community-Based Programs to Deliver Effective Treatments. Programs to support caregivers can be delivered individually or in groups by community health workers or experienced caregivers. Strain, possibly associated with BPSD, should trigger more intensive interventions that include psychological assessment and depression treatment for the caregiver, respite care, and caregiver education and training. Such interventions could be incorporated into horizontally constructed, community-based programs that address the generic needs of frail, dependent, older people and their caregivers, whether these needs arise from cognitive, mental, or physical disorders. Recent evidence has demonstrated the effectiveness of delivery of Internet–based caregiver interventions (Czaja and Rubert 2002; Marziali and Garcia 2011).

Dementia: Cost-Effectiveness of Interventions

The estimated worldwide societal cost of dementia exceeded US$818 billion dollars in 2015 (Prince and others 2015). Direct costs include health service use and institutionalization; the indirect costs include those associated with inability to work and caregiver care. Both kinds of costs impose significant financial burdens on individuals, families, and societies. Informal care costs are proportionally highest in LMICs, while the direct costs for social care account for over half the costs in HICs (Prince and others 2015). Several studies, most in HICs, have evaluated the cost effectiveness of interventions in dementia. Particular challenges in such studies are the heterogeneity in etiology of dementia and the capture of cost-effectiveness in patients with milder forms of cognitive impairment.

Screening
A study in the Republic of Korea, where there is a nationwide early detection program for dementia, showed that the cost per quality-adjusted life year gained from early screening ranged from US$24,150 to US$35,661, depending on the age group. The probability of screening being cost-effective was highest in the group over age 75 years in a wide range of willingness to pay (WTP) (Yu and others 2015). The most cost-effective benefit of disease modifying therapies has been seen in moderate to severe dementia (Plosker and Lyseng-Williamson 2005).

Pharmacotherapy
Available pharmacoeconomic data from Europe and the United States support the use of memantine as a cost-effective treatment. Two cost-effectiveness analyses of memantine in moderate-to-severe Alzheimer's disease have been conducted in Finland and the United Kingdom; patient progression was simulated through health states related to dependency, residential setting, and cognitive function (Francois and others 2004; Jones and others 2004). Memantine reduced total societal costs by US$1,090 per patient per month, compared with no pharmacological treatment, over 28 weeks in a resource utilization and cost analysis conducted alongside a pivotal trial in patients in the United States with moderate-to-severe Alzheimer's disease (Wimo and others 2003). Results were primarily driven by reductions in total caregiver costs, which included the opportunity cost of time spent in caregiving tasks, and in direct nonmedical costs, which included the cost of care in a nursing home or similar institution.

An analysis in Canada found that treatment with rivastigmine yielded savings in the direct cost of caring for patients with Alzheimer's disease that exceed the cost of the drug after two years of treatment (Hauber and others 2000). In a 20-year Markov cohort model of disease modifying treatment in Alzheimer's disease based on a Swedish population, the sensitivity analysis implied no cost savings with disease modifying therapy, but most options indicated cost effectiveness verses the chosen WTP (Skoldunger and others 2013). In another study evaluating treatment with cholinesterase inhibitors or memantine for those with mild to moderate vascular dementia, donepezil 10 mg orally daily was found to be the most cost-effective treatment (Wong and others 2009).

Other Therapies
In terms of nonpharmacologic therapies, cognitive stimulation therapy has been shown to be cost-effective for people with mild-to moderate dementia when delivered biweekly over 7 weeks though was found to have modest effects when continued for longer when added to administration of acetylcholinesterase inhibitors (D'Amico and others 2015). An exercise intervention was found to have

the potential to be cost-effective when considering behavioral and psychological symptoms but did not appear cost-effective when considering quality-adjusted life year gains. The START (STrAtegies for RelaTives) study, a randomised controlled trial to determine the clinical effectiveness and cost-effectiveness of a manual-based coping strategy program in promoting the mental health of carers of people with dementia, found the intervention to be cost-effective with respect to caregiver and patient outcomes, and National Institute for Health and Care Excellence (NICE) thresholds (Livingston and other 2014). In a health economic analysis of resource costs and costs of formal care on a psychosocial intervention for family caregivers of persons with dementia, those in the intervention group reported higher quality of life while their spouse was living at home (Dahlrup and others 2014).

Conclusions

Research for early diagnosis is important in view of the future availability of treatments that are likely to be more efficacious in the early stages of the disease, when diagnosis is more difficult. At present, there are no disease-modifying pharmacological treatments for dementia, and medications to treat symptoms appear to have limited efficacy (Birks 2006; McShane, Areosa Sastre, and Minakaran 2006). The ambitious goal to identify a cure for Alzheimer's disease by 2025, which was announced by world political leaders in 2013 during the G8 meeting in London, underscores the recognition of dementia as a global health threat and priority. However, the quest for a cure should not drain resources from research on modifiable risk factors, which remains crucial for prevention, to potentially delay the symptomatic onset or slow the disease progression. The first WHO Ministerial Conference on Global Action Against Dementia was held in March 2015 to foster awareness of the public health and economic challenges posed by dementia and improve the understanding of the roles and responsibilities of Member States and stakeholders; it led to a Call for Action supported by conference participants. Indeed, a broad public health approach to address the complex challenges of dementia is extremely important.

HEADACHE DISORDERS

The three headache disorders of particular public health importance are migraine, TTH, and MOH. Collectively, these three are the third most common cause of disability in populations throughout the world (Murray and others 2012; Steiner and others 2015; Stovner and others 2007; Vos and others 2012).

Headache disorders are the most frequent cause of consultation in primary care and neurology practice; it prompts many visits to internists; ear, nose, and throat specialists; ophthalmologists; dentists; psychologists; and proponents of a wide variety of complementary and alternative medical practices (WHO 2011). Headache is a common presenting symptom in emergency departments. The consequences of recurring migraine include pain, disability, diminished productivity, financial losses, and impaired quality of life. Therefore, although headache rarely signals serious underlying illness, its causal association with personal burdens of pain, disability, and diminished quality of life makes it a major contributor to ill health.

Definitions

Migraine

Migraine is a disorder commonly beginning in puberty and often lasting throughout life. Episodic attacks have a frequency of once or twice a month on average, but this may vary widely, subject to lifestyle and environmental factors. In women, prevalence is higher because of a hormonally-driven association with menstruation. Headache, nausea, and photophobia are the most characteristic attack features. In some attacks, about 10 percent overall, and in only one-third of people with migraine, headache is preceded by aura symptoms, most commonly visual. The headache itself, lasting for hours to two to three days, is typically moderate or severe and unilateral, pulsating, and aggravated by routine physical activity (International Headache Society 2013). Chronic migraine, with headache attacks on 15 or more days per month and/or loss of episodicity, is a particularly disabling form (Natoli and others 2010).

Tension-Type Headache

TTH is a highly variable disorder, commonly beginning in the teenage years and reaching peak levels for people in their 30s. It lacks the specific features and associated symptoms of migraine, with headache usually mild or moderate, generalized, and described as pressure or tightness (International Headache Society 2013).

Medication-Overuse Headache

MOH is earning recognition as a disorder of major public health importance for three reasons: it is an attribute of migraine or (less often) TTH; it is highly disabling at individual levels; and it is iatrogenic and avoidable. MOH affects between 1 and 2 percent of the general population (Westergaard and others 2014), up to 67 percent of the chronic headache population, and 30–50 percent of patients seen in specialized headache centers (Evers, Jensen, and European Federation of

Neurological Societies 2011). The cause is chronic excessive use of medications taken initially to treat episodic headache (Diener and Limmroth 2004). The overuse of all such medications is associated with this problem, although the mechanism through which it develops undoubtedly varies among drug classes (Steiner and others 2007).

Epidemiology and Burden of Disease

Estimating the global burden of headache disorders is a challenging task, given data paucity for many LMICs, variations in methodologies in epidemiological studies, and variation of cultural attitudes related to the reporting of complaints. Much of the world's population lives in countries where headache prevalence and burden are incompletely known (Stovner and others 2007). Regardless, estimations have been done and show that the global one-year prevalence of migraine constitutes 14.7 percent and TTH 20.8 percent of adults ages 18–65 (Murray and others 2012). The prevalence of all types of headache occurring on 15 or more days per month (including chronic migraine, chronic TTH, and MOH) is 3 percent (Stovner and others 2007). Although the prevalence of migraine is markedly lower in Asia (Stovner and others 2007) and was thought to be so in Africa, a study in Zambia has indicated a high one-year prevalence (22.9 percent), coupled with very high prevalences of headache on 15 or more days a month (11.5 percent) and probable MOH (7.1 percent), with considerable economic impact (Mbewe and others 2015).

Interventions

Worldwide, at least 50 percent of headaches are self-treated, even in high-income countries (HICs) (WHO 2011). Professional health care, when needed, should be provided in primary care settings for the majority of cases (WHO 2011), and guidelines for the management of headache disorders in these settings are available (Steiner and others 2007). History and examination should take due note of warning features that might suggest an underlying condition (Steiner and others 2007).

Many instruments, including the HALT questionnaire, are available to assess the burden of headache symptoms on individual patients. (Steiner and Martelletti 2007). Realistic goals of management include understanding that primary headaches cannot be cured but can be managed effectively. We focus our further treatment discussions on migraine.

Self-Management

Stress is a common predisposing factor for migraine. Improving the ability to cope is an alternative treatment approach, but the role of psychological therapies in migraine management is unclear. Most research has focused on high-end intensive treatment of individual cases of disabling and refractory headache, which has limited relevance to public health. Yet there is potential for low-cost delivery of group behavioral training, and even some very limited evidence of benefit (Mérelle and others 2008). This approach could be further explored in LMICs.

Obesity is a risk factor for migraine, especially for frequent migraine (Evans and others 2012). Regular exercise and keeping fit can be beneficial. A study among obese adolescents with migraine found a significant improvement in headache in those who participated in a 12-month weight-loss program (Evans and others 2012).

Pharmacological Interventions

Guidelines recommend a stepped-care approach commencing with acute treatment using simple analgesics (aspirin or one of several other nonsteroidal anti-inflammatory drugs) (Steiner and others 2007). Good evidence demonstrates the efficacy and tolerability of aspirin (Kirthi, Derry and Moore 2013), ibuprofen (Rabbie, Derry and Moore 2013), and diclofenac potassium (Derry, Rabbie, and Moore 2013). The most desirable outcome of acute treatment is complete relief from pain within two hours, without recurrence or need for further medication and without adverse events. This outcome is not commonly experienced with simple analgesics alone.

The more easily achievable outcome referred to as *sustained headache relief* (SHR) is defined as reduction of pain to no worse than mild within two hours of treatment, also without recurrence or need for further medication. Mild pain is assumed not to be associated with disability, and SHR implies full functional recovery when functional impairment was present initially. Aspirin alone provides SHR in an estimated 39 percent of users (Kirthi, Derry and Moore 2013); this is a modest effect in the sense that it leaves 61 percent without this benefit but at the same time is among the most cost-efficient interventions to improve public health (Linde, Steiner, and Chisholm 2015). Aspirin has the advantages of being universally available and on the WHO essential medicines list (WHO 2013). Ibuprofen provides SHR in a somewhat higher estimated proportion of users (45 percent) (Rabbie, Derry, and Moore 2013), at variable but not always higher cost. Diclofenac is considerably more costly, without significantly greater efficacy

(Derry, Rabbie, and Moore 2013). It is argued that the anti-inflammatory effect is important in acute migraine treatment, and paracetamol is therefore rather less effective than aspirin (at the same cost) or other nonsteroidal anti-inflammatory drugs (Derry and Moore 2013; Steiner and others 2007).

Antiemetics should also be used in acute treatment, and should not be restricted to patients who are vomiting or likely to vomit. Nausea is one of the most aversive and disabling symptoms of a migraine attack and should be treated appropriately (Silberstein and others 2012). Gastric stasis is a feature of migraine; prokinetic antiemetics, such as domperidone or metoclopramide, enhance gastric emptying and promote the efficacy of oral analgesics in migraine.

The usual second step in management is still acute treatment, with the substitution or addition of specific anti-migraine therapy (Steiner and others 2007). Ergotamine tartrate remains in use in many countries (WHO 2011), but it is poorly bioavailable, is not highly effective, and has potential side effects. Of the triptan class of agents–which are specific anti-migraine medications–seven are available in many countries. They differ somewhat in their pharmacokinetics, and they are not identical in efficacy; however, the differences between them are small when set against the up to ten-fold price differences between sumatriptan (available in generic versions) and the other six. Sumatriptan is available in four formulations (oral, intranasal, rectal, and subcutaneous). Sumatriptan 50 mg orally provides SHR in an estimated 35 percent of users (Derry, Derry, and Moore 2012), much the same as aspirin; however, it has a different mode of action, and responses to each drug are independent. When sumatriptan is used on its own, its cost-effectiveness is at least two orders of magnitude lower than that of aspirin (Linde, Steiner, and Chisholm 2015); it is usually reserved as a second-line treatment for those who fail to respond to first-line treatments (Steiner and others 2007). In adults and children, regular use of acute medications at high frequency (more than two days per week) risks the development of MOH.

Prophylactic medications are used in step three to reduce the number of attacks occurring when acute therapy is inadequate (Steiner and others 2007). There is adequate or good evidence of efficacy and tolerability for propranolol (Linde and others 2013b), amitriptyline (Dodick and others 2009), valproate (as sodium valproate or valproic acid) (Linde and others 2013b), and topiramate (Diener and others 2004; Linde and others 2013a). To assess outcome as migraine attacks averted requires comparison with an untreated base line, which is available for propranolol (28 percent) (Linde, Steiner, and Chisholm 2015), amitriptyline (44 percent) (Linde,

Steiner, and Chisholm 2015). In an American Academy of Neurology review, divalproex sodium, sodium valproate, topiramate, metoprolol, propranolol, and timolol were found to be effective for migraine prevention (Silberstein and others 2012). In terms of cost, propranolol and amitriptyline are similar and very low, and topiramate is much higher; amitriptyline might be the choice of prophylactic drug when resource conservation is the key consideration (Linde, Steiner, and Chisholm 2015). However, the mode of action of these medications in migraine is unknown, and failure of response to one does not predict the failure of others (Steiner and others 2007), which might be tried when amitriptyline is ineffective and resources permit.

Alternative Therapies

Acupuncture and physical therapies, such as spinal manipulation, requiring direct one-to-one therapist-patient interaction, are highly resource intensive, and have questionable efficacy (Bronfort and others 2004; Linde and others 2009) to justify their recommendation. Even the limited benefits seen in clinical trials may not be replicated in the real world, where therapists operate under time constraints.

Public Education Programs

Public education programs can help to improve migraine outcomes. Lifestyle factors may predispose people to or aggravate migraine. Although the evidence is poor that modifying lifestyle is an effective way of controlling migraine, avoidance of trigger factors is a logical stratagem (Steiner and others 2007).

Public education about the increasing risk of migraine with obesity (Bronfort and others 2004) may achieve some benefits, because, unlike many other ill-health consequences of obesity, headache is experienced in the present. Public education also appears to offer the most effective means of controlling a potential epidemic of MOH as a consequence of mistreated migraine. Recent evidence from the Global Campaign against Headache (Mbewe and others 2015) suggests this may be a particular problem in LMICs where medications are relatively more affordable and available than health care. The initial effectiveness of simple analgesics encourages their further use, which is not problematic at low frequency. With increasing frequency comes greater reliance and increasing risk of MOH. Once MOH is established, medication overuse is likely to escalate.

The incremental health benefits obtained in LMICs from adding educational programs to the use of over-the-counter and prescription medications appear to be achievable at acceptable incremental costs (Linde, Steiner, and Chisholm 2015). Pharmacists can be a key source of information to the public about headache disorders, treatments, and the dangers of medication overuse, but only if this role is explicitly recognized in their reimbursement, and only if their advice is sought. Further, the cost-effectiveness of treatments may increase with public education programs to improve adherence to treatments (Linde, Steiner, and Chisholm 2015).

Interventions to Optimize Health Care Delivery
In a global survey, one-third of responding countries recommended improved organization and delivery of health care for headache so that care would be efficient and equitable (WHO 2011). The organization of services to achieve this goal is clearly a challenge, and no single solution may be appropriate in all settings. Most patients do not require specialist expertise or special investigations (Steiner and others 2007), and the three-tier service model developed by the Global Campaign against Headache for Europe (Steiner and others 2011) is highly adaptable. This model had been used as part of demonstration projects to structure headache services in China (Yu and others 2014), and in Sverdlovsk Oblast in the Russian Federation (Lebedeva and others 2013). Using the model, about 90 percent of patients are managed in first-level care, usually but not necessarily by physicians; 1 percent require specialist care that is necessarily hospital-based. The intermediate 9 percent do not require specialist care, but may have diagnostic or management difficulties that would benefit from second-level care. Provision of this level of care depends on resources and local health service organizations. Each level must maintain a gatekeeper role to higher levels to make the model work.

Countries that have invested in headache services have, paradoxically, generally done so by setting up specialist headache clinics. Worldwide, the proportion of headache patients seen by specialists is 10 percent (WHO 2011), indicating considerable scope for resource reallocation for the benefit of more patients if the levels below were better utilized. Pharmacists need to be formally integrated into health care systems.

Training Health Care Providers. The ability of first-level services to deliver effective care depends on the providers—physicians, clinical officers, or nurses—having the basic knowledge required. Evidence clearly indicates deficiencies, and better professional education ranked far above all other proposals for change in WHO's global survey (WHO 2011). Training first-level doctors in the management of migraine is likely to improve outcomes, as well as to increase the cost-effectiveness of prescription medications (Linde, Steiner,

and Chisholm 2015). Furthermore, such training might reduce waste, through reductions in the high rates of unnecessary investigations to support diagnosis (WHO 2011).

Cost-Effectiveness of Interventions
There is a lack of nationally conducted cost-effectiveness studies to inform resource allocation decisions for headache disorders in LMICs. However, a recent cost-effectiveness modeling analysis of migraine treatment was carried out for four countries–China (an upper-middle-income country), India (a lower-middle-income country), Russia (an HIC), and Zambia (a lower-middle-income country). The analysis concluded that acute treatment with aspirin generated a year of healthy life for less than US$100 (Linde, Steiner, and Chisholm 2015), making it among the most efficient interventions to improve population health. Cost-effectiveness analysis was not carried out for paracetamol specifically, because the only evidence of SHR came from 42 highly atypical patients in the United States (Linde, Steiner, and Chisholm 2015). When sumatriptan is used on its own for acute management of migraine, its cost-effectiveness is at least two orders of magnitude less favorable than that of aspirin, which indicates why sumatriptan is reserved as a second-line treatment for those who fail to respond to first-line treatments (Steiner and others 2007).

Prophylactic medications are less cost-effective than acute therapy with simple analgesics, but considerably more cost-effective than acute therapy with the combination of analgesics and triptans (when needed), but this may be true only if prophylactics are reserved for those with three or more attacks per month (Linde, Steiner, and Chisholm 2015). The addition of educational programs (posters and leaflets in pharmacies) for the use of over-the-counter and prescription medications appears to increase population health gain at an acceptable incremental cost, as does training providers (Linde, Steiner, and Chisholm 2015).

Conclusions
It is clear that investment in structured headache services, with their basis in primary care and supported by educational initiatives aimed at professionals and the public, is the way forward for most countries. Such services require resource reallocation which is easily justified economically. Importantly, services for migraine would simultaneously provide for the other common and disabling headache disorders. The gains

in population health achievable through effective headache management are substantial and independent of any recovery of indirect costs attributable to these disorders. The financial costs to society through lost productivity from migraine alone are enormous: more than €100 billion (US$100 billion) per year in the European Union (Linde and others 2012) and far higher than the health care expenditure on headache in any country (WHO 2011). Greater investment to treat migraine effectively through well-organized health services supported by education may well be cost-saving overall (WHO 2011).

CONCLUSIONS AND RECOMMENDATIONS

Epilepsy, dementia, and headache disorders represent a significant burden on global health. Not only are these conditions prevalent, but they are associated with significant disability, poor psychosocial outcomes, and substantial economic costs.

Innovative health care management approaches are required in LMICs because of the lack of specialist care. Some of these approaches are discussed, but few have been subjected to cost-effectiveness evaluations. Further data collection is needed in many areas of global neurology, including epidemiological studies, needs assessments, and cost-effectiveness analyses.

For all three of these conditions, pharmacotherapies have advanced considerably in the past two decades, but these options are regrettably limited in LMICs. Indeed, the treatment gap for these conditions is substantial, driven by patient and health system factors, which are unlikely to improve without education of the public and health care professionals, legislation, and anti-stigma interventions. Fortunately, attitudes and knowledge about the burden of epilepsy, dementia, and migraine are starting to improve, and such progress can help reduce the treatment gap and enhance psychosocial outcomes for those suffering from these conditions. Ultimately, however, increased financial investments and legislative changes are required to improve neurological care in LMICs.

NOTE

World Bank Income Classifications as of July 2014 are as follows, based on estimates of gross national income (GNI) per capita for 2013:

- Low-income countries (LICs) = US$1,045 or less
- Middle-income countries (MICs) are subdivided:
  a) lower-middle-income = US$1,046 to US$4,125
  b) upper-middle-income (UMICs) = US$4,126 to US$12,745
- High-income countries (HICs) = US$12,746 or more.

REFERENCES

Aboulafia-Brakha, T., D. Suchecki, F. Gouveia-Paulino, R. Nitrini, and R. Ptak. 2014. "Cognitive-Behavioural Group Therapy Improves a Psychophysiological Marker of Stress in Caregivers of Patients with Alzheimer's Disease." *Aging Mental Health* 18 (6): 801–08.

Aguirre, E., R. T. Woods, A. Spector, and M. Orrell. 2013. "Cognitive Stimulation for Dementia: A Systematic Review of the Evidence of Effectiveness from Randomised Controlled Trials." *Ageing Research Reviews* 12 (1): 253–62.

Akpan, M. U., E. E. Ikpeme, and E. O. Utuk. 2013. "Teachers' Knowledge and Attitudes towards Seizure Disorder: A Comparative Study of Urban and Rural School Teachers in Akwa Ibom State, Nigeria." *Nigerian Journal of Clinical Practice* 16 (3): 365–70.

Asadi-Pooya, A. A., and M. R. Sperling. 2008. "Strategies for Surgical Treatment of Epilepsies in Developing Countries." *Epilepsia* 49 (3): 381–85.

Ba-Diop, A., B. Marin, M. Druet-Cabanac, E. B. Ngougou, C. R. Newton, and P. M. Preux. 2014. "Epidemiology, Causes, and Treatment of Epilepsy in Sub-Saharan Africa." *The Lancet Neurology* 13 (10): 1029–44. doi:10.1016 /S1474-4422(14)70114-0.

Bahar-Fuchs, A., L. Clare, and B. Woods. 2013. "Cognitive Training and Cognitive Rehabilitation for Mild to Moderate Alzheimer's Disease and Vascular Dementia." *Cochrane Database of Systematic Reviews* 6: CD003260. PubMed PMID:23740535.

Baird, R. A., S. Wiebe, J. R. Zunt, J. J. Halperin, G. Gronseth, and others. 2013. "Evidence-Based Guideline: Treatment of Parenchymal Neurocysticercosis: Report of the Guideline Development Subcommittee of the American Academy of Neurology." *Neurology* 80 (15): 1424–29. doi:10.1212 /WNL.0b013e31828c2f3e.

Banerjee, P. N., D. Filippi, and W. Allen Hauser. 2009. "The Descriptive Epidemiology of Epilepsy—A Review." *Epilepsy Research* 85 (1): 31–45. doi:10.1016/j.eplepsyres .2009.03.003.

Benamer, H. T., and D. G. Grosset. 2009. "A Systematic Review of the Epidemiology of Epilepsy in Arab Countries." *Epilepsia* 50 (10): 2301–04. doi:10.1111/j.1528-1167.2009.02058.x.

Berg, A. T., S. F. Berkovic, M. J. Brodie, J. Buchhalter, J. H. Cross, and others. 2010. "Revised Terminology and Concepts for Organization of Seizures and Epilepsies: Report of the ILAE Commission on Classification and Terminology, 2005–2009." *Epilepsia* 51 (4): 676–85. doi:EPI2522 [pii].10.1111/j.1528-1167.2010.02522.x.

Berg, A. T., S. R. Levy, F. M. Testa, and R. D'Souza. 2009. "Remission of Epilepsy after Two Drug Failures in Children: A Prospective Study." *Annals of Neurology* 65 (5): 510–19. doi:10.1002/ana.21642.

Bhalla, D., B. Godet, M. Druet-Cabanac, and P. M. Preux. 2011. "Etiologies of Epilepsy: A Comprehensive Review." *Expert Review of Neurotherapeutics* 11 (6): 861–76. doi:10.1586 /ern.11.51.

Birbeck, G. L., J. A. French, E. Perucca, D. M. Simpson, H. Fraimow, and others. 2012. "Evidence-Based Guideline: Antiepileptic

Drug Selection for People with HIV/AIDS: Report of the Quality Standards Subcommittee of the American Academy of Neurology and the Ad Hoc Task Force of the Commission on Therapeutic Strategies of the International League Against Epilepsy." *Neurology* 78 (2): 139–45. doi:10.1212/WNL.0b013e31823efcf8.

Birks, J. 2006. "Cholinesterase Inhibitors for Alzheimer's Disease." *Cochrane Database Systematic Reviews* 25 (1): CD005593.

Bradley, P. M., and B. Lindsay. 2008. "Care Delivery and Self-Management Strategies for Adults with Epilepsy." *Cochrane Database of Systematic Reviews* (1): CD006244. doi:10.1002/14651858.CD006244.pub2.

Bronfort, G., N. Nilsson, M. Haas, R. Evans, C. H. Goldsmith, and others. 2004. "Non-Invasive Physical Treatments for Chronic/Recurrent Headache." *Cochrane Database of Systematic Reviews* (3): CD001878.

Burneo, J. G., J. Tellez-Zenteno, and S. Wiebe. 2005. "Understanding the Burden of Epilepsy in Latin America: A Systematic Review of Its Prevalence and Incidence." *Epilepsy Research* 66 (1–3): 63–74. doi:S0920-1211(05)00138-5 [pii]10.1016/j.eplepsyres.2005.07.002.

Burton, K. J., J. Rogathe, R. Whittaker, K. Mankad, E. Hunter, and others. 2012. "Epilepsy in Tanzanian Children: Association with Perinatal Events and Other Risk Factors." *Epilepsia* 53 (4): 752–60. doi:10.1111/j.1528-1167.2011.03395.x.

Cameron, A., A. Bansal, T. Dua, S. R. Hill, S. L. Moshe, and others. 2012. "Mapping the Availability, Price, and Affordability of Antiepileptic Drugs in 46 Countries." *Epilepsia* 53 (6): 962–69. doi:10.1111/j.1528-1167.2012.03446.x.

Cheuk, D. K., and V. Wong. 2014. "Acupuncture for Epilepsy." *Cochrane Database of Systematic Reviews* (5): CD005062. doi:10.1002/14651858.CD005062.pub4.

Chisholm, D., and WHO-CHOICE. 2005. "Cost-Effectiveness of First-Line Antiepileptic Drug Treatments in the Developing World: A Population-Level Analysis." *Epilepsia* 46 (5): 751–59.

Chomba, E. N., A. Haworth, E. Mbewe, M. Atadzhanov, P. Ndubani, and others. 2010. "The Current Availability of Antiepileptic Drugs in Zambia: Implications for the ILAE/WHO 'Out of the Shadows' Campaign." *American Journal of Tropical Medicine and Hygiene* 83 (3): 571–74. doi:10.4269/ajtmh.2010.10-0100.

Cross, J. H. 2013. "New Research with Diets and Epilepsy." *Journal of Child Neurology* 28 (8): 970–74. doi:10.1177/0883073813487593.

Czaja, S. J., and M. P. Rubert. 2002. "Telecommunications Technology as an Aid to Family Caregivers of Persons with Dementia." *Psychosomatic Medicine* 64 (3): 469–76.

Dahlrup, B., E. Nordell, K. Steen Carlsson, and S. Elmståhl. 2014. "Health Economic Analysis on a Psychosocial Intervention for Family Caregivers of Persons with Dementia." *Dementia and Geriatric Cognitive Disorders* 37 (3–4): 181–95.

Derry, C. J., S. Derry, and R. A. Moore. 2012. "Sumatriptan (Oral Route of Administration) for Acute Migraine Attacks in Adults." *Cochrane Database of Systematic Reviews* 2 Article No. CD008615. doi:10.1002/14651858.CD008615.pub2.

Derry, S., and R. A. Moore. 2013. "Paracetamol (Acetaminophen) with or without an Antiemetic for Acute Migraine Headaches in Adults." *Cochrane Database of Systematic Reviews* (4): CD008040. doi:10.1002/14651858.CD008040.pub3.

Derry, S., R. Rabbie, and R. A. Moore. 2013. "Diclofenac with or without an Antiemetic for Acute Migraine Headaches in Adults." *Cochrane Database Systematic Reviews* (4): CD008783.

Deudon, A., N. Maubourguet, X. Gervais, E. Leone, P. Brocker, and others. 2009. "Non-Pharmacological Management of Behavioural Symptoms in Nursing Homes." *International Journal of Geriatric Psychiatry* (12): 1386–95. doi:10.1002/gps.2275.

Dias, A., M. E. Dewey, J. D'Souza, R. Dhume, D. D. Motghare, K. S. Shaji, and others. 2008. "The Effectiveness of a Home Care Program for Supporting Caregivers of Persons with Dementia in Developing Countries: A Randomised Controlled Trial from Goa, India." *PLoS One* 3 (6): e2333. doi:10.1371/journal..pone.0002333.

Diener, H. C., and V. Limmroth. 2004. "Medication-Overuse Headache: A Worldwide Problem." *The Lancet Neurology* 3 (8): 475–83.

Diener, H. C., P. Tfelt-Hansen, C. Dahlof, M. J. Lainez, G. Sandrini, S. J. Wang, W. Neto, U. Vijapurkar, A. Doyle, D. Jacobs, and M. S. Group. 2004. "Topiramate in Migraine Prophylaxis: Results from a Placebo-Controlled Trial with Propranolol as an Active Control." *Journal of Neurology* 251 (8): 943–50. doi:10.1007/s00415-004-0464-6.

Diop, A. G., D. C. Hesdorffer, G. Logroscino, and W. A. Hauser. 2005. "Epilepsy and Mortality in Africa: A Review of the Literature." *Epilepsia* 46 (Suppl. 11): 33–35. doi:10.1111/j.1528-1167.2005.00405.x.

Dodick, D. W., F. Freitag, J. Banks, J. Saper, J. Xiang, and others. 2009. "Topiramate versus Amitriptyline in Migraine Prevention: A 26-Week, Multicenter, Randomized, Double-Blind, Double-Dummy, Parallel-Group Noninferiority Trial in Adult Migraineurs." *Clinical Therapeutics* 31 (3): 542–59. doi:10.1016/j.clinthera.2009.03.020.

Donaldson, C., and A. Burns. 1999. "Burden of Alzheimer's Disease: Helping the Patient and Caregiver." *Journal of Geriatric Psychiatry Neurology* 12 (1): 21–28.

Evans, R. W., M. A. Williams, A. M. Rapoport, and B. L. Peterlin. 2012. "The Association of Obesity with Episodic and Chronic Migraine." *Headache* 52 (4): 663–71. doi:10.1111/j.1526-4610.2012.02114.x.

Evers, S., R. Jensen, and European Federation of Neurological Societies. 2011. "Treatment of Medication Overuse Headache—Guideline of the EFNS Headache Panel." *European Journal of Neurology* 18 (9): 1115–21. doi:10.1111/j.1468-1331.2011.03497.x.

Fiest, K. M., G. L. Birbeck, A. Jacoby, and N. Jette. 2014. "Stigma in Epilepsy." *Current Neurology and Neuroscience Reports* 14 (5): 444. doi:10.1007/s11910-014-0444-x.

Fisher, R. S., C. Acevedo, A. Arzimanoglou, A. Bogacz, J. H. Cross, and others. 2014. "ILAE Official Report: A Practical Clinical Definition of Epilepsy." *Epilepsia* 55 (4): 475–82. doi:10.1111/epi.12550.

Fitzsimons, M., C. Normand, J. Varley, and N. Delanty. 2012. "Evidence-Based Models of Care for People with Epilepsy." *Epilepsy & Behavior* 23 (1): 1–6. doi:10.1016/j.yebeh.2011.10.019.

Folstein, M., S. Folstein, and P. R. McHugh. 1973. "Clinical Predictors of Improvement after Electroconvulsive Therapy of Patients with Schizophrenia, Neurotic Reactions, and Affective Disorders." *Biological Psychiatry* 7 (2): 147–52.

Forsgren, L., E. Beghi, A. Oun, and M. Sillanpaa. 2005. "The Epidemiology of Epilepsy in Europe—A Systematic Review." *European Journal of Neurology* 12 (4): 245–53. doi:10.1111/j.1468-1331.2004.00992.x.

Francois, C., H. Sintonen, R. Sulkava, and B. Riva. 2004. "Cost Effectiveness of Memantine in Moderately Severe to Severe Alzheimer's Disease: A Markov Model in Finland." *Clinical Drug Investigations* 24 (7): 373–84.

Ganguli, M., V. Chandra, M. I. Kamboh, J. M. Johnston, H. H. Dodge, and others. 2000. "Apolipoprotein E Polymorphism and Alzheimer Disease: The Indo-US Cross-National Dementia Study." *Arch Neurology* 57 (6): 824–30.

Gavrilova, S. I., C. P. Cerri, N. Mikhaylova, O. Sokolova, S. Banerjee, and others. 2009. "Helping Carers to Care—The 10/66 Dementia Research Group's Randomized Control Trial of a Caregiver Intervention in Russia." *International Journal of Geriatric Psychiatry* 24 (4): 347–54.

Glauser, T., E. Ben-Menachem, B. Bourgeois, A. Cnaan, C. Guerreiro, and others. 2013. "Updated ILAE Evidence Review of Antiepileptic Drug Efficacy and Effectiveness as Initial Monotherapy for Epileptic Seizures and Syndromes." *Epilepsia* 54 (3): 551–63. doi:10.1111/epi.12074.

Grant, I, C. L. McKibbin, M. J. Taylor, P. Mills, J. Dimsdale, M. Ziegler, and T. L. Patterson. 2003. "In-Home Respite Intervention Reduces Plasma Epinephrine in Stressed Alzheimer Caregivers." *American Journal of Geriatric Psychiatry* 11 (1): 62–72.

Hauber, A. B., A. Gnanasakthy, and J. A. Mauskopf. 2000. "Savings in the Cost of Caring for Patients with Alzheimer's Disease in Canada: An Analysis of Treatment with Rivastigmine." *Clinical Therapeutics* (4): 439–51.

Henry, G., D. Williamson, and R. R. Tampi. 2011. "Efficacy and Tolerability of Antidepressants in the Treatment of Behavioral and Psychological Symptoms of Dementia, a Literature Review of Evidence." *American Journal of Alzheimer's Disease and Other Dementias* 26 (3): 169–83.

Hitiris, N., R. Mohanraj, J. Norrie, and M. J. Brodie. 2007. "Mortality in Epilepsy." *Epilepsy and Behavior* 10 (3): 363–76.

Institute for Quality and Efficiency in Health Care. 2014. https://www.iqwig.de/en/home.2724.html.

International Headache Society. 2013. "The International Classification of Headache Disorders, 3rd edition (beta version)." *Cephalalgia* 33 (9): 629–808. doi:10.1177/0333102413485658.

Jette, N., A. Y. Reid, and S. Wiebe. 2014. "Surgical Management of Epilepsy." *Canadian Medical Association Journal [Journal de l'Association medicale canadienne].* doi:10.1503/cmaj.121291.

Jette, N., and E. Trevathan. 2014. "Saving Lives by Treating Epilepsy in Developing Countries." *Neurology* 82 (7): 552–53. doi:10.1212/WNL.0000000000000133.

Jette, N., and S. Wiebe S. 2015. "Health Economics Issues." In *Long-Term Outcomes of Epilepsy Surgery in Adults and Children*, first edition, edited by K. Malmgren, S. Baxendale, and H. Cross. Springer.

Jones, R. W., P. McCrone, and C. Guilhaume. 2004. "Cost Effectiveness of Memantine in Alzheimer's Disease: An Analysis Based on a Probabilistic Markov Model From a UK Perspective." *Aging* 21 (9): 607–20.

Kale, R. 2002. "Global Campaign against Epilepsy: The Treatment Gap." *Epilepsia* 43 (Suppl. 6): 31–33.

Kales, H. C., L. N. Gitlin, C. G. Lyketsos, and Detroit Expert Panel on Assessment and Management of Neuropsychiatric Symptoms of Dementia. 2014. "Management of Neuropsychiatric Symptoms of Dementia in Clinical Settings: Recommendations from a Multidisciplinary Expert Panel." *Journal of the American Geriatrics Society* 62 (4): 762–69. doi:10.1111/jgs.12730.

Kales, H. C., H. M. Kim, K. Zivin, M. Valenstein, L. S. Seyfried, and others. 2012. "Risk of Mortality among Individual Antipsychotics in Patients with Dementia." *The American Journal of Psychiatry* 169 (1): 71–79. doi:10.1176/appi.ajp.2011.11030347.

Kim, L. G., T. L. Johnson, A. G. Marson, and D. W. Chadwick. 2006. "Prediction of Risk of Seizure Recurrence after a Single Seizure and Early Epilepsy: Further Results from the MESS Trial." *The Lancet Neurology* 5 (4): 317–22. doi:10.1016/S1474-4422(06)70383-0.

Kirthi, V., S. Derry, and R. A. Moore. 2013. "Aspirin with or without an Antiemetic for Acute Migraine Headaches in Adults." *Cochrane Database Systematic Reviews* (4): CD008041. doi:10.1002/14651858.CD008041.pub3.

Koppel, B. S., J. C. Brust, T. Fife, J. Bronstein, S. Youssof, and others. 2014. "Systematic Review: Efficacy and Safety of Medical Marijuana in Selected Neurologic Disorders: Report of the Guideline Development Subcommittee of the American Academy of Neurology." *Neurology* 82 (17): 1556–63. doi:10.1212/WNL.0000000000000363.

Kukull, W. A., R. Higdon, J. D. Bowen, W. C. McCormick, L. Teri, and others. 2002. "Dementia and Alzheimer Disease Incidence: A Prospective Cohort Study." *Archives of Neurology* 59 (11): 1737–46.

Kwan, P., A. Arzimanoglou, A. T. Berg, M. J. Brodie, H. W. Allen, and others. 2010. "Definition of Drug Resistant Epilepsy: Consensus Proposal by the Ad Hoc Task Force of the ILAE Commission on Therapeutic Strategies." *Epilepsia* 51 (6): 1069–77.

Kwan, P., and M. J. Brodie. 2000. "Early Identification of Refractory Epilepsy." *The New England Journal of Medicine* 342 (5): 314–19.

Langfitt, J. T. 1997. "Cost-Effectiveness of Anterotemporal Lobectomy in Medically Intractable Complex Partial Epilepsy." *Epilepsia* 38 (2): 154–63.

Langfitt, J. T., R. G. Holloway, M. P. McDermott, S. Messing, K. Sarosky, and others. 2007. "Health Care Costs Decline after Successful Epilepsy Surgery." *Neurology* 68 (16): 1290–98.

Launer, L. J., K. Andersen, M. E. Dewey, L. Letenneur, A. Ott, and others. 1999. "Rates and Risk Factors for Dementia and Alzheimer's Disease: Results from EURODEM Pooled Analyses. EURODEM Incidence Research Group and Work Groups. European Studies of Dementia." *Neurology* 52 (1): 78–84.

Lebedeva, E. R., J. Olesen, V. V. Osipova, L. I. Volkova, G. R. Tabeeva, and others. 2013. "The Yekaterinburg Headache Initiative: An Interventional Project, within the Global Campaign against Headache, to Reduce the Burden of Headache in Russia." *Journal of Headache and Pain* 14 (1): 101. doi:10.1186/1129-2377-14-101.

Leibson, C. L., K. H. Long, J. E. Ransom, R. O. Roberts, S. L. Hass, and others. 2015. "Direct Medical Costs and Source of Cost Differences across the Spectrum of Cognitive Decline: A Population-Based Study." *Alzheimer's Dement* 11 (8): 917–32. doi:10.1016/j.jalz.2015.01.007.

Leong, C. 2014. "Antidepressants for Depression in Patients with Dementia: A Review of the Literature." *Consultant Pharmacist* 29 (4): 254–63. doi:10.4140/TCP.n.2014.254.

Levin, C., and D. Chisholm. 2015. "Cost-Effectiveness and Affordability of Interventions, Policies, and Platforms for the Prevention and Treatment of Mental, Neurological, and Substance Use Disorders." In *Disease Control Priorities* (third edition): Volume 4, *Mental, Neurological, and Substance Use Disorders*, edited by V. Patel, D. Chisholm, T. Dua, R. Laxminarayan, and M. E. Medina-Mora. Washington, DC: World Bank.

Levy, R. G., P. N. Cooper, and P. Giri. 2012. "Ketogenic Diet and Other Dietary Treatments for Epilepsy." *Cochrane Database of Systematic Reviews* (3): CD001903. doi:10.1002/14651858.CD001903.pub2.

Linde, K., G. Allais, B. Brinkhaus, E. Manheimer, A. Vickers, and A. R. White. 2009. "Acupuncture for Migraine Prophylaxis." *Cochrane Database of Systematic Reviews* (1): CD001218. doi:10.1002/14651858.CD001218.pub2.

Linde, K., and K. Rossnagel. 2004. "Propranolol for Migraine Prophylaxis." *Cochrane Database of Systematic Reviews* (2): CD003225.

Linde, M., A. Gustavsson, L. J. Stovner, T. J. Steiner, J. Barré, and others. 2012. "The Cost of Headache Disorders in Europe: The Eurolight Project." *European Journal of Neurology* 19 (5): 703–11. doi:10.1111/j.1468-1331.2011.03612.x .Epub 2011 Dec 5.

Linde, M., W. M. Mulleners, E. P. Chronicle, and D. C. McCrory. 2013a. "Topiramate for the Prophylaxis of Episodic Migraine in Adults" *Cochrane Database of Systematic Reviews* 6: CD010611. doi:10.1002/14651858.

———. 2013b. "Valproate (Valproic Acid or Sodium Valproate or a Combination of the Two) for the Prophylaxis of Episodic Migraine in Adults." *Cochrane Database of Systematic Reviews* 6: CD010611. doi:10.1002/14651858.

Linde, M., T. J. Steiner, and D. Chisholm. 2015. "Cost-Effectiveness Analysis of Interventions for Migraine in Four Low- and Middle-Income Countries." *Journal of Headache Pain* 18 (16): 15. doi:10.1186/s10194-015-0496-6.

Lindsay, B., and P. M. Bradley. 2010. "Care Delivery and Self-Management Strategies for Children with Epilepsy." *Cochrane Database of Systematic Reviews* (12): CD006245. doi:10.1002/14651858.CD006245.pub2.

Livingston, G., J. Barber, P. Rapaport, M. Knapp, M. Griffin, and others. 2014. "Long-Term Clinical and Cost-Effectiveness of Psychological Intervention for Family Carers of People with Dementia: A Single-Blind, Randomised, Controlled Trial." *Lancet Psychiatry* (7): 539–48. doi:10.1016/S2215-0366(14)00073-X. Epub 2014 Dec 3.

Lowenstein, D. H., B. K. Alldredge, F. Allen, J. Neuhaus, M. Corry, and others. 2001. "The Prehospital Treatment of Status Epilepticus (PHTSE) Study: Design and Methodology." *Controlled Clinical Trials* 22: 290–309.

Maayan, N., K. Soares-Weiser, and H. Lee. 2014. "Respite Care for People with Dementia and their Carers." *Cochrane Database of Systematic Reviews* (1): CD004396. doi:10.1002/14651858.CD004396.pub3.

Mac, T. L., D. S. Tran, F. Quet, P. Odermatt, P. M. Preux, and others. 2007. "Epidemiology, Aetiology, and Clinical Management of Epilepsy in Asia: A Systematic Review." *The Lancet Neurology* 6 (6): 533–43.

Martín-Carrasco, M., M. F. Martín, C. P. Valero, P. R. Millán, C. I. García, and others. 2009. "Effectiveness of a Psychoeducational Intervention Program in the Reduction of Caregiver Burden in Alzheimer's Disease Patients' Caregivers." *International Journal of Geriatric Psychiatry* 24 (5): 489–99.

Marziali, E., and L. J. Garcia. 2011. "Dementia Caregivers' Responses to 2 Internet-Based Intervention Programs." *American Journal of Alzheimer's Diseases and Other Dementias* 26 (1): 36–43.

Mbewe, E., P. Zairemthiama, R. Paul, G. L. Birbeck, and T. J. Steiner. 2015. "The Burden of Primary Headache Disorders in Zambia: National Estimates from a Population-Based Door-to-Door Survey." *Journal of Headache Pain* 16: 513.

Mbuba, C. K., A. K. Ngugi, C. R. Newton, and J. A. Carter. 2008. "The Epilepsy Treatment Gap in Developing Countries: A Systematic Review of the Magnitude, Causes, and Intervention Strategies." *Epilepsia* 49 (9): 1491–503. doi:10.1111/j.1528-1167.2008.01693.x.

McShane, R., A. Areosa Sastre, and N. Minakaran. 2006. "Memantine for Dementia." *Cochrane Database of Systematic Reviews* (2): CD003154.

Medina, M. T., R. L. Aguilar-Estrada, A. Alvarez, R. M. Duron, L. Martinez, and others. 2011. "Reduction in Rate of Epilepsy from Neurocysticercosis by Community Interventions: The Salama, Honduras Study." *Epilepsia* 52 (6): 1177–85. doi:10.1111/j.1528-1167.2010.02945.x.

Megiddo, I., A. Colson, D. Chisholm, T. Dua, A. Nandi, and others. 2016. "Health and Economic Benefits of Public Financing of Epilepsy Treatment in India: An Agent-Based Simulation Model." *Epilepsia*. 2016. Epub. doi:10.1111/epi.13294.

Mérelle, S. Y., M. J. Sorbi, L. J. van Doornen, and J. Passchier. 2008. "Lay Trainers with Migraine for a Home-based Behavioral Training: A 6-Month Follow-Up Study." *Headache* 48 (9): 1311–25.

Meyer, A. C., T. Dua, J. Ma, S. Saxena, and G. Birbeck. 2010. "Global Disparities in the Epilepsy Treatment Gap: A Systematic Review." *Bulletin of the World Health Organization* 88 (4): 260–66. doi:10.2471 /BLT.09.064147.

Murray, C. J., T. Vos, R. Lozano, M. Naghavi, A. D. Flaxman, and others. 2012. "Disability-Adjusted Life Years (DALYs) for 291 Diseases and Injuries in 21 Regions, 1990–2010: A Systematic Analysis for the Global Burden of Disease Study 2010." *The Lancet* 380 (9859): 2197–223. doi:10.1016 /S0140-6736(12)61689-4.

Natoli, J. L., A. Manack, B. Dean, Q. Butler, C. C. Turkel, and others. 2010. "Global Prevalence of Chronic Migraine: A Systematic Review." *Cephalalgia* 30 (5): 599–609. doi:10.1111/j.1468-2982.2009.01941.x.

Neligan, A., G. S. Bell, S. D. Shorvon, and J. W. Sander. 2010. "Temporal Trends in the Mortality of People with Epilepsy: A Review." *Epilepsia* 51 (11): 2241–46. doi:10.1111/j.1528-1167.2010.02711.x.

Newton, C. R., and H. H. Garcia. 2012. "Epilepsy in Poor Regions of the World." *The Lancet* 380 (9848): 1193–201. doi:10.1016/S0140-6736(12)61381-6.

Ngugi, A. K., C. Bottomley, G. Fegan, E. Chengo, R. Odhiambo, and others. 2014. "Premature Mortality in Active Convulsive Epilepsy in Rural Kenya: Causes and Associated Factors." *Neurology* 82 (7): 582–89. doi:10.1212 /WNL.0000000000000123.

Ngugi, A. K., C. Bottomley, I. Kleinschmidt, R. G. Wagner, A. Kakooza-Mwesige, and others. 2013. "Prevalence of Active Convulsive Epilepsy in Sub-Saharan Africa and Associated Risk Factors: Cross-Sectional and Case-Control Studies." *The Lancet Neurology* 12 (3): 253–63. doi:10.1016 /S1474-4422(13)70003-6.

Ngugi, A. K., S. M. Kariuki, C. Bottomley, I. Kleinschmidt, J. W. Sander, and others. 2011. "Incidence of Epilepsy: A Systematic Review and Meta-Analysis." *Neurology* 77 (10): 1005–12. doi:10.1212/WNL.0b013e31822cfc90.

Ornstein, K., J. E. Gaugler, L. Zahodne, and Y. Stern. 2014. "The Heterogeneous Course of Depressive Symptoms for the Dementia Caregiver." International Journal of Aging and Human Development 78 (2): 133–48.

Picard, C., F. Pasquier, O. Martinaud, D. Hannequin, and O. Godefroy. 2011. "Early Onset Dementia: Characteristics in a Large Cohort from Academic Memory Clinics." *Alzheimer Disease and Associated Disorders* 25 (3): 203–05. doi:10.1097/WAD.0b013e3182056be7.

Prince, M., D. Acosta, H. Chiu, M. Scazufca, M. Varghese, and others. 2003. "Dementia Diagnosis in Developing Countries: A Cross-Cultural Validation Study." *The Lancet* 361 (9361): 909–17.

Prince, M., E. Albanese, M. Guerchet, and M. Prina. 2014. *World Alzheimer's Report 2014. Dementia and Risk Reduction: An Analysis of Protective and Modifiable Factors.* London: Alzheimer's Disease International.

Prince, M. J., F. Wu, Y. Guo, L. M. Gutierrez Robledo, M. O'Donnell, and others. 2015. "The Burden of Disease in Older People and Implications for Health Policy and Practice." *The Lancet* 385 (9967): 549–62. doi:10.1016 /S0140-6736(14)61347-7.

Rabbie, R., S. Derry, and R. A. Moore. 2013. "Ibuprofen with or without an Antiemetic for Acute Migraine Headaches in Adults." *Cochrane Database of Systematic Reviews* (4): CD008039. doi:10.1002/14651858.CD008039.pub3.

Reitz, C., C. Brayne, and R. Mayeux. 2011. "Epidemiology of Alzheimer Disease." *Nature Reviews Neurology* 7 (3): 137–52. doi:10.1038/nrneurol.2011.2.

Richardson, T. J., S. J. Lee, M. Berg-Weger, and G. T. Grossberg. 2013. "Caregiver Health: Health of Caregivers of Alzheimer's and Other Dementia Patients." *Current Psychiatry Reports* 15 (7): 367. doi:10.1007/s11920-013-0367-2.

Schiller, Y., and Y. Najjar. 2008. "Quantifying the Response to Antiepileptic Drugs: Effect of Past Treatment History." *Neurology* 70 (1): 54–65. doi:10.1212/01 .wnl.0000286959.22040.6e.

Selwood, A,. K. Johnston, C. Katona, C. Lyketsos, and G. Livingston. 2007. "Systematic Review of the Effect of Psychological Interventions on Family Caregivers of People with Dementia. *Journal of Affective Disorders* 101 (1–3): 75–89.

Semah, F., M. C. Picot, C. Adam, D. Broglin, A. Arzimanoglou, and others. 1998. "Is the Underlying Cause of Epilepsy a Major Prognostic Factor for Recurrence?" *Neurology* 51 (5): 1256–62.

Silberstein, S. D., S. Holland, F. Freitag, D. W. Dodick, C. Argoff, and E. Ashman. 2012. "Quality Standards Subcommittee of the American Academy of Neurology and the American Headache Society. Evidence-Based Guideline Update: Pharmacologic Treatment for Episodic Migraine Prevention in Adults: Report of the Quality Standards Subcommittee of the American Academy of Neurology and the American Headache Society." *Neurology* 78 (17): 1337–45. doi:10.1212/WNL.0b013e3182535d20.

Sköldunger, A., K. Johnell, B. Winblad, and A. Wimo. 2013. "Mortality and Treatment Costs Have a Great Impact on the Cost-Effectiveness of Disease Modifying Treatment in Alzheimer's Disease: A Simulation Study." *Current Alzheimer Research* 10 (2): 207–16.

Steiner, T. J., F. Antonaci, R. Jensen, M. J. A. Lainez, M. Lanteri-Minet, and others. 2011. "Recommendations for Headache Service Organisation and Delivery in Europe." *Journal of Headache Pain* 12 (4): 419–26.

Steiner, T. J., G. L. Birbeck, R. H. Jensen, Z. Katsarava, L. J. Stovner, and P. Martelletti. 2015. "Headache Disorders Are Third Cause of Disability Worldwide." *Journal of Headache Pain* 6: 58. doi:10.1186/s10194-015-0544-2.

Steiner, T. J., and P. Martelletti 2007. "Aids for Management of Common Headache Disorders in Primary Care." *Journal of Headache Pain* (Suppl. 1): S2.

Steiner, T. J., K. Paemeleire, R. Jensen, D. Valade, L. Savi, and others. 2007. "European Principles of Management of Common Headache Disorders in Primary Care." *Journal of Headache Pain* 8 (Suppl. 1): S3–47.

Stovner, L., K. Hagen, R. Jensen, Z. Katsarava, R. Lipton, and others. 2007. "The Global Burden of Headache: A Documentation of Headache Prevalence and Disability Worldwide." *Cephalalgia* 27 (3): 193–210.

Tam-Tham, H., M. Cepoiu-Martin, P. E. Ronksley, C. J. Maxwell, and B. R. Hemmelgarn. 2013. "Dementia Case Management and Risk of Long-Term Care Placement: A Systematic Review and Meta-Analysis." *International Journal of Geriatric Psychiatry* 28 (9): 889–902.

Tan, L., L. Tan, H. F. Wang, J. Wang, C. C. Tan, and others. 2015. "Efficacy and Safety of Atypical Antipsychotic Drug Treatment for Dementia: A Systematic Review and Meta-Analysis." *Alzheimer's Research and Therapy* 7 (1): 20. doi:10.1186/s13195-015-0102-9.

Tanner, J. A., B. S. Black, D. Johnston, E. Hess, J. M. Leoutsakos, and others. 2015. "A Randomized Controlled Trial of a Community-Based Dementia Care Coordination Intervention: Effects of MIND at Home on Caregiver Outcomes." *American Journal of Geriatric Psychiatry* 23 (4): 391–402. doi:10.1016/j.jagp.2014.08.00.

Van Mierlo, L. D., F. J. Meiland, H. G. Van der Roest, and R. M. Droes. 2012. "Personalised Caregiver Support: Effectiveness of Psychosocial Interventions in Subgroups of Caregivers of People with Dementia." *International Journal of Psychiatry* 27 (1): 1–14. doi:10.1002/gps.2694. Epub 2011.

Vos, T., A. D. Flaxman, M. Naghavi, R. Lozano, C. Michaud, and others. 2012. "Years Lived with Disability (YLDs) for 1160 Sequelae of 289 Diseases and Injuries 1990–2010: A Systematic Analysis for the Global Burden of Disease Study 2010." *The Lancet* 380 (9859): 2163–96. doi:10.1016/S0140-6736(12)61729-2.

Westergaard, M. L., E. H. Hansen, C. Glümer, J. Olessen, and R. H. Jensen. 2014. "Definitions of Medication-Overuse Headache in Healthy Lifestyle Behaviour and Stress in Chronic Headache: Results from a Population-Based Studies and Their Implications in Prevalence Estimates: A Systematic Review." *Cephalalgia* 34: 409–25.

WHO (World Health Organization). 2004. *Atlas: Country Resources for Neurological Disorders.* Geneva: WHO.

———. 2006. *Neurological Disorders: Public Health Challenges.* Geneva: WHO.

———. 2009a. *Report of the WHO Expert Consultation on Foodborne Trematode Infections and Taeniasis/Cysticercosis.* Geneva: WHO.

———. 2009b. *mhGAP Intervention Guide for Mental, Neurological, and Substance Use Disorders in Non-Specialized Health Settings.* Geneva: WHO.

———. 2011. *Lifting the Burden: The Global Campaign to Reduce the Burden of Headache.* Geneva: WHO.

———. 2012. *Dementia-A Public Health Priority.* Geneva: WHO.

———. 2013. http://www.who.int/selection_medicines/committees/expert/20/EML_2015_FINAL_amended_AUG2015.pdf?ua=1.

———. 2015. *First WHO Ministerial Conference on Global Action Against Dementia.* Geneva: WHO.

Wiebe, S., and N. Jette. 2012. "Pharmacoresistance and the Role of Surgery in Difficult to Treat Epilepsy." *Nature Reviews. Neurology* 8 (12): 669–77. doi:10.1038/nrneurol. 2012.181.

Wimo, A., B. Winblad, A. Stoffler, Y. Wirth, and H J. Mobius. 2003. "Resource Utilisation and Cost Analysis of Memantine in Patients with Moderate to Severe Alzheimer's Disease." *Pharmacoeconomics* 21 (5): 327–50.

Wohlgemut, J., C. Dewey, M. Levy, and F. Mutua. 2010. "Evaluating the Efficacy of Teaching Methods Regarding Prevention of Human Epilepsy Caused by Taenia Solium Neurocysticercosis in Western Kenya." *American Journal of Tropical Medicine and Hygiene* 82 (4): 634–42. doi:10.4269/ajtmh.2010.09-0404.

Wong, C. L., N. Bansback, P. E. Lee, and A. H. Anis. 2009. "Cost-Effectiveness: Cholinesterase Inhibitors and Memantine in Vascular Dementia." *Canadian Journal of Neurological Sciences* 36 (6): 735–39.

Woods, B., E. Aguirre, A. E. Spector, and M. Orrell. 2012. "Cognitive Stimulation to Improve Cognitive Functioning in People with Dementia." *Cochrane Database of Systematic Reviews* 2: CD005562. PubMed PMID:22336813.

Woods, B., A. Spector, C. Jones, M. Orrell, and S. Davies. 2005. "Reminiscence Therapy for Dementia." *Cochrane Database of Systematic Reviews* (2): CD001120.

Yu, S. Y., T. J. Lee, S. H. Jang, J. W. Han, T. H. Kim, and K. W. Kim. 2015. "Cost-Effectiveness of Nationwide Opportunistic Screening Program for Dementia in South Korea." *Journal of Alzheimer's Disease* 44 (1): 195–204. doi:10.3233/JAD-141632.

Yu, S., M Zhang, J. Zhou, R. Liu, Q. Wan, and Y. Li. 2014. "Headache Care in China." *Headache* 54: 601–09.

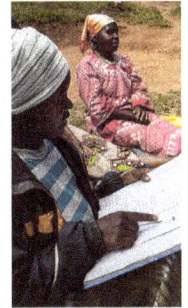

Chapter **6**

Illicit Drug Dependence

Louisa Degenhardt, Emily Stockings, John Strang,
John Marsden, and Wayne D. Hall

INTRODUCTION

In 2012, by various estimates, 165 million to 315 million people ages 15–64 years worldwide used illicit drugs, including those in the following categories (UNODC 2013):[1]

- *Cannabis products.* Marijuana, hashish, and bhang are the most widely used drugs, with an estimated 181 million users (129 million to 230 million) constituting 3.9 percent of the global population ages 15–64 years.
- *Amphetamine-type stimulants (ATSs).* The next most widely used illicit drugs are stimulants such as cocaine; methamphetamine; drugs with stimulant and hallucinogenic properties, such as MDMA (3,4-methylenedioxy-N-methylamphetamine), or ecstasy; and novel psychoactive substances,[2] with an estimated 34 million users worldwide (14 million to 53 million), including 17 million cocaine users (14 million to 21 million), and 20 million MDMA users (10 million to 29 million).
- *Illicit opioids.* An estimated 17 million persons use heroin or opium; 32 million use any illicit opioid, including diverted pharmaceutical opioids, such as methadone or morphine (28 million to 36 million).

Scope of the Chapter

This chapter is concerned with cannabis, amphetamine, and opioid dependence. The chapter identifies disease control priorities for illicit drug dependence in low- and middle-income countries (LMICs). First, we describe patterns of dependence and the disease burden (mortality, morbidity, and societal economic costs) attributable to dependence, by global region. Second, we summarize evidence on the effectiveness of interventions to reduce illicit drug dependence and the harm caused by such dependence. Finally, we consider the extent to which research on illicit drug dependence in high-income countries (HICs) is relevant to disease control priorities in LMICs.

In undertaking the reviews for this chapter, we relied on previous systematic reviews of the epidemiology of drug use, dependence, and health consequences (Degenhardt and Hall 2012), many of which were conducted for the Global Burden of Disease (GBD) 2010 study (Degenhardt, Whiteford, and others 2013). Our review of interventions drew heavily on our previous work reviewing effective interventions for illicit drug use and dependence (Strang and others 2012). We updated these with a review-of-reviews approach, whereby we conducted a systematic review of reviews of interventions to address illicit drug use and dependence.

Definition of Illicit Drug Dependence

The health risks of illicit drug use increase with the frequency and quantity of use and route of administration. The International Classification of Diseases (ICD) defines *harmful use* if there is evidence that substance use is causing physical or psychological harm; it defines

Corresponding author: Louisa Degenhardt, Ph.D., National Drug and Alcohol Research Centre, UNSW Australia, l.degenhardt@unsw.edu.au.

drug dependence if three or more indicators of dependence are present for at least one month within the past year (WHO 1993).

The *Diagnostic and Statistical Manual of Mental Disorders, 4th edition (DSM-4)* used a similar classification for *substance abuse* and *substance dependence* (APA 2000). However, the fifth edition *(DSM-5)* defines a *substance use disorder* if two of 11 criteria grouped under impaired control, social impairment, risky use, and pharmacological dependence are present; it categorizes the severity along a continuum of mild, moderate, and severe disorders, based on the number of criteria present (APA 2013).

NATURAL HISTORY OF DEPENDENCE

Onset of illicit drug use typically occurs in the mid- to late teens and peaks in the early to late 20s; few users continue beyond age 40 years (Degenhardt, Whiteford, and others 2013). The percentage of illicit drug users who transit from use to dependence ranges from 9 percent for cannabis to 20–25 percent for users of psychostimulants and heroin (Lopez-Quintero and others 2011). Cannabis use accounts for 80 percent of illicit drug use worldwide; the dependence risk is lower, and the morbidity attributable to its use is smaller, than for other drugs (Degenhardt, Whiteford, and others 2013).

The lag time from illicit drug use to dependence is shorter than that observed for substances such as nicotine and alcohol (Behrendt and others 2009). Dependence can occur within 1.5–2 years of cocaine and opioid use and within three years of cannabis use (Florez-Salamanca and others 2013; Wu and others 2011).

The 2010 rates of cannabis and opioid dependence were higher in HICs than LMICs; cocaine use and dependence rates were highest in North America and tropical and southern Latin America (Degenhardt, Bucello, Calabria, and others 2011). Amphetamine dependence rates, however, appear to be highest in Southeast Asia and Australasia (Degenhardt, Baxter, and others 2014).

Risk Factors

Risk factors often coexist and are similar across the different categories of illicit drugs, as well as across global regions (Degenhardt and others 2010):

- *Social and contextual factors:* low socioeconomic status, early substance-use onset, and social norms that are tolerant of alcohol and other drug use

- *Family factors:* poor quality of parent-child interaction and relationships, parental conflict, and parental and sibling drug use
- *Individual factors:* male gender; having an externalizing disorder, such as attention-deficit hyperactivity disorder or conduct disorders in early childhood; sensation- and novelty-seeking personality traits; and low education levels
- *Peer group factors:* association with antisocial or drug-dependent peers, which is one of the strongest risk factors for illicit drug dependence in adolescence and which operates independently of social, contextual, family, and individual factors.

Consequences

Mortality

Mortality rates for heavy users of opioids, amphetamines, and cocaine are 3–14 times higher across the lifespan than for the general population (Degenhardt, Bucello, Mathers, and others 2011; Stenbacka, Leifman, and Romelsjo 2010). In 2011, an estimated 211,000 people died from drug-related causes, mostly younger users whose deaths were primarily preventable (UNODC 2013).

Based on the type of drug dependence, studies have found the following risk correlations:

- *Heroin.* Long-term heroin users have a substantially increased risk of premature death from drug overdose, violence, suicide, and alcohol-related causes (Degenhardt, Charlson, and others 2014).
- *Amphetamines.* Amphetamine-related deaths typically are associated with cardiac failure and cerebral vascular accidents (Darke and others 2008).
- *Cocaine.* Cocaine dependence is associated with elevated risks of intentional and accidental injuries (Blow and others 2011). Cocaine-related deaths are usually related to cardiovascular complications, brain hemorrhage, stroke, and kidney failure (Restrepo and others 2009).
- *Cannabis.* Cannabis dependence is associated with significant disability burden, including the precipitation of psychosis in vulnerable people (Bloomfield and others 2013).

HIV and Hepatitis Infection

In 2010, injecting drug use accounted for almost two million years of life lost (YLLs) globally as a risk from HIV infection (Degenhardt, Whiteford, and others 2013). Injecting drug use has been a major driver of HIV epidemics in LMICs (Mathers and others 2010).

Hepatitis B and C infection is highly prevalent globally among people who inject drugs (Nelson and others 2011). Chronic infection occurs in 75 percent of infections, and 3–11 percent of chronic hepatitis C virus (HCV) carriers develop liver cirrhosis within 20 years. The risk of HIV and hepatitis C infection is elevated among non-injecting drug users; psychostimulants such as crack cocaine and amphetamine disinhibit users and facilitate riskier sexual activity and increase the risk of HIV infection (Volkow and others 2007). Among men who have sex with men, amphetamines (specifically, crystal methamphetamine) may be used to enhance sexual encounters, increasing the risk of HIV infection from unprotected anal intercourse (Rajasingham and others 2012).

Criminal Activity

The relatively few adults who become dependent on heroin have a disproportionate criminal impact on their communities. The average heroin user engages in criminal behavior 40–60 percent of the time that he or she is not incarcerated or in treatment (Ball, Shaffer, and Nurco 1983); the most common offenses include drug dealing and property crimes (Degenhardt, Larney, and others 2013).

Economic Losses

The production, distribution, and consumption of illicit drugs result in significant economic costs affecting consumers, families, industries, societies, and governments. For example, there is a strong correlation between unemployment and drug use in HICs and LMICs. Illicit drug use limits the affected individuals' chances of entering or remaining in the workforce and is linked to low productivity and accidents. Drug-taking employees in the United States are absent three times more often, are three to four times more likely to be involved in a workplace accident, and file approximately five times more workers' compensation claims than non-drug-taking employees (UNDCP 1998). There are opportunity costs of the expenditures used to treat illicit drug dependence, prevent crime, enforce laws, and process drug-dependent offenders in the judicial system. For example, the economic cost of drug abuse was estimated at 2 percent of gross domestic product in Australia (Collins and Lapsley 2007).

Trends

Global trends are difficult to estimate because drug use is routinely tracked only in a minority of HICs; assessments of trends in other countries often rely on indirect indicators, such as law enforcement data on drug seizures, demand for treatment, and overdose deaths.

Consumption Trends

Despite reported increases in the global number of illicit substance users, other indicators such as area under drug cultivation, production, manufacture, and seizures suggest that consumption (about 167 million to 315 million users) has remained relatively stable since 2010 (UNODC 2013). The illicit market for ATSs appears to be growing, with global increases in seizures, particularly in Africa and Mexico (see UNODC 2013). Cocaine markets appear to be shifting from the United States and Western Europe to Asia. Heroin availability, use, and overdose also appear to be increasing in Asia and East and West Africa and the United States. Afghanistan saw large increases in heroin availability and an increased net cultivation of 36 percent from 2012 to 2013, and a 140 percent increase in estimated regular users from 2005 to 2009 (UNODC 2009).

Of particular concern is the large increase in dependence on pharmaceutical opioids, such as oxycodone, methadone, hydrocodone, and fentanyl. In the United States, the annual incidence of pharmaceutical opioid abuse rose by almost 300 percent from 1990 (628,000 initiates) to 2001 (2.4 million) (U.S. Department of Health and Human Services 2012); treatment admissions and death rates due to overdose increased from 1999 to 2008 (CDC 2012). Similarly large increases in pharmaceutical opioid prescriptions and abuse have been reported in Australia, Estonia, Finland, and New Zealand (UNODC 2013).

Burden of Disease Trends

The GBD 2010 study found that disability-adjusted life years (DALYs) from drug use disorders rose 52 percent, from 13.1 million in 1990 to 20.0 million in 2010 (Degenhardt, Whiteford, and others 2013). Population growth accounted for 28 percent and increased prevalence for 22 percent of the increase in this period. The overall opioid dependence burden increased by 74 percent from 1990 to 2010, amounting to almost four million additional DALYs in 2010 (Degenhardt, Charlson, and others 2014). Much of the drug-related increase in DALYs can be attributed to population growth; one exception is opioid dependence, in which 56 percent of the total increase in DALYs was attributable to increased prevalence.

INTERVENTIONS AND POLICIES: EFFECTIVENESS AND COVERAGE

Research on the effectiveness and cost-effectiveness of policies and interventions for control of illicit drug use has varied in quantity and quality and largely comes from a few HICs, although recent research has assessed these interventions in LMICs.

Population Platform Interventions

Interventions to reduce the availability of illicit drugs and discourage their use include legal and regulatory approaches, such as prohibitions on the manufacture, sale, and use of opioid drugs for nonmedical purposes; law enforcement of these sanctions through fines and imprisonment; and restricted availability of medically prescribed drugs, such as opioids, to prevent their diversion to the black market. Interventions to increase public health and awareness include educational campaigns, delivered via the mass media or school-based drug education programs, about the health risks of drug use (table 6.1).

Control of the Supply of Illicit Drugs

Precursor Chemical Control. Precursor chemical regulation has produced some major supply interruptions (Cunningham, Liu, and Callaghan 2013).[3] However, the impacts are not always predictable, and drug supply interruptions have been relatively short lived (ONDCP 2008).

Law Enforcement. The most popular interventions in many countries have been law enforcement approaches focusing on drug interdiction and enforcement of sanctions against the possession, use, and sale of illicit drugs

(Strang and others 2012). Although there is limited evidence on the effectiveness of these expensive strategies (Kuziemko and Levitt 2004), these interventions work to reduce drug use and harm, including fatal and nonfatal heroin overdoses (Day and others 2004), as well as drug-related emergency room visits (Dave 2006), by increasing the price of illicit drugs. Alternative development programs in source countries do not seem to reduce availability or increase prices in destination countries (Babor and others 2010).

However, supply interruptions often arise from a convergence of circumstances that is difficult to reproduce by design in different regions and drug markets. Accordingly, it is difficult to assess the cost-effectiveness of supply reduction via expensive, high-level law enforcement strategies (Shanahan, Degenhardt, and Hall 2004). Nor have street-level law enforcement activities proven effective in the long run, as the markets are usually displaced elsewhere, causing more harm to some groups of drug users. For example, heroin shortages have been linked with marked increases in cocaine and amphetamine injection and incident HCV infection (Strang and others 2012).

Prescription Monitoring Programs. The evidence on control of pharmaceutical opioid misuse has been dominated by HICs. Control of pharmaceutical opioid misuse

Table 6.1 Summary of Population Platforms and Recommended Interventions for Illicit Drug Dependence

Universal prevention and health promotion	Evidence level	CEA available?	Notes
Legislation and regulation			
Precursor chemical control	May be effective	No	Some impact, short-term; some consequences difficult to predict
High-level law enforcement	May be effective	No	Difficult to know if or when effect will occur; may be short-lived
Street-level law enforcement	Inconclusive	No	May have short-term, localized effect but leads to compensatory increases elsewhere
Prescription monitoring programs	May be effective	No	Poorly studied to date; may have some impact, although misuse of other medications may occur
Information and awareness			
Mass media campaigns	Inconclusive	No	Limited research with inconsistent results, with some showing negative and others positive impacts on drug attitudes and use
Intersector collaboration			
Imprisonment	Inconclusive	No	No evidence suggesting drug use is reduced on release, although decreased use during imprisonment
Drug testing for offenders	May be effective	No	Encouraging observational evidence from U.S. states where this has been introduced
Court-mandated treatment	Inconclusive	No	Includes mandated treatment and drug courts

Note: CEA = cost-effectiveness analysis.

likely differs in LMICs, where opioids such as morphine are less readily available because of excessive enforcement of regulations to prevent their misuse. HICs have attempted to reduce increases in the use, misuse, and diversion of pharmaceutical opioids by implementing controlled-substance laws, prescription monitoring systems, and clinical guidelines against overprescribing (Compton and Volkow 2006).

However, extramedical users may obtain pharmaceutical opioids in several ways, for example, doctor shopping, informal sharing and trading of medications between peers and family members (Fischer, Bibby, and Bouchard 2010), larger-scale diversion via thefts (Inciardi and others 2007), and proliferation of online pharmacies (Littlejohn and others 2005) that limit the beneficial effects of prescription systems. Restrictions on one class of prescription drug may increase the use of another class; these measures can also restrict access by those who have a legitimate medical need for them (Strang and others 2012).

Public Awareness Campaigns
Populationwide mass media campaigns to deliver information and expand public awareness have not had consistent impacts on use (Ferri and others 2013; Wakefield, Loken, and Hornik 2010).

Criminal Justice Platforms
Imprisonment. One consequence of the focus on law enforcement is that imprisonment for drug or property offenses is the most common intervention (Strang and others 2012). Although imprisonment is not an effective way to reduce drug dependence (Manski, Pepper, and Petrie 2001), constructive health interventions, such as hepatitis B vaccinations, can be provided in this setting (Farrell, Strang, and Stover 2010).

Studies examining the effect of cannabis decriminalization (Room and others 2010) have been methodologically weak, often simply comparing the prevalence of cannabis use before and after changes in the law. This area remains controversial; only weak evidence exists that tougher sanctions reduce either criminal offending in general or drug use in particular (Strang and others 2012).

Drug Testing of Offenders. Research has yielded increasing evidence that sure, immediate, and modest sanctions for positive drug tests substantially reduce drug use among individuals under criminal justice supervision (Kleiman 2009), but controlled evaluations have been limited. Typically, this evidence applies to offenders who have been released into the community before trial or who are on probation or parole, and sanctions can include 24 hours of imprisonment.

Court-Mandated Treatment. Court-mandated treatment refers to treatment entered under legal coercion by persons who have been charged with or convicted of an offense to which their drug dependence has contributed. Such treatment is most often provided as an alternative to imprisonment—and usually with the threat of imprisonment if the person fails to comply with treatment (Hall, Farrell, and Carter 2014).

Research into the effectiveness of court-mandated treatment is largely limited to observational studies in the United States of offenders entering treatment under various forms of legal coercion, including methadone maintenance treatment (MMT). Early evidence of the effectiveness of such treatment comes from a study in the United States that showed that among illicit drug offenders, a much greater reduction in heroin use and substantially lower incarceration rates were found among those enrolled in opioid substitution therapy (OST) in the year after release from prison (Dole and others 1969). Some more recent observational studies support these findings (Anglin 1988; Young, Fluellen, and Belenko 2004), but others do not (Klag, O'Callaghan, and Creed 2005).

Formal drug courts are another alternative to suspended sentences or diversion programs; in the short term, they can reduce future criminal offending and drug use more than conventional courts. However, few randomized controlled trials have been conducted to evaluate these (Brown 2010), and there are few studies of the costs and cost-effectiveness of any of these criminal justice interventions. Of the 69 relevant studies conducted in Australia and the United States between 1980 and 2004 (Perry and others 2009), only one reported cost-effectiveness data (Schoenwald and others 1996), suggesting that the cost of treatment was nearly offset by the savings incurred by reducing days incarcerated.

Community Platform Interventions
Workplace Drug Testing
Drug testing has been increasingly used in workplace settings, such as athletics, criminal justice, mining, the military, government agencies, and health services. Urine sampling is considered the gold standard (Phan and others 2012) because of the accuracy, speed, ease of administration, and limited invasiveness required. There have been limited evaluations of the impact of mandatory drug testing in the workplace; some supportive

evidence is available from programs in the United States that have used drug testing with doctors and airline pilots (DuPont and others 2009).

School-Based Prevention Programs

Schools provide a popular setting for prevention programs, because of the ready access to young adults and the ease of intervention delivery. Evidence of the effectiveness of school-based interventions varies widely. Reviews of randomized controlled evaluations suggest that psychosocial interventions may have some benefit (Faggiano and others 2014), but no evidence indicates that interventions that only target knowledge and awareness of negative consequences of illicit drug use are effective (Strang and others 2012).

Drug Education. An example of a widely used but ineffective drug education program in the United States was the Drug Abuse Resistance Education (DARE) program, in which police officers gave classroom advice on the dangers of drug use. Rigorous study showed that DARE neither prevented nor delayed drug use (Ennett and others 1994). Similarly, evaluation of a populationwide mass media campaign targeted at youths ages 9–18 years to prevent cannabis use also showed that it had no effect and possibly increased use (Hornik and others 2008).

Skills Training. School-based interventions targeting social skills are effective in reducing drug use and have positive effects in other domains, including reducing internalizing and externalizing disorders.[4] The Strengthening Families Program, targeting youths ages 10–14 years and their parents, is an evidence-based family skills training program that has been shown to reduce drug abuse and other problem behaviors (Strang and others 2012). The Good Behavior Game, a classroom behavior management approach for children ages 5–7 years that originated in the United States and that has been tested worldwide, has shown positive outcomes up to 15 years after the intervention (Kellam, Reid, and Balster 2008). Economic analyses suggest that these early-age interventions are cost-effective because substantial lifetime benefits are realized from even modestly lower rates of early drug or alcohol use (Caulkins and others 2002).

Early Intervention with At-Risk Youth. There is limited, low-quality, and inconsistent evidence about the effectiveness of school-based drug testing among high school students (Shek 2010). The evidence on the impact of psychosocial interventions for young people using substances or at risk of doing so is limited and inconsistent (Strang and others 2012).

Self-Help and Mutual Aid Groups

Self-help and mutual aid groups are run by recovering drug users, typically using adaptations of the 12-step principles of Alcoholics Anonymous. The groups include Narcotics Anonymous, Cocaine Anonymous, and Marijuana Anonymous. A mutual aid approach called Self-Management and Recovery Training (SMART Recovery) offers an alternative choice for group-based rehabilitation without the 12-step approach, especially for those who are either unwilling or unable to use 12-step groups (Horvath 2000).

Some individuals use these groups as their sole support for abstinence; others use them in combination with professional counseling and other strategies (Freimuth 2000). Although self-help is probably the most common type of intervention delivered globally for drug abuse, until recently there have been few scientific studies of its effectiveness. Observational and quasi-experimental evidence suggests that participation in Narcotics Anonymous is associated with continued abstinence, lower health care costs, and improvement in other areas of functioning (Gossop, Stewart, and Marsden 2008; Strang and others 2012) (table 6.2).

Health Care Platform Interventions

Community-Level Care

Community-based strategies can potentially reduce harms related to illicit drug use, especially blood-borne virus (BBV) transmission and opioid overdoses. These strategies include OST, overdose prevention education, emergency response education, and supervised injecting facilities (SIFs) (table 6.3).

Access to Treatment. Consistent evidence from observational studies and randomized trials shows that the risk of death from overdose is substantially reduced in individuals while they receive OST compared with their risk when not receiving OST (Degenhardt, Bucello, Mathers, and others 2011). Maximizing OST provision to drug users in the community, in prison (Larney, Gisev, and others 2014), and after release from prison (Degenhardt, Larney, and others 2014) will have demonstrable population-level effects on overdose mortality.

Overdose Prevention Education. Polydrug use increases the chances of fatal overdose, particularly the concurrent use of opioids and other drugs that depress the central nervous system, like benzodiazepine and alcohol (Warner-Smith and others 2001). Educating people who use opioids, particularly by injection, about these dangers and the risks of injecting alone or on the

Table 6.2 Summary of Community Platforms and Recommended Interventions for Illicit Drug Dependence

Selective prevention and health promotion, by platform	Evidence level	CEA available?	Notes
Workplaces			
Drug testing	Limited	No	Evidence from programs for employees with identified substance use problems
Schools			
Drug testing	Inconclusive	No	Inconsistent, poor evidence
Drug education	Sufficient	No	Not effective; substance use possibly even increased
Skills and psychosocial interventions with primary school children	Sufficient	Yes	Strengthening Families Program
			Good Behavior Game: long-term effects up to 15 years post-intervention
Skills training with adolescents	Inconclusive	No	Short-term effects at best; no effect found by some studies
Early intervention with at-risk youth	Limited	No	Limited, low-quality evidence with inconsistent findings; small, short-term effects found by some studies, but no effects found by others
Community			
Self-help groups	Limited	No	Narcotics Anonymous, Cocaine Anonymous, Marijuana Anonymous, SMART Recovery (amphetamines): limited RCT evidence and selection bias likely in observational studies

Note: CEA = cost-effectiveness analysis; RCT = randomized controlled trial; SMART Recovery = Self-Management and Recovery Training.

streets, where assistance in case of overdose is limited, might reduce the risk of overdose (McGregor and others 2001).[5] However, the effectiveness of these strategies has not been rigorously evaluated.

Naloxone and Other Emergency Responses. Another strategy is to improve bystander responses to opioid overdoses by encouraging drug users who witness overdoses to seek medical assistance and use simple but effective resuscitation techniques until help arrives (Wagner and others 2010). This approach includes the distribution of naloxone to opioid injectors and their peers. Naloxone is a narcotic antagonist that rapidly reverses the effects of acute narcosis, including respiratory depression, sedation, and hypotension.[6] An increasing number of jurisdictions have been implementing such programs, although evaluations have largely been observational (Tobin and others 2009).

Supervised Injecting Facilities. SIFs are located in areas where injecting drug users are concentrated, typically in areas with large, open drug markets. The goal is to reduce drug overdose deaths and BBV infections among injectors who inject in public places. SIFs have potential community impact but exist in a limited number of locations, only 61 cities in eight countries (Hedrich, Kerr, and Dubois-Arber 2010; Kerr and others 2007).

Although models differ, all SIFs provide sterile injecting equipment and a hygienic environment where pre-obtained drugs can be injected.

Observational evaluations in Vancouver and Sydney have suggested that SIFs attract risky injectors, facilitate safe-injection education, reduce syringe sharing, and increase referral and entry into withdrawal management and drug treatment. Although reviews suggest that drug use does not change among clients or among drug injectors in the areas where SIFs are located (Kerr and others 2007; MSIC Evaluation Committee 2003), the evidence of their impact on HIV transmission is uncertain (Kimber and others 2010). However, reducing the risk among the most vulnerable injecting drug users may increase the effectiveness of other interventions.

Primary Health Care
Screening and Brief Intervention. Some evidence suggests that a single brief intervention in a clinical setting can reduce illicit drug use (Baker and others 2005; Humeniuk and others 2012), although a recent systematic review concluded that further studies were needed (Young and others 2014). Brief interventions from prescribers, such as tailored written letters to patients or consultations, reduced heavy benzodiazepine use up to six months after intervention (Mugunthan, McGuire, and Glasziou 2011).

Table 6.3 Summary of Health and Social Care Interventions and Recommendations for Illicit Drug Dependence

Intervention, by platform	Evidence level	CEA available?	Notes
Community-based care			
Emergency naloxone provision (opioid overdose)	Limited	No	Becoming increasingly implemented, but evidence limited to observational evaluation
Supervised injecting facilities	Limited	No	No clear impact on drug use per se (not the intent)
Primary health care			
Screening and brief intervention	Limited	No	Some evidence of short-term reduction in drug use, but further studies needed
Specialist health care			
Detoxification and withdrawal	Limited	No	Not effective as stand-alone postwithdrawal treatment
Naltrexone-accelerated withdrawal alone	Limited	No	Not effective as stand-alone postwithdrawal treatment
Medication for cannabis withdrawal alone	Limited	No	Reduces withdrawal symptoms; no difference in long-term reduction in cannabis use
Residential rehabilitation	Limited	No	Some level II and III studies[a]
Brief psychological intervention			
CBT for cannabis dependence	Sufficient	No	Short-term, modest impact
CBT for opioid dependence	Sufficient	No	As an adjunct to OST
CBT for psychostimulant dependence	Sufficient	No	Short-term, modest impact
Acupuncture	Inconclusive	No	Low-quality studies; no clear evidence of effect (cocaine and opioid dependence)
Medications for heroin and other opioid dependence			
BMT	Sufficient	Yes	Reduces risk of overdose and opioid use
MMT	Sufficient	Yes	Reduces risk of overdose and opioid use
HMT	Sufficient	No	Expensive; not first-line OST
Oral naltrexone	Sufficient	No	Effectiveness limited by poor adherence
Implant or sustained-release naltrexone	Limited	No	Potential for improved adherence, but insufficient evidence
Medications for cannabis dependence	Limited	No	Some limited benefits identified with symptomatic medications; preliminary evidence for cannabis antagonists
Medications for cocaine dependence	Sufficient	No	Not efficacious
Medications for psychostimulant dependence	Sufficient	No	Weak efficacy in trials; no evidence of effectiveness

Note: BMT = buprenorphine maintenance treatment; CBT = cognitive behavioral therapy; CEA = cost-effectiveness analysis; HMT = supervised injectable heroin maintenance treatment; MMT = methadone maintenance treatment; OST = opioid substitution therapy.

a. Level II studies refer to randomized controlled trials; level III studies refer to well-designed, pseudo-randomized controlled trials, cohort studies, case-control studies, or interrupted time-series studies.

Specialist Health Care

Detoxification and Withdrawal. Detoxification centers provide supervised withdrawal from a drug of dependence with the aim of minimizing the severity of withdrawal symptoms. Detoxification is not a treatment, but it is the intervention that dependent users seek most often. It provides users with a respite from use, an occasion to reconsider their drug use, and a potential prelude to abstinence-based treatment. Detoxification has minimal, if any, enduring impact on dependence on its own (Mattick and Hall 1996).

Residential Rehabilitation. Residential rehabilitation can be a therapeutic community (TC) model that typically involves residency for six months and a 12-step approach, often after 28 days of residential treatment followed by community engagement in a network of 12-step groups or a faith-based approach (for example, Christian rehabilitation houses), with the aim of abstinence from all opioid and other illicit drugs. These approaches often encourage patients to become involved in self-help groups, such as Narcotics Anonymous. They use group and psychological interventions to help users remain abstinent.

There have been few successful randomized controlled trials for TCs or outpatient drug counseling (Vanderplasschen and others 2013). TCs are more demanding of drug users and are less successful than OST in attracting and retaining drug users in treatment. Nevertheless, TCs substantially reduce drug use and crime in those who remain in treatment for at least three months (Smith, Gates, and Foxcroft 2006). TCs may be more effective if they are used in combination with legal coercion to ensure that drug users stay in treatment long enough to benefit from it (Gerstein and Harwood 1990).

Psychosocial Interventions.

Brief Intervention. Brief interventions have been found to be effective when provided through outreach services, such as needle and syringe programs. Behavioral family- and couple-based interventions have produced better abstinence rates in treatment and at follow-up (Strang and others 2012).

Cognitive Behavioral Therapy. Cognitive behavioral therapy, particularly short-term treatments provided in three to six outpatient sessions, have resulted in modest abstinence rates of 20–40 percent at the end of treatment, but high relapse rates and more modest abstinence rates after 12 months. Psychosocial treatments for cocaine and amphetamine dependence have limited effectiveness and high rates of relapse after treatment (NICE 2007; Strang and others 2012).

Contingency Management. Contingency management is a behavioral reinforcement approach that uses incentives, such as vouchers or clinic benefits, to improve adherence to treatment and duration of abstinence (Budney and others 2006). The benefits of treatment depend on the magnitude of reward. This form of intervention may work best for people with more severe dependence on cocaine (Petry and others 2004). Contingency management also improves completion of hepatitis B vaccination among opioid-dependent people (Weaver and others 2014).

Medications for Heroin and Other Opioid Dependence.

Methadone Maintenance. Once-daily oral MMT is the most common form of drug substitution worldwide that is more effective than a placebo (Mattick and others 2014). Large observational studies have found that patients in MMT decreased their heroin use and criminal activity while in treatment. MMT substantially reduces HIV transmission through needle sharing, and it is the best-supported form of OST in terms of retention in treatment and reduction of heroin use (Gowing, Hickman, and Degenhardt 2013; Mattick and others 2014).

Buprenorphine Maintenance. Buprenorphine is a mixed agonist-antagonist opioid receptor modulator that has partial agonist effects similar to those of morphine while also blocking the effects of pure agonists like heroin. In high doses, its effects can last up to three days, and its antagonist effects substantially reduce the risk of overdose and abuse. Meta-analyses of controlled trials of buprenorphine have found it to be effective in the treatment of heroin dependence (Mattick and others 2014).

Morphine Maintenance. Other opioid medications have been used as OST medications with success, such as supervised OST with long-acting morphine (Mathers and others 2010).

Supervised Injectable Heroin Maintenance. Supervised injectable heroin maintenance treatment (HMT) has been evaluated in a series of trials as a second-line treatment for chronic heroin users who have repeatedly failed to respond to oral forms of opioid maintenance. Reviews suggest that HMT can increase well-being and reduce heroin use and criminal activity; it may potentially reduce mortality. The risk of serious adverse events, however, means that HMT should be reserved for those who have failed in other treatments and should be provided under medical supervision (Ferri, Davoli, and Perucci 2011).

Naltrexone Maintenance. Naltrexone completely blocks the effects of any opiate, such as heroin. From a clinical perspective, however, oral naltrexone has been disappointing because of patient nonadherence (Minozzi and others 2011). This finding has led to two very different approaches to improving adherence: (a) behavioral strategies to improve adherence and the use of contingency management strategies, such as rewards for adherence, and (b) the development of long-acting naltrexone formulations (implant or slow-release injection). The evidence for the effectiveness of these approaches remains limited (Larney, Gowing, and others 2014).

Medications for Cannabis Dependence. No effective maintenance pharmacotherapies exist for cannabis dependence (Danovitch and Gorelick 2012); no pharmacotherapies have been approved for cannabis withdrawal. Only limited benefits are documented from trials of symptomatic medications, including antidepressants (Carpenter and others 2009); mood stabilizers, including lithium (Winstock, Lea, and Copeland 2009); and the α_2-adrenergic agonist lofexidine (Haney and others 2008).

Oral delivery of synthetic delta-9-tetrahydrocannabinol reduced a subset of cannabis withdrawal symptoms in laboratory (Haney and others 2004) and outpatient settings (Vandrey and others 2013). Nabiximols (Sativex), a cannabis agonist, has been found in a randomized controlled trial to significantly reduce the severity of cannabis withdrawal-related effects, including irritability, depression, and cannabis cravings, compared with a placebo (Allsop and others 2014).

Medications for Psychostimulant Dependence. Despite substantial investment in research, no effective pharmacological treatments have emerged for cocaine dependence (Amato and others 2011) or for amphetamine or methamphetamine dependence (Brensilver, Heinzerling, and Shoptaw 2013). Weak evidence indicates the efficacy of oral dexamphetamine maintenance (Galloway and others 2011; Longo and others 2010).

COST-EFFECTIVENESS OF INTERVENTIONS FOR ILLICIT DRUG DISORDERS

There is evidence of the cost-effectiveness of a few interventions (tables 6.1–6.3), but there is a paucity of information to support resource allocation to different drug policies. This lack of evidence can be attributed in part to challenges in identifying and measuring the costs and effects of supply-side strategies or policies, such as the high-level enforcement of sanctions against illicit drug possession, use, and sale (Shanahan, Degenhardt, and Hall 2004), or criminal justice interventions (NICE 2007). The paucity of information also mirrors the modest level of evidence on the cost-effectiveness of many of the interventions reviewed in this chapter. A final reason is the shortage of technical capacity to undertake these studies, particularly in LMICs.

Cost-effectiveness evidence is mainly available for substitution or maintenance treatment of opioid dependence using methadone or buprenorphine (Simoens and others 2006). One or two studies have also assessed the costs and consequences of school-based life skills programs on future illicit drug use (see, for example,

Caulkins and others 1999). Since these economic analyses have been conducted almost exclusively in HICs, their relevance to lower-resource contexts is limited. Nevertheless, the studies have demonstrated that these interventions represent reasonable value for money in these settings. In Australia, for example, MMT and buprenorphine maintenance treatment (BMT) were shown to produce increases in heroin-free days at an acceptable and not significantly different level of cost-effectiveness (Doran 2005; Harris, Gospodarevskaya, and Ritter 2005).

A cost-effectiveness analysis of MMT and BMT was conducted in LMICs as part of the second edition of *Disease Control Priorities in Developing Countries* (Hall and others 2006). This analysis found that MMT was a more cost-effective option than BMT, with a year of healthy life generated for less than US$1,000 in the lower prevalence settings (including Sub-Saharan Africa) and for US$1,000–US$10,000 elsewhere. In LMICs, where HIV is being spread by injecting drug users, MMT programs can be an effective and cost-effective strategy for prevention, as indicated in a study in Belarus, where the average cost per HIV infection averted was less than US$500 (Kumaranayake and others 2004).

IMPLICATIONS FOR LOW- AND MIDDLE-INCOME COUNTRIES

Most of the research on drug dependence, its disease burden, and its societal harm has been conducted in HICs. To translate these findings into disease control priorities for LMICs, we examine three sets of issues: country-specific variations in illicit drug use and disease burden, countries' health care infrastructure and capacity, and varying cultural attitudes toward drug problems and treatments.

Issues for Assessment

Illicit Drug Use and Disease Burden
Countries differ in the scale of illicit drug use and the disease burden. This variation may reflect differences in the prevalence of injecting versus non-injecting opioid and stimulant use; users' access to health services for treating overdoses, BBVs, and other complications of drug use; access to preventive interventions for HIV and other BBV infections, such as needle and syringe programs (Mathers and others 2010); and the extent to which illicit drug use is concentrated in socially disadvantaged groups. Many LMICs lack the research infrastructure to assess the use of illicit drugs and its harm and to evaluate the effectiveness of interventions.

Health Care Infrastructure and Capacity

Societal wealth and the extent of health care infrastructure affect the capacity of countries to respond to illicit drug dependence. For example, a country's capacity to provide OST is affected by the cost of opioid drugs and the nonexistence of infrastructure to deliver OST effectively and safely. This infrastructure would include, for example, specialist drug treatment centers; trained medical, nursing, and pharmacy staff; and a drug regulatory system. In HICs, the treatment delivery infrastructure includes medically trained staff and community-based pharmacists to prescribe and dispense these drugs and control systems for the distribution of substitute opioids that minimize diversion and illicit use. There is little evidence to suggest the level of minimal infrastructure necessary to deliver these treatments safely and effectively is available in LMICs.

Medical versus Moral Models of Addiction

A society's response to illicit drug use is affected by cultural attitudes and beliefs, including the dominant views on illicit drug use and the governing cultural images of drug dependence (Gerstein and Harwood 1990). A critical determinant is the relative dominance of moral and medical understandings of drug dependence.

A moral model of addiction sees drug use as largely voluntary and addiction as an excuse for bad behavior that allows drug users to continue without assuming responsibility for their conduct (Szasz 2003). According to the moral view, drug users who offend against the criminal code should be imprisoned (Szasz 2003). A medical model of addiction recognizes that some users lose control over their use and develop a mental or physical disorder—an addiction—that requires specific treatment to become and remain abstinent (Leshner 1997).

The competition between the medical and moral perspectives is not resolved in either HICs or LMICs. These competing views affect the societal preference for and acceptability of certain interventions, especially OST and abstinence-oriented approaches (Cohen 2003).

Research Needs

HICs and LMICs need better estimates of the prevalence of dependence. LMICs, in particular, need well-designed prospective studies of mortality and morbidity among illicit drug users, especially in countries with high rates of HIV infection and recent substantial increases in drug-related problems.

LMICs also need randomized controlled trials and economic and outcome evaluations of treatments for illicit drug dependence. Comparative data on efficacy and cost-effectiveness are essential to judge the applicability of findings in HICs to LMICs. The research needs to include LMIC-specific evaluation of a range of interventions, including self-help, abstinence-based approaches, and oral OST.

It is particularly important to assess the effectiveness and safety of treatment delivery modifications in LMICs that lack the quality of health care infrastructure found in HICs. Such studies may also identify novel and cheaper ways to deliver these treatments in lower-resource settings.

Potential New Treatments

New treatments and improved forms of existing treatments could improve the modest outcomes of treatment for illicit drug dependence. Technological advances are enabling researchers to develop ultra-long-acting implants or injectable depot formulations of drugs. These might overcome, at least in part, the major problem of poor medication adherence and dropout.

OST trials are exploring the potential for greater therapeutic gain using depot buprenorphine lasting at least a month, implant buprenorphine lasting at least six months, and ultra-long-lasting formulations of the opiate antagonist naltrexone as either depot injections (lasting a month) or implant (lasting several months).

Additional benefit might come from exploring existing medications or new formulations that are not yet widely considered in the addiction treatment field. For example, several European countries have prescribed slow-release morphine as an alternative opioid maintenance treatment.

Finally, health care providers could deliver existing treatments less expensively, thereby reaching a larger proportion of opioid-dependent people. Buprenorphine maintenance treatment is equally effective whether given in a first-level facility or a third-level facility in Australia (Gibson and others 2003).

CONCLUSIONS AND RECOMMENDATIONS

Illicit drug use contributes to premature mortality and morbidity on a global scale. The substantial economic costs include the health care costs of managing dependence; treating drug overdoses; and addressing the complications of BBV infections, such as HIV and hepatitis C. Illicit drug dependence also generates substantial externalities that the burden of disease estimates do not include, principally, high law enforcement costs in dealing with drug dealing, property crime, and loss of public amenities (such as clean, pleasant, and quality public infrastructure and environments).

The most popular interventions in HICs have involved law enforcement to interdict drug supply and arrest individuals for the possession, use, and sale of opioid drugs. Consequently, imprisonment for drug or property offenses is the primary intervention for most users. Treatment interventions hold the greatest promise for long-term effectiveness.

The most commonly available interventions for dependence have been medically supervised detoxification and drug-free (abstinence) approaches. OST is available in many countries, but coverage is typically poor (Mathers and others 2010). Opioid antagonists have a niche role in the maintenance treatment of opioid dependence, but suffer from poor compliance and probably increase the risk of overdose on return to heroin use. Their efficacy may improve with the development of long-acting depot formulations, but the evidence remains limited (Larney, Gowing, and others 2014; Lobmaier and others 2008).

Most of the limited research on the effectiveness and cost-effectiveness of interventions for illicit opioid dependence has been conducted in HICs. Three broad sets of issues affect the way in which these findings can be translated into disease control priorities in LMICs:

- Countries will differ in the scale of illicit drug use and the burden that it causes.
- Societal wealth and health care infrastructure will affect the capacity of LMIC societies to respond to illicit drug dependence.
- Countries' responses will be affected by cultural preferences for moral and medical understandings of drug dependence.

Multiple interventions have been shown to have an impact on illicit drug use and dependence, ranging from preventive interventions with young people to medication-assisted interventions with people who are opioid dependent. The challenge is to ensure that these efficacious interventions are delivered to scale, while minimizing the use of interventions that are not effective.

1. Illicit drugs are defined as those covered by international drug control treaties such as the Single Convention on Narcotic Drugs (United Nations General Assembly 1972).
2. "Novel psychoactive substances" refer to psychoactive substances not under international control that pose a health threat. They include substances such as ketamine, synthetic cannabinoids in various herbal mixtures, piperazines (such as N-benzylpiperazine [BZP]), products marketed as "bath salts" (cathinone-type substances such as mephedrone and methylenedioxypyrovalerone [MDPV]), and various phenethlamines (UNODC 2013).
3. "Precursor chemicals" refer to chemicals that are used in the manufacture of illicit drugs such as cocaine (for example, potassium permanganate, ethyl ether, and hydrochloric acid), heroin (acetic anhydride, ammonium chloride, ergot alkaloids, and lysergic acid), and ATSs (ephedrine and pseudoephedrine). Control measures for such chemicals typically involve regulations on their sale and distribution domestically and internationally, often requiring chemical producers to register with drug enforcement agencies and keep records of sales and customers. Communication and intelligence-gathering platforms (such as the Precursors Incident Communication System) are also used to alert governments of suspicious shipments, seizures, and actual and attempted diversions of precursors, and to identify emerging precursors (INCB 2014).
4. "Internalizing disorders" are mental disorders where the persons suffering from the disorder keep the problem to themselves, or "internalize it." Common examples include depression, withdrawal, and anxiety. "Externalizing disorders" are mental disorders that comprise negative behaviors that are directed toward the external environment (such as aggression and violence), including attention-deficit hyperactivity disorder, conduct disorder, and oppositional defiant disorder (APA 2000).
5. "Polydrug use" refers to the use of more than one drug or type of drug by an individual, consumed at the same time or sequentially. Polydrug use has several functions, including maximizing drug effects, balancing or controlling negative effects, and substituting the sought-after effects of a primary drug when supply is low (WHO 1993).
6. A narcotic antagonist is a receptor antagonist that binds to narcotic receptors, effectively preventing the body from responding to narcotics.

NOTES

World Bank Income Classifications as of July 2014 are as follows, based on estimates of gross national income (GNI) per capita for 2013:

- Low-income countries (LICs) = US$1,045 or less
- Middle-income countries (MICs) are subdivided:
  a) Lower-middle-income = US$1,046 to US$4,125
  b) Upper-middle-income (UMICs) = US$4,126 to US$12,745
- High-income countries (HICs) = US$12,746 or more.

REFERENCES

Allsop, D., J. Copeland, N. Lintzeris, A. Dunlop, M. Montebello, and others. 2014. "A Randomized Controlled Trial of Nabiximols (Sativex®) as an Agonist Replacement Therapy during Cannabis Withdrawal." *JAMA Psychiatry* 71 (3): 281–91.

Amato, L., S. Minozzi, P. P. Pani, R. Solimini, S. Vecchi, and others. 2011. "Dopamine Agonists for the Treatment of Cocaine Dependence." *Cochrane Database of Systematic Reviews* 12: CD003352. doi:http://dx.doi.org/10.1002/14651858.CD003352.pub3.

Anglin, M. D. 1988. "The Efficacy of Civil Commitment in Treating Narcotic Drug Addiction." In *Compulsory Treatment of Drug Abuse: Research and Clinical Practice*, edited by C. G. Leukefeld and F. M. Tims, 8–34. Rockville, MD: National Institute on Drug Abuse.

APA (American Psychiatric Association). 2000. *Diagnostic and Statistical Manual of Mental Disorders: DSM-IV-TR*. 4th ed., text revision. Washington, DC: APA.

———. 2013. *Diagnostic and Statistical Manual of Mental Disorders*. 5th ed. Washington, DC: APA.

Babor, T. F., J. Caulkins, G. Edwards, B. Fischer, D. Foxcroft, and others, eds. 2010. *Drug Policy and the Public Good*. Oxford: Oxford University Press.

Baker, A., N. K. Lee, M. Claire, T. J. Lewin, T. Grant, and others. 2005. "Brief Cognitive Behavioural Interventions for Regular Amphetamine Users: A Step in the Right Direction." *Addiction* 100 (3): 367–78.

Ball, J. C., J. W. Shaffer, and D. N. Nurco. 1983. "The Day-to-Day Criminality of Heroin Addicts in Baltimore—A Study in the Continuity of Offence Rates." *Drug and Alcohol Dependence* 12 (2): 119–42.

Behrendt, S., H. U. Wittchen, M. Hofler, R. Lieb, and K. Beesdo. 2009. "Transitions from First Substance Use to Substance Use Disorders in Adolescence: Is Early Onset Associated with a Rapid Escalation?" *Drug and Alcohol Dependence* 99 (1–3): 68–78. doi:10.1016/j.drugalcdep.2008.06.014.

Bloomfield, M. A., C. J. Morgan., A. Egerton, S. Kapur, H V. Curran, and others. 2013. "Dopaminergic Function in Cannabis Users and Its Relationship to Cannabis-Induced Psychotic Symptoms." *Biological Psychiatry* 75 (6): 470–78. doi:10.1016/j.biopsych.2013.05.027.

Blow, F. C., M. A. Walton, K. L. Barry, R. L. Murray, R. M. Cunningham, and others. 2011. "Alcohol and Drug Use among Patients Presenting to an Inner-City Emergency Department: A Latent Class Analysis." *Addict Behaviors* 36 (8): 793–800. doi:10.1016/j.addbeh.2010.12.028.

Brensilver, M., K. G. Heinzerling, and S. Shoptaw. 2013. "Pharmacotherapy of Amphetamine-Type Stimulant Dependence: An Update." *Drug and Alcohol Review* 32 (5): 449–60. doi:10.1111/dar.12048.

Brown, R. T. 2010. "Systematic Review of the Impact of Adult Drug-Treatment Courts." *Translational Research: The Journal of Laboratory and Clinical Medicine* 155 (6): 263–74. doi:http://dx.doi.org/10.1016/j.trsl.2010.03.001.

Budney, A. J., B. A. Moore, H. L. Rocha, and S. T. Higgins. 2006. "Clinical Trial of Abstinence-Based Vouchers and Cognitive-Behavioral Therapy for Cannabis Dependence." *Journal of Consulting and Clinical Psychology* 74 (2): 307.

Carpenter, K. M., D. McDowell, D. J. Brooks, W. Y. Cheng, and F. R. Levin. 2009. "A Preliminary Trial: Double-Blind Comparison of Nefazodone, Bupropion-SR, and Placebo in the Treatment of Cannabis Dependence." *American Journal on Addictions* 18 (1): 53–64. doi:10.1080/10550490802408936.

Caulkins, J. P., R. L. Pacula, S. M. Paddock, and J. Chiesa. 2002. *School-Based Drug Prevention: What Kind of Drug Use Does It Prevent?* Santa Monica, CA: RAND.

Caulkins, J. P., C. P. Rydell, S. S. Everingham, J. Chiesa, and S. Bushway. 1999. *An Ounce of Prevention, a Pound of Uncertainty: The Cost-Effectiveness of School-Based Drug Prevention Program*. Santa Monica, CA: RAND.

CDC (Centers for Disease Control and Prevention). 2012. "Community-Based Opioid Overdose Prevention Programs Providing Naloxone—United States, 2010." *Morbidity and Mortality Weekly Report* 61 (6): 101.

Cohen, J. 2003. "The Next Frontier for HIV/AIDS: Myanmar." *Science* 301 (5640): 1650–55.

Collins, D., and H. Lapsley. 2007. "The Costs of Tobacco, Alcohol and Illicit Drug Use to Australian Society in 2004/05." *National Drug Strategy Monograph*. Canberra: Commonwealth Department of Health and Ageing.

Compton, W. M., and N. D. Volkow. 2006. "Major Increases in Opioid Analgesic Abuse in the United States: Concerns and Strategies." *Drug and Alcohol Dependence* 81 (2): 103–7.

Cunningham, J. K., L.-M. Liu, and R. C. Callaghan. 2013. "Essential ('Precursor') Chemical Control for Heroin: Impact of Acetic Anhydride Regulation on US Heroin Availability." *Drug and Alcohol Dependence* 133 (2): 520–28. doi:http://dx.doi.org/10.1016/j.drugalcdep.2013.07.014.

Danovitch, I., and D. A. Gorelick. 2012. "State of the Art Treatments for Cannabis Dependence." *Psychiatric Clinics of North America* 35 (2): 309–26. doi:10.1016/j.psc.2012.03.003.

Darke, S., S. Kaye, R. McKetin, and J. Duflou. 2008. "Major Physical and Psychological Harms of Methamphetamine Use." *Drug and Alcohol Review* 27: 253–62.

Dave, D. M. 2006. "The Effects of Cocaine and Heroin Price on Drug-Related Emergency Department Visits." *Journal of Health Economics* 25: 311–33.

Day, C., L. Degenhardt, S. Gilmour, and W. Hall. 2004. "Effects of Reduction in Heroin Supply on Injecting Drug Use: Analysis of Data from Needle and Syringe Programmes." *British Medical Journal* 329 (7463): 428–29. doi:10.1136/bmj.38201.410255.55.

Degenhardt, L., A. Baxter, Y.-Y. Lee, W. Hall, G. E. Sara, and others. 2014. "The Epidemiology and Burden of Disease Attributable to Psychostimulant Dependence: Findings from the Global Burden of Disease Study 2010." *Drug and Alcohol Dependence* 137 (4): 36–47.

Degenhardt, L., C. Bucello, B. Calabria, P. Nelson, A. Roberts, and others. 2011. "What Data Are Available on the Extent of Illicit Drug Use and Dependence Globally? Results of Four Systematic Reviews." *Drug and Alcohol Dependence* 117: 85–101. doi:10.1016/j.drugalcdep.2010.11.032.

Degenhardt, L., C. Bucello, B. Mathers, C. Briegleb, H. Ali, and others. 2011. "Mortality among Problematic Users of Heroin and Other Illicit Opioids: A Systematic Review and Meta-Analysis of Cohort Studies." *Addiction* 106 (1): 32–51. doi:10.1111/j.1360-0443.2010.03140.x.

Degenhardt, L., F. Charlson, B. Mathers, W. Hall, A. Flaxman, and others. 2014. "The Global Epidemiology and Burden of Disease Attributable to Opioid Dependence: Findings from the Global Burden of Disease Study 2010." *Addiction* 109 (8): 1320–33. doi:10.1111/add.12551.

Degenhardt, L., L. Dierker, W. Chiu, M. Medina-Mora, Y. Neumark, and others. 2010. "Evaluating the Drug Use 'Gateway' Theory Using Cross-National Data: Consistency and Associations of the Order of Initiation of Drug Use among Participants in the WHO World Mental Health Surveys." *Drug and Alcohol Dependence* 108 (1): 84–97.

Degenhardt, L., and W. Hall. 2012. "Extent of Illicit Drug Use and Dependence, and Their Contribution to the Global Burden of Disease." *The Lancet* 379 (9810): 55–70.

Degenhardt, L., S. Larney, N. Gisev, J. Trevena, J. Kimber, and others. 2013. "Engagement with the Criminal Justice System among Opioid Dependent People: Retrospective Cohort Study." *Addiction* 108 (12): 2152–65.

Degenhardt, L., S. Larney, J. Kimber, N. Gisev, M. Farrell, and others. 2014. "The Impact of Opioid Substitution Therapy on Mortality Post-Release from Prison: Retrospective Data Linkage Study." *Addiction* 109 (8): 1306–17. doi:10.1111/add.12536.

Degenhardt, L., H. A. Whiteford, A. J. Ferrari, A. J. Baxter, F. J. Charlson, and others. 2013. "Global Burden of Disease Attributable to Illicit Drug Use and Dependence: Findings from the Global Burden of Disease Study 2010." *The Lancet* 382 (9904): 1564–74. doi:10.1016/s0140-6736(13)61530-5.

Dole, V. P., J. W. Robinson, J. Orraca, E. Towns, P. Searcy, and others. 1969. "Methadone Treatment of Randomly Selected Criminal Addicts." *The New England Journal of Medicine* 280 (25): 1372–75. doi:10.1056/nejm196906192802502.

Doran, C. M. 2005. "Buprenorphine, Buprenorphine/Naloxone and Methadone Maintenance: A Cost-Effectiveness Analysis." *Expert Review of Pharmacoeconomics and Outcomes Research* 5 (5): 583–91. doi:http://dx.doi.org/10.1586/14737167.5.5.583.

DuPont, R. L., A. T. McLellan, W. L. White, L. J. Merlo, and M. S. Gold. 2009. "Setting the Standard for Recovery: Physicians' Health Programs." *Journal of Substance Abuse Treatment* 36 (2): 159–71.

Ennett, S. T., N. S. Tobler, C. L. Ringwalt, and R. L. Flewelling. 1994. "How Effective Is Drug Abuse Resistance Education? A Meta-Analysis of Project DARE Outcome Evaluations." *American Journal of Public Health* 84 (9): 1394–401.

Faggiano, F., S. Minozzi, E. Versino, and D. Buscemi. 2014. "Universal School-Based Prevention for Illicit Drug Use." *Cochrane Database of Systematic Reviews (Online)* 12: CD003020. doi:10.1002/14651858.CD003020.pub3.

Farrell, M., J. Strang, and H. Stover. 2010. "Hepatitis B Vaccination in Prisons: A Much-Needed Targeted Universal Intervention." *Addiction* 105 (2): 189–90. doi:10.1111/j.1360-0443.2009.02781.x.

Ferri, M., E. Allara, A. Bo, A. Gasparrini, and F. Faggiano. 2013. "Media Campaigns for the Prevention of Illicit Drug Use in Young People." *Cochrane Database of Systematic Reviews (Online)* 6: CD009287. doi:10.1002/14651858.CD009287.pub2.

Ferri, M., M. Davoli, and C. A. Perucci. 2011. "Heroin Maintenance for Chronic Heroin-Dependent Individuals." *Cochrane Database of Systematic Reviews* (12): CD003410. doi:http://dx.doi.org/10.1002/14651858.CD003410.pub4.

Fischer, B., M. Bibby, and M. Bouchard. 2010. "Non-Medical Use and Diversion of Psychotropic Prescription Drugs in North America: A Review of Sourcing Routes and Control Measures." *Addiction* 105: 2062–70.

Florez-Salamanca, L., R. Secades-Villa, D. S. Hasin, L. Cottler, S. Wang, and others. 2013. "Probability and Predictors of Transition from Abuse to Dependence on Alcohol, Cannabis, and Cocaine: Results from the National Epidemiologic Survey on Alcohol and Related Conditions." *The American Journal of Drug and Alcohol Abuse* 39 (3): 168–79. doi:10.3109/00952990.2013.772618.

Freimuth, M. 2000. "Integrating Group Psychotherapy and 12-Step Work: A Collaborative Approach." *International Journal of Group Psychotherapy* 50 (3): 297–314.

Galloway, G. P., R. Buscemi, J. R. Coyle, K. Flower, J. D. Siegrist, and others. 2011. "A Randomized, Placebo-Controlled Trial of Sustained-Release Dextroamphetamine for Treatment of Methamphetamine Addiction." *Clinical Pharmacology and Therapeutics* 89 (2): 276–82. doi:10.1038/clpt.2010.307.

Gerstein, D. R., and H. Harwood, eds. 1990. *Treating Drug Problems.* Volume 1, *A Study of Effectiveness and Financing of Public and Private Drug Treatment Systems.* Washington, DC: National Academies Press.

Gibson, A. E., C. M. Doran, J. R. Bell, A. Ryan, and N. Lintzeris. 2003. "A Comparison of Buprenorphine Treatment in Clinic and Primary Care Settings: A Randomised Trial." *Medical Journal of Australia* 179 (1): 38–42.

Gossop, M., D. Stewart, and J. Marsden. 2008. "Attendance at Narcotics Anonymous and Alcoholics Anonymous Meetings, Frequency of Attendance and Substance Use Outcomes after Residential Treatment for Drug Dependence: A 5-Year Follow-Up Study." *Addiction* 103 (1): 119–25.

Gowing, L. R., M. Hickman, and L. Degenhardt. 2013. "Mitigating the Risk of HIV Infection with Opioid Substitution Treatment." *Bulletin of the World Health Organization* 91 (2): 148–49.

Hall, W., C. Doran, L. Degenhardt, and D. Shepard. 2006. "Illicit Opiate Abuse." In *Disease Control Priorities in Developing Countries*, 2nd ed., edited by D. T. Jamison, J. G. Breman, A. R. Measham, G. Alleyne, M. Claeson, D. B. Evans, P. Jha, A. Mills, and P. Musgrove, 907–32. Washington, DC: World Bank and Oxford University Press.

Hall, W., M. Farrell, and A. Carter. 2014. "Compulsory Treatment of Addiction in the Patient's Best Interests: More Rigorous Evaluations Are Essential." *Drug and Alcohol Review* 33 (3): 268–71.

Haney, M., C. L. Hart, S. K. Vosburg, S. D. Comer, S. C. Reed, and others. 2008. "Effects of THC and Lofexidine in a Human Laboratory Model of Marijuana Withdrawal and Relapse." *Psychopharmacology* 197 (1): 157–68.

Haney, M., C. L. Hart, S. K. Vosburg, J. Nasser, A. Bennett, and others. 2004. "Marijuana Withdrawal in Humans: Effects of Oral THC or Divalproex." *Neuropsychopharmacology* 29 (1): 158–70.

Harris, A. H., E. Gospodarevskaya, and A. J. Ritter. 2005. "A Randomised Trial of the Cost Effectiveness of Buprenorphine as an Alternative to Methadone Maintenance

Treatment for Heroin Dependence in a Primary Care Setting." *Pharmacoeconomics* 23 (1): 77–91.

Hedrich, D., T. Kerr, and F. Dubois-Arber. 2010. "Drug Consumption Facilities in Europe and Beyond." In *Harm Reduction: Evidence, Impacts and Challenges*, edited by T. Rhodes and D. Hedrich. Scientific Monograph Series 10. Lisbon: European Monitoring Centre for Drugs and Drug Addiction.

Hornik, R., L. Jacobsohn, R. Orwin, A. Piesse, and G. Kalton. 2008. "Effects of the National Youth Anti-Drug Media Campaign on Youths." *American Journal of Public Health* 98 (12): 2229.

Horvath, A. T. 2000. "Smart Recovery®: Addiction Recovery Support from a Cognitive-Behavioral Perspective." *Journal of Rational-Emotive and Cognitive-Behavior Therapy* 18 (3): 181–91.

Humeniuk, R., R. Ali, T. Babor, M. L. O. Souza Formigoni, R. B. de Lacerda, and others. 2012. "A Randomized Controlled Trial of a Brief Intervention for Illicit Drugs Linked to the Alcohol, Smoking and Substance Involvement Screening Test (ASSIST) in Clients Recruited from Primary Health Care Settings in Four Countries." *Addiction* 107 (5): 957–66.

INCB (International Narcotics Control Board). 2014. "Precursor Chemicals Frequently Used in the Illicit Manufacture of Narcotic Drugs and Psychotropic Substances." *International Narcotics Control Board*. Vienna: United Nations.

Inciardi, J., H. L. Surratt, S. Kurtz, and T. J. Cicero. 2007. "Mechanisms of Prescription Drug Diversion among Drug-Involved Club- and Street-Based Populations." *Pain Medicine* 8: 171–83.

Kellam, S. G., J. Reid, and R. L. Balster. 2008. "Effects of a Universal Classroom Behavior Program in First and Second Grades on Young Adult Outcomes." *Drug and Alcohol Dependence* 95 (Suppl. 1): S5–S28.

Kerr, T., J. Kimber, K. DeBeck, and E. Wood. 2007. "The Role of Safer Injection Facilities in the Response to HIV/AIDS among Injection Drug Users." *Current HIV/AIDS Reports* 4 (4): 158–64.

Kimber, J., N. Palmateer, S. Hutchinson, M. Hickman, D. Goldberg, and T. Rhodes. 2010. "Harm Reduction among Injecting Drug Users—Evidence of Effectiveness." In *Harm Reduction: Evidence, Impacts and Challenges*, edited by T. Rhodes and D. Hedrich, chapter 5. Lisbon: European Monitoring Centre for Drugs and Drug Addiction.

Klag, S., F. O'Callaghan, and P. Creed. 2005. "The Use of Legal Coercion in the Treatment of Substance Abusers: An Overview and Critical Analysis of Thirty Years of Research." *Substance Use and Misuse* 40 (12): 1777–95.

Kleiman, M. A. R. 2009. *When Brute Force Fails: Strategy for Crime Control*. Princeton, NJ: Princeton University Press.

Kumaranayake, L., P. Vickerman, D. Walker, S. Samoshkin, V. Romantzov, and others. 2004. "The Cost-Effectiveness of HIV Preventive Measures among Injecting Drug Users in Svetlogorsk, Belarus." *Addiction* 99 (12): 1565–76. doi:10.1111/j.1360-0443.2004.00899.x.

Kuziemko, I., and S. D. Levitt. 2004. "An Empirical Analysis of Imprisoning Drug Offenders." *Journal of Public Economics* 88: 2043–66.

Larney, S., N. Gisev, M. Farrell, T. Dobbins, J. Kimber, and others. 2014. "Opioid Substitution Therapy as a Strategy to Reduce Deaths in Prison: Retrospective Cohort Study." *BMJ Open* 4 (e004666). doi:10.1136/bmjopen-2013-004666.

Larney, S., L. Gowing, R. P. Mattick, M. Farrell, W. Hall, and others. 2014. "A Systematic Review and Meta-Analysis of Naltrexone Implants for the Treatment of Opioid Dependence." *Drug and Alcohol Review* 33 (2): 115–28.

Leshner, A. I. 1997. "Addiction Is a Brain Disease, and It Matters." *Science* 278 (5335): 45–47.

Littlejohn, C., A. Baldacchino, F. Schifano, and P. Deluca. 2005. "Internet Pharmacies and Online Prescription Drug Sales: A Cross-Sectional Study." *Drugs: Education, Prevention and Policy* 12: 75–80.

Lobmaier, P., H. Kornor, N. Kunoe, and A. Bjørndal. 2008. "Sustained-Release Naltrexone for Opioid Dependence." *Cochrane Database of Systematic Reviews* (2): CD006140. doi:10.1002/14651858.CD006140.pub2.

Longo, M., W. Wickes, M. Smout, S. Harrison, S. Cahill, and others. 2010. "Randomized Controlled Trial of Dexamphetamine Maintenance for the Treatment of Methamphetamine Dependence." *Addiction* 105 (1): 146–54. doi:10.1111/j.1360-0443.2009.02717.x.

Lopez-Quintero, C., D. S. Hasin, J. P. de Los Cobos, A. Pines, S. Wang, and others. 2011. "Probability and Predictors of Remission from Life-Time Nicotine, Alcohol, Cannabis or Cocaine Dependence: Results from the National Epidemiologic Survey on Alcohol and Related Conditions." *Addiction* 106 (3): 657–69. doi:10.1111/j.1360-0443.2010.03194.x.

Manski, C. F., J. V. Pepper, and C. V. Petrie. 2001. *Informing America's Policy on Illegal Drugs: What We Don't Know Keeps Hurting Us*. Washington, DC: National Academies Press.

Mathers, B. M., L. Degenhardt, H. Ali, L. Wiessing, M. Hickman, and others. 2010. "HIV Prevention, Treatment, and Care Services for People Who Inject Drugs: A Systematic Review of Global, Regional, and National Coverage." *The Lancet* 375 (9719): 1014–28. doi:10.1016/s0140-6736(10)60232-2.

Mattick, R. P., C. Breen, J. Kimber, and M. Davoli. 2014. "Buprenorphine Maintenance versus Placebo or Methadone Maintenance for Opioid Dependence." *Cochrane Database of Systematic Reviews* 2: CD002207. doi:10.1002/14651858.CD002207.pub4.

Mattick, R. P., and W. Hall. 1996. "Are Detoxification Programmes Effective?" *The Lancet* 347 (8994): 97–100.

McGregor, C., R. Ali, P. Christie, and S. Darke. 2001. "Overdose among Heroin Users: Evaluation of an Intervention in South Australia." *Addiction Research and Theory* 9 (5): 481–501.

Minozzi, S., L. Amato, S. Vecchi, M. Davoli, U. Kirchmayer, and others. 2011. "Oral Naltrexone Maintenance Treatment for Opioid Dependence." *Cochrane Database of Systematic Reviews* (4): CD001333. doi:10.1002/14651858.CD001333.pub4.

MSIC Evaluation Committee. 2003. *Final Report of the Evaluation of the Sydney Medically Supervised Injecting Centre*. Sydney: University of New South Wales.

Mugunthan, K., T. McGuire, and P. Glasziou. 2011. "Minimal Interventions to Decrease Long-Term Use of

Benzodiazepines in Primary Care: A Systematic Review and Meta-Analysis." *British Journal of General Practice* 61 (590): e573–78.

Nelson, P. K., B. M. Mathers, B. Cowie, H. Hagan, D. Des Jarlais, and others. 2011. "Global Epidemiology of Hepatitis B and Hepatitis C in People Who Inject Drugs: Results of Systematic Reviews." *The Lancet* 378 (9791): 571–83. doi:10.1016/s0140-6736(11)61097-0.

NICE (National Institute for Health and Care Excellence). 2007. *Drug Misuse: Psychosocial Interventions (CG51—Clinical Guideline 51)*. London: NICE.

ONDCP (Office of National Drug Control Policy). 2008. *Efforts to Control Precursor Chemicals*. Washington, DC: Executive Office of the President of the United States.

Perry, A. E., Z. Darwin, C. Godfrey, C. McDougall, J. Lunn, and others. 2009. "The Effectiveness of Interventions for Drug-Using Offenders in the Courts, Secure Establishments and the Community: A Systematic Review." *Substance Use and Misuse* 44 (3): 374–400. doi:http://dx.doi.org/10.1080/10826080802347560.

Petry, N. M., J. Tedford, M. Austin, C. Nich, K. M. Carroll, and others. 2004. "Prize Reinforcement Contingency Management for Treating Cocaine Users: How Low Can We Go, and With Whom?" *Addiction* 99 (3): 349–60.

Phan, H. M., K. Yoshizuka, D. J. Murry, and P. J. Perry. 2012. "Drug Testing in the Workplace." *Pharmacotherapy: The Journal of Human Pharmacology and Drug Therapy* 32 (7): 649–56. doi:http://dx.doi.org/10.1002/j.1875-9114.2011.01089.x.

Rajasingham, R., M. J. Mimiaga, J. M. White, M. M. Pinkston, R. P. Baden, and others. 2012. "A Systematic Review of Behavioral and Treatment Outcome Studies among HIV-Infected Men Who Have Sex with Men Who Abuse Crystal Methamphetamine." *AIDS Patient Care STDS* 26 (1): 36–52. doi:10.1089/apc.2011.0153.

Restrepo, C. S., C. A. Rojas, S. Martinez, R. Riascos, A. Marmol-Velez, and others. 2009. "Cardiovascular Complications of Cocaine: Imaging Findings." *Emergency Radiology* 16 (1): 11–19. doi:10.1007/s10140-008-0762-x.

Room, R., B. Fischer, W. Hall, S. Lenton, and P. Reuter. 2010. *Cannabis Policy: Moving beyond Stalemate*. Oxford, U.K.: Oxford University Press.

Schoenwald, S., D. Ward, S. Henggeler, S. Pickrel, and H. Patel. 1996. "Multisystemic Therapy Treatment of Substance Abusing or Dependent Adolescent Offenders: Costs of Reducing Incarceration, Inpatient, and Residential Placement." *Journal of Child and Family Studies* 5 (4): 431–44. doi:10.1007/BF02233864.

Shanahan, M., L. Degenhardt, and W. Hall. 2004. *Estimating the Economic Consequences of Reduced Heroin Supply in Australia 2000–2003*. NDARC Technical Report 195. Sydney: National Drug and Alcohol Research Centre, University of New South Wales.

Shek, D. T. L. 2010. "School Drug Testing: A Critical Review of the Literature." *The Scientific World Journal* 10: 356–65. doi:http://dx.doi.org/10.1100/tsw.2010.31.

Simoens, S., A. Ludbrook, C. Matheson, and C. Bond. 2006. "Pharmaco-Economics of Community Maintenance for Opiate Dependence: A Review of Evidence and Methodology." *Drug and Alcohol Dependence* 84 (1): 28–39. doi:10.1016/j.drugalcdep.2005.12.009.

Smith, L. A., S. Gates, and D. Foxcroft. 2006. "Therapeutic Communities for Substance Related Disorder." *Cochrane Database of Systematic Reviews (Online)* (1): CD005338. doi:10.1002/14651858.CD005338.pub2.

Stenbacka, M., A. Leifman, and A. Romelsjo. 2010. "Mortality and Cause of Death among 1,705 Illicit Drug Users: A 37-Year Follow-Up." *Drug and Alcohol Review* 29 (1): 21–27. doi:10.1111/j.1465-3362.2009.00075.x.

Strang, J., T. Babor, J. Caulkins, B. Fischer, D. Foxcroft, and others. 2012. "Drug Policy and the Public Good: Evidence for Effective Interventions." *The Lancet* 379 (9810): 71–83.

Szasz, T. 2003. *Ceremonial Chemistry: The Ritual Persecution of Drugs, Addicts, and Pushers*. Syracuse, NY: Syracuse University Press.

Tobin, K. E., S. G. Sherman, P. Beilenson, C. Welsh, and C. A. Latkin. 2009. "Evaluation of the Staying Alive Programme: Training Injection Drug Users to Properly Administer Naloxone and Save Lives." *International Journal of Drug Policy* 20 (2): 131–36.

UNDCP (United Nations International Drug Control Programme). 1998. *Economic and Social Consequences of Drug Abuse and Illicit Trafficking*. Vienna: UNDCP.

United Nations General Assembly. 1972. *1972 Protocol Amending the Single Convention on Narcotic Drugs, 1961*. Vienna: United Nations Office on Drugs and Crime.

UNODC (United Nations Office on Drugs and Crime). 2009. *Drug Use in Afghanistan: 2009 Survey*. Vienna: UNODC.

———. 2013. *World Drug Report 2013*. Vienna: United Nations.

U.S. Department of Health and Human Services. 2012. *Results from the 2012 National Survey on Drug Use and Health: Summary of National Findings*. Rockville, MD: Center for Behavioral Health Statistics and Quality.

Vanderplasschen, W., K. Colpaert, M. Autrique, R. C. Rapp, S. Pearce, and others. 2013. "Therapeutic Communities for Addictions: A Review of Their Effectiveness from a Recovery-Oriented Perspective." *The Scientific World Journal* 2013 (427817). doi:http://dx.doi.org/10.1155/2013/427817.

Vandrey, R., M. L. Stitzer, M. Z. Mintzer, M. A. Huestis, J. A. Murray, and others. 2013. "The Dose Effects of Short-Term Dronabinol (Oral THC) Maintenance in Daily Cannabis Users." *Drug and Alcohol Dependence* 128 (1–2): 64–70. doi:10.1016/j.drugalcdep.2012.08.001.

Volkow, N. D., G. J. Wang, J. S. Fowler, F. Telang, M. Jayne, and others. 2007. "Stimulant-Induced Enhanced Sexual Desire as a Potential Contributing Factor in HIV Transmission." *The American Journal of Psychiatry* 164 (1): 157–60. doi:10.1176/appi.ajp.164.1.157.

Wagner, K. D., T. W. Valente, M. Casanova, S. M. Partovi, B. M. Mendenhall, and others. 2010. "Evaluation of an Overdose Prevention and Response Training Programme for Injection

Drug Users in the Skid Row Area of Los Angeles, CA." *International Journal of Drug Policy* 21 (3): 186–93.

Wakefield, M. A., B. Loken, and R. C. Hornik. 2010. "Use of Mass Media Campaigns to Change Health Behaviour. (review). (104 refs.)." *The Lancet* 376 (9748): 1261–71.

Warner-Smith, M., S. Darke, M. Lynskey, and W. Hall. 2001. "Heroin Overdose: Causes and Consequences." *Addiction* 96 (8): 1113–25.

Weaver, T., N. Metrebian, J. Hellier, S. Pilling, V. Charles, and others. 2014. "Use of Contingency Management Incentives to Improve Completion of Hepatitis B Vaccination in People Undergoing Treatment for Heroin Dependence: A Cluster Randomised Trial." *The Lancet* 384: 153–63.

WHO (World Health Organization). 1993. *The ICD-10 Classification of Mental and Behavioural Disorders: Diagnostic Criteria for Research.* Geneva: WHO.

Winstock, A. R., T. Lea, and J. Copeland. 2009. "Lithium Carbonate in the Management of Cannabis Withdrawal in Humans: An Open-Label Study." *Journal of Psychopharmacology* 23 (1): 84–93.

Wu, L. T., G. E. Woody, C. Yang, P. Mannelli, and D. G. Blazer. 2011. "Differences in Onset and Abuse/Dependence Episodes between Prescription Opioids and Heroin: Results from the National Epidemiologic Survey on Alcohol and Related Conditions." *Substance Abuse and Rehabilitation* 2011 (2): 77–88. doi:10.2147/sar.s18969.

Young, D., R. Fluellen, and S. Belenko. 2004. "Criminal Recidivism in Three Models of Mandatory Drug Treatment." *Journal of Substance Abuse Treatment* 27 (4): 313–23. doi:http://dx.doi.org/10.1016/j.jsat.2004.08.007.

Young, M. M., A. Stevens, J. Galipeau, T. Pirie, C. Garritty, and others. 2014. "Effectiveness of Brief Interventions as Part of the Screening, Brief Intervention and Referral to Treatment (SBIRT) Model for Reducing the Nonmedical Use of Psychoactive Substances: A Systematic Review." *Systematic Reviews* 3: 50. doi:10.1186/2046-4053-3-50.

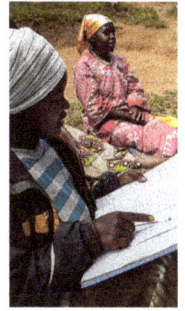

Chapter 7

Alcohol Use and Alcohol Use Disorders

María Elena Medina-Mora, Maristela Monteiro,
Robin Room, Jürgen Rehm, David Jernigan,
Diego Sánchez-Moreno, and Tania Real

INTRODUCTION

Alcohol is one of the most important risk factors for premature mortality and disability. Premature mortality disproportionately affects low- and middle-income countries (LMICs) (WHO 2011a); more than 85 percent of all deaths attributable to alcohol occur in these nations (Room and others 2013; WHO 2011a). This chapter updates the chapter on alcohol in *Disease Control Priorities in Developing Countries*, 2nd ed. (DCP2) (Rehm and others 2006), with new scientific evidence for interventions based on population, community, and individuals, with an emphasis on evidence from LMICs.

Alcoholic beverages vary with respect to their raw material, method of production, alcohol content, and presentation. Beverages are usually classified as *fermented* or *distilled*. In addition to the alcohol that appears in official statistics, many countries have a substantial amount of *unrecorded alcohol,* which may include illegally produced or smuggled alcohol products, but also surrogate alcohol (nonbeverage alcohol not officially intended for human consumption) and legal but unrecorded alcohol products (Lachenmeier, Sarash, and Rehm 2009).

Role of Industry

The alcohol industry is diverse and includes beer, wine, and spirits producers and importers, as well as bars, restaurants, and often stores that sell alcohol. Alcohol is an important contributor to business opportunities and jobs in the hospitality and retail sectors and a source of revenues for governments. It also plays an important role in commercial activity linked to the hospitality industry, such as hotels and airlines, and the advertising industry.

In recent years, a few large corporations have dominated the international alcohol market, particularly the beer and spirits sectors. In 2009, global companies produced 67 percent of the world's commercially brewed beer; "the big four" corporations produced 50 percent—AB InBev, SABMiller, Heineken, and Carlsberg (Impact Databank 2011). A similar trend has been observed in the spirits sector, with Diageo and Pernod Ricard managing some of the world's leading brands (Babor and others 2010). These companies are headquartered in high-income countries (HICs), which are the leading exporters of alcoholic beverages, but about 95 percent of alcoholic beverages are produced locally (WHO 1999).

The size of these corporations allows them to devote considerable resources, directly or indirectly, to promote the industry's policy interests. For example, the alcohol producers and their nonprofit organizations are involved in collecting, funding, and providing scientific evidence to inform the public, as well as sponsoring prevention activities (Zhang and Monteiro 2013), especially those known to have no or small effects on behavior

Corresponding author: María Elena Medina-Mora, Instituto Nacional de Psiquiatría Ramón de la Fuente (Ramón de la Fuente National Institute of Psychiatry), México; medinam@imp.edu.mx.

(Babor, Robaina, and Jernigan 2014). These activities challenge the public health sector and governments to respond with public health strategies to minimize the adverse health and societal consequences of the expanding global markets in alcoholic beverages (Babor and others 2010).

The high level of globalization has significant effects on markets. Transnational companies own the formulas and grant licenses to local subsidiaries. Most product development targets external markets, and advertising is usually produced externally. Transnational companies, supported by these economic advantages, are dynamic promoters of modifications in local drinking practices, including the types and quantity of beverages consumed (Room, Jernigan, Carlini, Gmel, and others 2013; Room, Jernigan, Carlini, Gureje, and others 2002).

Public Health Considerations

The substantial health and societal costs of alcohol consumption outweigh its economic benefits and contribute to the view of public health professionals that alcohol cannot be considered an "ordinary commodity" (Babor and others 2010). Special policies are needed to curb the consequences of harmful use, especially in LMICs where the burden is higher.

This public health perspective has received little attention in international negotiations concerning trade agreements and in resolutions of disputes under those agreements (Room, Jernigan, Carlini, Gmel, and others 2013; Room, Jernigan, Carlini, Gureje, and others 2002). This lack of attention reduces the ability of LMICs to ensure the internal regulation of markets (Grieshaber-Otto, Schacter, and Sinclair 2006; Zhang and Monteiro 2013). Governments in LMICs are deterred or forced to abandon alcohol controls as a result of trade disputes; for example, Thailand faces opposition from some World Trade Organization members to its proposed graphic warning labels on containers of alcohol sold within its borders (O'Brien 2013).

ALCOHOL-RELATED DISORDERS

Patterns of Alcohol Use, Alcohol Use Disorders, and Fetal Alcohol Spectrum Disorders

Alcohol is a major contributor to mortality, morbidity, and injuries. It is a causal factor in more than 60 diseases, including liver cirrhosis and cardiovascular disease, and it is involved in the etiology of more than 200 other conditions, such as neuropsychiatric conditions and diabetes mellitus. It also affects other people through the risky behavior and inattention of drinkers while intoxicated, resulting in acts of violence, driving while impaired, inconsistent family environments affecting normal child development, and workplace absenteeism (WHO 2014a).

An additional and increasingly significant consequence of maternal drinking during pregnancy is fetal alcohol syndrome (FAS), a pattern of retarded growth and development, both neuropsychological and physical, with typical facial dysmorphic features, that is found is some children exposed to alcohol in utero. A spectrum of physical and neurodevelopmental abnormalities, which includes FAS, that is attributed to the effects of alcohol on the fetus, is termed fetal alcohol syndrome disorders (FASD). The level of maternal alcohol consumption required to produce FASD, which has yet to be established, is influenced by genetic and other maternal and fetal characteristics (Gray, Mukherjee, and Rutter 2009; May and Gossage 2011).

Alcohol's impact on disease and injury is associated with two dimensions: the overall volume consumed and the drinking patterns of how the volume is distributed by drinking. Heavy drinking episodes have particularly damaging effects. The consequences associated with a high volume of drinking or recurrent heavy drinking occur through three mechanisms: toxic and other effects on organs and tissues, behavior during intoxication, and alcohol dependence and other alcohol-induced mental disorders (APA 2013; WHO 1992, 2013a).

The Burden

Patterns of Alcohol Use and Trends

One of the most commonly used indicators of overall alcohol consumption and comparison by location is per capita consumption. Although it is the best estimate available, it contains a substantial element of uncertainty, which increases where there are large proportions of unrecorded production, which is more common in LMICs.

Globally, per capita alcohol consumption in 2012 was an estimated 6.2 liters of pure alcohol by persons ages 15 years and older (WHO 2014a); 24.8 percent is consumed as unrecorded alcohol (Lachenmeier, Sarash, and Rehm 2009; WHO 2014a).

In general, HICs have the highest levels of per capita consumption and often the highest prevalence of heavy episodic drinking. The prevalence of heavy episodic drinking among adolescents ages 15–19 years mirrors that of the adult population, with the highest rates in the World Health Organization (WHO) regions of Europe, the Americas, and the Western Pacific (WHO 2014a).

Altogether, women drink less than men and have a lower prevalence of alcohol use disorders (AUDs);

in 2010, 52.3 percent of men and 71.1 percent of women did not drink alcohol in the previous year (WHO 2014a). Weekly heavy episodes are also more prevalent among men than women, 21.5 percent and 5.7 percent, respectively (WHO 2014a). Despite these lower rates of consumption, women in LMICs suffer greater social consequences per liter consumed, since this activity is often seen as inconsistent with their traditional roles (Medina-Mora 2001). The highest regional prevalence of AUDs for women was in the Americas; the highest regional prevalence for men was in Europe (WHO 2014a).

Global per capita consumption of alcohol is increasing, driven particularly by increases in China and India, as well as the Americas. The five-year trend in the WHO regions of Africa and Europe is stable, although some countries in these regions report significant reductions (WHO 2014a).

Consequences

Estimations made by the WHO indicate that the proportion of deaths attributable to alcohol (5.9 percent) is higher than the proportion observed for HIV/AIDS (2.8 percent), violence (0.9 percent), and tuberculosis (1.7 percent). Alcohol plays a prominent role in liver cirrhosis, oral cavity and pharynx cancer, pancreatitis, and laryngeal and esophageal cancer. Alcohol also plays a role in intentional injuries from interpersonal violence, self-harm and poisoning, and unintentional injuries and falls. Harmful use and dependence ranged from 0.1 to 3.4 percent (WHO 2014b).

Mortality. The Global Burden of Disease Study 2010 project (Murray and others 2012) estimated that alcohol as a risk factor increased from 1,988,502 deaths in 1990 to 2,735,511 in 2010, a (crude) increase of 37.6 percent. According to Lim and others (2012), alcohol is the leading risk factor for death in Eastern Europe, Andean Latin America, and southern Sub-Saharan Africa, and worldwide for people ages 15–49 years.

Disability-Adjusted Life Years. The WHO estimated the proportion of disability-adjusted life years accounted for by alcohol as a cause. Neuropsychiatric disorders rank first (24.6 percent of all disability-adjusted life years), mainly caused by AUDs, followed by unintentional injuries (20.4 percent), and cardiovascular diseases and diabetes collectively (15.5 percent). Globally, AUDs occur among 7.2 percent of men and 1.3 percent of women (WHO 2014a).

It has also been estimated that in LMICs, most of the harm is related to hazardous or harmful drinking rather than to alcohol dependence. This behavior is not often identified and treated within the first level of care; treatment for alcohol dependence is usually provided in specialized clinics. This situation calls for a shift of focus to cost-effective early interventions (Benegal, Chand, and Obot 2009).

Unintentional Injuries and Violence. Social consequences are also salient. Road traffic injuries cost LMICs an estimated 1 to 2 percent of their gross domestic product (GDP) (WHO 2014a).

Harmful alcohol use is a major contributor to violence. The alcohol-attributable portion of total violent deaths is approximately 30.0 percent: 32.5 percent in men, and 20.1 percent in women (WHO 2011a). Many perpetrators consume alcohol prior to assaults, with rates reported in special studies varying from 35 percent in the United States to 50 percent in China. Men are more likely than women to drink alcohol and to be perpetrators and victims of alcohol-related violence. For suicide, 11 percent of global mortality is attributed to alcohol, ranging from 2 percent in the Middle East and North Africa to 31 percent in Europe and Central Asia.

Injuries and social consequences are particularly related to patterns of drinking. A Patterns of Drinking score developed by Rehm and others (2003) measures this as a reflection of how people drink, a separate dimension of what total volume of alcohol they drink. Given the predominance of men among those drinking heavily in many cultures, the score may be predominantly comparing men's patterns of drinking (Gmel and others 2007). The score reflects how much of total consumption occurs on intoxicated occasions. The score includes the usual quantity of consumption, whether there is festive drinking, the proportion of events when drinkers get drunk, the proportion of drinkers who drink daily or nearly daily, and the proportion who drink with meals and in public places. Two attributes, drinking with meals and drinking daily or almost daily, are scored negatively, as reducing risk per liter. Low-risk patterns (risk score lower than 3) are usually found in upper-middle-income countries and HICs; more than 95 percent of LMICs have a risk score of at least 3 (WHO 2014a).

Disparate Burden. Within countries, there are generally more drinkers, more drinking occasions, and more drinkers with low-risk drinking patterns in the highest socioeconomic groups, and more abstainers in the lowest socioeconomic groups (WHO 2014a). However, drinkers in the lower socioeconomic groups are more likely to drink at higher levels of risk, with high quantities per drinking occasion (Room, Jernigan, Carlini, Gmel, and others 2013; Room, Jernigan, Carlini, Gureje, and others 2002), and they are more vulnerable to the consequences, at least partly reflecting their lower resources to cope with consequences and pay for treatment.

Many LMICs have higher alcohol-attributable mortality rates than HICs, despite the higher consumption in HICs. This can be explained by the fact that the harm derived from each liter of alcohol consumed is much greater because of a riskier pattern of alcohol consumption, a larger proportion of use of unrecorded alcohol, and the types of disorders with which alcohol is associated, with unintentional injuries the most salient (Room, Jernigan, Carlini, Gmel, and others 2013; Room, Jernigan, Carlini, Gureje, and others 2002). In a lower-income country, the built environment—for example, roads and footpaths—tends to offer less protection from injuries.

Societal Responses

Societies have used different strategies to cope with alcohol-related problems, depending on the specific ways in which the problem has been conceptualized. Strategies vary from total to partial bans on alcohol and from highly regulated markets to infrequent enforcement of the few existing regulations. Policies based on a combination of alcohol control and medical traditions—including normative measures to control availability and promote a safe environment for drinkers and the general population, as well as the prevention and treatment of the disorder—have had significant success in holding down rates of problems in HICs (Babor and others 2010). In LMICs, except those with a strong religious tradition that rejects drinking, the situation appears more challenging and offers few mitigating factors. Controls on the alcohol market that existed in many countries have been swept away, often by mandates from international aid agencies for market deregulation or privatization or as a result of trade disputes under free-trade agreements (Room, Jernigan, Carlini, Gureje, and others 2002). In many cultures, drunkenness is often tolerated, and regulations are not widespread; nevertheless, important lessons can be drawn from experiences where intervention measures have been used.

CHOICE OF INTERVENTIONS

The interventions in this chapter were identified with reference to a standardized matrix developed at a meeting of the volume editors and lead authors. The matrix divides interventions into three main groups:

- Population platform interventions, including universal prevention (IOM 1998)
- Community platform interventions
- Health care platform interventions.

This mapping exercise updates the DCP2 chapter on alcohol (Rehm and others 2006) and draws on three key

previous exercises that reviewed the existing evidence (Babor and others 2010; Room, Jernigan, Carlini, Gmel, and others 2013; Room, Jernigan, Carlini, Gureje, and others 2002; WHO 2008, 2011b).

The search process consisted of an electronic review of the following databases: Medline (1994–2013), Embase (1994–2013), PsycINFO (1966–2013), Ovid (1970–2013), National Institute on Drug Abuse Database, SciELO (1994–2013), EBSCO (1994–2013), ISI Web of Knowledge (1994–2013), National Institute for Health and Care Excellence evidence search, Global Information System on Alcohol and Health, CINAHL, and Mental Health Gap Action Programme (mhGAP). The review resulted in identifying 42 articles; 21 additional records were identified through other sources. Of the 63 articles screened, 18 were excluded because they did not use a robust design; 45 were selected and assessed for eligibility, but three were excluded because of methodological limitations (Moher and others 2009).

Population-based interventions are usually evaluated by before-and-after population surveys, analyses of archival and official statistics, time-series analyses, qualitative research, and quasi-experimental studies. Quasi-experimental studies involve before-and-after measurements of communities or jurisdictions exposed to the intervention, compared with similar communities or jurisdictions where the intervention has not been implemented.

Natural experiments take advantage of the implementation of a new policy to test the effects; accordingly, they lack the random assignment of communities to the interventions being tested and so provide a lower level of evidence. Randomized controlled trials (RCTs), considered the gold standard for evaluating the effect of health interventions, are rarely used to test population-based interventions (Babor and others 2010). Although individual-based interventions are more suitable for RCTs, they must meet rigid standards to be considered robust (Guyatt and others 2011).

Interventions at a populationwide level that do not use experimental methodology were assessed using less stringent criteria, so quasi-experiments and natural experiments were rated as very good (+++) or good (++), depending on the strategies for data analysis. Time-series analysis or statistical modeling were considered to have a *very good* level of evidence. Other strategies, such as key informants or reports where information was lacking, were rated as *limited* + and not included in the analysis.

Community and health and social care interventions were assessed using primarily the Grading of Recommendations Assessment, Development and Evaluation (GRADE) guidelines. Using these, RCTs are regarded as having high quality (very good +++). When only some criteria included in the GRADE guidelines were used, the rank was lower (*good* ++). Studies with limitations in the methods (the sample size or follow-up period assessment), inconsistencies (low reliability due to low variable control), lack of directedness (use of surrogate variables), or imprecision (confidence intervals not reported) were ranked as having a lower level of evidence (*limited* +). Only articles rated as very good or good were included in this review.

POPULATION PLATFORM INTERVENTIONS

Reducing the Availability of Alcohol

To control the physical availability of alcohol, governments need to be able to control its production, distribution, and sale. This control can be achieved by prohibition, monopolization, or other measures grouped in three clusters:

- Limiting the availability by means of taxes and minimum prices
- Limiting advertising and promotion
- Constraining access by licensing producers and wholesalers and retailers: when and where beverages can be available, to whom can they be sold, and how they can be sold.

Licensing systems facilitate the enforcement of regulations, the assessment of the origin of the alcohol, the determination of whether it has been legally produced and sold, and the collection of taxes. Settings in which unrecorded alcohol is highly available require additional controls. The following section describes evidence for these measures by region; tables 7.1, 7.2, and 7.3 provide additional information.

Prohibition, Rationing, and Partial Bans

Bans on sales, when effectively enforced, have proved effective in reducing consumption and harm. However, evidence suggests that these measures encourage the black market, which is difficult and expensive to eliminate (Lachenmeier, Taylor, and Rehm 2011). Several experiments on prohibitions and bans have been conducted in recent years, showing a reduction in use, followed by an increase when controls were abolished (Room, Jernigan, Carlini, Gmel, and others 2013; Room, Jernigan, Carlini, Gureje, and others 2002).

Indigenous Communities. Margolis and others (2011) studied four remote Australian Indigenous communities; three implemented prohibition, and the fourth allowed low-alcohol beer within licensed premises. Serious injury rates declined in all four communities. Similar results were observed in the First Nation Communities in Canada (Gliksman, Rylett, and Douglas 2007). The remoteness of the communities studied is likely to have enhanced the effectiveness of the intervention.

Table 7.1 Population-Based Interventions to Reduce Alcohol Availability

Population	Type of study	Main results
Prohibition, rationing, and partial bans		
Indigenous communities/*Australia and Canada*	Doctor service data, quasi-experimental (+++)	Prohibition and allowance of low-alcohol beer at licensed premises reduced serious injury (Gliksman, Rylett, and Douglas 2007; Margolis and others 2011).
Latin America/*Venezuela, RB*	National statistics, quasi-experimental time-series analysis, modeling (++)	Restriction intervention ("dry laws") reduced use and accidents (Herrera and others 2009).
Taxation		
East Asia/*Thailand*	Data from alcohol producers, national alcohol use surveys and statistics; theoretical evaluation, simulation and empirical analysis; price elasticity analysis; quasi-experimental, time lapse analysis (+++)	Taxation on distilled spirits led to a reduction in overall consumption (Chaiyasong and others 2011; Sornpaisarn, Shield, and Rehm 2012); prevented the onset of drinking among youth (ages 15–24 years) (Sornpaisarn and others 2013; *but* use of beer rose as a substitution effect (Chaiyasong and others 2011).
East Asia and Pacific/*China, Thailand;* Central and South Asia/*Turkey and India;* Sub-Saharan Africa/*Kenya, Tanzania*	Systematic review, PRISMA (+++)	Twelve studies showed evidence of a link between alcohol prices or taxation and consumption in LMICs; unrecorded alcohol was not considered (Sornpaisarn and others 2013).

Note: LMICs = low- and middle-income countries; PRISMA = Preferred Reporting Items for Systematic Reviews and Meta-Analyses; ++ = good; +++ = very good.

Table 7.2 Restrictions on Alcohol Sale and Advertising: Density, Hours, Days, and Locations

Population	Type of study	Main results
Indigenous communities/ *Australia*	Data from admissions to local hospitals, women's refugee centers, sobering-up shelters, and police records; time-series analysis, quasi-experimental (+++)	After two years of constraints on the days, hours, and amounts of different beverages allowed for sale, annual per capita consumption of pure alcohol (19.4 percent) and hospital admissions declined (Gray and others 2000).
Latin America and the Caribbean/ *Brazil, Colombia, and Peru*	Police records; time-lapse analysis on homicides; linear regression analysis, quasi-experimental (+++)	A significant reduction in violence was reported in Brazil following the implementation of a municipal law preventing the sale of alcohol after 11 p.m., followed by a public information campaign (Duailibi and others 2007). Similar results have been observed through restrictions on alcohol service hours in cities in Colombia (Sánchez and others 2011) and Peru (Málaga and others 2012).

Note: +++ = very good.

Table 7.3 Law Enforcement Measures to Reduce Impaired Driving

Population	Type of study	Main results
East Asia and Pacific/*China*	Serial cross-sectional telephone surveys; time-lapse analysis; liquor sales; quasi-experimental (+++)	Random breath tests reduced impaired driving rates (Kim and others 2013).
		Arrests of impaired drivers who exceeded blood alcohol limits were associated with a reduction in fatal accidents in Taiwan, China (Chang and Yeh 2004).
Latin America and the Caribbean/*Brazil*	Representative sample of trauma care centers; time-series analysis, quasi-experimental (+++)	Low blood alcohol rates reduced traffic injuries and deaths (Andreuccetti and others 2011).

Note: +++ = very good.

Latin America and the Caribbean. The impact of partial bans on alcohol consumption on traffic accidents and injuries was evaluated in República Bolivariana de Venezuela during one week of national holidays (Herrera and others 2009). During the week the law was in effect, alcohol use was reduced and fewer accidents were reported.

Alternative solutions to prohibition include measures to regulate the alcohol market. Evidence has shown that alcohol consumption and related problems decrease when accessibility is diminished (for example, by pricing alcohol higher than other products) and consumption is more difficult (for example, by limiting the hours of sale). Alcohol prices may be increased through taxes, curbing consumption problems while increasing government revenues. Evidence has shown that this measure impacts heavy drinkers (defined as an average of more than 20 grams of pure alcohol per day for women and more than 40 grams for men) and light to moderate drinkers (less than 20 grams for women and less than 40 grams men), as well as younger and older drinkers (underage and legal age) (Babor and others 2010).

Taxation

The effects of taxation can be measured by price elasticity, which reflects the change in consumption in relation to the size of the price increase (percentage of change in quantity purchased/percentage change in price); an elasticity of less than –1.0 indicates that demand is relatively responsive to changes in price or is "elastic." Elasticities between –1.0 and 0 indicate that the demand is less responsive to prices or is "inelastic" (NIAAA 2000). An inelastic response to a tax increase may still have positive public health effects.

Evidence, mostly from HICs, shows a range of elasticities from –0.3 for the beverage ranked first in the target population's preferences to –1.5 for the one ranked last (Rehm and others 2003). Accordingly, an elasticity of –0.3 with respect to a tax on alcohol means that consumption will be reduced 3 percent by a 10 percent tax increase, while the alcohol tax revenue for the government will rise by 6.7 percent.

Latin America and the Caribbean. In Mexico, the price elasticity of demand was near –0.2 (Galindo, Robles, and Medina-Mora 2012); in República Bolivariana de Venezuela, the price elasticity was quite low, between −0.074 and −0.058 (Herrera and others 2009).

East Asia and Pacific. In China, using data from the China Health and Nutrition Surveys for 1993, 1997, 2000, 2004, and 2006 in nine provinces in China, the price elasticity was virtually zero for beer and only −0.12 for liquor (Tian and Liu 2011). A previous estimate derived from household surveys conducted in 1993 and 1998 in three main cities and one province of China found elasticities of −0.51 for wine coolers, −0.85 for beer, and −1.39 for wine (Pan, Fang, and Malaga 2006). Using time-series data for consumption and retail prices in Taiwan, China, the price elasticity for alcohol was −0.771 (Lee and others 2010).

A study conducted in Thailand showed the effectiveness of two taxation approaches (Sornpaisarn, Shield, and Rehm 2012). One tax schedule is based on *alcohol content,* aimed at discouraging harmful patterns by promoting beverages with low alcohol content, suitable for contexts with a high prevalence of current drinkers. The other tax scheme is estimated as a *function of price,* which increases taxes on beverages consumed by heavy drinkers and potential new drinkers. Since the first scheme has the potential risk of promoting consumption in abstainers who are a large segment of the population in LMICs (WHO 2013a), a combination of both measures is proposed, together with interventions designed to control the promotion of alcoholic beverages.

East Asia and Pacific, South Asia, and Sub-Saharan Africa. In a systematic literature review and meta-analysis, Sornpaisarn and others (2013) found 12 studies with evidence of the link between alcohol prices or taxation and consumption in LMICs (China, India, Kenya, Tanzania, Thailand, and Turkey), although unrecorded alcohol was not considered. Elasticity estimates were −0.64 (95% confidence interval [CI]: −0.80 to −0.48) for total alcohol consumption, −0.50 (95% CI: −0.78 to −0.21) for beer consumption, and −0.79 (95% CI: −1.09 to −0.49) for consumption of other alcoholic beverages. They concluded that the price elasticity of demand for alcohol in LMICs is similar to that in HICs, and suggested more research was needed on the association between alcohol price or taxation and alcohol-related harm and drinking initiation in LMICs.

Control of the Unrecorded Market
Quantitative studies of the effects of policy options for controlling the unrecorded market are scarce. The main concern for controling unrecorded alcohol is that it can undercut the effects of regulatory measures by offering people an alternative. Some successful control examples include the centuries-old requirement of official sealing labels over corks or stoppers; this measure has been widely used, and the attendant threat to withdraw the liquor license of any place caught using untaxed alcohol has been effective (Lachenmeier, Rehm, and Gmel 2007).

Another concern about unrecorded alcohol is its potential toxic effects. Although according to Lachenmeier, Rehm, and Gmel (2007) the contribution of these effects to mortality is still unclear, because of their public health importance some measures to reduce harm can be included in policies. For example, such measures could include abolishing denatured alcohol; abolishing the use of methanol, which is a simple form of alcohol closely related to ethanol and found in unregistered alcoholic beverages, but more toxic (Pincock and ABC Health & Wellbeing 2013); or treating products not intended for human consumption with bittering agents to prevent people from using them (Lachenmeier, Rehm, and Gmel 2007). For example, recently in Mexico, after an increase in the number of seizures of unrecorded alcohol, a new regulation was issued requiring that all ethyl alcohol and methanol produced in the country be mapped to the primary manufacturing process. This regulation prevents diversions to informal channels, where unrecorded alcohol can be mixed with alcoholic beverages. The regulation prohibits the sale of alcohol in bulk and the incorporation of methanol as a raw product in beverages (CSG 2014).

Following a review of policy options for regulating unrecorded alcohol, Lachenmeier, Taylor, and Rehm (2011) classified policies in:

- *Reducing health risks*: prohibiting the toxic compounds that are used to denature alcohol and substituting them with substances with acceptable toxic profiles, for example, via the use of bittering agents, to prevent accidental deaths
- *Reducing cross-border shopping*: narrowing tax differences between unrecorded and recorded beverages or introducing stricter controls
- *Limiting illegal trade and counterfeiting*: implementing tax stamps and electronic surveillance systems for the alcohol trade.

These authors also suggested that the introduction of education campaigns could increase awareness of the risks associated with drinking illegal alcohol. They concluded that the most problematic category was the control of home and small-scale artisanal production; the most promising option was to offer financial incentives to producers to ensure registration and quality control. There is a need for further research in countries with different cultures and traditions (Lachenmeier, Taylor, and Rehm 2011).

Minimum Prices and Bans on Discounts and Promotions

Evidence in HICs suggests that price discounts—such as happy hours and grocery store promotions—increase consumption and that higher prices for distilled spirits shift consumption to beverages with lower alcohol content, resulting in lower total intake. Enforcing minimum prices for a standard unit of alcohol is one of the most effective ways to reduce alcohol-related problems (Babor and others 2010). No evidence is available for LMICs.

Restrictions on Density, Hours, Days, Locations of Sale, and Advertising

Control of the physical availability of alcohol through measures such as restricting the hours, days, and locations of sale; limiting the density of concentration of retail drinking establishments and off-sales stores (shops licensed to sell alcoholic beverages for consumption off the premises); and establishing a minimum legal purchase age have diminished alcohol use and related problems in HICs (Babor and others 2010).

Although such measures have also been implemented in LMICs, only a few impact studies have been identified in these settings.

Latin America and the Caribbean. A significant reduction in violence was reported in Brazil following the implementation of a municipal law preventing the sale of alcohol after 11 p.m. Enactment of this law was followed by a public information campaign, the law was strictly enforced, and the measure was assessed by an interrupted time-series analysis. The results suggest that the law prevented an estimated 319 homicides over three years (Duailibi and others 2007). Similar results have been observed through restrictions on alcohol service hours in cities in Colombia (Sánchez and others 2011) and Peru (Málaga and others 2012).

Indigenous Communities. Some studies are available for indigenous groups within HICs. A study conducted in Tennant Creek in the Northern Territory, Australia, assessed the effectiveness of interventions and community attitudes toward increased restrictions on the availability of alcohol that included constraints on the days, hours, and amounts of different beverages allowed for sale. After two years, annual per capita consumption of pure alcohol declined by 19.4 percent,

accompanied by declines in hospital admissions (Gray and others 2000).

In HICs that have banned advertising, an econometric analysis showed that these measures had only a modest effect on alcohol use (Rehm and others 2006). However, other research indicates that banning advertising, accompanied by taxation and availability restriction, combine to constitute the best buy in reducing alcohol-related problems (WHO 2014a). Research on restrictions on advertising has not been replicated in LMICs. However, research from Taiwan, China, has replicated findings from HICs showing that exposure to alcohol marketing is associated with greater likelihood of initiation and persistence of drinking among youth (Chang and others 2014).

Countermeasures to Alcohol-Impaired Driving

The harmful consequences of alcohol can be curbed by risk-reducing measures, such as drinking and impaired driving countermeasures. Impaired driving laws, when accompanied by strategies for reinforcing them, such as regular random breath testing of drivers, have been shown to reduce the number of fatal and nonfatal traffic injuries. These strategies modify the drinking practices of high-risk alcohol users and protect other members of the population, such as passengers, other drivers, and pedestrians.

- Various blood alcohol concentration (BAC) limits are in place globally. Setting and enforcing legislation on BAC limits of 0.05 grams per deciliter (g/dL) can lead to significant reductions in alcohol-related crashes (Babor and others 2010). Setting lower BAC limits (0.02 g/dL or less) or zero tolerance is recommended for inexperienced drivers and young adults as an effective means of reducing crashes related to impaired driving; HICs are more likely to have these laws in place than LMICs. These laws are more effective when random breath testing for all drivers is conducted, and when drivers perceive a high likelihood of being arrested if they break the law (WHO 2013b).
- Rehm and others (2006) estimated that random breath testing could reduce fatalities between 6 and 10 percent if partially implemented, and up to 18 percent if implementation were extended. For nonfatal injuries, they calculated a reduction of 15 percent. However, these estimates are based on information obtained from HICs, where road infrastructure and driving patterns may significantly differ from those in LMICs.
- A related measure—sobriety checkpoints—has a high level of research support, with a robust, although lower, level of evidence of effectiveness in HICs (Babor and others 2010).

- Administrative license suspension for driving under the effects of alcohol, allowing licensing authorities to suspend a driver's license without a court hearing at the time of the offense or shortly after, has a good level of evidence; when punishment is swift, effectiveness is increased, particularly in countries where it is consistently applied (Babor and others 2010). Evidence in LMICs is scarce.

East Asia and Pacific. Studies conducted in China found that random breath tests and the perceived potential legal consequences of conviction reduced impaired driving rates (Kim and others 2013). The arrest of intoxicated drivers on BAC limits and enforcement were associated with a reduction of fatal accidents involving impaired driving in Taiwan, China (Chang and Yeh 2004).

Latin America and the Caribbean. In Brazil, low BAC rates reduced traffic injuries and deaths (Andreuccetti and others 2011).

COMMUNITY PLATFORM INTERVENTIONS

The impact of this measure is generally evaluated in terms of knowledge and attitudes. The most common target group is young drinkers; school-based interventions are one of several education and persuasion initiatives tested.

Indigenous Communities

The effectiveness of web-based alcohol screening versus web-based screening and a brief intervention for reducing hazardous drinking was tested in Maori university students, an indigenous population from New Zealand. The study used a parallel, double-blind, multisite RCT with a five-month follow-up assessment. The results indicated that the web-based screening and brief intervention reduced hazardous and harmful drinking among non-help-seeking respondents (Kypri and others 2013).

Babor and others (2010) concluded from their review that the effects of the interventions on the onset of drinking and on drinking problems are equivocal and minimal. Evidence shows that classroom education may increase knowledge and change attitudes, but it has no long-term effect on drinking behavior. Similar results were observed in college students exposed to a multicomponent program comprising mass media campaigns and impaired driving campaigns, warning labels, and social marketing.

Family-Based Interventions

Family interventions have improved communication skills, parental supervision of children and adolescents, the setting of rules and norms, and modeling behavior within families, yet have little impact on behavior on their own. In LMICs, some interventions have been implemented to help families cope with members who have developed disorders, but the research designs used to evaluate interventions for substance use disorders have not included clinical trials (Natera and others 2011; Tiburcio and Guillermina 2003). Outcomes are more compelling when family programs are combined with the other measures described in this chapter (Babor and others 2010).

Mass Media Campaigns

Awareness initiatives include mass media campaigns. When combined with policies and regulatory controls, awareness campaigns can help to increase public support for policy measures and compliance with laws and regulations. Warning labels related to drinking during pregnancy have been introduced in HICs and LMICs. A review of published literature testing the effectiveness of alcohol warning levels in the prevention of FASD in Canada, France, New Zealand, and the United States showed that although alcohol warning labels are popular, their effectiveness in changing behavior is limited (Thomas and others 2014). FASD, whether complete or incomplete, is a growing problem that warrants further attention. There is insufficient evidence, even in HICs; however, studies show that warning labels, when delivered through channels that are perceived to be useful, can be beneficial and can influence behavior if they are part of a comprehensive strategy (Wilkinson and Room 2009).

The mhGAP (WHO 2008) recommends advising women who are pregnant, breastfeeding, or planning to become pregnant to avoid alcohol completely, and offering social support services for those who require additional assistance (WHO 2014b). Treatment in some cases could be helpful.

Studies in South Africa show that treatment using case management interventions to reduce alcohol intake among high-risk pregnant women had positive effects. The effects included stopping drinking, changing drinking behavior reflected in reduced Alcohol Use Disorders Identification Test scores, and reducing problem drinking (Maraisa and others 2011) (table 7.4).

HEALTH CARE PLATFORM INTERVENTIONS

Screening and Brief Interventions

Key elements of brief interventions include feedback, responsibility, advice, strategies, empathy, and self-efficacy. Strong evidence supports clinically significant effects on drinking behavior and related problems

Table 7.4 Community-Based Interventions: School and Family Interventions and Media Campaigns

Population	Type of study	Main results
Indigenous communities/*Maori in New Zealand*	Parallel, double-blind, multisite RCT with a five-month follow-up assessment (+++)	Web-based screening and brief intervention reduced hazardous and harmful drinking among non-help-seeking respondents (Kypri and others 2013).
South Africa	Pragmatic cluster randomized trial with no evidence of a diagnostic test used in the assessment phase (++)	Treatment using case management interventions to reduce alcohol intake among high-risk pregnant women reduced risk (Maraisa and others 2011; Rendall-Mkosi and others 2013).

Note: RCT = randomized controlled trial; ++ = good; +++ = very good.

(Diaz and others 2011; Nagel and others 2009). The mhGAP Intervention Guide (WHO 2011b) identifies three levels of interventions with individual problematic drinkers:

- Screening and brief interventions by trained primary health care professionals
- Early identification and treatment of AUDs in primary health care
- Referral and supervisory support by specialists.

The WHO mhGAP action plan promotes scaling up services for mental, neurological, and substance use disorders, with more cases treated at the first level of care (WHO 2008). The program is based on a review and evaluation of the strength of the evidence to submit recommendations for action. Psychosocial support was found to be more effective than no treatment, while motivational interviewing and motivation enhancement were possibly more effective than standard psychosocial treatment involving families and friends (mainly spouses), or no treatment, or individual counseling.

Evidence in LMICs is widespread and consistent, showing positive results (table 7.5).

Medical and Social Detoxification, Treatment, Follow-Up, and Referral

The recent evidence for LMICs is consistent with what had previously been reported (Patel and others 2007) (table 7.6).

The mhGAP recommends referral from first-level care and supervisory support by specialists for patients with established alcohol dependence. The recommended actions include the planning of cessation of alcohol consumption and detoxification; if necessary, the treatment of withdrawal symptoms with diazepam; the use of medications to prevent relapses, such as naltrexone, acamprosate, or disulfuram; and the assessment and

Table 7.5 Screening and Brief Interventions in Low- and Middle-Income Countries

Site	Main results
Thailand (++)	Motivational interviewing was tested in low-resource settings (Noknoy and others 2010; Segatto and others 2011).
China (+++)	Counseling was supported with health promotion booklets (Tsai and others 2009).
Brazil (+++)	Brief advice was provided on cognitive behavioral interventions (Marques and Formigoni 2001).
Mexico (++)	Motivation therapy showed a greater reduction of alcohol use compared with cognitive behavioral therapy (Diaz and others 2011).
Indigenous communities/ *Australia* (++)	Brief psycho-educational intervention that included motivational care planning, problem solving, and impulse management showed significant benefits, compared with a control group (Nagel and others 2009).
Kenya (++)	Intervention was among people with HIV/AIDS (Papas and others 2010).

Note: ++ = good; +++ = very good; HIV/AIDS = human immunodeficiency virus and acquired immune deficiency syndrome.

treatment of comorbidity and possible referral to self-help groups (WHO 2008).

Self-Help and Support Groups

Mutual help and self-help organizations for those interested in reducing or ceasing drinking have been an important part of the social response to alcohol in many societies. Given that many religions forbid or discourage drinking, adherence to a religious congregation or group often carries with it an expectation of mutual help to stop drinking. In many social groups in Latin America and the Caribbean, joining a Protestant sect has often been a way out of sociocultural expectations of heavy drinking, particularly for

Table 7.6 Medical and Social Detoxification, Treatment, Follow-Up, and Referral

Site	Main results
Brazil (++)	There were no significant differences between naltrexone versus placebo during detoxification (Castro and Laranjeira 2009).
	Acamprosate was superior to a placebo in supporting abstinence in men undergoing treatment (Baltieri and Guerra de Andrade 2003).
Iran (++)	Naltrexone demonstrated better results than placebo when used as a maintenance treatment for a 12-week period (Ahmadi and Ahmadi 2002).
India (++)	Lorazepam and chlordiazepoxide showed similar efficacy in reducing the symptoms of alcohol withdrawal (Kumar, Andrade, and Murthy 2009).

Note: ++ = good.

men (Butler 2006; Eber 2001). Many mutual help groups that are not affiliated with particular religions or that are entirely secular have formed in different countries (Room, Jernigan, Carlini, Gmel, and others 2013; Room, Jernigan, Carlini, Gureje, and others 2002). The most well-known and widespread is Alcoholics Anonymous, which has proved adaptable to many cultural settings (Eisenbach-Stangl and Rosenqvist 1998; Mäkelä 1991).

Affiliation with Alcoholics Anonymous and similar groups is not considered a form of formal treatment—although some groups have affiliations with treatment institutions—and incorporating mutual help groups into a treatment system is likely to undercut their effectiveness. The principles of voluntary mutual help organizations often do not allow random-assignment clinical trials to test their effectiveness; consequently, not much research has been conducted on the impact of these groups (Ferri, Amato, and Davoli 2006; Terra and others 2007). However, survey results support the important role of these groups; 71 percent of the countries included in WHO's *Atlas on Substance Use* (2010) reported the presence of Alcoholics Anonymous.

Latin America and the Caribbean. In Mexico according to a National Household Survey (Medina-Mora and others 2012), 44 percent of persons in treatment for alcohol problems reported being affiliated with self-help groups, while only 35 percent received professional treatment. A study conducted in a nonprobabilistic sample of 192 members of Alcoholics Anonymous found that the level of affiliation or involvement with the organization was negatively related to relapse; with more involvement, mean participation time was higher, and activities related to service were more frequent. Most of the

nonrelapsed subjects were sponsors helping newcomers, practiced the 12 steps more often, and reported spiritual awakening experiences more frequently (Gutiérrez and others 2007; Gutiérrez and others 2009).

The WHO (2011b) makes a standard recommendation—that indicates that it can be offered to the majority of patients but might not be applicable to all cases—for nonspecialist health care workers to be encouraged to familiarize themselves with locally available self-help groups. These groups should offer services at no cost to patients, and they should provide support for recovery and new social connections unrelated to drinking. Relatives of patients with alcohol dependence should be encouraged to participate in appropriate self-help groups for families, so that they can better understand their relatives' conditions and support their recovery.

COST-EFFECTIVENESS OF INTERVENTIONS

The addition of a cost component or economic dimension to health impact assessment introduces the opportunity to identify alcohol prevention and control strategies that have better or worse value for money. For example, devoting scarce resources to interventions that do not discernibly reduce ill-health caused by the consumption of alcohol—as is the case for information and education—is a clear case of investing in interventions that are not cost-effective. At the other end of the spectrum, in contrast, imposition and enforcement of taxation policies offers an example of a highly cost-effective public health intervention that costs relatively little to implement but reaps substantial health returns.

The available body of economic evidence to inform decisions around these alcohol control measures in LMICs remains modest and is based on a modeling approach that relies on data from higher-income settings for some of its inputs. Rehm and others (2006) reported on the comparative cost-effectiveness of a group of interventions—enactment of legislation on drinking and driving, random breath testing, taxation of alcoholic beverages, reduced hours of sale, and advertising bans—in East Asia and Pacific, Latin America and the Caribbean, South Asia, and Sub-Saharan Africa. Increased taxation was the most cost-effective strategy, although it may have a regressive impact on the incidence of alcohol consumption if accompanied by a rise in an already high level of unrecorded consumption. The authors found reductions from 2 to 4 percent in the incidence of high-risk alcohol use, depending on regional drinking patterns. The strategy of reducing the hours of sale produced a modest reduction of 1.5–3.0 percent in the incidence of high-risk drinking, together with a 1.5–4.0 percent reduction in alcohol-related traffic fatalities.

The overall conclusion from this study was that countries with a high prevalence of high-risk drinking should begin with taxation, because in such contexts it appears to have the largest impact for the fewest resources. In settings where high-risk drinking is less of a public health burden, other strategies that restrict the supply or promotion of alcoholic beverages appear to be promising and relatively cost-effective mechanisms, although there is a clear need for greater empirical support of their efficacy. In Mexico, a combination of interventions yielded the best results, with higher taxation (by 50 percent) ranked first (Medina-Mora and others 2010). Tax increases were also the measure recommended in India (Mahal 2000). Banning advertising, in conjunction with taxation and restrictions on availability, is considered the best combination of measures (WHO 2014b).

In terms of individual-level measures, trial-based economic evaluations have been conducted in HICs, the results of which have been used to model expected costs and health gains in LMICs (Chisholm and others 2004; Rehm and others 2006). Although found to be the most costly intervention to implement, brief interventions also lead to a large health gain in the population as a result of an estimated 13–34 percent reduction in consumption among high-risk drinkers, making it a relatively cost-effective measure.

The relative cost-effectiveness of these alcohol control and prevention measures is further discussed and reviewed in chapter 12 in this volume (Levin and Chisholm 2015).

CHALLENGES AND OPPORTUNITIES

Challenges for LMICs

Alcohol is responsible for a high proportion of the global burden of disease. Although drinkers in LMICs consume relatively smaller quantities of alcohol compared with drinkers in HICs, those in LMICs are more adversely affected. They tend to drink high quantities of alcohol per occasion, increasing the negative effects on health as well as increasing the rates of intentional and unintentional injuries.

The challenge of implementing a health-oriented alcohol policy is high, especially in LMICs, with higher burdens and fewer mitigating factors for harm, such as those derived from a temperance tradition that supports control over availability and limits quantities of alcohol intake. The public health perspective has received little attention in international negotiations affecting alcohol markets (Casswell and Thamarangsi 2009; Grieshaber-Otto, Schacter, and Sinclair 2006; Zeigler 2006). Financial aid to LMICs from international agencies has often

been conditioned on market deregulation, which has diminished controls on alcohol sales. In many countries, drunkenness is often tolerated, awareness of the consequences of alcohol is limited, multinational alcohol industry interests have been politically influential, and resources to fund policy measures to reduce the societal burden are scarce.

In settings in which alcohol use is well established, prohibition has not proved to be an effective way to curb the problem. The most promising alternatives are measures that increase the cost of alcoholic beverages and reduce the availability, accompanied by efforts to reduce unrecorded alcohol. Public health campaigns may be needed to increase awareness of the seriousness of alcohol problems in society and build support for intervention measures.

Measures to Control Price
- Market regulation, prevention, and treatment have been identified as strategies of choice for diminishing alcohol-related harm.
- Price discounts can increase consumption. Although research on the policy impact is scarce, evidence from HICs supports the use of minimum prices for a standard unit of alcohol as one of the most effective ways to reduce alcohol-related problems.
- Tax increases have proven to be cost-effective, independent of the level of income, even in countries with relatively low price elasticity.

Control of Alcohol Availability
Measures to control the availability of alcohol are typically adopted as part of a system of alcohol control that includes licensing sellers. Enforcement of the licensing regime is accomplished most efficiently in civil rather than criminal law. These measures include restricting the hours, days, and locations of sale; the density of the concentration of on-premises and retail drinking establishments; and the exposure to the intoxicating effects of alcohol. Although these measures have been implemented in LMICs, only a few studies have been identified in these contexts regarding a significant reduction in violence; no evidence is available on the level of enforcement of regulations.

Unrecorded Alcohol
Research shows that in LMICs where unrecorded alcohol is widely available, the strategy of tax increases needs to be accompanied by reductions in the supply and sales of unrecorded alcohol. Strategies to control the unregulated market can include regulating or raising the cost of nonbeverage alcohol products (such as mouthwashes and cleaning agents) that are used as substitute

beverages, narrowing the tax gap between beverages, introducing stricter controls to reduce cross-border shopping, and implementing tax stamps and electronic surveillance systems of alcohol trade sites to limit illegal trade and counterfeiting. Education campaigns could increase awareness of the risks associated with drinking illegal alcohol. The most promising option for the control of home and small-scale artisanal production is to offer financial incentives to producers to ensure registration and quality control.

Other Opportunities

Other substantial opportunities exist to reduce the burden of alcohol when the political will to do so exists.

Alcohol-Impaired Driving Laws

Impaired driving laws and strategies for reinforcing them influence the rates of fatal and nonfatal traffic injuries by modifying the drinking practices of high-risk alcohol users. These measures also protect others affected by the behavior of drinkers. BAC limits of 0.05 g/dL can lead to significant reductions in alcohol-related crashes, particularly if accompanied by enforcement.

Interventions to Reduce the Risk of FASD

Although alcohol warning labels are popular, their effectiveness in changing behavior is unknown. More positive results have been linked to treatment interventions to reduce alcohol intake among high-risk pregnant women.

Advertising Bans

Bans on advertising, a measure not widely tested across cultures or in LMICs, have at least a modest effect on alcohol use. Producers and sellers tend to transfer their advertising budgets to promotions that fall outside the bans. Effects may be greater in young and abstaining populations. Implementation of such bans is generally inexpensive and can be included in the package of interventions. Such packages that include banning advertising, accompanied by higher taxation and availability restrictions, constitute the best buy in reducing problems related to alcohol use (WHO 2014b).

School-and Family-Based Interventions

The effects of school-based interventions on the onset of drinking and drinking problems, if not accompanied by effective interventions aimed at the general population, are equivocal and minimal. Evidence shows that classroom education may increase knowledge and change attitudes, but it has no demonstrated long-term effect on drinking behavior. Family interventions have proved to change communication skills within the family, yet have little impact on behavior on their own. More promising outcomes are obtained from programs that combine this approach with alcohol regulations.

Screening and Brief Interventions

Screening and brief interventions by trained primary health care professionals, early identification and treatment of AUDs in primary health care settings, and referral and supervisory support by specialists have been widely tested in LMICs and have demonstrated clinically significant effects in reducing drinking behavior and related problems.

Treatment of Withdrawal

Treatment of withdrawal symptoms—a potential life-threatening condition that can occur when a person reduces or stops drinking after a period of heavy drinking—is recommended as a prerequisite to treatment of alcohol dependence. The quality of evidence on the effectiveness of medications for the treatment ranges from low to very low. Psychosocial support has been found to be more effective than no treatment. Motivational interviewing and motivation and motivation enhancement were more effective than standard psychosocial treatment involving families and friends (mainly spouses), and more effective than no treatment or individual counseling. Referral and supervisory support by specialists for patients with established alcohol dependence are a beneficial complement, as is the involvement of patients and their families in mutual help groups. Evidence suggests that packages that combine interventions are more promising and have added effects on curbing the alcohol problem.

Interventions for Alcohol Use during Pregnancy

Women who are pregnant, breastfeeding, or planning to become pregnant are recommended to avoid alcohol. Screening and brief interventions, detoxification and quitting programs, and management of infants exposed to alcohol tailored to the needs of the pregnant women and the infants should be included in the services provided.

Cost Analysis

The available body of economic evidence to inform decisions around alcohol *control measures* in LMICs, constituting *fiscal instruments*, *legal limits,* and *regulation*, remains modest. It is based on a modeling approach that relies on data from HICs for some inputs (involving effect sizes, for example). Although more research is needed, results from this approach support further action.

In terms of individual-level measures, brief interventions can result in substantial health gains. Although these measures are among the most costly interventions to implement, they can produce an estimated 13–34 percent reduction in consumption among high-risk drinkers, thereby making this type of measure relatively cost-effective. Evidence suggests that packages that combine interventions are more promising and have a greater effect on curbing the alcohol problem.

CONCLUSIONS

LMICs have a high burden of disease derived from alcohol use, medium-to-low levels of policy implementation for reducing alcohol use and consequences, insufficient evidence of the impact of measures to reduce the burden, and a paucity of research. The combination of these factors constitutes a compelling argument that more decisive action is needed by national and international organizations to reduce the burden derived from alcohol use, which is a preventable cause of death and disability. This chapter documents the urgent need to increase research support to assemble evidence, monitor progress, and reduce the gap between evidence, its application in communities, and its inclusion in policies (Barnes 2000).

NOTE

World Bank Income Classifications as of July 2014 are as follows, based on estimates of gross national income (GNI) per capita for 2013:

- Low-income countries (LICs) = US$1,045 or less
- Middle-income countries (MICs) are subdivided:
  a) Lower-middle-income = US$1,046 to US$4,125
  b) Upper-middle-income (UMICs) = US$4,126 to US$12,745
- High-income countries (HICs) = US$12,746 or more

REFERENCES

Ahmadi, J. and N. Ahmadi. 2002. "A Double Blind, Placebo-Controlled Study of Naltrexone in the Treatment of Alcohol Dependence." *German Journal of Psychiatry* 5 (4): 85–89.

Andreuccetti, G., H. B. Carvalho, C. J. Cherpitel, Y. Ye, J. C. Ponce, and others. 2011. "Reducing the Legal Blood Alcohol Concentration Limit for Driving in Developing Countries: A Time for Change? Results and Implications Derived from a Time-Series Analysis (2001–10) Conducted in Brazil." *Addiction* 106 (12): 2124–31.

APA (American Psychiatric Association). 2013. *Diagnostic and Statistical Manual of Mental Disorders (DSM-5)*. Washington, DC: APA. http://www.dsm5.org/Documents/Substance%20 Use%20Disorder%20Fact%20Sheet.pdf.

Babor, T. F., R. Caetano, S. Casswell, G. Edwards, N. Giesbrecht, and others 2010. *Alcohol: No Ordinary Commodity—Research and Public Health*. 2nd ed. New York: Oxford University Press.

Babor, T. F., K. Robaina, and D. Jernigan. 2014. "The Influence of Industry Actions to Increase Availability of Alcoholic Beverages in the African Region." *Addiction* 10 (4): 561–71.

Baltieri, D., and A. Guerra de Andrade. 2003. "Efficacy of Acamprosate in the Treatment of Alcohol-Dependent Outpatients." *Revista Brasileira de Psiquiatria* 25 (3): 156–59.

Barnes, H. M. 2000. "Collaboration in Community Action: A Successful Partnership between Indigenous Communities and Researchers." *Health Promotion International* 15 (1): 17–25.

Benegal, V., P. K. Chand, and I. S. Obot. 2009. "Packages of Care for Alcohol Use Disorders in Low- and Middle-Income Countries." *PLoS Medicine* 6 (10): e1000170.

Butler, B., ed. 2006. *Holy Intoxication to Drunken Dissipation: Alcohol among Quichua Speakers in Otavalo, Ecuador*. Albuquerque: University of New Mexico Press.

Casswell, S., and T. Thamarangsi. 2009. "Reducing Harm from Alcohol: Call to Action." *The Lancet* 373 (9682): 2247–57.

Castro, L. A., and R. Laranjeira. 2009. "A Double Blind, Randomized and Placebo-Controlled Clinical Trial with Naltrexone and Brief Intervention in Outpatient Treatment of Alcohol Dependence." *Jornal Brasileiro de Psiquiatria* 58 (2): 79–85.

Chaiyasong, S., S. Limwattananon, C. Limwattananon, T. Thamarangsi, V. Tangchareonsathien, and others. 2011. "Impacts of Excise Tax Raise on Illegal and Total Alcohol Consumption: A Thai Experience." *Drug: Education Prevention and Policy* 18 (2): 90–99.

Chang, H. L., and C. C. Yeh. 2004. "The Life Cycle of the Policy for Preventing Road Accidents: An Empirical Example of the Policy for Reducing Drunk Driving Crashes in Taipei." *Accident Analysis and Prevention* 36 (5): 809–18.

Chang, F. C., C. M. Lee, P. H. Chen, C. H. Chiu, N. F. Miao, and others. 2014. "Using Media Exposure to Predict the Initiation and Persistence of Youth Alcohol Use in Taiwan." *International Journal of Drug Policy* 25 (3): 386–92.

Chisholm, D., J. Rehm, M. Van Ommeren, and M. Monteiro. 2004. "Reducing the Global Burden of Hazardous Alcohol Use: A Comparative Cost-Effectiveness Analysis." *Journal of Studies on Alcohol* 65 (6): 782–93.

CSG (Consejo de Salubridad General). 2014. "Acuerdo que Establece las Medidas para la Venta y Producción de Alcohol Etílico y Metanol." Diario Oficial de la Federación, Secretaría de Gobernación, Mexico.

Diaz, A., L. R. Diaz, A. C. Rodríguez, A. Diaz, H. Fernández, and others. 2011. "Eficacia de un programa de intervenciones terapéuticas en estudiantes universitarios diagnosticados con dependencia al alcohol." *Salud Mental* 34 (3): 185–94.

Duailibi, S., W. Ponicki, J. Grube, I. Pinsky, R. Laranjeira, and others. 2007. "The Effect of Restricting Opening Hours on Alcohol-Related Violence." *American Journal of Public Health* 97 (12): 2276–80.

Eber, C. 2001. "'Take My Water': Liberation through Prohibition in San Pedro Chenalho, Chiapas, Mexico." *Social Science and Medicine* 53 (2): 251–62.

Eisenbach-Stangl, I., and P. Rosenqvist, eds. 1998. *Diversity in Unity: Studies of Alcoholics Anonymous in Eight Societies.* Publication No. 33. Helsinki: Nordic Council for Alcohol and Drug Research Publication No. 33. http://www .nordicwelfare.org/PageFiles/5230/33publikation.pdf.

Ferri, M., L. Amato, and M. Davoli. 2006. "Alcoholics Anonymous and Other 12-Step Programmes for Alcohol Dependence." *Cochrane Database of Systematic Reviews* (3): CD005032.

Galindo, L. M., R. Robles, and M. E. Medina-Mora. 2012. "El Consumo de Alcohol en México, externalidades negativas y el uso de impuestos en el contexto de las elasticidades, ingreso y precio de la demanda." In *Alcohol y Políticas Públicas*, edited by M. E. Medina-Mora. Mexico City: El Colegio Nacional.

Gliksman, L., M. Rylett, and R. R. Douglas. 2007. "Aboriginal Community Alcohol Harm Reduction Policy (ACAHRP) Project: A Vision for the Future." *Substance Use and Misuse* 42 (12–13): 1851–66.

Gmel, G., R. Room, H. Kuendig, and S. Kuntsche. 2007. "Detrimental Drinking Patterns: Empirical Validation of the Pattern Values Score of the Global Burden of Disease 2000 Study in 13 Countries." *Journal of Substance Use* 12 (5): 337–58.

Gray, D., S. Saggers, D. Atkinson, B. Sputore, and D. Bourbon. 2000. "Beating the Grog: An Evaluation of the Tennant Creek Liquor Licensing Restrictions." *Australian and New Zealand Journal of Public Health* 24 (1): 39–44.

Gray, R., R. A. S. Mukherjee, and M. Rutter. 2009. "Alcohol Consumption during Pregnancy and Its Effects on Neurodevelopment: What Is Known and What Remains Uncertain." *Addiction* 104 (8): 1270–73.

Grieshaber-Otto, J., N. Schacter, and S. Sinclair. 2006. "Dangerous Cocktail: International Trade Treaties, Alcohol Policy, and Public Health." Report prepared for the World Health Organization, Geneva.

Gutiérrez, R., P. Andrade, A. Jiménez, and F. Juárez. 2007. "La espiritualidad y su relación con la recuperación del alcohol- ismo en integrantes de Alcohólicos Anónimos (AA)." *Salud Mental* 30 (4): 62–68.

Gutiérrez, R., P. Andrade, A. Jiménez, G. Saldívar, and F. Juárez. 2009. "Alcohólicos Anónimos (AA): Aspectos relacionados con la adherencia (afiliación) y diferencias entre recaídos y no recaídos." *Salud Mental* 32 (5): 427–33.

Guyatt, G. H., A. D. Oxman, S. Sultan, P. Glasziou, E. A. Akl, and others. 2011. "GRADE Guidelines: 9. Rating Up the Quality of Evidence." *Journal of Clinical Epidemiology* 64 (12): 1311–16.

Herrera, N., B. Reif, A. Suárez, and M. Malo. 2009. *El Alcohol y las Políticas Públicas en Venezuela: Dos Estudios Caracas Organización Panamericana de la Salud.* file:///C:/Users /trealq/Downloads/El_alcohol_y_las_Politicas_Publicas _Venezuela.pdf.

Impact Databank. 2011. *The Global Drinks Market: Impact Databank Review and Forecast, 2010 Edition.* New York: M. Shanken Communications.

IOM (Institute of Medicine). 1998. *Bridging the Gap between Practice and Research: Forging Partnerships with Community-Based Drug and Alcohol Treatment*, edited by M. G. S. Lamb and D. McCarty. Committee on Community-Based Drug Treatment, IOM. Washington, DC: National Academies Press. http://www.nap.edu/catalog/6169.html.

Kim, J. H., A. H. Wong, W. B. Goggins, J. Lau, and S. M. Griffiths. 2013. "Drink Driving in Hong Kong: The Competing Effects of Random Breath Testing and Alcohol Tax Reductions." *Addiction* 108 (7): 1217–28.

Kumar, C., C. Andrade, and P. Murthy. 2009. "A Randomized, Double-Blind Comparison of Lorazepam and Chlordiazepoxide in Patients with Uncomplicated Alcohol Withdrawal." *Journal of Studies on Alcohol and Drugs* 70 (3): 467–74.

Kypri, K., J. McCambridge, T. Vater, S. Bowe, J. Saunders, and others. 2013. "Web-Based Alcohol Intervention for Māori University Students: Double-Blind, Multi-Site Randomized Controlled Trial." *Addiction* 108 (2): 331–38.

Lachenmeier, D., J. Rehm, and G. Gmel. 2007. "Surrogate Alcohol: What Do We Know and Where Do We Go?" *Alcoholism-Clinical and Experimental Research* 31 (10): 1613–24.

Lachenmeier, D. W., B. Sarash, and J. Rehm. 2009. "The Composition of Alcohol Products from Markets in Lithuania and Hungary, and Potential Health Consequences: A Pilot Study." *Alcohol and Alcoholism* 44 (1): 93–102.

Lachenmeier, D. W., B. J. Taylor, and J. Rehm. 2011. "Alcohol Under the Radar: Do We Have Policy Options Regarding Unrecorded Alcohol?" *International Journal of Drug Policy* 22 (2): 153–60.

Lee, J. M., M. G. Chen, T. C. Hwang, and C. Y. Yeh. 2010. "Effect of Cigarette Taxes on the Consumption of Cigarettes, Alcohol, Tea and Coffee in Taiwan." *Public Health* 124: 429–36.

Levin, C., and D. Chisholm. 2015. "Cost and Cost-Effectiveness of Interventions, Policies, and Platforms for the Prevention and Treatment of Mental, Neurological, and Substance Use Disorders." In *Disease Control Priorities* (third edition): Volume 4, *Mental, Neurological, and Substance Use Disorders*, edited by V. Patel, D. Chisholm, T. Dua, R. Laxminarayan, and M. E. Medina-Mora. Washington, DC: World Bank.

Lim, S. S., T. Vos, A. D. Flaxman, G. Danaei, K. Shibuya, and others. 2012. "A Comparative Risk Assessment of Burden of Disease and Injury Attributable to 67 Risk Factors and Risk Factor Clusters in 21 Regions, 1990–2010: A Systematic Analysis for the Global Burden of Disease Study 2010." *The Lancet* 380 (9859): 2224–60.

Mahal, A. 2000. "What Works in Alcohol Policy? Evidence from Rural India." *Economic and Political Weekly* 35: 3959–68.

Mäkelä, K. 1991. "Social and Cultural Preconditions of Alcoholics Anonymous (AA) and Factors Associated with the Strength of AA." *British Journal of Addiction* 86 (11): 1405–13.

Málaga, H., M. Huanuco, G. Agüero, and L. López. 2012. *Case Study on Alcohol Policy Development and Implementation.* Lima: Consultant Metropolitan Lima, City Hall.

Maraisa, S., E. Jordaanb, D. Viljoenc, L. Olivier, J. de Waalc, and others. 2011. "The Effect of Brief Interventions on the Drinking Behaviour of Pregnant Women in a High-Risk Rural South African Community: A Cluster Randomised Trial." *Early Child Development and Care* 181 (4): 463–74.

Margolis, S. A., V. A. Ypinazar, R. Muller, and A. Clough. 2011. "Increasing Alcohol Restrictions and Rates of Serious Injury in Four Remote Australian Indigenous Communities." *Medical Journal of Australia* 194 (10): 503–06.

Marques, A., and M. L. Formigoni. 2001. "Comparison of Individual and Group Cognitive-Behavioral Therapy for Alcohol and/or Drug-Dependent Patients." *Addiction* 96 (6): 835–46.

May, P., and P. Gossage. 2011. "Maternal Risk Factors for Fetal Alcohol Spectrum Disorders Not as Simple as It Might Seem." *Alcohol Research and Health* 34 (1): 15–26.

Medina-Mora, M. E. 2001. "Women and Alcohol in Developing Countries." *Salud Mental* 24 (2): 3–10.

Medina-Mora, M. E., I. García-Téllez, D. Cortina, R. Orozco, R. Robles, and others. 2010. "Estudio de costo-efectividad de intervenciones para prevenir el abuso de alcohol en México." *Salud Mental* 33 (5): 373–78.

Medina-Mora, M. E, J. A. Villatoro-Velázquez, C. Fleiz-Bautista, M. M. Téllez-Rojo, L. R. Mendoza-Alvarado, and others. 2012. *Encuesta Nacional de Adicciones 2011: Reporte de Alcohol.* México, D.F.: Instituto Nacional de Psiquiatría Ramón de la Fuente Muñiz. http://www.inprf.gob.mx.

Moher, D., A. Liberati, J. Tetzlaff, D. Altman, and PRISMA Group. 2009. "Preferred Reporting Items for Systematic Reviews and Meta-Analyses: The PRISMA Statement." *Annals of Internal Medicine* 151 (4): 264–70.

Murray, C., T. Vos, R. Lozano, A. Flaxman, C. Michaud, and others. 2012. "Disability-Adjusted Life Years (DALYs) for 291 Diseases and Injuries in 21 Regions, 1990–2010: A Systematic Analysis for the Global Burden of Disease Study 2010." *The Lancet* 380 (9859): 2197–223.

Nagel, T., G. Robinson, J. Condon, and T. Trauer. 2009. "Approach to Treatment of Mental Illness and Substance Dependence in Remote Indigenous Communities: Results of a Mixed Methods Study." *Australian Journal of Rural Health* 17 (4): 174–82.

Natera Rey, G., P. S. Medina Aguilar, F. Callejas Pérez, F. Juárez, and M. Tiburcio. 2011. "Efectos de una intervención a familiares de consumidores de alcohol en una región indígena en México." *Salud Mental* 34 (3): 195–201.

NIAAA (National Institute of Alcohol Abuse and Alcoholism). 2000. "Economic and Health Services Perspectives: Effects of Changes in Alcohol Prices and Taxes." In *10th Special Report to the U.S. Congress on Alcohol and Health*, 341–54. Highlights from current research. Washington, DC: NIAAA.

Noknoy, S., R. Rangsin, P. Saengcharnchai, U. Tantibhaedhyangkul, and J. McCambridge. 2010. "RCT of Effectiveness of Motivational Enhancement Therapy Delivered by Nurses for Hazardous Drinkers in Primary Care Units in Thailand." *Alcohol and Alcoholism* 45 (3): 263–70.

O'Brien, P. 2013. "Australia's Double Standard on Thailand's Alcohol Warning Labels." *Drug and Alcohol Review* 32 (1): 5–10.

Pan, S., C. Fang, and J. Malaga. 2006. "Alcoholic Beverage Consumption in China: A Censored Demand System Approach." *Applied Economics Letters* 13: 975–79.

Papas, R. K., J. E. Sidle, S. Martino, J. B. Baliddawa, R. Songole, and others. 2010. "Systematic Cultural Adaptation of Cognitive-Behavioral Therapy to Reduce Alcohol Use among HIV-Infected Outpatients in Western Kenya." *AIDS and Behavior* 14 (3): 669–78.

Patel, V., R. Aroya, S. Chatterjee, D. Chisholm, A. Cohen, and others. 2007. "Treatment and Prevention of Mental Disorders in Low-Income and Middle-Income Countries." *The Lancet* 370 (9591): 991–1005.

Pincock, S., and ABC Health & Wellbeing. 2013. "A Drink to Die For? Avoiding Methanol Poisoning." http://www.abc .net.au/health/features/stories/2013/09/10/3845522.htm.

Rehm, J., N. Rehn, R. Room, M. Monteiro, G. Gmel, and others. 2003. "The Global Distribution of Average Volume of Alcohol Consumption and Patterns of Drinking." *European Addiction Research* 9 (4): 147–56.

Rehm, J., C. Dan, R. Robin, and L. Alan. 2006. "Alcohol." In *Disease Control Priorities in Developing Countries*, 2nd ed., edited by D. T. Jamison, J. G. Bremen, A. R. Measham, G. Alleyne, M. Claeson, D. B. Evans, P. Jha, A. Mills, and P. Musgrove, chapter 47. Washington, DC: World Bank and Oxford University Press.

Rendall-Mkosi, K., N. Morojele, L. London, S. Moodley, C. Singh, and others. 2013. "A Randomized Controlled Trial of Motivational Interviewing to Prevent Risk for an Alcohol-Exposed Pregnancy in the Western Cape, South Africa." *Addiction* 108 (4): 725–32.

Room, R., D. Jernigan, B. Carlini, G. Gmel, O. Gureje, and others 2013. *El Alcohol y los países en desarrollo. Una perspectiva de salud pública.* México, D.F.: Organización Panamericana de la Salud, Fondo de Cultura Económica.

Room, R., D. Jerningan, B. Carlini, O. Gureje, K. Mäkelä, and others, 2002. *Alcohol in Developing Societies: A Public Health Approach.* Geneva: Finnish Foundation for Alcohol Studies, World Health Organization.

Sánchez, A., A. Villaveces, R. Krafty, P. Taeyoung, W. Harold, and others. 2011. "Policies for Alcohol Restriction and Their Association with Interpersonal Violence: A Time-Series Analysis of Homicides in Cali, Colombia." *International Journal of Epidemiology* 40 (4): 1037–46.

Segatto, M. L., S. Andreoni, R. D. E. Silva, A. Diehl, and I. Pinsky. 2011. "Brief Motivational Interview and Educational Brochure in Emergency Room Settings for Adolescents and Young Adults with Alcohol-Related Problems: A Randomized Single-Blind Clinical Trial." *Revista Brasileira de Psiquiatria* 33 (3): 225–33.

Sornpaisarn, B., K. Shield, J. Cohen, R. Schwartz, and J. Rehm. 2013. "Elasticity of Alcohol Consumption, Alcohol-Related Harms, and Drinking Initiation in Low- and Middle-Income Countries: A Systematic Review and Meta-Analysis." *The International Journal of Alcohol and Drug Research* 2 (1): 14.

Sornpaisarn, B., K. Shield, and J. Rehm. 2012. "Alcohol Taxation Policy in Thailand: Implications for Other Low- to Middle-Income Countries." *Addiction* 107 (8): 1372–84.

Terra, M. B., H. M. T. Barros, A. T. Stein, I. Figueira, L. D. Athayde, and others. 2007. "Predictors of Engagement in the Alcoholics Anonymous Group or to Psychotherapy among Brazilian Alcoholics—A Six-Month Follow-Up Study." *European Archives of Psychiatry and Clinical Neuroscience* 257 (4): 237–44.

Thomas, G., G. Gonneau, N. Poole, and J. Cook. 2014. "The Effectiveness of Alcohol Warning Labels in the Prevention of Fetal Alcohol Spectrum Disorder: A Brief Review." *International Journal of Alcohol and Drug Research* 3 (1): 91–103.

Tian, G., and F. Liu. 2011. "Is the Demand for Alcoholic Beverages in Developing Countries Sensitive to Price? Evidence from China." *International Journal of Environmental Research and Public Health* 8 (6): 2124–31.

Tiburcio, M., and N. Guillermina. 2003. "Evaluación de un modelo de intervención breve para familiares de usuarios de alcohol y drogas: Un estudio piloto." *Salud Mental* 26 (5): 33–42.

Tsai, Y. F., M. C. Tsai, Y. P. Lin, and C. Y. Chen. 2009. "Brief Intervention for Problem Drinkers in a Chinese Population: A Randomized Controlled Trial in a Hospital Setting." *Alcoholism: Clinical and Experimental Research* 33 (1): 95–101.

WHO (World Health Organization). 1992. *The ICD-10 Classification of Mental and Behavioral Disorders: Clinical Descriptions and Diagnostic Guidelines.* Geneva: WHO.

———. 1999. *Global Status Report on Alcohol 1999.* Geneva: WHO.

———. 2008. *mhGAP: Mental Health Gap Action Programme: Scaling Up Care for Mental, Neurological and Substance Use Disorders.* Geneva: WHO.

———. 2010. *Atlas on Substance Use: Resources for Prevention and Treatment of Substance Use Disorders.* Geneva: WHO.

———. 2011a. *Global Status Report on Alcohol and Health 2011.* Geneva: WHO.

———. 2011b. *mhGAP: Intervention Guide for Mental, Neurological and Substance Use Disorders in Non-Specialized Health Settings.* Geneva: WHO.

———. 2013a. *Additional Background Material on the Draft Comprehensive Mental Health Action Plan 2013–2020.* Geneva: WHO.

———. 2013b. *Global Status Report on Road Safety 2013: Supporting a Decade of Action.* Geneva: WHO.

———. 2014a. *Global Status Report on Alcohol and Health 2014.* Geneva: WHO.

———. 2014b. *Guidelines for the Identification and Management of Substance Use and Substance Use Disorders in Pregnancy.* Geneva: WHO.

Wilkinson, C., and R. Room. 2009. "Warning on Alcohol Containers and Advertisements: International Experience and Evidence on Effects." *Drug and Alcohol Review* 28 (4): 426–35.

Zeigler, D. W. 2006. "International Trade Agreements Challenge Tobacco and Alcohol Control Policies." *Drug and Alcohol Review* 25 (6): 567–79.

Zhang, C., and M. Monteiro. 2013. "Tactics and Practices of the Alcohol Industry in Latin America: What Can Policy Makers Do?" *International Journal of Alcohol and Drug Research* 2 (2): 75–81.

Chapter 8

Childhood Mental and Developmental Disorders

James G. Scott, Cathrine Mihalopoulos,
Holly E. Erskine, Jacqueline Roberts, and Atif Rahman

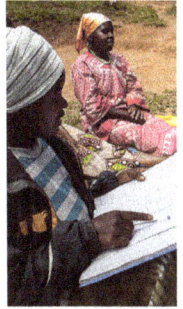

INTRODUCTION

Childhood mental and developmental disorders encompass neurodevelopmental, emotional, and behavioral disorders that have broad and serious adverse impacts on psychological and social well-being. Children with these disorders require significant additional support from families and educational systems; the disorders frequently persist into adulthood (Nevo and Manassis 2009; Polanczyk and Rohde 2007; Shaw and others 2012). These children are more likely to experience a compromised developmental trajectory, with increased need for medical and disability services, as well as increased risk of contact with law enforcement agencies (Fergusson, Horwood, and Lynskey 1993).

Childhood Mental and Behavioral Disorders

This chapter limits the discussion to the following five conditions: childhood anxiety disorders, attention-deficit hyperactivity disorder (ADHD), conduct disorder, autism, and intellectual disability (intellectual developmental disorder).

- *Anxiety disorders* are characterized by excessive or inappropriate fear, with associated behavioral disturbances that impair functioning (APA 2013). Children with anxiety disorders have clinical symptoms, such as excessive anxiety; severe physiological anxiety symptoms; behavioral disturbances, such as avoidance of feared objects; and associated distress or impairment (Beesdo, Knappe, and Pine 2009).
- *ADHD* is a neurodevelopmental disorder characterized by inattention and disorganization, with or without hyperactivity-impulsivity, causing impairment of functioning (APA 2013). ADHD persists into adulthood in approximately 20 percent of individuals (Polanczyk and Rohde 2007).
- *Conduct disorder* diagnosed in children under the age of 18 years is characterized by a pattern of antisocial behaviors that violate the basic rights of others or major age-appropriate societal norms.
- *Autism* is a neurodevelopmental disorder characterized by severe impairment in reciprocal social interactions and communication skills, as well as the presence of restricted and stereotypical behaviors.
- *Intellectual disability* is a generalized disorder that is characterized by significantly impaired cognitive functioning and deficits in two or more adaptive behaviors (APA 2013).

Scope of the Chapter

This chapter reviews interventions to reduce the prevalence of childhood mental and developmental disorders through the prevention, reduction, or remission

Corresponding author: James G. Scott, The University of Queensland Centre for Clinical Research, Queensland; Royal Brisbane and Women's Hospital, Queensland, Australia; james.scott@health.qld.gov.au.

of symptoms. The effectiveness of selected interventions is evidence based; these interventions have the potential to be delivered in low- and middle-income countries (LMICs). The chapter does not discuss childhood depression, because of the overlap in interventions with adult depression.

The chapter considers interventions in terms of delivery platforms rather than specific disorders. This choice is because of the very high comorbidity between childhood mental and developmental disorders (Bakare 2012; Rutter 2011). In addition, risk factors for childhood disorders are nonspecific and pluripotent. For example, children who are maltreated are at higher risk of a wide range of mental and developmental disorders (Benjet, Borges, and Medina-Mora 2010).

NATURE OF CHILDHOOD MENTAL AND DEVELOPMENTAL DISORDERS

Childhood mental and developmental disorders are an emerging challenge to health care systems globally. Two contributing factors are the increases in the proportion of children and adolescents in the populations of LMICs, which is a result of reduced mortality of children under age five years (Murray and others 2012), and the fact that the onset of many adult mental and developmental disorders occurs in childhood and adolescence (Kessler and others 2007).

Global Epidemiology and the Burden of Childhood Mental and Developmental Disorders

Ascertaining the global epidemiology of mental disorders is a difficult task, given the significant paucity of data for many geographical regions, as well as the cultural variations in presentation and measurement. These issues are exacerbated when investigating mental disorders in children, particularly in LMICs where other health concerns, such as infectious diseases, are priorities. The issue of data paucity was highlighted in the Global Burden of Disease Study 2010 (GBD 2010) (Whiteford and others 2013).

Epidemiologically, childhood mental disorders were relatively consistent across the 21 world regions defined by GBD 2010. However, these prevalence estimates were based on sparse data; some regions, such as Sub-Saharan Africa, have no data whatsoever for some disorders or no data for specific disorders in childhood. Although regional differences may exist, the lack of data makes them difficult to ascertain. The 12-month global prevalence of childhood mental disorders in 2010 is shown in table 8.1. ADHD, conduct disorder, and autism were more prevalent in males; females were more likely to

suffer from anxiety disorders. Anxiety disorders and ADHD were more common in adolescents compared with children.

Most children and adolescents with mental and developmental disorders were in South Asia, reflecting the high population in this region and the reduction in mortality of infants and young children (Murray and others 2012). The populations of LMICs tend to have higher proportions of children and adolescents than those of high-income countries (HICs). For example, 40 percent of the population in the least developed countries is younger than age 15 years, compared with 17 percent in more developed regions (United Nations 2011). Furthermore, population aging is occurring more slowly in LMICs, with some low-income countries predicted to have the youngest populations by 2050, given their high fertility rates (United Nations 2011). These trends mean that childhood mental and developmental disorders will increase in significance in LMICs. Furthermore, the continuing reductions in infant mortality caused by infectious diseases mean more children will reach adolescence where the prevalence of mental disorders increases and the onset of adult mental disorders occurs. This will challenge already limited mental health services in these countries.

Risk Factors for Childhood Mental and Developmental Disorders

The risk factors for childhood mental and developmental disorders shown in table 8.2 can be divided into lifelong and age-specific risk factors (Kieling and others 2011). The health of children is highly dependent on the health and well-being of their caregivers; the environments in which the children live (including home and school); and, as they transition into adolescence, the influence of their peers. The relative importance of a particular risk factor should be considered in terms of prevalence, strength of the association with an adverse outcome, and potential to reduce exposure to that risk factor (Scott and others 2014). Using these criteria, efforts to address maternal mental health problems and improve parenting skills have the greatest potential to reduce mental and developmental disorders in children.

Consequences of Childhood Mental and Developmental Disorders

The consequences of these disorders include the impact during childhood and the persistence of mental ill health into adult life. In childhood, the impact is broad, encompassing the individual suffering of children, as well as the negative effects on their families and peers. This impact may include aggression toward other children and

Table 8.1 Global Point Prevalence of Childhood Mental and Developmental Disorders by Gender and Total Number of Cases, 2010

| Age group | Anxiety disorders | | | ADHD | | | Conduct disorder | | | Autism | | |
	N (1,000,000)	Males (%)	Females (%)	N (1,000,000)	Males (%)	Females (%)	N (1,000,000)	Males (%)	Females (%)	N (1,000,000)	Males (%)	Females (%)
5–9 years	5.4	0.62 (0.55–0.70)	1.17 (1.04–1.32)	5.8	1.14 (1.31–1.52)	0.46 (0.43–0.50)	16.1	3.67 (3.24–4.18)	1.54 (1.38–1.73)	1.6	0.39 (0.37–0.42)	0.14 (0.13–0.14)
10–14 years	21.8	2.54 (2.26–2.90)	4.77 (4.31–5.32)	11.9	2.95 (2.75–3.17)	0.92 (0.86–0.98)	16.2	3.73 (3.42–4.05)	1.57 (1.45–1.71)	1.6	0.39 (0.37–0.41)	0.13 (0.13–0.14)
15–19 years	32.2	3.74 (3.33–4.16)	7.02 (6.38–7.85)	8.4	2.12 (1.98–2.26)	0.61 (0.57–0.65)	15.4	3.54 (3.17–3.96)	1.49 (1.34–1.68)	1.6	0.38 (0.36–0.41)	0.13 (0.13–0.14)

Source: Prevalence data from Whiteford and others 2013.

Note: ADHD = attention-deficit hyperactivity disorder; N = number. Values in parentheses are 95 percent confidence intervals.

Table 8.2 Risk Factors for Mental and Developmental Disorders in Children and Adolescents

Life-long	Preconception	Prenatal and perinatal	Infancy and early childhood	School-age children	Adolescence
Natural disasters	Unwanted pregnancy	Inadequate prenatal care	Maternal mental illness	Family, peer, or school problems	Family, peers, or inadequate parenting
Physical illness	Inadequate spacing of children	Complications during pregnancy	Early emotional deprivation	Maternal mental illness	Developmental and behavioral problems
Malnutrition	Adolescent pregnancy	Maternal cigarette and alcohol use	Inadequate stimulation	Bullying	Maternal mental illness
Illness or loss of caregivers	Consanguinity	In utero exposure to pesticides and other toxins	Inadequate parenting	Inadequate parenting	Substance misuse
Exposure to trauma, adversity, violence, or conflict		Birth hypoxia and other obstetric complications	Developmental and behavioral problems	Inadequacies of schools or teachers	Early sexual activity
Genetic background		Maternal difficulties adapting to pregnancy or arrival of newborn		Developmental and behavioral problems	Risk-taking behaviors
Toxins		Perinatal maternal mortality		Risk-taking behaviors	School problems
Immigrant status					

Source: Kieling and others 2011.

distraction of peers from learning. Children with mental and developmental disorders are at higher risk of mental and physical health problems in adulthood, as well as increased likelihood of unemployment, contact with law enforcement agencies, and need for disability support.

Trends in Childhood Mental and Developmental Disorders

GBD 2010 estimated burden across five time points (1990, 1995, 2000, 2005, and 2010) and found that the prevalence and burden of childhood mental disorders remained consistent between 1990 and 2010 (Erskine and others 2015). Although the rates may not have changed, population growth and aging have impacts on the burden of disease attributable to mental disorders in childhood. As the population of children increases globally, the burden of disease attributable to mental disorders in children will increase.

INTERVENTIONS FOR CHILDHOOD MENTAL AND DEVELOPMENTAL DISORDERS

Population Platform Interventions

Child and Adolescent Mental Health Policies and Plans
Few countries have developed national policies and plans to address mental and developmental disorders

in children. The World Health Organization (WHO) has published a modular package for governments, policy makers, and service planners, *Child and Adolescent Mental Health Policies and Plans*, to address this need (WHO 2005b). The guidelines recommend attention to a broad range of areas pertaining to childhood mental and developmental disorders (box 8.1). The provision of health services for children in isolation will not prevent mental and developmental disorders or have significant benefits for children with these disorders. Instead, an ecological approach that addresses problems in the systems around children (parents, family, and school) in combination with targeted interventions for children is necessary to make a meaningful difference (Kieling and others 2011).

Child Protection Legislation
Child maltreatment is a well-established risk factor for mental and developmental disorders in children (Benjet, Borges, and Medina-Mora 2010). Child maltreatment is defined as any form of physical or emotional ill-treatment, sexual abuse, neglect or negligent treatment, or commercial or other exploitation that results in actual or potential harm to a child's health, survival, development, or dignity in the context of a relationship of responsibility, trust, or power (Krug and others 2002). Legislation to address child maltreatment requires the support of well-integrated systems that

increase public awareness and enable incident reporting to a constituted authority with investigative and interventional expertise and the ability to prosecute (Svevo-Cianci, Hart, and Rubinson 2010). Limited evidence suggests that legislation to protect children living outside the family home in LMICs has benefits for their health and safety (Fluke and others 2012); however, further research is needed to determine the effectiveness of such legislation for children living with their families of origin.

Community Platform Interventions

Early Child Development

Attempts have been made to develop community- and primary care–based services in LMICs. Eickmann and others (2003) delivered a community-based psychosocial stimulation intervention to mothers in a study of 156 infants (age 12 months) in four towns in Brazil. The intervention consisted of 14 contacts (three workshops and 11 home visits) where mothers were taught the importance of play for children's development, how to make toys from disposable household items, and how to play and positively interact with their children. Children of mothers who received the intervention had significantly improved cognitive and motor development; the greatest effects were observed in infants whose development was mildly delayed. The authors proposed

the intervention could be delivered through local neighborhood groups run by mothers (Eickmann and others 2003).

Powell and others (2004) demonstrate that a psychosocial stimulation intervention could be delivered to infants in Jamaica by community health aid workers in a cluster randomized control trial of 139 mother-infant dyads where the infants were malnourished. The weekly home visits supporting maternal play with children showed that infants in the intervention group had improved overall development as well as improved hearing, speech, and hand-eye coordination. Health aid workers received two weeks of additional training to deliver the intervention, which was provided as part of an existing home visitation program for malnourished children (Powell and others 2004). A follow-up study 25 years later found that those Jamaican children who received early psychosocial stimulation had, on average, 25 percent increased earnings, suggesting long-term economic benefits to infants receiving this intervention (Gertler and others 2014). These studies show psychosocial stimulation is an effective intervention to support cognitive, language, and motor development in young children, conferring short- and long-term benefits, although mental health outcomes were not assessed.

The delivery of community-based interventions poses significant challenges, but the feasibility has been demonstrated in LMICs (Bauermeister and others 2006). Brazil, the Arab Republic of Egypt, Israel, and Lebanon implemented and evaluated a comprehensive community-based program with a package of interventions that could be adapted to different countries and localities based on the following:

- Amount of health care and school resources available
- Nature and severity of the types of problems in children
- Preferences and cultural factors that are important within communities.

Manuals were developed that enabled non-mental health professionals in areas with limited resources to deliver the interventions. The manuals consisted of education, parenting skills training, child training, and cognitive and behavioral therapy. These were adapted for local communities with attention to terminology, modifications to reduce stigma, and emphasis on culturally acceptable parenting skills. The feedback received from these sites indicates that the interventions were useful in helping children with internalizing and externalizing problems (Bauermeister and others 2006). Strategies to improve access to community-based interventions require investments in gatekeepers, such as parents, teachers, and general practitioners. Easy-to-read manuals and guides with culturally adapted strategies for the management of childhood mental disorders through nonspecialist primary care can be useful resources for practitioners seeking to develop services in such settings (Eapen, Graham, and Srinath 2012).

Most preventive interventions implemented in early childhood in LMICs target child development generally, rather than child mental health specifically. However, increasing evidence shows that some of these early interventions can benefit the mental health of children, with benefits maintained into adolescence and adulthood. In Jamaica, an early stimulation program for very undernourished children, which involved home visits over two years, reduced anxiety, depression, and attention deficit disorder, and enhanced self-esteem at ages 17–18 years (Walker and others 2010). In Mauritius, two years of high-quality preschool, from age three years, reduced conduct disorder and schizotypal symptoms at age 17 years and criminal offenses at age 23 years (Raine and others 2003). These benefits were greatest for children who were undernourished at age three years. Such interventions can be integrated with community-based maternal child health programs and should be prioritized in LMICs (Kieling and others 2011).

School-Based Interventions
Schools have a profound influence on children, families, and communities. School-based mental health services also have the potential to bridge the gap between need and utilization by reaching children who would otherwise not have access to these services. These settings could provide an ideal environment in which programs for child mental health can be integrated in a cost-effective, culturally acceptable, and nonstigmatizing manner (Patel, Aronson, and Divan 2013). However, the evidence for school-based interventions for childhood mental and developmental problems in LMICs is limited (Kieling and others 2011; Maulik and Darmstadt 2007).

In Jamaica, Baker-Henningham and others (2012) conducted a cluster randomized control trial of 225 children (ages 3–6 years) with high levels of emotional and behavioral problems, attending 24 community preschool centers. The study examined the effectiveness of teacher training in "The Incredible Years," a children's mental health program. The intervention led to significant reductions in conduct problems (effect size [ES] = 0.42) and increased friendship skills (ES = 0.74). School attendance and parent-reported behavior at home also improved

(Baker-Henningham and others 2012). This study demonstrates that school-based interventions in a middle-income country are effective and feasible in reducing behavioral problems in young children.

Bullying or peer victimization is a specific form of aggression defined as "a form of aggression in which one or more children repeatedly and intentionally intimidate, harass, or physically harm a victim" (Vreeman and Carroll 2007). The long-term impacts of bullying behavior are serious; children who are victims, bullies, or both have elevated rates of psychiatric disorders in childhood and early adulthood (Copeland and others 2013). Accordingly, the prevention of peer victimization in schools is an important strategy to reduce the occurrence of mental disorders and other adverse consequences in children and adults.

Different approaches to reducing bullying behavior have been assessed in the literature. In one systematic review, Vreeman and Carroll (2007) grouped the interventions into three main types: curriculum interventions, whole-of-school approaches, and social and behavioral skills training. Whole-of-school approaches have been found to be effective; these approaches use a multidisciplinary approach that includes combinations of school rules and sanctions, classroom curriculum, teacher training, individual counseling, and conflict resolution training. In a meta-analysis, Ttofi and Farrington (2011) found that school-based anti-bullying programs can reduce bullying by about 20 percent, with greater effects observed in interventions that adopt more of a whole-of-school approach. However, very few, if any, evaluations of interventions to prevent bullying have been conducted in LMICs.

Further research is required to demonstrate the effectiveness of school-based interventions supporting children with autism and intellectual disability.

Voluntary Sector Programs
Agencies in the voluntary sector (those that are nongovernment and not for-profit) have traditionally played an important role in raising awareness of the issues faced by children with mental health difficulties and their families, as well as in reducing the associated stigma. In some countries, the voluntary sector provides the bulk of child mental health services. However, the evidence base for such interventions is poor, largely because of the absence of research support for program evaluation. The magnitude of mental health problems affecting children and the absence of policies to guide service development are significant barriers to coordinated service provision and evaluation of voluntary sector programs for children in LMICs (Omigbodun 2008; Patel and Thara 2003).

Health Care Platform Interventions

Screening and Community Rehabilitation for Developmental Disorders

Providing early interventions to children with developmental disorders may optimize their developmental outcomes (Sonnander 2000). Screening is necessary to identify children in need of these resource-intensive interventions. Screening instruments for LMICs need to be culturally acceptable and have sound psychometric properties that have been validated in the local context (Robertson and others 2012). Instruments developed for screening children for developmental disorders in HICs (such as Denver II) may not be appropriate (Gladstone and others 2008). For example, items assessing whether a child can cut using scissors or catch a bouncing ball may be inappropriate if these resources are unavailable in the community or if parents do not model or encourage these activities. A systematic review identified instruments that have been used for the developmental screening of young children in LMICs (Robertson and others 2012). Two of the screening tools identified as useful were the Ten Questions (TQ) screen (Belmont 1986; Zaman and others 1990) and the ACCESS portfolio (Wirz and others 2005).

The TQ screen (box 8.2) is a brief questionnaire administered to parents of children ages two to nine years. Five questions assess cognitive ability; two questions assess movement ability; one question addresses any history of seizures; one assesses vision; and one assesses hearing. The items require a dichotomous response of yes-no and ask about the skills that children will acquire in any culture. They ask parents to compare their children to other children in their community (Belmont 1986; Zaman and others 1990). The TQ was included as a disability module in the third round of the United Nations Children's Fund Multiple Indicator Cluster Survey, and administered to almost 200,000 children across 18 countries (Gottlieb and others 2009). The TQ is a sensitive tool that identifies 80–100 percent of children with developmental disorders; however, it has a low specificity, necessitating a second stage to examine those children who screen positive (Durkin and others 1994).

Administration of the ACCESS portfolio provides screening of children with developmental disorders, as well as simple advice to parents. Community health workers (CHWs) in Sri Lanka and Uganda used the ACCESS portfolio to assess children younger than age three years whose mothers had expressed concerns. The CHWs' assessments of delay had an 82 percent accuracy in children older than age two years, compared with those identified by medical or allied health staff, although the sensitivity and specificity of the instrument were not measured. The ACCESS portfolio raised awareness of developmental disorders in communities, and CHWs and parents reported it to be helpful (Wirz and others 2005).

Box 8.2

Ten Questions Screen

1. Compared with other children, did the child have any serious delay in sitting, standing, or walking?
2. Compared with other children, does the child have difficulty seeing, either in the daytime or night?
3. Does the child appear to have difficulty hearing?
4. When you tell the child to do something, does he/she seem to understand what you are saying?
5. Does the child have difficulty in walking or moving his/her arms, or does he/she have weakness and/or stiffness in the arms or legs?
6. Does the child sometimes have fits, become rigid, or lose consciousness?
7. Does the child learn to do things like other children his/her age?
8. Does the child speak at all (can he/she make himself/herself understood in words, can he/she say any recognizable words)?
9. *For children ages three to nine years, ask:* Is the child's speech in any way different from normal (not clear enough to be understood by people other than his/her immediate family)?
   For children age two years, ask: Can he/she name at least one object (for example, an animal, a toy, a cup, a spoon)?
10. Compared with other children of his/her age, does the child appear in any way mentally backward, dull, or slow?

Source: Zaman and others 1990.

Two significant issues arise following the identification of children with developmental disorders. The first involves the stigma associated with these diagnoses in some countries and cultures. The second is the limited evidence for the effectiveness of community-based rehabilitation for children with intellectual disabilities and autism in LMICs. These issues do not necessarily indicate that interventions are ineffective, but rather that further evaluation is required (Hastings, Robertson, and Yasamy 2012; Robertson and others 2012).

Parenting Skills Training

Parenting skills training aims to enhance or support the parental role through education and training, thereby improving emotional and behavioral outcomes for children. A meta-analysis identified four components of parenting skills training that were particularly effective. Increasing positive parent-child interactions, teaching parents how to communicate emotionally with their children, teaching parents the use of time out as a means of discipline, and supporting parents to consistently respond to their children's behaviors had the largest effects on reducing externalizing behaviors in children (Kaminski and others 2008).

Several systematic reviews have demonstrated the effectiveness of parenting skills training in reducing internalizing and externalizing problems in children (Furlong and others 2013; Kaminski and others 2008), as well as in reducing the risk of unintentional childhood injuries (Kendrick and others 2007) and improving the mental health of parents (Barlow and others 2014). Childhood disruptive and externalizing behaviors may persist into adolescence, affecting peers, schools, and communities (Fergusson, Horwood, and Lynskey 1994). Furthermore, although many externalizing behaviors diminish as individuals mature through adolescence, life course persistence of antisocial behaviors is more likely in those with childhood-onset conduct problems (Moffitt and others 2002). A meta-analysis of group-based parenting skills training for parents of children with conduct problems showed moderate effect sizes with a standardized mean difference in conduct problems of −0.53 (95 percent confidence interval [CI]: −0.72 to −0.34) as assessed by parents (Furlong and others 2013). Therefore, parenting skills interventions can reduce or prevent the onset of childhood mental disorders and subsequent adverse health and social outcomes.

The evidence for the effectiveness of parenting skills training comes from studies conducted in HICs (Furlong and others 2013). A systematic review of parenting interventions in LMICs reported that most studies examined educational or physical outcomes (Mejia, Calam, and

Sanders 2012). However, eight studies examined interventions to prevent or reduce emotional and behavioral problems in children. The following outcomes were assessed:

- Infant attachment (Cooper and others 2009)
- Maternal understanding and attitude about child development (Jin and others 2007; Klein and Rye 2004; Rahman and others 2009)
- Mother-child interaction (Klein and Rye 2004; Wendland-Carro, Piccinini, and Millar 1999)
- Child abuse (Aracena and others 2009; Oveisi and others 2010)
- Reductions in child behavioral problems (Fayyad and others 2010).

The mean effect size of the parenting skills training across the eight studies was large (Cohen's d = 0.81) (Mejia, Calam, and Sanders 2012); benefits persisted in the follow-up studies, which were as long as 18 months in a study in South Africa (Cooper and others 2009) and six years in a study in Ethiopia (Klein and Rye 2004). Thus, emerging evidence from available research suggests parenting skills training is a feasible and effective intervention in LMICs. The extensive research base available from HICs requires integration with knowledge acquired from studies conducted in LMICs for the development of culturally appropriate parenting skills training.

Maternal Mental Health Interventions

Poor maternal mental health is a risk factor for children's physical, cognitive, and socioemotional development (Deave and others 2008; Feldman and others 2009; Glasheen, Richardson, and Fabio 2010; Grace, Evindar, and Stewart 2003; Grigoriadis and others 2013; Grote and others 2010; Hamadani and others 2012; Wachs, Black, and Engle 2009; Wan and others 2007); the impact continues into adolescence and adulthood (Murray and others 2011; Pearson and others 2013). Interventions that target maternal mental health problems, especially in the perinatal period and early infancy, are important for child mental health and need to be incorporated into primary care.

Perinatal mental disorders can be divided into *common mental disorders* (including depression and anxiety disorders) and *severe mental disorders* (schizophrenia and bipolar disorder). Two meta-analyses have reported that the prevalence of common mental disorders in women in LMICs is between 15.6 percent during pregnancy and 19.8 percent postpartum (Fisher and others 2012; Parsons and others 2012). Maternal depression is the most prevalent condition—and has the largest public health impact (Rahman, Surkan, and others 2013).

A recent systematic review identified 16 longitudinal studies of adolescent mental and developmental health outcomes of children of mothers who had postnatal depression. Increased risk of cognitive delays in the children was the most consistent finding, with some studies also reporting that children of mothers with postnatal depression had increased risk of internalizing and externalizing symptoms and increased general psychopathology (Sanger and others 2015). Accordingly, treatment of maternal mental health problems can reduce suffering in the mother while potentially preventing mental and developmental disorders in the children.

Postnatal depression is the condition for which interventions are most amenable to integration into primary care and maternal and child health platforms (Rahman, Surkan, and others 2013). Such integration requires task-shifting strategies, supported by the development of training curricula and treatment packages that bundle skills that are logically grouped together for content, training, and operational use (Patel and others 2013).

These interventions also require a change in the approach of mental health specialists, as well as health policy and planning specialists—a shift of focus from a model that is specialist and center based to a model that is primary care and community based. Integrated treatment programs, in which health and social care providers are supported to manage common mental health problems, offer a chance to treat the whole person. This approach is more patient centered and is often more effective than one in which mental, physical, and reproductive health problems are addressed separately without effective communication among providers (Patel and others 2013).

Maternal and child health workers are well-positioned to adopt comprehensive approaches to care, which is particularly important for children because their psychosocial well-being is closely linked to the mental health of their parents and the quality of their family and school environments. Maternal and child health workers have knowledge of community resources and health, social, and education services, and they can better respond to the specific needs of local communities. In Pakistan, the Canadian "Learning through Play" program was adapted and taught through one-day workshops to women in the Lady Health Workers program, members of the local community who deliver preventive maternal and child health care. A cluster randomized trial demonstrated that an evidence-based program for maternal mental health and child development can be delivered through existing local health workers in an LMIC (Rahman, Surkan, and others 2013).

In Chile, a multicomponent intervention for postnatal depression was evaluated in a randomized control trial of 230 women. The intervention consisted of group education about illness and symptoms, problem-solving strategies for mothers, and structured pharmacotherapy when required, delivered through existing local primary care clinics. Compared with those who received treatment as usual, mothers with depression had significant improvements. This study demonstrates the efficacy and feasibility of delivering care to mothers with postnatal depression in an LMIC (Rojas and others 2007).

Participatory women's groups are also a viable model of intervention for postnatal depression. Improvements in maternal and infant health were achieved in a study of 19,030 births in rural India through monthly participatory groups facilitated by peers. The study involved the identification of maternal and neonatal health problems, identification of solutions, and implementation and evaluation of strategies in partnership with local health services (Tripathy and others 2010). This study demonstrates the feasibility and effectiveness of participatory women's groups in reducing postnatal depression in a very poorly resourced region of India.

Much of the research on psychological and psychosocial interventions for maternal depression has been conducted in HICs (Sockol, Epperson, and Barber 2011). Substantial evidence indicates that such interventions are effective in reducing depressive symptoms within the first year postpartum (relative risk = 0.70, 95 percent CI: 0.60 to 0.81) (Dennis and Hodnett 2007). Over the past decade, evidence of the effectiveness of interventions led by non-mental health specialists (for example, by nurses, health visitors, or midwives) has increased (Crockett and others 2008; Lumley and others 2006; MacArthur and others 2003; Morrell and others 2009; Roman and others 2009).

In LMICs, the public health importance of maternal mental health has led to increased research on interventions. A review and meta-analysis identified 13 trials that included 20,092 participants (Rahman, Fisher, and others 2013). In all these studies, the intervention was delivered by supervised, nonspecialist health and community workers; in many of the studies, the intervention was integrated into a primary care platform. Compared with routine care, the evidence suggests significant benefits for mothers and children from the interventions tested. The pooled effect size for maternal depression was 0.38 (95 percent CI: −0.56 to −0.21). Where assessed, the benefits to children included improved mother-infant interaction, better cognitive development, reduced diarrheal episodes, and increased rates of immunization.

Cognitive Behavioral Therapy

Cognitive behavioral therapy (CBT) is a psychological intervention used for the management of anxiety disorders in children. The components of CBT for children consist of cognitive interventions and behavioral strategies. The cognitive interventions teach children to recognize their anxious feelings and the somatic experiences that accompany anxiety (for example, breathlessness and palpitations), identify the anxious thoughts that are associated with the anxious feelings, develop alternative thoughts (for example, positive self-talk) and other coping strategies, and evaluate the differences in their emotions after using the coping strategies. The behavioral interventions include relaxation training, modeling behaviors, and graded exposure to anxiety-provoking stimuli.

A meta-analysis of 41 studies examined the effectiveness of CBT compared with waitlist control, treatment as usual, and other interventions (James and others 2013). Compared with waitlist controls, CBT had a large effect on reducing anxiety diagnoses and symptoms, with a standarized mean difference of –0.98 (95 percent CI: –1.21 to –0.74). However, these studies were conducted in outpatient clinics in HICs; none of the included studies were from LMICs.

The evidence for the effectiveness of CBT in LMICs is very limited; two studies evaluate the effectiveness of this intervention. In Zambia, local lay counselors delivered trauma-focused CBT to the families of 58 children and adolescents between the ages of 5 and 18 years who had moderate to severe trauma symptoms. The intervention was provided to the families of the children and achieved significant reductions in the severity of trauma symptoms, as well as the feelings of shame. Although there was no control group, this study demonstrates the potential feasibility of delivering trauma-focused CBT in LMICs (Murray, Dorsey, and others 2013; Murray, Familiar, and others 2013).

In a study in Brazil, clinical psychologists delivered 14 sessions of group-based CBT, with two concurrent parental sessions, to 28 children ages 10–13 years who were suffering from anxiety disorders. Twenty children (71 percent) completed the treatment; there was a reduction in symptoms, with a moderate to large effect size (Cohen's d between 0.59 and 2.06), depending on the outcome measure used (De Souza and others 2013). These studies provide preliminary evidence of the feasibility of CBT-based interventions for anxiety disorders in LMICs; however, further research is needed.

Medications for ADHD

Pharmacotherapy has the strongest evidence for reducing behavioral problems and improving the attention and educational performance of children with ADHD (Benner-Davis and Heaton 2007; Greenhill and others 2002; Prasad and others 2013). The dispensing of stimulant medications is increasing in HICs (Hollingworth and others 2011; McCarthy and others 2012), but no studies have examined whether these trends exist in LMICs. The wide recognition in HICs of the problems of stimulant medication diversion and misuse has resulted in recommendations for increased monitoring and regulations (Kaye and Darke 2012). Therefore, although stimulant medications are very effective treatments for ADHD, the potential difficulties with obtaining comprehensive assessments of the children to ensure accurate diagnosis and the high likelihood of diversion and misuse in the absence of regulatory systems limit the feasibility of the widespread use of stimulant medications in LMICs.

Specialist Health Care

Medications for Conduct Disorder. Parenting interventions are the best treatments for younger children with disruptive behavioral disorders, such as oppositional defiant disorder and conduct disorder. However, the use of pharmacotherapy can assist in the treatment of adolescents with conduct disorder. Recent evidence has suggested that the use of pharmacologic agents—in particular, second-generation antipsychotics—is increasing (Pringsheim and Gorman 2012) in children and adolescents with conduct disorder.

Although the use of such agents is increasing, the evidence base is not necessarily strong. Reasonably strong evidence supports the use, particularly in the short term, of second-generation antipsychotics, especially risperidone, in young people with borderline intelligence quotients (IQs) (Duhig, Saha, and Scott 2013). However, the evidence in young people with a normal IQ is not strong. Other agents have also been evaluated in such children, including stimulants and lithium (Ipser and Stein 2007). Psychopharmacological therapy in young people with conduct disorder needs to be carefully monitored and only introduced within the setting of specialist care (Ipser and Stein 2007). Its routine use, particularly in LMICs, is not recommended.

Psychosocial Treatments for Conduct Disorder. Psychosocial treatments have been evaluated for children and adolescents with conduct disorder and other disruptive behaviors, including cognitive behavioral intervention (CBI), problem-solving skills therapy (PSST), and multisystem therapy.

- *Cognitive behavioral intervention.* The goal of CBI is to train children in altering their dysfunctional (aggressive) cognitive processes. Generally, such interventions have been found to be effective in children with disruptive behaviors, with effect sizes observed of approximately 0.67 (Sukhodolsky, Kassinove, and Gorman 2004). A meta-analysis of CBI and parenting interventions and CBI for the treatment of youth with antisocial behavior problems (a common sequalae of conduct disorder) found that the effect size was 0.47 for parenting interventions and 0.35 for CBI (McCart and others 2006). This review concluded that parent training appeared to have greater impacts on younger children and CBI was more effective for adolescents.

- *Problem-solving skills therapy*. PSST is an individual-based intervention for children and adolescents that focuses on changing the way children interact with the significant others in their lives. The existing evaluations of this type of therapy were conducted in the 1990s (Kazdin, Siegel, and Bass 1992). These studies have shown the therapy to be largely efficacious and incrementally supportive of the therapeutic effects of parent training (Handwerk and others 2012). PSST has also been found to be effective as an adjunctive treatment for conduct disorder. The evidence suggests that PSST can complement parenting interventions and increase the effectiveness of parenting interventions incrementally (Handwerk and others 2012). The evidence for adapting PSST to various cultures is limited, and further research is required before this intervention can be recommended in LMICs.

- *Multisystem therapy*. Multisystem therapy is a comprehensive intervention targeting adolescents with disruptive behaviors. It is a highly intensive therapy based on the use of different types of therapies deemed appropriate by individual therapists. The existing evaluations of this therapy, including meta-analyses, have demonstrated its efficacy, particularly in adolescents with more serious delinquency tendencies (Curtis, Ronan, and Borduin 2004). However, the therapy's highly intensive nature may render it unsuitable as an intervention in LMICs.

Handwerk and others (2012) provide an excellent summary of the literature on interventions targeting conduct disorders. The overall recommendations include parent training, particularly for parents of younger children, with the choice of intervention format largely a matter of personal and health system preference. The evidence base for CBI is not as extensive as that for parenting interventions; the effect sizes appear to be small to modest. Notably, the augmentation of parenting interventions with CBI appears to be particularly promising. Furthermore, CBI interventions seem to have more efficacy in adolescents.

COST-EFFECTIVENESS ANALYSES

The evidence base for the cost-effectiveness of interventions targeting children and adolescents is considerably more modest than that for adults. In a systematic review of the literature that included studies published up to 2009, Kilian and others (2010) found 19 studies of the cost-effectiveness of psychiatric interventions targeting children and adolescents. Few studies use a cost-utility analysis framework, whereby outcomes are expressed as generic indices combining mortality and morbidity; a common example of such an outcome is quality-adjusted life years (QALYs). The advantage of cost-utility analysis is that value-for-money judgments can be made, since thresholds of good value can be specified for QALYs in different health care settings (Drummond and others 2005). Moreover, interventions can be compared within and across different disorder categories.

Studies of pharmacological interventions for ADHD have largely found such interventions to be cost-effective (King and others 2006), with existing studies finding that such interventions fall below commonly accepted thresholds of value for money in HICs (such as £30,000/QALY[1]). Studies that have evaluated uncertainty around the point estimates have found such conclusions to be robust (Donnelly and others 2004). Evaluations of behavioral interventions find such interventions to be cost-effective; for example, Dretzke and others (2005) find that parenting interventions for conduct disorder are cost-effective. However, sensitivity testing around this estimate shows that the results could change dramatically depending on model assumptions. Mihalopoulos and others (2007) find that modest improvements in the symptoms of conduct disorder can be associated with considerable cost-savings that outweigh the cost of implementing the parenting intervention in an Australian setting. No identified studies have evaluated the cost-effectiveness of interventions in LMICs.

In conclusion, the evidence base of the cost-effectiveness of interventions targeting children and adolescents with mental disorders is still in its infancy. The reasons for this include the limitations of the use of generic outcome indexes, such as QALYs, in children with mental disorders, as well as the difficulties in assessing costs. Future research to fill this evidence gap is urgently needed.

CONCLUSIONS

Childhood mental and developmental disorders globally account for a significant health and societal burden. The evidence base for interventions to prevent and treat mental and developmental disorders in LMICs is limited.

Table 8.3 Summary of Recommendations for Interventions for Childhood Mental and Developmental Disorders

Intervention	Childhood disorders/problems	Supporting evidence in LMICs
Perinatal interventions, for example, screening for congenital hypothyroidism	Intellectual disability	Existing screening is in more than 30 countries, including LMICs.
Population-based interventions targeting maternal alcohol use	Intellectual disability and other delays associated with fetal alcohol spectrum disorder	One case control study demonstrates effectiveness and feasibility (Chersich and others 2012).
Psychosocial stimulation of infants and young children	Developmental delays in infants younger than 3 years	RCTs demonstrate excellent effectiveness and feasibility.
School-based life skills training to build social and emotional competencies in children and adolescents	Behavioral problems in pre-school children (ages 3 to 6 years)	One RCT in Jamaica shows effectiveness and feasibility.
Screening with TQ or the ACCESS portfolio	Developmental disorders in children and adolescents	Feasibility demonstrated may be useful in assessing the needs of a community.
Parenting skills training	Emotional and behavioral problems; developmental disorders	Meta-analysis of multiple studies demonstrates effectiveness and feasibility for reducing emotional and behavioral problems with a large effect size (0.81).
Maternal mental health interventions	Emotional and behavioral problems and developmental delays in children	Meta-analysis of multiple studies demonstrates effectiveness and feasibility with a moderate effect size (0.38).
Cognitive and behavioral therapy	Anxiety, post-traumatic stress disorder	Evidence is limited to two small RCTs.

Note: LMICs = low- and middle-income countries; RCT = randomized control trial; TQ = Ten Questions screen.

Future implementation of programs to address childhood mental and developmental disorders in LMICs should be evaluated. Other evidence-based key recommendations for interventions are summarized in table 8.3.

As the evidence presented in this chapter indicates, key interventions that have the potential to reduce mental and developmental disorders in childhood are parenting skills training that includes psychosocial stimulation, teacher training with "The Incredible Years" program, and maternal mental health interventions. The evidence suggests that these can be feasibly delivered in LMICs, and that they have a strong efficacy in HICs. CBT for anxiety disorders has a strong evidence base in HICs, but much more work is needed to demonstrate the feasible delivery of this intervention in LMICs. Pharmacotherapy requires specialist care and assessment that limits use in LMICs.

The screening of children for developmental disorders is possible in LMICs; however, the evidence for intervening once autism or intellectual disability has been identified is limited. Similarly, child protection and reduction of bullying in schools are important preventive strategies for childhood mental disorders. The systems required for child protection are complex and require collaboration across sectors and significant government investment. Further research on interventions to protect children is urgently required in LMICs. Reducing bullying in schools may prevent mental disorders in childhood and later in life; however, there are no data to show effective programs in LMICs.

The widespread implementation and evaluation of parenting skills training, including psychosocial stimulation and maternal mental health interventions, is recommended in all countries to achieve a meaningful reduction in the global prevalence and burden of childhood mental and developmental disorders.

NOTES

World Bank Income Classifications as of July 2014 are as follows, based on estimates of gross national income (GNI) per capita for 2014:

- Low-income countries (LICs) = US$1,045 or less
- Middle-income countries (MICs) are subdivided:
  a) lower-middle-income = US$1,046 to US$4,125
  b) upper-middle-income = US$4,126 to US$12,745
- High-income countries (HICs) = US$12,746 or more.

1. This is a standard cutoff for cost-effectiveness used in the United Kingdom, comparable to the US$50,000 threshold commonly used.

REFERENCES

APA (American Psychiatric Association). 2013. *Diagnostic and Statistical Manual of Mental Disorders*. 5th ed. Arlington, VA: American Psychiatric Publishing.

Aracena, M., M. Krause, C. Perez, M. J. Mendez, L. Salvatierra, and others. 2009. "A Cost-Effectiveness Evaluation of a Home Visit Program for Adolescent Mothers." *Journal of Health Psychology* 14: 878–87.

Bakare, M. O. 2012. "Attention Deficit Hyperactivity Symptoms and Disorder (ADHD) among African Children: A Review of Epidemiology and Co-Morbidities." *African Journal of Psychiatry [Le Journal Africain de Psychiatrie]* 15: 358–61.

Baker-Henningham, H., S. Scott, K. Jones, and S. Walker. 2012. "Reducing Child Conduct Problems and Promoting Social Skills in a Middle-Income Country: Cluster Randomised Controlled Trial." *British Journal of Psychiatry* 201: 101–8.

Barlow, J., N. Smailagic, N. Huband, V. Roloff, and C. Bennett. 2014. "Group-Based Parent Training Programmes for Improving Parental Psychosocial Health." *Cochrane Database of Systematic Reviews* 5: CD002020.

Bauermeister, J. J., C. Y. So, P. S. Jensen, O. Krispin, A. S. El Din, and others. 2006. "Development of Adaptable and Flexible Treatment Manuals for Externalizing and Internalizing Disorders in Children and Adolescents." *Revista Brasileira de Psiquiatria* 28: 67–71.

Beesdo, K., S. Knappe, and D. S. Pine. 2009. "Anxiety and Anxiety Disorders in Children and Adolescents: Developmental Issues and Implications for DSM-V." *Psychiatric Clinics of North America* 32: 483–524.

Belfer, M. L., and S. Saxena. 2006a. "The Treatment of Child and Adolescent Mental Health Problems in Primary Care: A Systematic Review." *Family Practice* 18: 373–82.

————. 2006b. "WHO Child Atlas Project." *The Lancet* 367: 551–52.

Belmont, L. 1986. "Screening for Severe Mental Retardation in Developing Countries: The International Pilot Study of Severe Childhood Disability." In *Science and Technology in Mental Retardation*, edited by J. Berg, 389–95. London: Methuen.

Benjet, C., G. Borges, and M. E. Medina-Mora. 2010. "Chronic Childhood Adversity and Onset of Psychopathology during Three Life Stages: Childhood, Adolescence and Adulthood." *Journal of Psychiatric Research* 44: 732–40.

Benner-Davis, S., and P. C. Heaton. 2007. "Attention Deficit and Hyperactivity Disorder: Controversies of Diagnosis and Safety of Pharmacological and Nonpharmacological Treatment." *Current Drug Safety* 2: 33–42.

Chersich, M. F., M. Urban, L. Olivier, L. A. Davies, C. Chetty, and others. 2012. "Universal Prevention Is Associated with Lower Prevalence of Fetal Alcohol Spectrum Disorders in Northern Cape, South Africa: A Multicentre Before-After Study." *Alcohol and Alcoholism* 47: 67–74.

Cooper, P. J., M. Tomlinson, L. Swartz, M. Landman, C. Molteno, and others. 2009. "Improving Quality of Mother-Infant Relationship and Infant Attachment in Socioeconomically Deprived Community in South Africa: Randomised Controlled Trial." *British Medical Journal* 338: b974.

Copeland, W. E., D. Wolke, A. Angold, and E. J. Costello. 2013. "Adult Psychiatric Outcomes of Bullying and Being Bullied by Peers in Childhood and Adolescence." *Journal of the American Medical Association* 70: 419–26.

Crockett, K., C. Zlotnick, M. Davis, N. Payne, and R. Washington. 2008. "A Depression Preventive Intervention for Rural Low-Income African-American Pregnant Women at Risk for Postpartum Depression." *Archives of Women's Mental Health* 11: 319–25.

Curtis, N. M., K. R. Ronan, and C. M. Borduin. 2004. "Multisystemic Treatment: A Meta-Analysis of Outcome Studies." *Journal of Family Psychology* 18: 411–19.

De Souza, M. A., G. A. Salum, R. B. Jarros, L. Isolan, R. Davis, and others. 2013. "Cognitive-Behavioral Group Therapy for Youths with Anxiety Disorders in the Community: Effectiveness in Low and Middle Income Countries." *Behavioural and Cognitive Psychotherapy* 41: 255–64.

Deave, T., J. Heron, J. Evans, and A. Emond. 2008. "The Impact of Maternal Depression in Pregnancy on Early Child Development." *An International Journal of Obstetrics and Gynaecology* 115: 1043–51.

Dennis, C. L., and E. Hodnett. 2007. "Psychosocial and Psychological Interventions for Treating Postpartum Depression." *Cochrane Database of Systematic Reviews* 4: CD006116.

Donnelly, M., M. M. Haby, R. Carter, G. Andrews, and T. Vos. 2004. "Cost-Effectiveness of Dexamphetamine and Methylphenidate for the Treatment of Childhood Attention Deficit Hyperactivity Disorder." *Australian and New Zealand Journal of Psychiatry* 38: 592–601.

Dretzke, J., E. Frew, C. Davenport, J. Barlow, S. Stewart-Brown, and others. 2005. "The Effectiveness and Cost-Effectiveness of Parent Training/Education Programmes for the Treatment of Conduct Disorder, Including Oppositional Defiant Disorder, in Children." *Health Technology Assessment* 9: iii, ix–x, 1–233.

Drummond, M., M. Sculpher, G. Torrance, B. O'Brien, and G. Stoddart. 2005. *Methods for the Economic Evaluation of Health Care Programmes*. 3rd ed. Oxford: Oxford University Press.

Dua, T., C. Barbui, N. Clark, A. Fleischmann, V. Poznyak, and others. 2011. "Evidence-Based Guidelines for Mental, Neurological, and Substance Use Disorders in Low- and Middle-Income Countries: Summary of WHO Recommendations." *PLoS Medicine* 8: e1001122.

Duhig, M. J., S. Saha, and J. G. Scott. 2013. "Efficacy of Risperidone in Children with Disruptive Behavioural Disorders." *Journal of Paediatrics and Child Health* 49: 19–26.

Durkin, M. S., L. L. Davidson, P. Desai, Z. M. Hasan, N. Khan, and others. 1994. "Validity of the Ten Questions Screened for Childhood Disability: Results from Population-Based Studies in Bangladesh, Jamaica, and Pakistan." *Epidemiology* 5: 283–89.

Eapen, V., P. Graham, and S. Srinath. 2012. *Where There Is No Child Psychiatrist: A Mental Healthcare Manual.* London: Royal College of Psychiatrists.

Eickmann, S. H., A. C. Lima, M. Q. Guerra, M. C. Lima, P. I. Lira, and others. 2003. "Improved Cognitive and Motor Development in a Community-Based Intervention of Psychosocial Stimulation in Northeast Brazil." *Developmental Medicine and Child Neurology* 45: 536–41.

Erskine, H. E., T. E. Moffitt, W. E. Copeland, E. J. Costello, A. J. Ferrari, and others. 2015. "A Heavy Burden on Young Minds: The Global Burden of Mental and Substance Use Disorders in Children and Youth." *Psychological Medicine* 45: 1551–63.

Fayyad, J. A., L. Farah, Y. Cassir, M. M. Salamoun, and E. G. Karam. 2010. "Dissemination of an Evidence-Based Intervention to Parents of Children with Behavioral Problems in a Developing Country." *European Child and Adolescent Psychiatry* 19: 629–36.

Feldman, R., A. Granat, C. Pariente, H. Kanety, J. Kuint, and others. 2009. "Maternal Depression and Anxiety across the Postpartum Year and Infant Social Engagement, Fear Regulation, and Stress Reactivity." *Journal of the American Academy of Child and Adolescent Psychiatry* 48: 919–27.

Fergusson, D. M., L. J. Horwood, and M. T. Lynskey. 1993. "The Effects of Conduct Disorder and Attention Deficit in Middle Childhood on Offending and Scholastic Ability at Age 13." *Journal of Child Psychology and Psychiatry and Allied Disciplines* 34: 899–916.

———. 1994. "The Childhoods of Multiple Problem Adolescents: A 15-Year Longitudinal Study." *Journal of Child Psychology and Psychiatry and Allied Disciplines* 35: 1123–40.

Fisher, J., M. Cabral de Mello, V. Patel, A. Rahman, T. Tran, and others. 2012. "Prevalence and Determinants of Common Perinatal Mental Disorders in Women in Low- and Lower-Middle-Income Countries: A Systematic Review." *Bulletin of the World Health Organization* 90: 139G–149G.

Fluke, J. D., P. S. Goldman, J. Shriberg, S. D. Hillis, K. Yun, and others. 2012. "Systems, Strategies, and Interventions for Sustainable Long-Term Care and Protection of Children with a History of Living Outside of Family Care." *Child Abuse and Neglect* 36: 722–31.

Furlong, M., S. McGilloway, T. Bywater, J. Hutchings, S. M. Smith, and others. 2013. "Cochrane Review: Behavioural and Cognitive-Behavioural Group-Based Parenting Programmes for Early-Onset Conduct Problems in Children Aged 3 to 12 Years (Review)." *Evidence-Based Child Health* 8: 318–692.

Gertler, P., J. Heckman, R. Pinto, A. Zanolini, C. Vermeersch, and others. 2014. "Labor Market Returns to an Early Childhood Stimulation Intervention in Jamaica." *Science* 344: 998–1001.

Gladstone, M. J., G. A. Lancaster, A. P. Jones, K. Maleta, E. Mtitimila, and others. 2008. "Can Western Developmental Screening Tools Be Modified for Use in a Rural Malawian Setting?" *Archives of Disease in Childhood* 93: 23–29.

Glasheen, C., G. A. Richardson, and A. Fabio. 2010. "A Systematic Review of the Effects of Postnatal Maternal Anxiety on Children." *Archives of Women's Mental Health* 13: 61–74.

Gottlieb, C. A., M. J. Maenner, C. Cappa, and M. S. Durkin. 2009. "Child Disability Screening, Nutrition, and Early Learning in 18 Countries with Low and Middle Incomes: Data from the Third Round of UNICEF's Multiple Indicator Cluster Survey (2005–06)." *The Lancet* 374: 1831–39.

Grace, S. L., A. Evindar, and D. E. Stewart. 2003. "The Effect of Postpartum Depression on Child Cognitive Development and Behavior: A Review and Critical Analysis of the Literature." *Archives of Women's Mental Health* 6: 263–74.

Greenhill, L. L., S. Pliszka, M. K. Dulcan, W. Bernet, V. Arnold, and others. 2002. "Practice Parameter for the Use of Stimulant Medications in the Treatment of Children, Adolescents, and Adults." *Journal of the American Academy of Child and Adolescent Psychiatry* 41: 26S–49S.

Grigoriadis, S., E. H. VonderPorten, L. Mamisashvili, G. Tomlinson, C. L. Dennis, and others. 2013. "The Impact of Maternal Depression during Pregnancy on Perinatal Outcomes: A Systematic Review and Meta-Analysis." *Journal of Clinical Psychiatry* 74: e321–41.

Grote, N. K., J. A. Bridge, A. R. Gavin, J. L. Melville, S. Iyengar, and others. 2010. "A Meta-Analysis of Depression during Pregnancy and the Risk of Preterm Birth, Low Birth Weight, and Intrauterine Growth Restriction." *Archives of General Psychiatry* 67: 1012–24.

Hamadani, J. D., F. Tofail, A. Hilaly, F. Mehrin, S. Shiraji, and others. 2012. "Association of Postpartum Maternal Morbidities with Children's Mental, Psychomotor and Language Development in Rural Bangladesh." *Journal of Health, Population and Nutrition* 30: 193–204.

Handwerk, M., C. Field, A. Dahl, and J. Malmberg. 2012. "Conduct, Oppositional Defiant, and Disruptive Behaviour Disorders." In *Handbook of Evidence-Based Practice in Clinical Psychology: Volume One Child and Adolescent Disorders*, edited by P. Sturmey and M. Hersen, 267–302. Hoboken, NJ: John Wiley and Sons.

Hastings, R. P., J. Robertson, and M. T. Yasamy. 2012. "Interventions for Children with Pervasive Developmental Disorders in Low- and Middle-Income Countries." *Journal of Applied Research in Intellectual Disabilities* 25: 119–34.

Hollingworth, S. A., L. M. Nissen, S. S. Stathis, D. J. Siskind, J. M. Varghese, and others. 2011. "Australian National Trends in Stimulant Dispensing: 2002–2009." *Australian and New Zealand Journal of Psychiatry* 45: 332–36.

Ipser, J., and D. J. Stein. 2007. "Systematic Review of Pharmacotherapy of Disruptive Behavior Disorders in Children and Adolescents." *Psychopharmacology* 191: 127–40.

James, A. C., G. James, F. A. Cowdrey, A. Soler, and A. Choke. 2013. "Cognitive Behavioural Therapy for Anxiety Disorders in Children and Adolescents." *Cochrane Database of Systematic Reviews* 6: CD004690.

Jin, X., Y. Sun, F. Jiang, J. Ma, C. Morgan, and others. 2007. "'Care for Development' Intervention in Rural China: A

Prospective Follow-Up Study." *Journal of Developmental and Behavioral Pediatrics* 28: 213–18.

Jordans, M. J., W. A. Tol, I. H. Komproe, D. Susanty, A. Vallipuram, and others. 2010. "Development of a Multi-Layered Psychosocial Care System for Children in Areas of Political Violence." *International Journal of Mental Health Systems* 4: 15.

Kaminski, J. W., L. A. Valle, J. H. Filene, and C. L. Boyle. 2008. "A Meta-Analytic Review of Components Associated with Parent Training Program Effectiveness." *Journal of Abnormal Child Psychology* 36: 567–89.

Kaye, S., and S. Darke. 2012. "The Diversion and Misuse of Pharmaceutical Stimulants: What Do We Know and Why Should We Care?" *Addiction* 107: 467–77.

Kazdin, A. E., T. C. Siegel, and D. Bass. 1992. "Cognitive Problem-Solving Skills Training and Parent Management Training in the Treatment of Antisocial Behavior in Children." *Journal of Consulting and Clinical Psychology* 60: 733–47.

Kendrick, D., J. Barlow, A. Hampshire, L. Polnay, and S. Stewart-Brown. 2007. "Parenting Interventions for the Prevention of Unintentional Injuries in Childhood." *Cochrane Database of Systematic Reviews* 3: CD006020.

Kessler, R. C., G. P. Amminger, S. Aguilar-Gaxiola, J. Alonso, S. Lee, and others. 2007. "Age of Onset of Mental Disorders: A Review of Recent Literature." *Current Opinion in Psychiatry* 20: 359–64.

Kieling, C., H. Baker-Henningham, M. Belfer, G. Conti, I. Ertem, and others. 2011. "Child and Adolescent Mental Health Worldwide: Evidence for Action." *The Lancet* 378: 1515–25.

Kilian, R., C. Losert, A.-L. Park, D. McDaid, and M. Knapp. 2010. "Cost-Effectiveness Analysis in Child and Adolescent Mental Health Problems: An Updated Review of the Literature." *International Journal of Mental Health Promotion* 12: 45–57.

King, S., S. Griffin, Z. Hodges, H. Weatherly, C. Asseburg, and others. 2006. "A Systematic Review and Economic Model of the Effectiveness and Cost-Effectiveness of Methylphenidate, Dexamfetamine and Atomoxetine for the Treatment of Attention Deficit Hyperactivity Disorder in Children and Adolescents." *Health Technology Assessment* 10: 1–162.

Klein, P. S., and H. Rye. 2004. "Interaction-Oriented Early Intervention in Ethiopia: The MISC Approach." *Infants and Young Children* 17: 350–54.

Krug, E. G., J. A. Mercy, L. L. Dahlberg, and A. B. Zwi. 2002. "The World Report on Violence and Health." *The Lancet* 360: 1083–88.

Lancet Global Mental Health Group, D. Chisholm, A. J. Flisher, C. Lund, V. Patel, and others. 2007. "Scale Up Services for Mental Disorders: A Call for Action." *The Lancet* 370: 1241–52.

Lumley, J., L. Watson, R. Small, S. Brown, C. Mitchell, and others. 2006. "PRISM (Program of Resources, Information and Support for Mothers): A Community-Randomised Trial to Reduce Depression and Improve Women's Physical Health Six Months after Birth [ISRCTN03464021]." *BMC Public Health* 6: 37.

MacArthur, C., H. R. Winter, D. E. Bick, R. J. Lilford, R. J. Lancashire, and others. 2003. "Redesigning Postnatal Care: A Randomised Controlled Trial of Protocol-Based Midwifery-Led Care Focused on Individual Women's Physical and Psychological Health Needs." *Health Technology Assessment* 7: 1–98.

Maulik, P. K., and G. L. Darmstadt. 2007. "Childhood Disability in Low- and Middle-Income Countries: Overview of Screening, Prevention, Services, Legislation, and Epidemiology." *Pediatrics* 120 (Suppl. 1): S1–55.

McCart, M. R., P. E. Priester, W. H. Davies, and R. Azen. 2006. "Differential Effectiveness of Behavioral Parent-Training and Cognitive-Behavioral Therapy for Antisocial Youth: A Meta-Analysis." *Journal of Abnormal Child Psychology* 34: 527–543.

McCarthy, S., L. Wilton, M. L. Murray, P. Hodgkins, P. Asherson, and others. 2012. "The Epidemiology of Pharmacologically Treated Attention Deficit Hyperactivity Disorder (ADHD) in Children, Adolescents and Adults in UK Primary Care." *BMC Pediatrics* 12: 78.

Mejia, A., R. Calam, and M. R. Sanders. 2012. "A Review of Parenting Programs in Developing Countries: Opportunities and Challenges for Preventing Emotional and Behavioral Difficulties in Children." *Clinical Child and Family Psychology Review* 15: 163–75.

Mihalopoulos, C., M. R. Sanders, K. M. Turner, M. Murphy-Brennan, and R. Carter. 2007. "Does the Triple P-Positive Parenting Program Provide Value for Money?" *The Australian and New Zealand Journal of Psychiatry* 41: 239–46.

Moffitt, T. E., A. Caspi, H. Harrington, and B. J. Milne. 2002. "Males on the Life-Course-Persistent and Adolescence-Limited Antisocial Pathways: Follow-Up at Age 26 Years." *Development and Psychopathology* 14: 179–207.

Morrell, C. J., P. Slade, R. Warner, G. Paley, S. Dixon, and others. 2009. "Clinical Effectiveness of Health Visitor Training in Psychologically Informed Approaches for Depression in Postnatal Women: Pragmatic Cluster Randomised Trial in Primary Care." *British Medical Journal* 338: a3045.

Morris, J., M. Belfer, A. Daniels, A. Flisher, L. Ville, and others. 2011. "Treated Prevalence of and Mental Health Services Received by Children and Adolescents in 42 Low- and Middle-Income Countries." *Journal of Child Psychology and Psychiatry and Allied Disciplines* 52: 1239–46.

Murray, L., A. Arteche, P. Fearon, S. Halligan, I. Goodyer, and others. 2011. "Maternal Postnatal Depression and the Development of Depression in Offspring Up to 16 Years of Age." *Journal of the American Academy of Child and Adolescent Psychiatry* 50: 460–70.

Murray, L. K., S. Dorsey, S. Skavenski, M. Kasoma, M. Imasiku, and others. 2013. "Identification, Modification, and Implementation of an Evidence-Based Psychotherapy for Children in a Low-Income Country: The Use of TF-CBT in Zambia." *International Journal of Mental Health Systems* 7: 24.

Murray, L. K., I. Familiar, S. Skavenski, E. Jere, J. Cohen, and others. 2013. "An Evaluation of Trauma Focused Cognitive Behavioral Therapy for Children in Zambia." *Child Abuse and Neglect* 37: 1175–85.

Murray, C. J., T. Vos, R. Lozano, M. Naghavi, A. D. Flaxman, and others. 2012. "Disability-Adjusted Life Years (DALYs) for 291 Diseases and Injuries in 21 Regions, 1990–2010: A Systematic Analysis for the Global Burden of Disease Study 2010." *The Lancet* 380: 2197–223.

Nevo, G. A., and K. Manassis. 2009. "Outcomes for Treated Anxious Children: A Critical Review of Long-Term Follow-Up Studies." *Depression and Anxiety* 26: 650–60.

Omigbodun, O. 2008. "Developing Child Mental Health Services in Resource-Poor Countries." *International Review of Psychiatry* 20: 225–35.

Oveisi, S., H. E. Ardabili, M. R. Dadds, R. Majdzadeh, P. Mohammadkhani, and others. 2010. "Primary Prevention of Parent-Child Conflict and Abuse in Iranian Mothers: A Randomized-Controlled Trial." *Child Abuse and Neglect* 34 (3): 206–13.

Parsons, C. E., K. S. Young, T. J. Rochat, M. L. Kringelbach, and A. Stein. 2012. "Postnatal Depression and Its Effects on Child Development: A Review of Evidence from Low- and Middle-Income Countries." *British Medical Bulletin* 101: 57–79.

Patel, V., L. Aronson, and G. Divan. 2013. *A School Counsellor's Casebook*. Delhi: Byword Books.

Patel, V., G. S. Belkin, A. Chockalingam, J. Cooper, S. Saxena, and others. 2013. "Grand Challenges: Integrating Mental Health Services into Priority Health Care Platforms." *PLoS Medicine* 10: e1001448.

Patel, V., and R. Thara. 2003. *Meeting Mental Health Needs in Developing Countries: NGO Innovations in India*. New Delhi: Sage.

Pearson, R. M., J. Evans, D. Kounali, G. Lewis, J. Heron, and others. 2013. "Maternal Depression during Pregnancy and the Postnatal Period: Risks and Possible Mechanisms for Offspring Depression at Age 18 Years." *Journal of the American Medical Association Psychiatry* 70: 1312–19.

Polanczyk, G., and L. A. Rohde. 2007. "Epidemiology of Attention-Deficit/Hyperactivity Disorder across the Lifespan." *Current Opinion in Psychiatry* 20: 386–92.

Powell, C., H. Baker-Henningham, S. Walker, J. Gernay, and S. Grantham-McGregor. 2004. "Feasibility of Integrating Early Stimulation into Primary Care for Undernourished Jamaican Children: Cluster Randomised Controlled Trial." *BMJ* 329: 89.

Prasad, V., E. Brogan, C. Mulvaney, M. Grainge, W. Stanton, and others. 2013. "How Effective Are Drug Treatments for Children with ADHD at Improving On-Task Behaviour and Academic Achievement in the School Classroom? A Systematic Review and Meta-Analysis." *European Child and Adolescent Psychiatry* 22: 203–16.

Pringsheim, T., and D. Gorman. 2012. "Second-Generation Antipsychotics for the Treatment of Disruptive Behaviour Disorders in Children: A Systematic Review." *Canadian Journal of Psychiatry [Revue Canadienne de Psychiatrie]* 57: 722–27.

Rahman, A., J. Fisher, P. Bower, S. Luchters, T. Tran, and others. 2013. "Interventions for Common Perinatal Mental Disorders in Women in Low- and Middle-Income Countries: A Systematic Review and Meta-Analysis." *Bulletin of the World Health Organization* 91: 593–601.

Rahman, A., Z. Iqbal, C. Roberts, and N. Husain. 2009. "Cluster Randomized Trial of a Parent-Based Intervention to Support Early Development of Children in a Low-Income Country." *Child: Care, Health and Development* 35: 56–62.

Rahman, A., P. J. Surkan, C. E. Cayetano, P. Rwagatare, and K. E. Dickson. 2013. "Grand Challenges: Integrating Maternal Mental Health into Maternal and Child Health Programmes." *PLoS Medicine* 10: e1001442.

Raine, A., K. Mellingen, J. Liu, P. Venables, and S. A. Mednick. 2003. "Effects of Environmental Enrichment at Ages 3–5 Years on Schizotypal Personality and Antisocial Behavior at Ages 17 and 23 Years." *American Journal of Psychiatry* 160: 1627–35.

Robertson, J., C. Hatton, E. Emerson, and M. T. Yasamy. 2012. "The Identification of Children with, or at Significant Risk of, Intellectual Disabilities in Low- and Middle-Income Countries: A Review." *Journal of Applied Research in Intellectual Disabilities* 25: 99–118.

Rojas, G., R. Fritsch, J. Solis, E. Jadresic, C. Castillo, and others. 2007. "Treatment of Postnatal Depression in Low-Income Mothers in Primary-Care Clinics in Santiago, Chile: A Randomised Controlled Trial." *The Lancet* 370: 1629–37.

Roman, L. A., J. C. Gardiner, J. K. Lindsay, J. S. Moore, Z. Luo, and others. 2009. "Alleviating Perinatal Depressive Symptoms and Stress: A Nurse-Community Health Worker Randomized Trial." *Archives of Women's Mental Health* 12: 379–91.

Rutter, M. 2011. "Research Review: Child Psychiatric Diagnosis and Classification: Concepts, Findings, Challenges and Potential." *Journal of Child Psychology and Psychiatry and Allied Disciplines* 52: 647–60.

Sanger, C., J. E. Iles, C. S. Andrew, and P. G. Ramchandani. 2015. "Associations between Postnatal Maternal Depression and Psychological Outcomes in Adolescent Offspring: A Systematic Review." *Archives of Women's Mental Health* 18: 147–62.

Scott, J. G., S. E. Moore, P. D. Sly, and R. E. Norman. 2014. "Bullying in Children and Adolescents: A Modifiable Risk Factor for Mental Illness." *Australian and New Zealand Journal of Psychiatry* 48: 209–12.

Shaw, M., P. Hodgkins, H. Caci, S. Young, J. Kahle, and others. 2012. "A Systematic Review and Analysis of Long-Term Outcomes in Attention Deficit Hyperactivity Disorder: Effects of Treatment and Non-Treatment." *BMC Medicine* 10: 99.

Sockol, L. E., C. N. Epperson, and J. P. Barber. 2011. "A Meta-Analysis of Treatments for Perinatal Depression." *Clinical Psychology Review* 31: 839–49.

Sonnander, K. 2000. "Early Identification of Children with Developmental Disabilities." *Acta Paediatrica Supplement* 89: 17–23.

Sukhodolsky, D., H. Kassinove, and B. Gorman. 2004. "Cognitive-Behavioural Therapy for Anger in Children and Adolescents: A Meta-Analysis." *Aggression and Violent Behaviour* 9: 247–69.

Svevo-Cianci, K. A., S. N. Hart, and C. Rubinson. 2010. "Protecting Children from Violence and Maltreatment: A Qualitative Comparative Analysis Assessing the Implementation of U.N. CRC Article 19." *Child Abuse and Neglect* 34: 45–56.

Tripathy, P., N. Nair, S. Barnett, R. Mahapatra, J. Borghi, and others. 2010. "Effect of a Participatory Intervention with Women's Groups on Birth Outcomes and Maternal Depression in Jharkhand and Orissa, India: A Cluster-Randomised Controlled Trial." *The Lancet* 375: 1182–92.

Ttofi, M. M., and D. P. Farrington. 2011. "Effectiveness of School-Based Programs to Reduce Bullying: A Systematic and Meta-Analytic Review." *Journal of Experimental Criminology* 7: 27–56.

United Nations. 2011. *World Population Prospects: The 2010 Revision*. New York: United Nations.

Vreeman, R. C., and A. E. Carroll. 2007. "A Systematic Review of School-Based Interventions to Prevent Bullying." *Archives of Pediatric and Adolescent Medicine* 161: 78–88.

Wachs, T. D., M. M. Black, and P. L. Engle. 2009. "Maternal Depression: A Global Threat to Children's Health, Development, and Behavior and to Human Rights." *Child Development Perspectives* 3: 51–59.

Walker, S. P., S. M. Chang, N. Younger, and S. M. Grantham-McGregor. 2010. "The Effect of Psychosocial Stimulation on Cognition and Behaviour at 6 Years in a Cohort of Term, Low-Birthweight Jamaican Children." *Developmental Medicine and Child Neurology* 52: e148–54.

Wan, M. W., M. P. Salmon, D. M. Riordan, L. Appleby, R. Webb, and others. 2007. "What Predicts Poor Mother-Infant Interaction in Schizophrenia?" *Psychological Medicine* 37: 537–46.

Wendland-Carro, J., C. A. Piccinini, and W. S. Millar. 1999. "The Role of an Early Intervention on Enhancing the Quality of Mother-Infant Interaction." *Child Development* 70: 713–21.

Whiteford, H. A., L. Degenhardt, J. Rehm, A. J. Baxter, A. J. Ferrari, and others. 2013. "Global Burden of Disease Attributable to Mental and Substance Use Disorders: Findings from the Global Burden of Disease Study 2010." *The Lancet* 382: 1575–86.

WHO (World Health Organization). 2005a. *Atlas of Child and Adolescent Mental Health Resources*. Geneva: WHO.

———. 2005b. *Mental Health Policy and Service Guidance Package: Child and Adolescent Mental Health Policies and Plans*. Geneva: WHO.

———. 2008. *WHO Mental Health Gap Action Programme (mhGAP)*. http://www.who.int/mental_health/mhgap/en.

Wirz, S., K. Edwards, J. Flower, and A. Yousafzai. 2005. "Field Testing of the ACCESS Materials: A Portfolio of Materials to Assist Health Workers to Identify Children with Disabilities and Offer Simple Advice to Mothers." *International Journal of Rehabilitation Research* 28: 293–302.

Zaman, S. S., N. Z. Khan, S. Islam, S. Banu, S. Dixit, and others. 1990. "Validity of the 'Ten Questions' for Screening Serious Childhood Disability: Results from Urban Bangladesh." *International Journal of Epidemiology* 19: 613–20.

Chapter **9**

Suicide

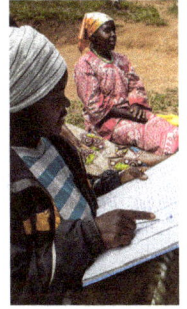

Lakshmi Vijayakumar, Michael R. Phillips,
Morton M. Silverman, David Gunnell,
and Vladimir Carli

INTRODUCTION

An estimated 804,000 deaths by suicide occurred globally in 2012 (WHO 2014a). Of these, 75.5 percent were in low- and middle-income countries (LMICs), which have limited resources to address the issue. The reasons for suicides are multifactorial, but suicides are preventable.

Suicide is operationally defined for the purpose of this chapter as the deliberate act of killing oneself. *Suicide attempt* describes any nonfatal suicidal behavior, such as intentional self-inflicted poisoning, injury, or self-harm. The inclusion of deliberate self-harm (DSH) within the definition of suicide attempt is potentially controversial, because it includes some acts carried out without suicidal intent. Nevertheless, suicide intent can be difficult to ascertain. Accordingly, the approach in this chapter follows that used by the World Health Organization (WHO) and classifies DSH under *suicide attempt*.

EPIDEMIOLOGY OF SUICIDE IN LMICs

The WHO report on suicide (WHO 2014a) provides the most up-to-date estimates of the global burden of suicide, but it is important to keep in mind the limitations of these data. The report uses vital registration data provided by countries and recorded in

the WHO mortality database to generate estimates of cause-specific mortality globally—the Global Health Estimates (GHE). However, many countries, particularly LMICs, do not have high-quality vital registration systems; 78 of the 140 LMICs do not have any vital registration system at all. Most estimates of suicide rates in LMICs are based on subnational reports, which may not be nationally representative, and modeling algorithms. The number and quality of the subnational studies have increased and these modeling algorithms have improved, but serious questions remain about the accuracy of the estimated suicide rates. This problem is most evident in the WHO Africa and Eastern Mediterranean regions, where 98 and 75 percent, respectively, of estimated suicides occur in countries with no vital registration system.

The GHE estimates (WHO 2014b) provide the best available *estimates* of the number and demographic characteristics of suicides in 2012 for 197 countries and territories. The WHO report provides global and regional estimates and country-specific results for 172 of the 194 member states that have populations greater than 300,000. The estimates and results can help to inform the discussions of decision makers in LMICs interested in reducing suicides, but independent assessments of the accuracy and reliability of the estimates in specific jurisdictions are needed.

Corresponding author: Lakshmi Vijayakumar, Sneha, Voluntary Health Services, Chennai, India; Center for Youth Mental Health, University of Melbourne, Australia; lakshmi@vijayakumars.com.

Suicide Mortality

WHO reports that 804,000 suicide deaths occurred globally in 2012. The demographic characteristics and regional distribution of suicides, and the changes in suicide rates between 2000 and 2012, are shown in table 9.1 and figure 9.1. Substantial differences exist in the rates and characteristics of suicide between LMICs and high-income countries (HICs) as well as among LMICs in the six WHO regions. To facilitate the comparison of rates between regions and countries, the rates reported here per 100,000 population are all standardized to the age distribution of the global population in 2012.

Overall Suicide Rates

The 2012 age-adjusted suicide rate in HICs (12.7) was slightly higher than that in LMICs (11.2); over 75 percent of all global suicides occur in LMICs, given their larger proportion of the global population. Among LMICs, the region-specific suicide rate in the six regions varies over a threefold range (from 6.1 to 17.7); the country-specific rate varies over a 100-fold range, from 0.44 in the Syrian Arab Republic to 44.2 in Guyana.

Suicide Rates by Gender

The suicide rate among males in HICs is higher than among males in LMICs, 19.9 versus 13.7, respectively; the suicide rate among females in HICs is lower than among females in LMICs (5.7 versus 8.7). This results in a substantially lower male-to-female ratio of suicide rates in LMICs (1.6) than HICs (3.5). Suicides among females account for 43 percent of all suicides in LMICs, and 22 percent in HICs. However, the comparison of all HICs to all LMICs obscures region-specific differences. For example, the male-to-female ratios in LMICs in Europe and the Americas are higher (not lower) than in HICs.

Suicide Rates by Age

Figure 9.2 shows the gender by age pattern of suicide for several regions in 2012. All regions have low rates in those younger than age 15 years and relatively high rates in those over age 70 years. The suicide rate by gender between ages 15 and 69 years varies by region. In most regions, rates among males are much higher than among females in all age groups other than the very young; however, in the Eastern Mediterranean and Western Pacific regions, male and female suicide rates are comparable in all age groups. The Africa region has a peak in suicide rates among young men, which is not seen in other regions, while the South-East Asia region has a peak in suicide rates among young women that is much more muted or absent in other regions.

The mean age of suicide in HICs is higher than in LMICs, 50.4 versus 42.0 years, respectively, a difference largely accounted for by the difference in the median ages of the populations. Despite the higher rates of suicide in the elderly, for males and females in LMICs, over 63 percent of all suicides occur in individuals ages 15–49 years.

Relative Importance of Suicide as a Cause of Death

Suicide accounted for 1.7 percent of all deaths in HICs and 1.4 percent in LMICs in 2012, making suicide the 11th most important cause of death in HICs and the 17th most important cause in LMICs. Among ages 15–29 years in LMICs, suicide accounts for 7.9 percent of all deaths and is the third most important cause of death; among persons ages 30–49 years, suicide accounts for 3.4 percent of all deaths and is the seventh most important cause of death. Another measure of the public heath importance of suicide is that it is the most important type of intentional violent death (which includes suicides, murders, and war-related deaths): in LMICs, suicide accounts for 44 percent of all violent deaths in males and 70 percent of all violent deaths in females.

Changes in Suicide Rates, 2000–12

The WHO report highlights the volatility of suicide rates. From 2000 to 2012, the absolute number of suicides in LMICs dropped by 11 percent, and the suicide rate dropped by 30 percent.

As shown in figure 9.1, among LMICs in the six regions, the percent change in suicide rates ranged from a drop of 58 percent in the Western Pacific, largely driven by the drop in rates in China (Wang, Chan, and Yip 2014), to an increase of 1.5 percent in the Africa region. In 54 (44 percent) of the 123 LMICs with populations greater than 300,000, the rate increased by more than 10 percent; in 22 countries (18 percent), the rate decreased by more than 10 percent. Given these rapid changes in suicide rates for the majority of LMICs, policies and programs to reduce suicides need to be based on recent information about suicide in the target community. The use of before versus after changes in suicide rates is not a reliable method for assessing the effectiveness of prevention initiatives.

Suicide Attempts

Prior suicide attempt is one of the strongest predictors of subsequent death by suicide, so monitoring the rate, demographic pattern, and methods of suicide attempts is a key component of suicide prevention efforts. However, there is a lack of high-quality data on suicide attempts in LMICs.

Table 9.1 Estimated Incidence and Characteristics of Suicide in HICs and LMICs, based on WHO Global Health Estimates

Region	Number of suicides in 2012 (thousands)	Global suicides (%)	Age-adjusted suicide rate in 2012 (per 100,000)			M:F ratio	Mean age of suicide	All deaths due to suicide (%)	Rank of suicide as a cause of death in 2012			Change in number of suicides from 2000 to 2012 (%)	Change in age-adjusted suicide rate from 2000 to 2012 (%)		
			Male + female	Male	Female				Male + female	Male	Female		Male + female	Male	Female
Global[a]	804	100.0	11.4	15.0	8.0	1.87	44.1	1.44	15	13	22	-9.0	-26.3	-22.8	-32.2
HICs[a]	197	24.5	12.7	19.9	5.7	3.49	50.4	1.69	11	9	21	-2.9	-14.3	-17.5	-4.5
LMICs[a]	607	75.5	11.2	13.7	8.7	1.57	42.0	1.37	17	17	21	-10.8	-29.7	-24.2	-36.7
LMICs in six WHO regions															
Africa	61	7.6	10.0	14.4	5.8	2.47	37.6	0.66	24	27	37	38.0	1.5	2.0	0.7
Americas	35	4.3	6.1	9.8	2.7	3.61	40.4	1.02	22	15	33	17.5	-6.8	-7.0	-6.3
Eastern Mediterranean	30	3.7	6.4	7.5	5.2	1.45	39.7	0.77	27	27	26	32.0	-1.2	3.9	-7.2
Europe	35	4.3	12.0	20.0	4.9	4.08	45.3	1.35	11	8	22	-30.3	-37.9	-38.3	-37.2
South-East Asia	314	39.1	17.7	21.6	13.9	1.55	36.7	2.28	11	11	12	9.5	-10.8	-5.7	-17.4
Western Pacific	131	16.3	7.5	7.2	7.9	0.91	57.0	1.16	13	16	11	-46.6	-57.7	-55.9	-59.1

Note: HICs = high-income countries; LMICs = low- and middle-income countries; WHO = World Health Organization.
a. Global figures, overall HIC figures, and overall LMIC figures include data for three territories that are not member states: Puerto Rico and Taiwan, China, are included with HICs; the West Bank and Gaza is included with LMICs. The figures for LMICs in the six WHO regions only include WHO member states.

Figure 9.1 Percent Change in Age-Adjusted Suicide Rate in Different Regions of the World from 2000 to 2012 Based on WHO Global Health Estimates

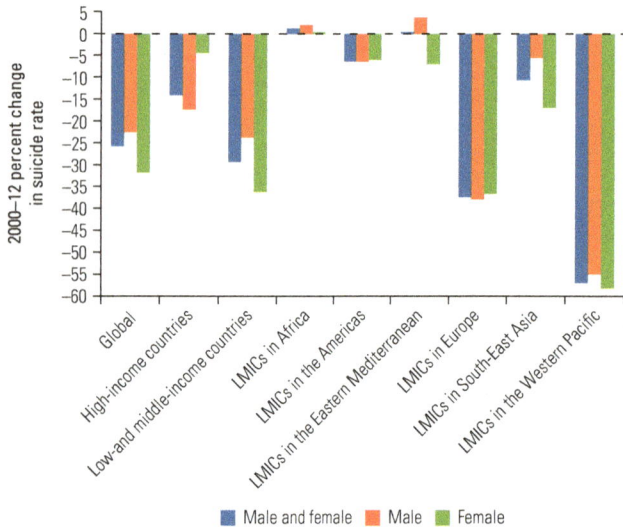

Note: LMICs = low- and middle-income countries; WHO = World Health Organization.

There are two sources of data for suicide attempts: self-reports from community surveys and reports from emergency departments of general hospitals (where most suicide attempts that receive medical care are treated). For the majority of the survey data and emergency department data about suicide attempts available from LMICs, the lack of standardized methods for identifying suicide attempts, methodological limitations, or unknown representativeness of the sample limit their usefulness.

One notable exception is the World Mental Health Survey, which collected self-reported data on suicide attempts from nationally representative samples in nine HICs, four middle-income countries (MICs), and one low-income country (LIC) (Kessler and Ustun 2008). Based on the results of this survey, of persons 18 years of age or older from 2001 to 2007, the self-reported one-year prevalence of suicide attempt is 0.03 per 100,000 for males and females in HICs, 0.03 for males and 0.06 for females in MICs, and 0.04 for males and females in LICs. Combining this very crude result from a small number of countries with the estimated global suicide rate in

Figure 9.2 Suicide Rates by Gender and Age for Selected Regions, Based on WHO Global Health Estimates, 2012

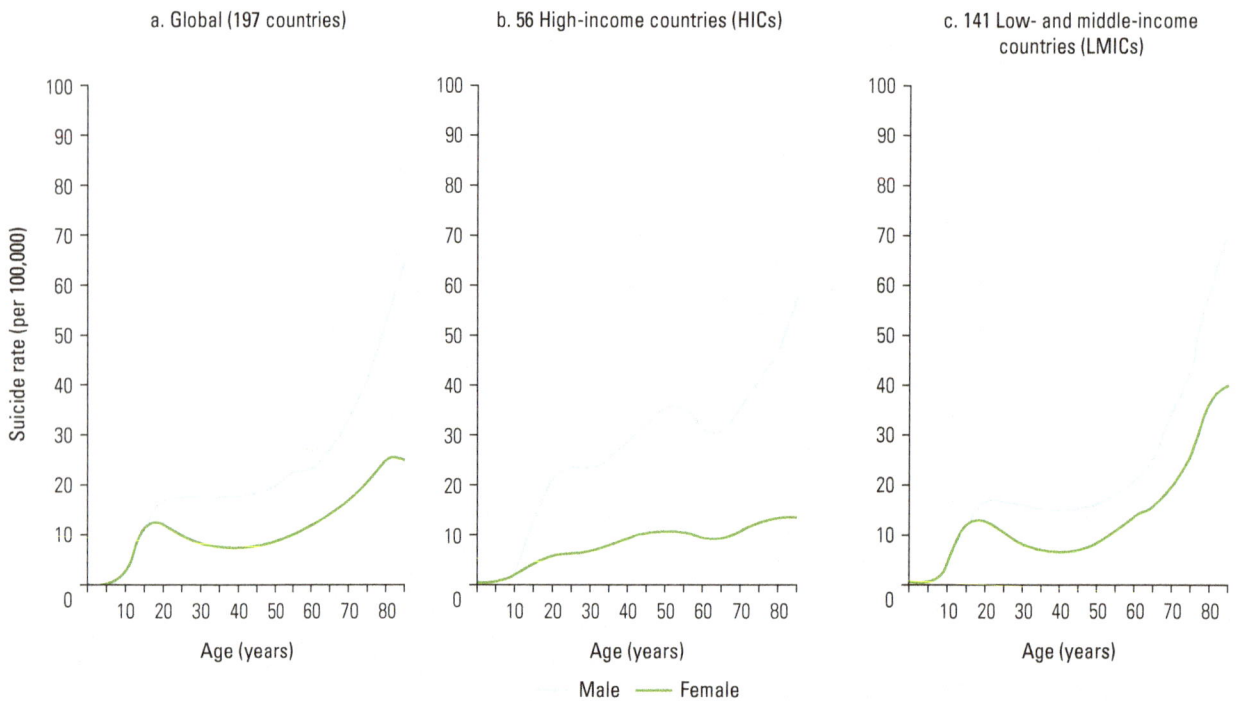

a. Global (197 countries)

b. 56 High-income countries (HICs)

c. 141 Low- and middle-income countries (LMICs)

Male ——— Female

figure continues next page

Figure 9.2 (continued)

d. 46 LMICs in WHO Africa region

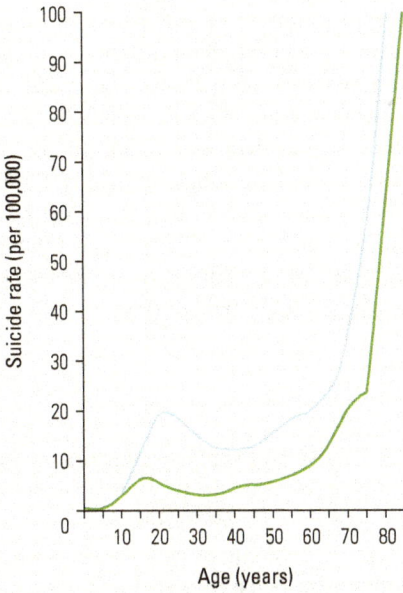

e. 26 LMICs in WHO Americas region

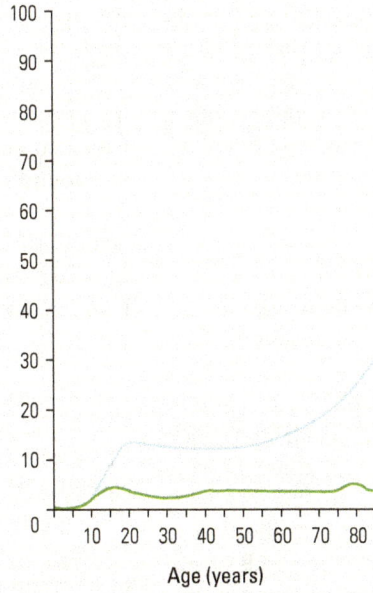

f. 16 LMICs in WHO Eastern Mediterranean region

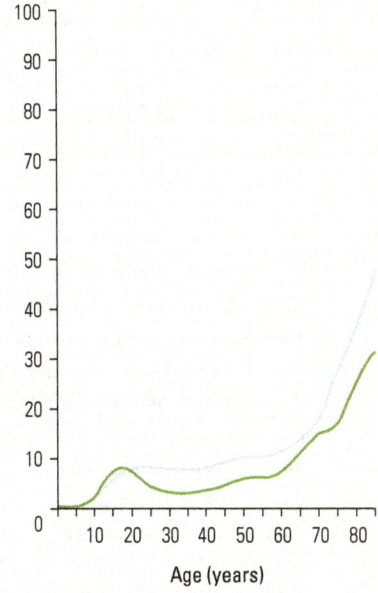

g. 20 LMICs in WHO Europe region

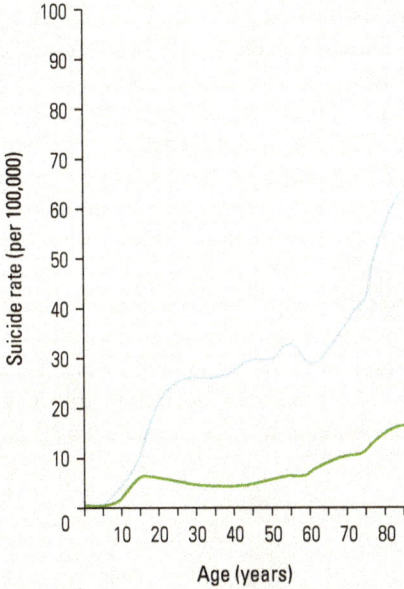

h. 11 LMICs in WHO South-East Asia region

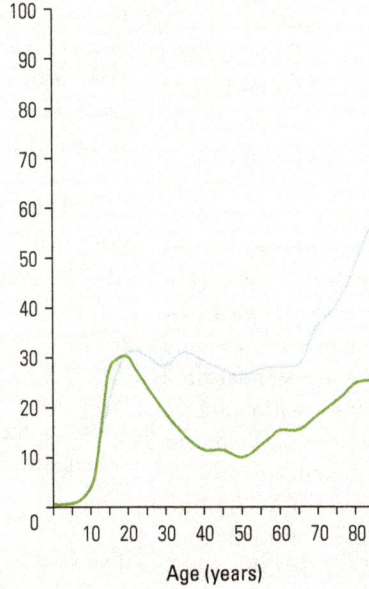

i. 21 LMICs in WHO Western Pacific region

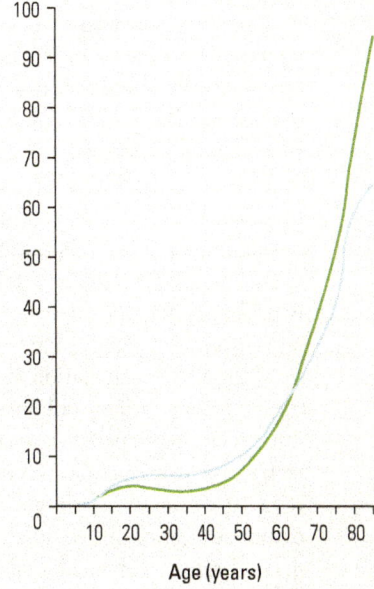

Male — Female

Note: The countries included in each region are listed in annex 2 of WHO 2014a. HICs = high-income countries; LMICs = low- and middle-income countries; WHO = World Health Organization.

persons ages 18 years or older (15.4), globally there are about 20 self-reported suicide attempts for each death by suicide in persons ages 18 or older; this amounts to 15 million suicide attempts worldwide each year.

The limited nationally representative data available from HICs suggest that the case-fatality of medically treated suicide attempts is greater for males than females for all methods and increases with age, but it is unknown whether this pattern is also true in LMICs (WHO 2014a).

Methods of Suicide and Suicide Attempts

Collecting information about the methods used in fatal and nonfatal suicidal behavior, the demographic profile of individuals who use different methods, and the case-fatality of the different methods is an important component of a comprehensive suicide prevention plan. Unfortunately, only a minority of countries provides method-specific data when reporting mortality data to WHO, although International Classification of Diseases-10 (ICD-10) codes exist for all methods of suicide. Of the 140 LMICs, only 36 provided data on suicide methods at any time after 2005, and these countries only accounted for 11 percent of all suicides in LMICs in 2012.

In the absence of national-level data from WHO, it is necessary to consider reviews of subnational data. A systematic review (Gunnell, Eddleston, and others 2007) of the global literature from 1990 to 2007 estimated that about 30 percent of all suicides worldwide are caused by pesticide self-poisoning, most of which occur in LMICs, particularly in rural areas where residents practice small-scale agriculture and have easy access to pesticides. Based on this result, pesticide ingestion is the most common method of suicide globally. However, it is probable that the choice of method varies greatly by region, gender, age, urban versus rural residence, and over time, so each nation must develop standardized methods for routinely obtaining this information to help inform country-specific and community-specific means restriction strategies. For countries that already provide ICD-10 cause of death mortality data to WHO, this could be accomplished relatively easily by mandating that all reports of accidental deaths include the corresponding X-code.

Role of Surveillance in Suicide Prevention in LMICs

The available evidence suggests that substantial cross-national variation in the rates, demographic profile, and methods of suicide and attempted suicide is the rule rather than the exception. Other reports also indicate large differences in suicide rates between different geographic regions of large LMICs, like China (Phillips and others 2002) and India (Patel and others 2012). Some of these differences can be attributed to limitations or biases in the reporting of suicides, but most of the reported differences reflect real differences in suicide rates. Given the magnitude of these differences, policy makers and planners should be cautious when transposing a prevention strategy from HICs to LMICs, from one nation to another, or even from one region to another in a country. Development and ongoing quality control of registry systems that monitor the changing rates, demographic profile, and methods of fatal and nonfatal suicidal behavior in the country or region is essential for planning and implementing interventions.

RISKS AND PROTECTIVE FACTORS IN LMICs

The identification of risk and protective factors is a key component of any prevention strategy and guides the development of appropriate interventions. Risk factors can be present in different categories—individual, relationships, community, society, and health system—that can have multiple points of overlap (WHO 2014a). There are several theoretical ways to conceptualize how risk factors influence suicidal behaviors. One approach to conceptualize risk factors is to view their influence as being proximal versus distal. Proximal risk factors include psychiatric disorder, physical disorder, psychosocial life crisis, availability of means, and exposure to models of suicide. Distal risk factors include genetic susceptibility/loading, personality characteristics such as impulsivity or aggression, early traumatic events, and neurobiological disturbances such as serotonin dysfunction (Hawton and van Heeringen 2009).

There are also different patterns of risk across the lifespan. For example, risk factors for the elderly differ from those for adolescents and young adults. What is universal is that the greater the number of risk factors present, the greater is the likelihood of a range of suicidal behaviors (Phillips and others 2002).

Risk Factors

The relative importance of certain risk factors differs by country and region, such as age of onset of a psychiatric disorder, religious orientation and practice, geographical location, age ranges, and gender distribution. Even within a region, national and intranational differences exist in the prevalence of risk factors; any listing of risk factors may not apply to all LMICs, even in the same region.

Risk factors are variable over time and may be influenced by the rapidity of change occurring within a country or region, such as by the increasing global influence of the Internet, migration from rural to urban areas, and movement of ethnic populations (Malakouti and others 2015). For example, in Chile, from 1998 to 2011, the age range with the highest suicide rates changed, from 40–59 years between 1998 and 2006 to 25–39 years between 2006 and 2009 (Otzen and others 2014). Qualitative studies are needed to identify culturally relevant risk factors and to understand how risk factors may be connected to suicidal behaviors in different sociocultural contexts (Mars and others 2014).

A review of risk factors reported that the profiles in LMICs differed from HICs in some respects, while certain risks were universal (Phillips and others 2002; Vijayakumar and others 2005). In Africa, reported risk factors were similar for suicide and suicide attempts, and included interpersonal difficulties, mental and physical health problems, socioeconomic problems, and drug and alcohol use and abuse (Mars and others 2014).

In a recent review of 17 published studies from Latin America and the Caribbean, the main risk factors for suicide attempts included major depressive disorder, family dysfunction, and prior suicide attempt; the main risk factors for death by suicide were male gender and major depressive disorder. Although the methodological quality of most of the studies was low, the authors concluded that the majority of relevant risk factors for suicide and suicide attempts in the region were similar to those observed in Western societies, but they were different from those reported in Eastern societies (Teti and others 2014).

Risk factors that appear to be universal include youth or old age, a mental disorder, low socioeconomic standing, substance use, and previous suicide attempts. Mental disorders occupy a premier position in the matrix of causation, although their relative contribution to suicide differs across countries. Loss, interpersonal conflict, suicide bereavement, chronic pain, chronic illness, and intimate partner violence increase the risk of suicide when they are associated with one another or when they are associated with another high-risk condition.

Recent stressful life events play a role in HICs and LMICs, although their nature may differ. For example, agents such as social change are more important in LMICs (Vijayakumar and others 2005). Access to means heightens risk in HICs and LMICs, but the specific means used may vary. Regional and national suicide rates vary in relation to geographic preferences for, and access to, high-lethality methods (Yip and others 2012).

Proximal Risk Factors

Mental Disorders and Alcohol Misuse

The classic method of investigating characteristics of individuals who have died by suicide is through a psychological autopsy, involving interviews with key informants and examination of official records (Hawton and others 1998). This approach has shown that in many HICs, psychiatric disorders are present in about 80–90 percent of people who kill themselves and contribute 47–74 percent to population risk of suicide (Cavanagh and others 2003; Cheng and others 2000). Affective disorder is the most common psychiatric disorder, followed by substance (especially alcohol) misuse and schizophrenia. A study based on the Global Burden of Disease 2010 stated that the relative risk of suicide in an individual with major depressive disorder was 19.9 (odds ratio (OR) = 9.5–41.7); with schizophrenia, 12.6 (OR = 11.0–14.5); and with alcohol dependence, 9.8 (OR = 9.0–10.7) (Ferrari and others 2014).

Psychological autopsy studies reveal that 40 percent of suicides in China, 35 percent in India, and 37 percent in Sri Lanka had a diagnosis of depression (Abeyasinghe and Gunnell 2008; Phillips and others 2002; Vijayakumar and Rajkumar 1999). However, a study in Pakistan found that 73 percent had depressive disorder (Khan and others 2008). In LMICs, the role of mental disorders is accorded less importance; equal or more importance is given to other sociocultural and environmental factors. Although their absolute level of risk is somewhat lower in LMICs, people with depression, mental disorders, or alcohol abuse or dependence are at a higher risk of suicide (WHO 2012).

Alcohol misuse, particularly dependence, is strongly associated with suicide risk in HICs and LMICs. The severity of the disorder, aggression, impulsivity, and hopelessness seem to predispose to suicide. Life events, stressors, and depression are not necessarily mutually exclusive, although they may be located at different points along the pathway to suicide.

Physical Disorders

Suicide is associated with several physical disorders. In a study from Nigeria (Chikezie and others 2012), 34.7 percent of HIV/AIDS patients versus 4.0 percent of controls expressed suicidal ideation in the preceding month, with 9.3 percent attempting suicide in the six months prior to the study.

Psychosocial Life Crises

Poverty, low education, social exclusion, gender disadvantage, conflict, and disasters are the major social determinants of mental health in LMICs (Patel 2007);

these factors are also associated with suicide. In Turkey, from 1990 to 2010, economic problems, relationship problems, and educational failure were the most common reasons for suicide (Oner, Yenilmez, and Ozdamar 2015). In Brazil, from 1980 to 2006, the most dominant sociodemographic characteristics of those who died by suicide were low educational level and single status (Lovisi and others 2009). Another study from Brazil found that income inequality represents a community-level risk factor for suicide rates (Machado, Rasella, and Dos Santos 2015).

Urban versus Rural Locations
Globally, suicide rates are higher in urban than in rural areas, but these can vary across countries by age and gender. In LMICs, living in a rural area increases risk. In China, the suicide rates are three times higher in rural areas than urban areas (Cao and others 2000; Phillips and others 2002); in Sri Lanka, the rural suicide rate is twice that of urban areas (Jayasinghe and de Silva 2003); and in India, about 90 percent of the suicides occur in rural areas (Gajalakshmi and Peto 2007; Joseph and others 2003).

Availability of Means and Methods
When a person is contemplating suicide, access to specific methods might be the factor that leads from suicidal thoughts and plans to action.

The easy availability of highly lethal methods is a significant factor in suicides in LMICs. As many as 30 percent of global suicide deaths might involve ingestion of pesticides (Gunnell, Eddleston, and others 2007). This situation is compounded by the limited availability of appropriate health care services and professionals, and by the complexity of managing pesticide overdoses that lead to increased fatalities.

In Turkey, from 1990 to 2010, the most common suicide method was hanging, and men used firearms more frequently than women did (Oner, Yenilmez, and Ozdamar 2015). In Brazil, the most common methods were hanging, firearms, and poisoning (Lovisi and others 2009). In Africa, the most frequently used methods of suicide were hanging and pesticide poisoning (Mars and others 2014).

In a systematic review and meta-analysis of the most common methods of suicide in the Eastern Mediterranean region, the pooled proportions of hanging, self-immolation, and poisoning were 39.7, 17.4, and 20.3 percent, respectively (Morovatdar and others 2013). More females died by self-immolation than males (29.4 percent versus 11.3 percent); more males died by hanging than females (38.8 percent versus 26.3 percent); and more females died by poisoning than males (32.0 percent versus 19.0 percent).

Exposure to Models
Risk of suicidal behavior can be influenced by exposure to similar behavior by other people.

A substantial body of evidence indicates that certain types of media reporting and portrayal of suicidal behavior can influence suicide and self-harm in the general population (Pirkis and Blood 2010). Newspaper reporting of suicides can be particularly influential if it is sensational, if it includes dramatic headlines and pictures, if it reports methods of suicide in detail, and if the subject is a celebrity (Stack 2003).

One of the most distressing features of suicide in LMICs is the frequent occurrence of suicide pacts and family suicides, which constitute an estimated 1 percent of suicides. Family suicides are often a suicide-homicide, in which the adults murder their children prior to their own suicide. These suicides are frequently driven by debt, poverty, and other social issues rather than by depression or mental disorders (Gupta and Gambhir Singh 2008; Vijayakumar and Thilothammal 1993).

Distal Risk Factors
Several biological systems might be involved in suicidal behavior, particularly with regard to the serotonin, noradrenalin, and hypo-thalamic-pituitary-adrenal axis systems (Mann 2003).

Family history of suicide increases the risk at least twofold, particularly in girls and women, independent of family psychiatric history (Qin, Agerbo, and Mortensen 2003). Studies from India (OR = 1.33; confidence interval (CI) = 0.59–3.09) (Vijayakumar and Rajkumar 1999) and China (OR = 3.9; CI = 2.4–6.3) (Phillips and others 2002) corroborate these findings.

History of Suicide Attempts
A history of self-harm or suicide attempts is seen as a very strong risk factor. Studies from China, India, and Sri Lanka reveal that around one-third of those who died by suicide had made a prior suicide attempt (Abeysinghe and Gunnell 2008; Phillips and others 2002; Vijayakumar and Rajkumar 1999).

Early Traumatic Events
Childhood adversities, including physical, emotional, and sexual abuse, have been associated with higher risk for suicide. A highly significant relationship between domestic violence and suicidal ideations has been found in many LMICs, with 48 percent of women in Brazil, 61 percent in the Arab Republic of Egypt, 64 percent in India, 11 percent in Indonesia, and 28 percent in the Philippines reporting suicidal ideations and domestic violence (WHO 2001).

In a study of the relationship between childhood trauma and current suicide risk in 1,380 individuals ages 14–35 years, in the city of Pelotas, Brazil (Barbosa and others 2014), suicide risk was associated with all types of childhood trauma. Suicide risk was increased in emotional neglect (OR = 3.7), physical neglect (OR = 2.8), sexual abuse (OR = 3.4), physical abuse (OR = 3.1), and emotional abuse (OR = 6.6).

Vulnerable Groups in LMICs

Women

Several social and cultural factors make women vulnerable, especially in LMICs in South Asia. These include the practice of arranged and often forced marriages that trap women in unwanted marriages; some opt for suicide as a means of escape. Young persons who love each other, but whose families disapprove of their relationship, may take their lives, either together or alone.

In Turkey, from 1990 to 2010, the number of suicides in females ages 15–24 years was significantly higher than in males. The leading reason for suicide in females was relationship problems (Oner, Yenilmez, and Ozdamar 2015).

Self-immolation, seen almost exclusively in LMICs (10–30 percent versus 0.06–1.00 percent in HICs), has emerged as a major cause of death and disability in parts of the Middle East and Central Asia, especially among young married Muslim women (Campbell and Guiao 2004). Self-immolation remains the only lethal means used more by women than men. In the Islamic Republic of Iran and in Pakistan, 81 percent of self-immolation is by women; in Sri Lanka, the rate is 79 percent; in India, it is 64 percent. Marital conflicts and failed love affairs were identified as the most common reasons (Ahmadi and others 2009).

Pressure on women to bear children soon after marriage, failure to become pregnant, and infertility carry severe social stigma, leading some women to resort to suicide. Domestic violence is fairly common; its practice is, to a large extent, socially and culturally condoned in many LMICs. In a population-based study on domestic violence, 9,938 women were studied in different parts of India and across sections of the society. An estimated 40 percent experienced domestic violence (Kumar and others 2005); 64 percent showed a significant correlation between domestic violence and suicidal ideation (WHO 2001). Domestic violence was found in 36 percent of suicides and was a major risk factor (OR = 6.82; CI = 4.02–11.94) (Gururaj and others 2004). However, relatively little is known about domestic violence as a risk factor across LMICs, and it is an important area for future research.

Youth

Many LMICs experience peaks in suicide rates among young adults. These peaks likely reflect a combination of factors, including the use of high-lethality methods in impulse (low intent) suicide attempts; relationship stresses and arranged marriages, particularly in young women; and the high incidence of impulsive suicide attempts in response to socioeconomic stressors, such as job loss, substantial disparities in incomes, and inability to meet role obligations in a changed environment following large-scale privatization and liberalization of the economy (Schlebusch 2005). The breakdown of the joint family system that had provided emotional support and stability was also an important contributing factor (Thara and Padmavati 2010).

Farmers

In Brazil, suicide risk was higher among agricultural workers than nonagricultural workers, elevated in regions that used more pesticides, and greatest in regions that produced more tobacco. These findings suggest that the combined effects of pesticide and tobacco exposure may be linked to higher suicide risk among agricultural workers (Krawczyk and others 2014). Farmer death from pesticide self-poisoning is very common in several LMICs, including China, Fiji, India, Indonesia, Sri Lanka, and Suriname (Phillips and others 2002; Vijayakumar and others 2005). A common reason includes falling into debt traps following crop failure. When this difficulty is coupled with the easy availability of a lethal means of suicide, the situation becomes particularly dangerous.

Refugees and Internally Displaced Persons

Refugee status, or seeking asylum, puts individuals at significant risk for suicide (Kalt and others 2013). More than 59 million people were displaced in 2014; 86 percent of these were in LMICs. The least-developed nations provided asylum to 3.6 million people (UNHCR 2014). Most refugees in LMICs are residents of refugee camps with poor infrastructure and limited services (McColl, McKenzie, and Bhui 2008).

Suicidal behavior in refugees is often not reported, because it is considered politically sensitive. A review suggests that the overall prevalence of suicidal behavior among refugees ranges from 3.4 percent to 34.0 percent (Vijayakumar and Jotheeswaran 2010). The results of a study of adults in refugee camps showed that 50 percent of the sample had serious psychological problems, with interventions often not available; suicidal thoughts were common among mothers (Rahman and Hafeez 2003). Children and adolescents formed an especially vulnerable group, since they constitute almost 50 percent of the world's internally displaced and refugee populations. Accordingly, it is essential to take steps to provide appropriate interventions (Reed and others 2012).

Sexual Minorities

In many LMICs, discrimination against sexual minorities, such as lesbians, gays, bisexuals, and transgenders, is ongoing, endemic, and systemic. This problem can lead to the continued experience of stressful life events, such as loss of freedom, rejection, stigmatization, and violence that can lead to suicidal behaviors (Haas and others 2011). There have been no studies that have compared suicide rates among sexual minorities in countries with or without social acceptance of alternative lifestyles.

Survivors of Suicide Loss

People bereaved by the suicide of loved ones or a close contact often experience significant emotional distress as a result of their loss. These feelings are often accompanied by feelings of stigma, loss of trust, and social isolation. Many survivors experience suicidal thoughts themselves.

Every year, an estimated four million people may be actively experiencing the aftermath of a suicide, many of them children, due to the high proportion of young married women in China and India who die by suicide. Many LMICs do not provide programs for survivors in any systematic way. Families in which suicide has occurred may be ostracized and isolated, and the marriage prospects of sisters and daughters of people who die by suicide may be marred (Khan and Prince 2003). These attitudes may affect the ways in which people respond to survivors and may reduce the likelihood that survivors seek what limited services might be available.

Protective Factors

The role of protective factors, such as resiliency, social support, self-esteem, problem-solving skills, and religious affiliation have not been as well studied as risk factors.

Strong Personal Relationships

The promotion and maintenance of healthy close relationships can increase resilience and act as a protective factor against the risk of suicide. In a study in Brazil, the protective factors for boys and girls included having good family relationships and feeling liked by friends and teachers, and these factors seemed beneficial (Anteghini and others 2001). Similarly, a survey of adolescents from nine Caribbean countries reported that strong connections with family and school provided the best protective factors (Blum and others 2003). Relationships are especially protective for adolescents and elderly persons, who have higher levels of dependency.

Religious and Spiritual Beliefs

Religious and strong cultural beliefs that discourage suicide are seen as major protective factors. The protective value of religion and spirituality probably arises in part from providing access to a socially cohesive and supportive community. Islam and Christianity, and specifically Catholicism, prohibit the taking of one's own life, and this prohibition can have a strong inhibitory effect on suicidal behavior. Data from Islamic countries and from countries in Latin America and the Caribbean that are predominantly Catholic bear this out; however, the strong stigma associated with suicide in these cultures may mean that underreporting is likely. The rates of suicide in Islamic countries are very low; for example, Saudi Arabia and Syria have a similar rate of 0.4 per 100,000 (WHO 2014a). Islam also prohibits alcohol consumption, a known risk factor for suicide.

A survey of young people from nine Latin American and Caribbean countries reported that attendance at religious services and connectedness with parents and school reduced risk behaviors (Blum and others 2003). A study from India revealed that religiosity acted as a strong protective factor against suicide (Vijayakumar 2002). Due to the lack of reliable data, the debate remains open as to whether it is the religious beliefs per se or the social connectedness that occurs in the context of religious involvement that is protective.

Positive Coping Strategies and Well-Being

Subjective personal well-being and effective positive coping strategies seem to be protective against suicide (Sisask and others 2008). However, ample debate remains regarding the international measures of national and individual well-being, making the relationship between well-being and suicide less than simple.

Use of upstream approaches, such as addressing risk and protective factors early in the life course, has the potential to shift the odds in favor of more adaptive outcomes. Moreover, upstream approaches may simultaneously impact a wide range of health and societal outcomes, such as suicide, substance abuse, violence, and crime (Jané-Llopis and others 2005).

Figure 9.3 provides a list of key risk factors for suicide aligned with their possible interventions.

SUICIDE PREVENTION IN LMICs

This section summarizes the evidence for suicide prevention in LMICs. It provides an overview of potential populationwide, community-based, and health and social care interventions and describes the development of national suicide prevention strategies.

Figure 9.3 Risk Factors and Possible Interventions

Key risk factors for suicide aligned with relevant interventions
(Lines reflect the relative importance of interventions at different levels for different areas of risk factors)

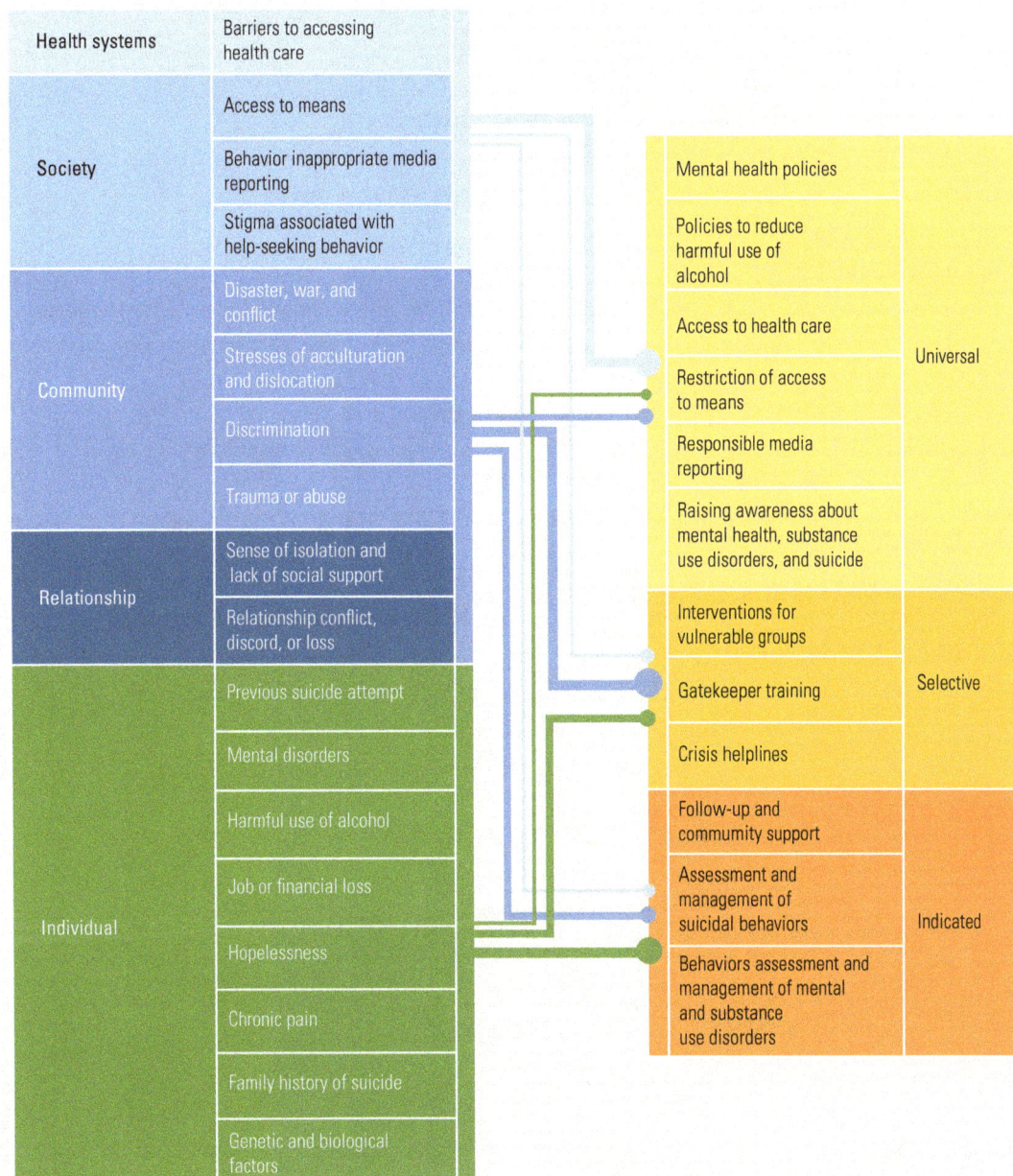

Source: WHO 2014a.

Suicide was once commonly viewed as a mental health problem that needed to be addressed primarily by clinical intervention, especially by the treatment of depression. Suicide is now recognized as a public health issue that should be addressed by social and public health programs, as well as clinical activities targeting mental disorders. Moreover, in LMICs, the availability of mental health professionals needed to deliver mental health interventions is often limited.

WHO has produced several documents on suicide prevention. Based on these documents and recent literature, table 9.2 highlights potential interventions in LMICs;

Table 9.2 Potential Interventions for Suicide in LMICs

Population platform interventions
Universal prevention and health promotion

Restrict the availability of toxic pesticides and other commonly used methods

Decriminalize suicide

Reduce the availability and excessive use of alcohol and illicit drugs

Work with national and local media organizations to limit inappropriate reporting of suicides

Conduct campaigns to reduce the stigma associated with suicide and mental disorders and to encourage help-seeking behavior

Provide adequate economic and welfare support to individuals who are unemployed, disabled, or destitute

Community platform interventions
Selective prevention and health promotion

NGOs: provide suicide hotlines and crisis centers, and promote social cohesion and interpersonal support in communities and families

Initiate school-based mental health promotion programs to enhance psychological resilience, problem-solving skills, and appropriate help-seeking behavior

Organize community-based safe storage activities for pesticides, other poisons, and medications

Provide gatekeeper training to teachers, people looking after refugees, police, social workers, practitioners of alternative systems of medicine, traditional healers, and other individuals who interact with suicidal individuals

Implement communitywide health promotion programs to encourage help-seeking for psychological problems and reduce alcohol and drug abuse, child abuse, and domestic violence

Health care platform interventions
Indicated (targeted) prevention and care for persons with mental, neurological, and substance disorders and their families

Conduct brief interventions for people who have attempted suicide

Train primary health care workers in the identification and management of individuals at high risk of suicidal behavior

Improve health care professionals' identification and treatment of depression and alcohol or drug abuse

Provide regular follow-up, social support, and (if appropriate) cognitive behavioral therapy or other psychological treatment to individuals who have attempted suicide

Improve the medical management of poisoning with pesticides and other poisons associated with high case-fatality

Establish services to support individuals bereaved by suicide (postvention services)

Note: Given the wide variability of suicidal behavior between and within countries, any interventions must be based on local conditions (for example, commonly used high-lethality methods); interventions from other countries or jurisdictions can be considered but should not be implemented prior to conducting a formal assessment of their local feasibility and appropriateness. However, many LMICs do not have quality vital registration systems to identify suicidal deaths, or community-based or hospital-based monitoring programs to identify suicide attempts. This deficit poses a serious dilemma for stakeholders in LMICs. It is not feasible to delay the initiation of suicide prevention activities until a comprehensive monitoring system of suicidal behavior is operational; it is appropriate to integrate monitoring in the target communities in parallel with the initiation of the intervention programs. LMICs = low- and middle-income countries; NGOs = nongovernmental organizations.

the relevance of these to a particular LMIC depends on its epidemiology of suicide, key risk factors, and social context, as well as the available resources in the country.

The evidence is of mixed quality; in some cases, it extrapolates from research in HICs. Furthermore, because of the low incidence of suicide, the evidence for several of the interventions comes from trials that have used suicide attempts, rather than suicide, as the primary outcome measure.

Some of the interventions highlighted in other chapters, such as those to reduce the incidence of alcohol misuse and depression, will help to decrease the incidence

of suicide. In this section, we consider interventions specific to suicidal behavior, such as restricting access to commonly used methods of suicide, and those to improve the mental health of the population in general, where an impact on suicide seems probable.

Population Platform Interventions

Restricting Access to Lethal Means

Research has demonstrated that one of the most effective approaches to reducing suicide is restricting access to highly lethal and commonly used methods (Mann and others 2005). Suicidal impulses are often short lived; if access to high-lethality methods is restricted, the impulse may pass or a less lethal method may be chosen. Most people who survive a suicide attempt do not go on to kill themselves.

Pesticide self-poisoning accounts for a high proportion of all suicides in LMICs. In Sri Lanka, where pesticide poisoning accounted for two-thirds of all suicides in the 1980s, a series of bans on the import of the most toxic pesticides was followed by a halving in suicide rates (Gunnell, Fernando, and others 2007). In recent years, China and the Republic of Korea have followed Sri Lanka's lead by banning some of the most toxic pesticides. Other methods of suicide potentially amenable to means-restriction interventions include gun control legislation and protective barriers at suicide hotspots.

Decriminalization

In a recent study, 25 of the 192 countries investigated had specific laws and punishments for attempted suicide (Mishara and Weisstub 2014). These countries are principally LMICs. The impacts of criminalizing suicide are the following:

- People may not present for care following a suicide attempt and so not receive the medical or psychological help they may require.
- It stigmatizes suicide and may discourage help-seeking.
- Police interrogation of people who have attempted suicide causes increased distress, shame, and guilt, and may lead to further suicide attempts.
- There may be gross underreporting of attempted suicides, leading to underestimation of the magnitude of the problem.

Changing the laws should result in improved help-seeking behavior, reduce stigmatization, provide better data, and save lives.

Alcohol and Drug Misuse

The contribution of alcohol and drug misuse to the burden of suicide varies from country to country depending on cultural norms. Evidence from HICs suggests that restricting alcohol availability by pricing or restrictions on purchasing may lead to reductions in suicide (Pridemore, Chamlin, and Andreev 2013), but this has not been evaluated in LMICs.

Media Reporting

Improving the portrayal of suicide in the media is an important component of suicide prevention. Sensational reporting can raise awareness (cognitive availability) of high-lethality suicide methods that, if popularized, may have an adverse impact on suicide rates (Chen and others 2014). Many LMICs do not have effective media regulatory bodies or media guidelines such as those developed by WHO (http://www.who.int/mental_health/prevention /suicide/resource_media.pdf). If poor reporting is an issue, it is important to work with national media organizations and journalists to develop local guidelines and provide regular feedback on their reporting.

Other Populationwide Interventions

Stigma. Many people who die by suicide have not sought help for their emotional distress. The stigma associated with mental disorder, the belief that nothing can be done, and, in some countries, the criminalization of suicide contribute to this reluctance to seek help. Media, school-based, and other campaigns to address this issue may promote appropriate help-seeking, although robust research evidence to support this approach is lacking (Dumesnil and Verger 2009).

Examination Stress. In many LMICs with fierce competition for places in higher education, examination failure is a recognized risk factor for suicide. In India, 1.8 percent of suicides were by students following failure in examinations (NCRB 2014). Similar patterns have been reported in Malaysia, Pakistan, and Sri Lanka. An example of good practice in this area is work by Sneha, a nongovernmental suicide prevention organization in India. Sneha worked with the media to raise awareness of the issue and undertook education and awareness training for parent associations. In Tamil Nadu, India, a new law came into effect in 2003 that allowed students who failed examinations to be able to retake them within one month and pursue higher studies without losing an academic year (Vijayakumar and Armson 2005). In 2004, there were 407 suicides due to examination failure (suicide rate 61.6 per 100,000 students), whereas in 2013 there were 277 suicides (suicide rate 24.7) among students in Tamil Nadu. Other states in India, including Andhra Pradesh and Maharashtra, have enacted similar laws.

Economic Issues. Poverty, debt, chronic ill-health, and low socioeconomic position are risk factors for suicide in LMICs (Knipe and others 2015). Adequate welfare provision for these more vulnerable members of society is important to reduce risk but poses a challenge to the struggling economies of many LMICs.

Community Platform Interventions

Services of Nongovernmental Organizations

Most LMICs do not have the financial or personnel resources to support suicide prevention programs, especially health care system–driven models. It has become imperative to develop low-cost interventions that can be delivered by lay volunteers or community health workers.

This enormous gap in mental health services has been the catalyst for the emergence of nongovernmental mental health organizations. Many African and South-East Asian countries have such organizations, often taking the form of suicide prevention centers, staffed largely by volunteers and operating as crisis centers or hotlines, providing free service in many LMICs. For example, the Beijing Suicide Research and Prevention Center in China established a national hotline and provides standardized training to other hotline services around the country.

The primary goal of these prevention centers is to provide emotional support to suicidal persons through befriending and counseling in person or by telephone. In many countries, as the primary or sole agency for suicide prevention, they have enlarged their perspectives by being proactive in rural and remote areas and in special populations. Although many innovative programs for raising awareness and increasing help-seeking behavior have been developed, most have not been evaluated (Vijayakumar and Armson 2005).

School-Based Interventions

There is mixed evidence concerning the effectiveness of school-based interventions for preventing suicide. In the largest randomized control trial (RCT) carried out to date—the Saving and Empowering Young Lives in Europe trial—mental health awareness and skills training reduced the incidence of suicidal thoughts and attempts among secondary school children (Wassermann and others 2015). More research is needed in this area in LMICs.

Safe Storage of Pesticides

Multiple projects have investigated approaches to restricting access to pesticides in farming communities in rural Asia. These include studies of lockable safe storage boxes in Sri Lanka (Hawton and van Heeringen 2009; Konradsen and others 2007) and a centralized community pesticide storage facility in southern India (Vijayakumar and others 2013). These approaches show some promise, although the possibility of adverse effects has been raised. A randomized trial of locked storage devices that is enrolling 200,000 people is underway in Sri Lanka (Pearson and others 2011).

Gatekeeper Training

A gatekeeper is anyone in a position to identify whether someone may be at risk of suicide. Gatekeepers include schoolteachers, people caring for refugees and victims of disaster, hospital emergency department staff, practitioners of traditional and alternative medicine, police, prison staff, and youth leaders. Training gives these individuals the skills to identify and respond to at-risk individuals (WHO 2012, 2014a).

Although research evidence to support this activity is limited to institutional settings (Mann and others 2005), it appears to be intuitively sensible and is valued by front-line personnel and communities.

Other Community Platform Interventions

Recently, there has been interest in multifaceted, community-based approaches to improving the identification and treatment of depression and reducing suicide. Hungary participated in the European Alliance against Depression Programme. The program includes four levels of intervention: general practitioner training workshops, a public information campaign, training community facilitators (gatekeepers), and interventions targeted at high-risk groups. Szekely and others (2013) report data from the intervention (population 77,000) and control (population 163,000) regions of Hungary; they find evidence of a significantly greater reduction in suicide in the intervention region compared with the control area.

A multifaceted suicide prevention program in a Brazilian municipality, the Program for Promotion of Life and Suicide Prevention, was designed to reduce suicide rates in the general population (Conte and others 2012). The components of the program included trying to break taboos and talking about death, improving and streamlining the process of care, and reorganizing work processes in the basic network. Although suicide rates fell in the municipality, the lack of comparison information from control areas means it is not possible to determine whether the reduction was due to the program or other influences.

Campaigns to reduce stigma associated with suicide and encourage help-seeking have been suggested as a population-level intervention; such campaigns may also be appropriately carried out by local communities. Activity might also focus on groups identified as being at high risk in the particular community, such as victims of domestic abuse, people who abuse alcohol, or those who engage in gambling.

An unusual intervention in the Islamic Republic of Iran used videos documenting the stories of self-immolation victims (Ahmadi and Ytterstad 2007). Young women from socioeconomically deprived groups who were identified as at high risk were targeted. There was some evidence of a beneficial effect on self-immolation and overall suicide attempts compared with a nonintervention city.

Such interventions need to be designed carefully to avoid possible unanticipated effects, such as glamorizing suicide.

Health Care Platform Interventions

Brief Intervention and Contact

Few interventions for people presenting to clinical services have been evaluated in LMICs. An exception is the WHO's multisite RCT of the provision of brief intervention and contact (BIC) to people who presented to hospital emergency departments in Brazil, China, India, the Islamic Republic of Iran, and Sri Lanka. BIC comprised a one-hour individual information session, as close to the time of discharge as possible, combined with periodic follow-up after discharge. The 18-month follow-up reported significantly fewer deaths from suicide in the intervention arm than the control arm (treatment as usual) (Fleischmann and others 2008), although surprisingly there was no impact on the incidence of repeat (nonfatal) suicide attempts (Bertolote and others 2010).

Another brief intervention that has attracted attention in recent years is mailing a series of supportive postcards to people in the 12 months after a suicide attempt. A recent systematic review found no strong evidence of an effect of this sort of intervention in studies largely carried out in HICs (Milner and others 2015). However, the one RCT conducted in an LMIC, the Islamic Republic of Iran (Hassanian-Moghaddam and others 2011), was more promising. The study showed a reduction in suicidal ideation, suicide attempts, and number of attempts at one-year follow-up. This trial should be replicated in other LMICs.

In China, intervention by messaging through mobile phones was piloted in 15 people who had attempted suicide; most participants considered the text message contacts an acceptable and useful form of help (Chen, Mishara, and Liu 2010). However, a subsequent three-arm RCT comparing telephone contact, cognitive therapy, and controls showed no evidence of a beneficial effect on repeated suicide attempts, depression scores, or quality of life at one-year follow-up, although loss to follow-up was high in all three treatment groups (Wei and others 2013).

Improving the Medical Management of Poisoning with Pesticides

The appropriate medical management of pesticide self-poisoning may reduce case-fatality. The WHO has produced guidelines on the clinical management of pesticide intoxication (WHO 2008); these guidelines should be reviewed by local health services. The guidelines cover training and initial and longer-term care, and include notes of caution about overuse of gastric lavage, the appropriate use of antidotes—for example, atropine for organophosphate poisoning—and careful attention to respiratory failure.

Disasters and Refugees

LMICs are particularly prone to natural disasters, war, and food shortages. These problems often result in large numbers of displaced people or refugees. These people are at heightened risk not only because of their displacement, but also because of the traumas, physical and psychological, they may have experienced. Those in contact with such individuals should be appropriately trained to be aware of their vulnerabilities and how to respond.

Monitoring and Reporting Systems

Reliable and timely information on the prevalence, demographic patterns, and methods employed in suicides and suicide attempts is essential for the development and monitoring of suicide prevention efforts (WHO 2012). It is essential to involve community and nongovernmental organizations at multiple levels to address this issue in terms of monitoring, reporting, and providing interventions.

A direct transference of the methodologies used in HICs is unlikely to be efficacious in LMICs. The significant differences in gender ratio, age structure, and methods for suicide between HICs and LMICs mean that interventions have to be suitably adapted to address local requirements and be consistent with local social and cultural practices.

National Suicide Prevention Strategies

A key step in acting to prevent suicide is to identify and engage the key national stakeholders in developing a national suicide prevention strategy. The Ministry of Health is the most appropriate body to lead strategy development.

Under the WHO Mental Health Action Plan 2013–2020, member states have committed to work toward the global target of reducing the suicide rate in countries by 10 percent by 2020. WHO has produced recommendations for suicide prevention interventions in several documents, including the Mental Health Global Action Program (WHO 2010a), *Public Health Action for the Prevention of Suicide* (WHO 2012), and *Preventing Suicide: A Global Imperative* (WHO 2014a), which provides evidence-based technical guidance to expand service provision in countries. Sadly, few LMICs have developed national prevention strategies. Malaysia and Sri Lanka are exceptions, although Sri Lanka's strategy is no longer operational. In India, suicide prevention is included in the country's national mental health program.

Although many risk factors for suicide are shared by all countries, their relative importance in determining the local incidence of suicide varies. The first step in informing priority areas for suicide prevention is to collect good quality, nationally representative data on the age- and gender-specific incidence of suicide, the methods used by those who take their lives, and the key risk factors. Guidelines by WHO to set up a surveillance system and the process to be followed can be accessed from the STEPwise approach to surveillance at http://www.who.int/chp/steps/en.

COST-EFFECTIVENESS OF PREVENTION EFFORTS

The cost of treating suicide attempts, particularly self-poisoning by pesticides in LMICs, is high (Sgobin and others 2015; Wickramasinghe and others 2009). Suicide prevention control measures may need to be tailored to the context of a specific country, taking into consideration the epidemiological, geographic, and gender distribution of suicide, political will, perceptions of stigma, legislation, and resource availability to deliver appropriately designed prevention programs. As such programs are developed, there will be a need to generate cost and cost-effectiveness information. Although there have been some promising interventions in LMICs, the evidence of cost-effectiveness remains sparse, and evidence on costs and cost-effectiveness from HICs may not be relevant (WHO 2010b). No economic evaluation was conducted for the multicountry RCT of BIC (Fleishmann and others 2008), but the clinical costs were equal to treatment as usual. Chapter 12 in this volume (Levin and others 2015) provides a review of costs and cost-effectiveness for mental health interventions more broadly.

CONCLUSIONS

Suicide is a major public health problem in LMICs. The magnitude of the problem and the paucity of resources in these countries necessitate a need for collaboration and cooperation across a variety of stakeholders to implement strategies that are culturally relevant and cost-effective. The huge variability in the prevalence, demographic patterns, and methods of suicide should be considered when making global cross-national prevention recommendations. LMICs need to adopt a process whereby they can decide on the interventions that are appropriate for their cultures and populations.

A substantial minority of individuals who attempt suicide or die by suicide in these settings does not have a mental disorder. Psychosocial and economic risk factors need to be acknowledged, and interventions need to be developed that target these factors. In LMICs, suicide prevention is more of a social and public health objective than a traditional mental health sector objective.

Before intervening, information about the prevalence, demographic patterns, and methods of suicide in the country or community is needed. Data from representative locations on the pattern of deaths is particularly important in countries without effective registry systems. Several evidence gaps exist. A more refined estimate of the burden and modeling that focuses on risk factor abatement, resilience enhancement, and intervention effects will effectively direct future suicide prevention activities.

NOTE

Portions of this chapter are based on work that will appear in the *International Handbook of Suicide Prevention, 2nd edition*, forthcoming from Wiley.

The authors are very grateful to Mr. Sujit John, Senior Research Coordinator, Schizophrenia Research Foundation, for his technical assistance in the preparation of the chapter.

World Bank Income Classifications as of July 2014 are as follows, based on estimates of gross national income (GNI) per capita for 2013:

- Low-income countries (LICs) = US$1,045 or less
- Middle-income countries (MICs) are subdivided:
  a) lower-middle-income = US$1,046 to US$4,125
  b) upper-middle-income (UMICs) = US$4,126 to US$12,745
- High-income countries (HICs) = US$12,746 or more.

REFERENCES

Abeyasinghe, R., and D. Gunnell. 2008. "Psychological Autopsy Study of Suicide in Three Rural and Semi-Rural Districts of Sri Lanka." *Social Psychiatry and Psychiatric Epidemiology* 43 (4): 280–85.

Ahmadi, A., R. Mohammadi, D. C. Schwebel, N. Yeganeh, A. Soroush, and S. Bazargan-Hejazi. 2009. "Familiar Risk Factors for Self Immolation: A Case Control Study." *Journal of Women's Health* 18 (7): 1025–31.

Ahmadi, A., and B. Ytterstad. 2007. "Prevention of Self-Immolation by Community-Based Intervention." *Burns* 33 (8): 1032–40.

Anteghini, M., H. Fonseca, M. Ireland, and R. W. Blum. 2001. "Health Risk Behaviors and Associated Risk and Protective Factors among Brazilian Adolescents in Santos, Brazil." *Journal of Adolescent Health* 28 (4): 295–302.

Barbosa, L. P., L. Quevedo, G. da Silva Gdel, K. Jansen, R. T. Pinheiro, and others. 2014. "Childhood Trauma and

Suicide Risk in a Sample of Young Individuals Aged 14–35 Years in Southern Brazil." *Child Abuse and Neglect* 38 (7): 1191–96.

Bertolote, J. M., A. Fleischmann, D. De Leo, M. R. Phillips, N. J. Botega, and others. 2010. "Repetition of Suicide Attempts. Data from Emergency Care Settings in Five Culturally Different Low- and Middle-Income Countries Participating in the WHO SUPRE-MISS Study." *Crisis* 31: 194–201.

Blum, R. W., L. Halcón, T. Beuhring, E. Pate, S. Campell-Forrester, and A. Venema. 2003. "Adolescent Health in the Caribbean: Risk and Protective Factors." *American Journal of Public Health* 93 (3): 456–60.

Campbell, E. A., and I. Z. Guiao. 2004. "Muslim Culture and Female Self-Immolation: Implications for Global Women's Health Research and Practice." *Health Care for Women International* 25 (9): 782–93.

Cao, W., T. Wu, T. An, and L. Li. 2000. "Study on the Mortality of Injury in the Chinese Population in Urban and Rural Areas from 1990 to 1997." *Zhonghua Liu Xing Bing Xue Za Zhi*. 21 (5): 327–29 [Chinese].

Cavanagh, J. T. O., A. J. Carson, M. Sharpe, and S. M. Lawrie. 2003. "Psychological Autopsy Studies of Suicide: A Systematic Review." *Psychological Medicine* 33: 395–405.

Chen, H., B. L. Mishara, and X. X. Liu. 2010. "A Pilot Study of Mobile Telephone Message Interventions with Suicide Attempters in China." *Crisis* 31 (2): 109–12.

Chen, Y.-Y., P. S. F. Yip, C. H. Chan, K.-W. Fu, S.-S. Chang, and others. 2014. "The Impact of a Celebrity's Suicide on the Introduction and Establishment of a New Method of Suicide in South Korea." *Archives of Suicide Research* 18: 221–22.

Cheng, A. T. A., T. H. H. Chen, C.-C. Chen, and R. Jenkins. 2000. "Psychosocial and Psychiatric Risk Factors for Suicide. Case-Control Psychological Autopsy Study." *British Journal of Psychiatry* 177: 360–65.

Chikezie, U. E., A. N. Otakpor, O. B. Kuteyi, and B. O. James. 2012. "Suicidality among Individuals with HIV/AIDS in Benin City, Nigeria: A Case-Control Study." *AIDS Care* 24 (7): 843–45.

Chisholm, D., K. A. Johansson, N. Raykar, I. Megiddo, A. Nigam, and others. 2015. "Moving Toward Universal Health Coverage for Mental, Neurological, and Substance Use Disorders: An Extended Cost-Effectiveness Analysis." In *Disease Control Priorities* (third edition): Volume 4, *Mental, Neurological, and Substance Use Disorders*, edited by V. Patel, D. Chisholm, T. Dua, R. Laxminarayan, and M. E. Medina-Mora. Washington, DC: World Bank.

Conte, M., S. N. Meneghel, A. G. Trindade, R. F. Ceccon, L. Z. Hesler, and others. 2012. "Suicide Prevention Program: Case Study in a Municipality in the South of Brazil." [In Portuguese.] *Cien Saude Colet* 17 (8): 2017–26.

Dumesnil, H., and P. Verger. 2009. "Public Awareness Campaigns about Depression and Suicide: Review." *Psychiatric Services* 60: 1203–13.

Ferrari, A. J., R. E. Norman, G. Freedman, A. J. Baxter, J. E. Pirkis, and others. 2014. "The Burden Attributable to Mental and Substance Use Disorders as Risk Factors for Suicide: Findings from the Global Burden of Disease Study 2010." *PloS One* 9 (4): e91936. doi:10.1371/journal.pone.0091936.

Fleischmann, A., J. M. Bertolote, D. Wasserman, D. De Leo, J. Bolhari, and others. 2008. "Effectiveness of Brief Intervention and Contact for Suicide Attempters: A Randomized Controlled Trial in Five Countries." *Bulletin of the World Health Organization* 86 (9): 703–09.

Gajalakshmi, V., and R. Peto. 2007. "Suicide Rates in Tamil Nadu, South India: Verbal Autopsy of 39,000 Deaths in 1997–98." *International Journal of Epidemiology* 36 (1): 203–07.

Gunnell, D., M. Eddleston, M. R. Phillips, and F. Konradsen. 2007. "The Global Distribution of Fatal Pesticide Self-Poisoning: Systematic Review." *BMC Public Health* 7 (1): 357.

Gunnell, D., R. Fernando, M. Hewagama, W. D. D. Priyangika, F. Konradsen, and M. Eddleston. 2007. "The Impact of Pesticide Regulations on Suicide in Sri Lanka." *International Journal of Epidemiology* 36 (6): 1235–42.

Gupta, B. D., and O. Gambhir Singh. 2008. "A Unique Trend of Murder-Suicide in the Jamnagar Region of Gujarat, India (A Retrospective Study of 5 Years)." *Journal of Forensic and Legal Medicine* 15 (4): 250–55.

Gururaj, G., M. K. Isaac, D. K. Subbakrishna, and R. Ranjani. 2004. "Risk Factors for Completed Suicides: A Case-Control Study from Bangalore, India." *Injury Control and Safety Promotion* 11 (3): 183–91.

Haas, A. P., M. Eliason, V. M. Mays, R. M. Mathy, S. D. Cochran, and others. 2011. "Suicide and Suicide Risk in Lesbian, Gay, Bisexual, and Transgender Populations: Review and Recommendations." *Journal of Homosexuality* 58 (1): 10–51.

Hassanian-Moghaddam, H., S. Sarjami, A.-A. Kolahi, and G. L. Carter. 2011. "Postcards in Persia: Randomised Controlled Trial to Reduce Suicidal Behaviours 12 Months after Hospital-Treated Self-Poisoning." *British Journal of Psychiatry* 198 (4): 309–16.

Hawton, K., L. Appleby, S. Platt, T. Foster, J. Cooper, and others. 1998. "The Psychological Autopsy Approach to Studying Suicide: A Review of Methodological Issues." *Journal of Affective Disorders* 50: 269–76.

Hawton, K., and K. van Heeringen. 2009. "Suicide." *The Lancet* 373: 1372–81. doi:10.1016 /S0140-6736 (09)60372-X.

Jané-Llopis, E., M. Barry, C. Hosman, and V. Patel. 2005. "Mental Health Promotion Works: A Review." *Promotion & Education* 12 (9): 9–25.

Jayasinghe, S., and D. de Silva. 2003. "Minimum Pesticide List for the Developing World." *The Lancet* 361 (9353): 259.

Joseph, A., S. Abraham, J. P. Muliyil, K. George, J. Prasad, and others. 2003. "Evaluation of Suicide Rates in Rural India Using Verbal Autopsies, 1994–9." *BMJ* 326 (7399): 1121–22.

Kalt, A., M. Hossain, L. Kiss, and C. Zimmerman. 2013. "Asylum Seekers, Violence and Health: A Systematic Review of Research in High-Income Host Countries." *American Journal of Public Health* 103 (3): e30–42.

Kessler, R., and T. B. Ustun, eds. 2008. *The WHO World Mental Health Surveys*. New York: Cambridge University Press.

Khan, M. M., S. Mahmud, M. S. Karim, M. Zaman, and M. Prince. 2008. "Case-Control Study of Suicide in Karachi, Pakistan." *British Journal of Psychiatry* 193 (5): 402–05.

Khan, M. M., and M. Prince. 2003. "Beyond Rates: The Tragedy of Suicide in Pakistan." *Tropical Doctor* 33 (2): 67–69.

Knipe, D. W., R. Carroll, K. H. Thomas, A. Pease, D. Gunnell, and C. Metcalfe. 2015. "Association of Socio-Economic Position and Suicide/Attempted Suicide in Low and Middle Income Countries in South and South-East Asia—A Systematic Review." *BMC Public Health* 15: 1055. doi:10.1186/s12889-015-2301-5.

Konradsen, F., R. Pieris, M. Weerasinghe, W. Van der Hoek, M. Eddleston, and A. H. Dawson. 2007. "Community Uptake of Safe Storage Boxes to Reduce Self-Poisoning from Pesticides in Rural Sri Lanka." *BMC Public Health* 7 (1): 13.

Krawczyk, N., A. Meyer, M. Fonseca, and J. Lima. 2014. "Suicide Mortality among Agricultural Workers in a Region with Intensive Tobacco Farming and Use of Pesticides in Brazil." *Journal of Occupational and Environmental Medicine* 56 (9): 993–1000.

Kumar, S., J. Lakshmanan, S. Saradha, and R. C. Ahuja. 2005. "Domestic Violence and Its Mental Health Correlates in Indian Women." *British Journal of Psychiatry* 187 (1): 62–67.

Lovisi, G. M., S. A. Santos, L. Legay, L. Abelha, and E. Valencia. 2009. "Epidemiological Analysis of Suicide in Brazil from 1980 to 2006." *Brazilian Journal of Psychiatry* 31 (2): S86–94.

Machado, D. B., D. Rasella, and D. N. Dos Santos. 2015. "Impact of Income Inequality and Other Social Determinants on Suicide Rate in Brazil." *PLoS One* 10 (4): e0124934.

Malakouti, S. K., F. Davoudi, S. Khalid, M. A. Asl, M. M. Khan, and others. 2015. "The Epidemiology of Suicide Behaviors among the Countries of the Eastern Mediterranean Region of WHO: A Systematic Review." *Acta Medica Iranica* 53 (5): 257–65.

Mann, J. J. 2003. "Neurobiology of Suicidal Behaviour." *Nature Review Neuroscience* 4: 819–28.

Mann, J. J., A. Apter, J. Bertolote, A. Beautrais, D. Currier, and others. 2005. "Suicide Prevention Strategies: A Systematic Review." *Journal of the American Medical Association* 294 (16): 2064–74.

Mars, B., S. Burrows, H. Hjelmeland, and D. Gunnell. 2014. "Suicidal Behaviour across the African Continent: A Review of the Literature." *BMC Public Health* 14 (14): 606. doi:10.1186/1471-2458-14-606.

McColl, H., K. McKenzie, and K. Bhui. 2008. "Mental Healthcare of Asylum-Seekers and Refugees." *Advances in Psychiatric Treatment* 14 (6): 452–59.

Milner, A. J., G. Carter, J. Pirkis, J. Robinson, and M. J. Spittal. 2015. "Letters, Green Cards, Telephone Calls and Postcards: Systematic Review and Meta-Analytic Review of Brief Contact Interventions for Reducing Self-Harm, Suicide Attempts and Suicide." *British Journal of Psychiatry* 206: 184–90.

Mishara, B. L., and D. N. Weisstub. 2014. "Suicide Laws: An International Review." *International Journal of Law and Psychiatry* (in press).

Morovatdar, N., M. Moradi-Lakeh, S. K. Malakouti, and M. Nojomi. 2013. "Most Common Methods of Suicide in Eastern Mediterranean Region of WHO: A Systematic Review and Meta-Analysis." *Archives of Suicide Research* 17 (4): 335–44.

NCRB (National Crime Research Bureau). 2014. *Accidental Deaths and Suicide in India*. Ministry of Home Affairs, Government of India, New Delhi.

Oner, S., C. Yenilmez, and K. Ozdamar. 2015. "Sex-Related Differences in Methods of and Reasons for Suicide in Turkey between 1990 and 2010." *Journal of International Medical Research* 43 (4): 483–93.

Otzen, T., A. Sanhueza, C. Manterola, and J. A. Escamilla-Cejudo. 2014. "Mortalidadporsuicidioen Chile: Tendenciasenlosanos 1998–2011" ["Trends in Suicide Mortality in Chile from 1998 to 2011"]. *Revista Medica de Chile* 142: 305–13.

Patel, V. 2007. "Mental Health in Low- and Middle-Income Countries." *British Medical Bulletin* 81 (1): 81–96.

Patel, V., C. Ramasundarahettige, L. Vijayakumar, J. S. Thakur, V. Gajalakshmi, and others. 2012. "Suicide Mortality in India: A Nationally Representative Survey." *The Lancet* 379 (9834): 2343–51.

Pearson, M., F. Konradsen, D. Gunnell, A. H. Dawson, R. Pieris, and others. 2011. "A Community-Based Cluster Randomised Trial of Safe Storage to Reduce Pesticide Self-Poisoning in Rural Sri Lanka: Study Protocol." *BMC Public Health* 21 (11): 879.

Phillips, M. R., G. Yang, Y. Zhang, L. Wang, H. Ji, and M. Zhou. 2002. "Risk Factors for Suicide in China: A National Case-Control Psychological Autopsy Study." *The Lancet* 360 (9347): 1728–36.

Pirkis, J., and R. W. Blood. 2010. "Suicide and the News and Information Media: A Critical Review." http://www.mindframe-media.info/__data/assets/pdf_file/0016/5164/Pirkis-and-Blood-2010,-Suicide-and-the-news-and-information-media.pdf.

Pridemore, W. A., M. B. Chamlin, and E. Andreev. 2013. "Reduction in Male Suicide Mortality Following the 2006 Russian Alcohol Policy: An Interrupted Time-Series Analysis." *American Journal of Public Health* 103: 2021–26.

Qin, P., E. Agerbo, and P. B. Mortensen. 2003 "Suicide Risk in Relation to Family History of Completed Suicide and Psychiatric Disorders. A Nested Case-Control Study." *Ugeskr Laeger* 165 (25): 2573–77 [original article in Danish].

Rahman, A., and A. Hafeez. 2003. "Suicidal Feelings Run High among Mothers in Refugee Camps: A Cross-Sectional Survey." *Acta Psychiatrica Scandinavica* 108 (5): 392–93.

Reed, R. V., M. Fazel, L. Jones, C. Panter-Brick, and A. Stein. 2012. "Mental Health of Displaced and Refugee Children Resettled in Low-Income and Middle-Income Countries: Risk and Protective Factors." *The Lancet* 379 (9812): 250–65.

Schlebusch, L. 2005. *Suicidal Behaviour in South Africa*. Pietermaritzburg, University of KwaZulu-Natal Press.

Sgobin, S. M., A. L. Traballi, N. J. Botega, and O. R. Coelho. 2015. "Direct and Indirect Cost of Attempted Suicide in a General Hospital: Cost-of-Illness Study." *Sao Paolo Medical Journal* 133 (3): 218–26. doi:10.1590/1516-3180.2014.8491808.

Sisask, M., A. Värnik, K. Kolves, K. Konstabel, and D. Wasserman. 2008. "Subjective Psychological Well-Being (Who-5) in Assessment of the Severity of Suicide Attempt." *Nordic Journal of Psychiatry* 62 (6): 431–35.

Stack, S. 2003. "Media Coverage as a Risk Factor in Suicide." *Journal of Epidemiology and Community Health* 57:238–40.

Szekely, A., B. K. Thege, R. Mergl, E. Birkas, S. Rozsa, and others. 2013. "How to Decrease Suicide Rates in Both Genders? An Effectiveness Study of a Community-Based Intervention (EAAD)." *PLoS One* 8 (9): e75081. doi:10.1371/journal.pone.0075081.

Teti, G. L., F. Rebok, S. M. Rojas, L. Grendas, and F. M. Daray. 2014. "Systematic Review of Risk Factors for Suicide and Suicide Attempt among Psychiatric Patients in Latin America and Caribbean." *Revista Panamericana de Salud Pública* 36 (2): 124–33.

Thara, R., and R. Padmavati. 2010. "Social Psychiatry in India." In *Principles of Social Psychiatry*, 2nd ed., edited by C. Morgan and D. Bhugra, 533–40. West Sussex: John Wiley and Sons Ltd.

UNHCR (United Nations High Commissioner for Refugees). 2014. "Global Trends." http://www.unhcr.org/statistic.

Vijayakumar, L. 2002. "Religion: A Protective Factor in Suicide." *Suicidology* 2: 9–12.

Vijayakumar, L., and S. Armson. 2005. "Volunteer Perspective on Suicides." In *Prevention and Treatment of Suicidal Behaviour*, edited by K. Hawton, 335–50. Oxford: Oxford University Press.

Vijayakumar, L., L. Jeyaseelan, S. Kumar, R. Mohanraj, S. Devika, and S. Manikandan. 2013. "A Central Storage Facility to Reduce Pesticide Suicides—A Feasibility Study from India." *BMC Public Health* 13 (1): 850.

Vijayakumar, L., S. John, J. Pirkis, and H. Whiteford. 2005. "Suicide in Developing Countries (2): Risk Factors." *Crisis* 26 (3): 112–19.

Vijayakumar, L., and A. T. Jotheeswaran. 2010. "Suicide in Refugees and Asylum Seekers." In *Mental Health of Refugees and Asylum Seekers*, edited by D. Bhugra, 195–210. Oxford, UK: Oxford University Press.

Vijayakumar, L., and S. Rajkumar. 1999. "Are Risk Factors for Suicide Universal? A Case Control Study in India." *Acta Psychitrica Scandinavica* 99: 407–11.

Vijayakumar, L., and N. Thilothammal. 1993. "Suicide Pacts." *Crisis: The Journal of Crisis Intervention and Suicide Prevention* 14 (1): 43–46.

Wang, C. W., C. L. Chan, and P. S. Yip. 2014. "Suicide Rates in China from 2002 to 2011: An Update." *Social Psychiatry and Psychiatric Epidemiology* 49: 929–41.

Wassermann, D., C. W. Hoven, C. Wasserman, M. Wall, R. Eisenberg, and others. 2015. "School-Based Suicide Prevention Programmes: The SEYLE Cluster-Randomised, Controlled Trial." *The Lancet* 385 (9977): 1536–44. doi:10.1016/S0140-6736(14)61213-7.

Wei, S., L. Liu, B. Bi, H. Li, J. Hou, and others. 2013. "An Intervention and Follow-Up Study Following a Suicide Attempt in the Emergency Departments of Four General Hospitals in Shenyang, China." *Crisis* 34 (2): 107–15.

WHO (World Health Organization). 2001. *The World Health Report 2001: Mental Health: New Understanding, New Hope.* Geneva: WHO.

———. 2008. *Clinical Management of Acute Pesticide Intoxication: Prevention of Suicidal Behaviours.* Geneva: WHO.

———. 2010a. *mhGAP Intervention Guide for Mental, Neurological, and Substance Use Disorders in Non-Specialized Health Settings.* Geneva: WHO.

———. 2010b. *Towards Evidence-Based Suicide Prevention Programmes.* Western Pacific Regional Office. Manila: WHO.

———. 2012. *Public Health Action for the Prevention of Suicide: A Framework.* Geneva: WHO.

———. 2014a. *Preventing Suicide: A Global Imperative.* Geneva: WHO.

———. 2014b. *Global Health Estimates: 1990–2012.* http://www.who.int/healthinfo/globalburdendisease/en.

Wickramasinghe, K., P. Steele, A. Dawson, D. Dharmaratne, A. Gunawardena, and others. 2009. "Cost to Government Health-Care Services of Treating Acute Self-Poisonings in a Rural District in Sri Lanka." *Bulletin of the World Health Organization* 87 (3): 180–85.

Yip, P. S. F., E. Caine, S. Yousuf, S.-S. Chang, K. S.-S. Chang, and Y.-Y. Chen. 2012. "Means Restriction for Suicide Prevention." *The Lancet* 379 (9834): 2393–99. doi:10.1016/S0140-6736(12)60521-2.

10

Population and Community Platform Interventions

Inge Petersen, Sara Evans-Lacko, Maya Semrau,
Margaret Barry, Dan Chisholm, Petra Gronholm,
Catherine O. Egbe, and Graham Thornicroft

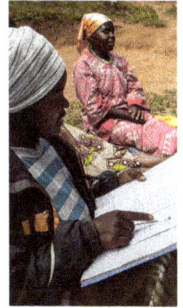

INTRODUCTION

Populationwide and community-level platforms are important for the delivery of mental, neurological, and substance use (MNS) interventions along the continuum of care. Certain interventions that promote mental health, prevent MNS disorders, and protect people are most appropriately delivered on a populationwide basis. Legislation, regulations, and public information campaigns are the common delivery channels of this platform.

Other interventions are best delivered by targeting a particular community setting or group in the community that shares a certain purpose. Community delivery channels include schools, workplaces, and neighborhoods and community groups.

Populationwide and community-level interventions often require coordinated efforts among different sectors, such as health, education, social development, labor, and criminal justice systems.

A third platform for delivering interventions—the health care system—is the subject of chapter 11 in this volume (Shidhaye, Lund, and Chisholm 2015).

KEY FINDINGS

Populationwide and community-level platforms are important for promotion and prevention interventions; identification and case detection; and, to a lesser degree, treatment, care, and rehabilitation. The evidence

presented in this chapter for each platform and delivery channel is structured around the core elements of the continuum of care (table 10.1).

Prevention interventions strive to prevent the onset, duration, and recurrence of MNS disorders; promotion interventions foster the positive mental health and well-being of the general population. Fairly good evidence is available from high-income countries (HICs) for interventions across these platforms and along the continuum of care, but the evidence base from low- and middle-income countries (LMICs) is far less robust. The chapter includes evidence from HICs and LMICs; identified best practice and good practice strategies are based on the best available evidence from both.

POPULATION-LEVEL PLATFORM

Populationwide interventions are rarely evaluated using the gold standard of randomized control trials (RCTs). More commonly used evaluation methods and approaches are quasi-experimental natural experiments, with before-and-after data obtained from archival analysis of official statistics or surveys, and comparisons with populations that have not been exposed to the intervention, where possible. Best-practice interventions were identified on the basis of existing quasi-experimental evidence from LMICs and evidence of cost-effectiveness (at least from HICs). Good-practice interventions were identified on the basis of emerging evidence in LMICs and assumptions that laws and regulations that are in

Corresponding author: Inge Petersen, University of KwaZulu Natal, Durban, Psychology, School of Applied Human Sciences, South Africa, peterseni@ukzn.ac.za.

Table 10.1 Matrix of Best-Practice and Good-Practice Interventions

Delivery platform	Promotion and primary prevention	Identification and case detection	Treatment, care, and rehabilitation
Population			
• Legislation and regulation	• Laws and regulations to reduce demand for alcohol use: taxes		• Mental health laws and regulations that are in line with the best practice and human rights standards
	• Laws and regulations to reduce demand for alcohol use; enforcement of BAC limits, advertising bans, and minimum ages		
	• Laws and regulations to restrict access to means of self-harm and suicide		
	• Child protection laws		
	• Laws and regulations promoting healthy lifestyles, for example, tobacco control		
	• Laws and regulations to promote improved control of neurocysticercosis		
• Information and awareness	• Mass public awareness campaigns		
Community			
• Workplace	• Integrating mental health promotion strategies, such as stress reduction and awareness of alcohol and drug misuse, into occupational health and safety policies		
• Schools	• Universal and targeted SEL programs for vulnerable children	• Identification and case detection in schools of children with MNS disorders	
	• Awareness programs		
• Neighborhood and community groups	• Parenting programs during infancy	• Training of gatekeepers, including community health workers, police, and social workers, in identification of MNS disorders, including self-harm	
	• Early childhood enrichment and preschool educational programs		
	• Parenting programs for children ages 2–14 years		

Note: Interventions in red indicate best practice; Interventions in black indicate good practice. BAC = blood alcohol concentration; MNS = mental, neurological, and substance use; SEL = social and emotional learning.

line with human rights standards would be protective. Additional interventions were identified on the assumption that addressing the known determinants of MNS disorders should promote mental health and lead to a reduction in MNS disorders, but these interventions were not recommended as good practice, given the lack of evidence of their effectiveness. The thorough review in this volume of the available evidence of the most effective and cost-effective interventions for the respective disorders was used as the evidence base, supplemented by a desk review of the best evidence where necessary (see online annex table 10A.) For further information on the cost-effectiveness of the mental health interventions referenced in this chapter, see chapter 12 in this volume (Levin and Chisholm 2015).

Legislation and Regulations for Promotion and Primary Prevention

Reducing Harmful Alcohol Use

The prevention of harmful alcohol use in adults provides benefits across diseases. It can help prevent the development of alcohol use disorder and unipolar depression, as well as other chronic diseases, such as cardiovascular disease, diabetes, and cirrhosis of the liver, and it can reduce the risk of contracting human immunodeficiency virus (HIV). It can also help with the prevention of accidental and intentional injuries or death (Rehm and others 2006).

Evidence from HICs and LMICs indicates that the most cost-effective strategy for reducing alcohol consumption is increased taxation or pricing of alcohol products, followed by bans on alcohol advertising, restrictions on access to alcohol, and enforcement of drinking-and-driving legislation (see chapter 7 in this volume, Medina-Mora and others 2015; and chapter 12 in this volume, Levin and Chisholm 2015). However, raising taxes is less effective in countries with lower levels of alcohol consumption; other targeted interventions, such as enforcing drunk driving legislation and brief screening and intervention, are more effective. Regulations may also be less effective in countries where alcohol can be easily acquired through the unregulated or black market or home brews (Rehm and others 2006). The cost of scaling up these interventions has been estimated for LMICs; implementation of a package of population-based demand reduction measures amounts to no more than US$0.25 per person (WHO 2011a).

Restricting Access to Means of Suicide

Suicide is one of the leading causes of premature deaths worldwide. Globally, the ingestion of pesticides, hanging, and use of firearms are among the most common methods (WHO 2014). Regulations restricting access to common, regional-specific, lethal means of suicide—such as firearm control legislation, restrictions on pesticides, and detoxification of domestic gas—have been shown to decrease rates of suicide in HICs and LMICs (van der Feltz-Cornelis and others 2011). Means restrictions require an understanding of the common methods used in different sectors of societies and countries, as well as the cooperation of different sectors (WHO 2014). The impact of the introduction of pesticide regulations on the reduction of suicides in Sri Lanka provides a case study of how this strategy has been effectively applied in LMICs (box 10.1). Cost-effectiveness modelling of such a pesticide ban in the Indian context has been undertaken for this volume (Nigam and others 2015).

Other Multisector Legislative and Regulatory Interventions

Other legislative and regulatory interventions to promote mental health and prevent the development of MNS disorders in children and adults in LMICs are included here based on evidence of the determinants, as well as emerging but promising evidence of the effectiveness, of the recommended interventions in LMICs.

Prenatal development and infancy is a particularly vulnerable period for the development of a wide range of MNS disorders. Possible interventions are suggested, based on evidence of the determinants of healthy development and MNS disorders during this stage. The assumption is that addressing these determinants would lead to a reduction in MNS disorders (Petersen and others 2014). However, the following interventions are not recommended as good practice, given the lack of evidence of effectiveness in LMICs:

- Regulations to improve obstetric and perinatal care to prevent birth trauma, given its association with physical and mental disabilities, notably epilepsy (see chapter 5 in this volume, Thakur and others 2015)
- Regulations to strengthen prenatal and postnatal immunization programs to prevent infectious diseases, such as HIV, as well as rubella and toxoplasmosis, which can impact cognitive development
- Regulations to increase access to micronutrients for vulnerable populations, including salt iodization programs to prevent iodine deficiency, which is associated with mental retardation during early infancy
- Regulations to promote folic acid food fortification and selective protein supplementation programs to promote healthy cognitive development.

During childhood, maltreatment is a risk factor for the development of MNS disorders. Some promising evidence from LMICs indicates that the enactment of child protection laws for children living outside the family has health and safety benefits for these children (Fluke and others 2012), although further research to assess the benefits for children within their families of origin is indicated. Such laws are, nevertheless, considered as good practice. Emerging evidence indicates

---

Box 10.1

Pesticide Regulations as an Intervention to Reduce Suicide: Sri Lanka

Self-poisoning with pesticide is the most common method of suicide in Sri Lanka, accounting for two-thirds of suicide deaths. The suicide rate in Sri Lanka reached a peak in 1995 at 47 deaths per 100,000 population. With the banning of all World Health Organization toxicity Class 1 pesticides in 1995 and the banning of endosulfan, a Class II toxicity pesticide, in 1998, the suicide rate halved from 1996 to 2005, with a reduction of 19,769 suicides, compared with 1986–95 (Gunnel and others 2007).

the protective influence of conditional cash transfers against poor cognitive and behavioral outcomes in vulnerable children (Fernald and Gunnar 2009; Lund and others 2011). Further research is, however, required before recommendations can be made.

Other multisector laws and regulations to promote mental health and prevent MNS disorders in children and adults include the following:

- *Restricting access to illicit drugs through laws and regulations preventing their sale, possession, and use.* However, the evidence on the effectiveness of such interventions in LMICs remains insufficient for them to be recommended as good practice (see chapter 6 in this volume, Degenhardt and others 2015).
- *Legislation to reduce traumatic brain injury and the consequent risk of epilepsy, such as through mandatory use of helmets by motorcyclists.* Evidence as to the effectiveness of this strategy for reducing epilepsy in LMICs is still required before it can be recommended as good practice (see chapter 5 in this volume, Thakur and others 2015).
- *Regulations to improve control of neurocysticercosis* (a common cause of epilepsy in LMICs) through deworming of humans, vaccination of pigs, improved sanitation, better meat inspection, and improved pig farming. Promising evidence is emerging from Honduras that these interventions can reduce epilepsy in hyperendemic populations (Medina and others 2011), and they are recommended as good practice.
- *Legislation against domestic violence as possible intervention*, given that risk factors for common mental disorders in women include interpersonal violence (Patel and others 2010). Some limited evidence from HICs suggests that such legislation reduces the chances of family or intimate partner violence (Dugan 2003). However, evidence from LMICs is required before it can be recommended as good practice.
- *Regulations promoting healthy lifestyles, given that risk for dementia in later life includes cardiovascular conditions.* These interventions are recommended as good practice (see chapter 5 in this volume, Thakur and others 2015).

Protecting Persons with MNS Disorders

The utility of national or state regulations and legislation and their effects on mental health promotion, prevention, treatment, care, and rehabilitation are more fully covered by policy guidelines than by evidence-based literature. The World Health Organization (WHO) and others have produced detailed guidance on the formulation of national strategies, national laws, human rights provisions, primary care integration and treatment guideline formulation, information systems, and suicide prevention (Hess and others 2004; Pinfold and others 2003; Swartz and others 2010; Thornicroft 2000; Watson and others 2004; WHO 2008, 2011b, 2012, 2013a); these issues are closely related to the growing field of implementation science (Tansella and Thornicroft 2009).

The WHO QualityRights Project has a toolkit to help countries assess and implement strategies to meet key standards in inpatient and outpatient mental health and social care facilities. These strategies are in alignment with the International Convention on the Rights of Persons with Disabilities (WHO 2012).

The objectives of the WHO QualityRights Project are as follows:

- Improving the quality of care and human rights conditions in mental health and social care facilities
- Changing attitudes and building capacity in service users, families, and health workers to understand and promote human rights and recovery
- Promoting the involvement of people with mental disabilities in advocacy work
- Reforming national policies and legislation to be in alignment with best-practice and international human rights standards.

Even without an evidence base to support such an initiative, it is reasonable to assume that up-to-date mental health laws and regulations that are in line with human rights standards, as outlined by the WHO QualityRights Project, should be readily accepted as good practice.

Information and Awareness Campaigns for Promotion and Primary Prevention

Information and public awareness campaigns employ broad strategies and messages to promote mental health literacy—defined as knowledge and beliefs about mental disorders to aid their recognition, management, and prevention (Jorm 2012)—as well as reduce stigma and discrimination. The campaigns disseminate information, for example, about signs and symptoms, locations where people may receive help, facts and figures about prevalence and risk factors, and evidence to combat stigmatizing beliefs. Multifaceted techniques to supplement traditional media outlets via lobbying of important stakeholder groups, facilitating grassroots activism, and mobilizing the public at popular events seem to be the most effective for encouraging prosocial behaviors, such as stigma reduction and help-seeking (Thornicroft and others, 2015).

Most information and awareness programs represent low-intensity interventions aimed at large numbers of people, often through print media, recordings, radio, television, cinema, mobile phones, and the Internet (Andreasen 2006; Clement and others 2013). Several examples of large-scale national efforts, and a growing evidence base, demonstrate their effectiveness in increasing knowledge about and recognition of MNS disorders (Jorm, Christensen, and Griffiths 2005), improving attitudes (Dunion and Gordom 2005; Evans-Lacko, Malcolm, and others 2013), and reducing discrimination in a cost-effective manner (Corker and others 2013; Evans-Lacko, Henderson, and others 2013; Henderson and others 2012; McCrone and others 2010; Thornicroft and others 2010; Thornicroft and others 2014). Although information and awareness programs often cover a broad range of MNS disorders, most focus on mental rather than neurological disorders. One RCT from Hong Kong SAR, China, however, showed that exposing individuals to information about dementia through vignettes led to a statistically significant reduction in stigma (Cheng and others 2011).

Several recent systematic reviews of the literature have examined the effectiveness of various types and components of anti-stigma interventions, including awareness programs aimed at the general public in HICs. A systematic review that focused on mass media strategies showed that such interventions may reduce prejudice, although fewer studies have investigated the effects of media strategies on discrimination (Clement and others 2013). A recent review by Corrigan and others (2012) examined anti-stigma approaches specific to mental illness and incorporated elements of education, protest, or contact. In-person contact interventions yielded the greatest effect in adults; education was most effective among adolescents. One challenge is to deliver these types of interventions on a mass scale to the public. Some evidence, using a pre-post research design, demonstrates the feasibility and effectiveness of achieving positive intergroup contact through large public events (Evans-Lacko and others 2012). Moreover, evidence supports the effectiveness of virtual contact via film or video; these types of interventions could be more cost-effective (Clement and others 2012), a finding that could be especially relevant for low-resource settings. For example, mobile phones and other technologies in LMICs might be explored as ways to increase access to information and awareness.

Evidence of the effectiveness of mass information programs in LMICs is limited. In 1996, the World Psychiatric Association initiated several national and regional efforts through the Open the Doors program (http://www.openthedoors.com/english/index.html) to reduce stigma, specifically in relation to people with schizophrenia (Warner 2005); however, evaluation of the program in LMICs is lacking. General lessons emphasize involving patients and caregivers in the development and evaluation of anti-stigma work, establishing a local network of committed institutions and individuals, and addressing stigma within health care through incorporating anti-stigma efforts into MNS services (Sartorius 2010; Stuart 2008).

The experiences and consequences of stigma vary across countries and cultures. Development and evaluation of anti-stigma interventions that are tailored and locally developed in LMICs are needed (Thornicroft and others 2015; Yang and others 2007).

Online interventions may represent a low-cost method of reaching individuals in LMICs. Many websites provide information on MNS disorders, but few studies have performed evaluations. One intervention in LMICs looked at whether an anti-stigma computer program would improve knowledge and attitudes and reduce social distance among university students in the Russian Federation (Finkelstein, Lapshin, and Wasserman 2008). Students were randomized to one of three groups: a computer program group, a reading group, or a control group. Participants were evaluated at baseline, immediately following the intervention, and six months later. Immediately following the intervention, knowledge, attitudes, and social distance improved among students in the reading and computer program groups. At the six-month follow-up, the reading group showed some improvement in attitudes; all stigma outcomes were significant in the computer program group.

Based on sufficient evidence from HICs and emerging promising evidence from LMICs, mass public awareness campaigns and, to a lesser extent, more targeted programs are recommended as good practice. For stigma reduction, in particular, more research, generating evidence of the effectiveness of social contact among the adult population and education-focused interventions among adolescents is recommended for HICs and LMICs. In LMICs in particular, more information is needed about how best to tailor existing interventions to local cultures, using available resources, and how best to reach key stakeholders—both targets and instigators of stigma—in these settings.

COMMUNITY-LEVEL PLATFORMS

Studies on interventions at the community-level platform in LMICs are limited; best-practice interventions were identified from the chapters on MNS disorders in this volume (chapter 6 in this volume, Degenhardt and others 2015; chapter 8 in this volume, Scott and others 2015) and supplemented by a desk review of available systematic reviews and trials in LMICs. Many of these interventions have a prevention and promotion focus, and the Assessing Cost-Effectiveness (ACE) prevention framework (Carter and others 2000) was used to evaluate effectiveness. The ACE grading system provides a single framework for the evaluation of evidence on clinical, public health, and behavioral interventions.

- *Sufficient evidence.* There is evidence of effectiveness as demonstrated by at least one systematic review of RCTs, as well as several good-quality RCTs or several high-quality pseudo-RCTs using alternate allocation or another method, or non-RCTs with comparative groups to exclude chance.
- *Limited evidence.* The effect is probably not due to chance, but bias cannot be ruled out as a possible explanation for the effect. We have classified this evidence as *promising*.
- *Inconclusive evidence.* There is no evidence of systematic reviews or RCTs, although there may be a few poor-quality pseudo-randomized non-RCTs with comparative groups or cohort studies.

Best-practice interventions were identified on the basis of two criteria:

- Evidence of their effectiveness based on sufficient evidence from LMICs, using the ACE framework, as well as their cost-effectiveness in HICs.
- Evidence of their feasibility in relation to cultural acceptability and capacity for scale-up in resource-constrained settings in LMICs.

Good-practice interventions were identified on the basis of sufficient evidence of their effectiveness in HICs and/or promising evidence of their effectiveness in LMICs, using the ACE framework.

Workplaces

Promotion and Primary Prevention
Workplace settings provide an ideal delivery channel for promotion and prevention interventions for adults. Evidence from HICs indicates that individual- and organization-level interventions improve and maintain mental health in the workplace. These interventions include screening and cognitive behavioral therapy (CBT) for pre-clinical symptoms of depression and anxiety to prevent the onset of these disorders (Nytro and others 2000; WHO 2000). However, the evidence base from LMICs is sparse.

Limited but promising evidence from LMICs of the effectiveness of primary prevention and promotion is provided by the SOLVE training package, developed by the International Labour Organization (Probst, Gold, and Caborn 2008). This training of trainers program provides human resource managers, trade unions, employers, and health professionals with the necessary knowledge and skills for integrating mental health promotion strategies, such as stress reduction and awareness of alcohol and drug misuse, into occupational health and safety policies and workplace action programs. The SOLVE program has been implemented in several countries, including China, India, Kenya, Malaysia, Namibia, the Philippines, South Africa, Sri Lanka, Swaziland, and Zambia. Preliminary evaluation of the original SOLVE program, with 268 participants in seven countries, using a pre-post test design, produced encouraging findings concerning knowledge gains following training (Probst, Gold, and Caborn 2008). However, more rigorous studies are needed to determine the long-term effectiveness and sustainability of this program across diverse workplace settings in LMICs. In view of the limited but promising evidence of the feasibility and impact of this program, such integrated mental health strategies in the workplace are considered as good practice.

Identification and Case Detection
Evidence on the identification and case detection of MNS disorders in the workplace could only be sourced from HICs. An evaluation of the APPRAND program in France provided evidence on individuals on sick leave who were screened by company health physicians and identified as having anxiety and depressive disorders and who received an awareness-raising and referral intervention. Those individuals displayed higher remission and recovery rates, compared with individuals in other centers who were not screened and who did not receive the intervention (Godard and others 2006). Positive effects have also been reported for a mental health first aid course in Australia that included training in screening for mental disorders (Kitchener and Jorm 2004).

For neurological disorders, positive outcomes have been reported in the United States for migraine and headache management programs that have included screening questionnaires and educational initiatives. These interventions resulted in an increase in the number of participants seeking help from physicians, an improvement in headache symptoms, a reduction in absenteeism among those affected, and a reduction in the cost burden to employers (Page and others 2009; Schneider and others 1999). No evidence for screening for MNS disorders in the workplace could be sourced from LMICs, and these interventions are not yet recommended.

Treatment, Care, and Rehabilitation

Interventions for the treatment, care, and rehabilitation of MNS disorders in the workplace have been effective in HICs. For people with common mental disorders, individual therapies rather than organizational interventions have been the most effective, in particular, CBT (BOHRF 2005; Hill and others 2007; Seymour 2010), either face to face or more questionably via computer software (Grime 2004; van der Klink and others 2001). To a lesser extent, exercise and relaxation interventions, such as aerobic or meditation sessions, have been beneficial (Graveling and others 2008). Independent case management by third-party specialists, such as labor experts or employment advisors, has shown a positive impact on people with common mental disorders when combined with psychological therapies, such as CBT (Seymour 2010). Multimodal interventions may be more effective than single interventions (BOHRF 2005). With respect to severe mental disorders (SMDs), sufficient evidence from HICs indicates the benefits of supported employment, for example, individual placement and support, in helping people obtain competitive employment (Crowther and others 2001; Dickson and Gough 2008; McDaid 2008).

For neurological disorders, a few studies have shown positive effects, although with mixed results, for educational and physical programs implemented in workplace settings in Finland and Italy to reduce headaches and neck and shoulder pain (Mongini and others 2012; Rota and others 2011; Sjögren and others 2005). Furthermore, an RCT in South Africa found that a workplace intervention consisting of workability assessments and workplace visits was able to facilitate return to work for stroke patients (Ntsiea 2013).

Overall, evidence from LMICs for the treatment, care, and rehabilitation of MNS disorders in the workplace is insufficient for recommendations to be made. Further research is recommended on the effectiveness of training in first-level management of acute symptoms, particularly CBT, for anxiety or depression (possibly combined with independent case management); supported employment for people with SMDs; and educational, physical, and return-to-work interventions for neurological disorders.

Schools

Promotion and Primary Prevention

Information and Awareness. Examples of robust evaluations of broad information and awareness interventions addressing MNS literacy are more available in HICs (Pinfold and others 2003; Swartz and others 2010; Watson and others 2004). In LMICs, only one study that was performed in rural secondary schools in Pakistan could be sourced. The intervention, led by health care professionals, involved a short training course for teachers, with a co-constructed educational program of lectures and several participatory activities. The study used an RCT evaluation and assessed changes in knowledge and attitudes four months after the start of the program. Improvements were noted among schoolchildren, parents, friends, and neighbors. In the control group, there were improvements only among schoolchildren and their friends (Rahman and others 1998).

For neurological disorders, only studies in HICs could be sourced. Hip Hop Stroke is an example of an information and awareness program for children (ages 8 to 12 years) from schools in a high-risk stroke neighborhood in the United States. Following the program, the children showed improved knowledge of stroke symptoms and behavioral intent to call 911 (Williams and others 2012). Given that promising evidence is emerging on the positive impact of information and awareness interventions in schools in LMICs, these programs are recommended as good practice. Further research on the impact of such interventions in schools is needed.

Social and Emotional Learning Interventions. Studies from HICs and LMICs indicate that life skills programs to build socioemotional competencies in children and adolescents (social and emotional learning [SEL] programs) can improve social and emotional functioning and academic performance in exposed children. The programs also reduce risk behavior, when combined with reproductive and sexual health and substance use education. Systematic reviews from HICs show that universal SEL interventions in primary and post-primary schools promote children's social and emotional functioning and academic performance in the long term (Durlak and others 2011; Lister-Sharp and others 1999; NICE 2009; Tennant and others 2007; Weare and Nind 2011; Wells, Barlow, and Stewart-Brown 2003).

In relation to substance abuse in particular, school-based interventions that target social skills more broadly in younger children have been found to have a greater positive effect than in high school–age children (see chapter 6 in this volume, Degenhardt and others 2015). Evidence from HICs also indicates that interventions that employ a whole-school approach are most effective and have helped to reduce bullying. In the whole-school approach, SEL is supported by a school ethos and a physical and social environment that is health-enabling and involves staff, students, parents, the school environment, and the local community. Bullying has been identified as a risk factor for the development of psychiatric disorders in bullies and their victims (see chapter 8 in this volume, Scott and others 2015).

A systematic review (Barry and others 2013) and other studies (De Villiers and van den Berg 2012; Mueller and others 2011; Smith and others 2008; Srikala and Kishore 2010) provide sufficient evidence of the beneficial effects of universal SEL programs in LMICs. These interventions can be feasibly delivered by teachers and school counselors through the integration of SEL into life orientation curricula, as demonstrated by the HealthWise program in South Africa (Smith and others 2008) (box 10.2). However, the quality of implementation and contextual issues can affect the impact of SEL interventions; teacher training, support, and supervision are needed, as is attention to the school environment (Caldwell and others 2012), suggesting that integration into a whole-school approach is preferred.

For high-risk children, targeted and indicated interventions that promote coping skills, resilience, and cognitive skills training have helped prevent the onset of anxiety, depression, and suicide in HICs (Clarke and others 1995; Jaycox and others 1994; Shucksmith and others 2007). Several RCTs of targeted interventions for vulnerable children have been conducted in LMICs (Fazel and others 2014). Some classroom-based interventions (CBIs) for vulnerable children, especially those orphaned by HIV or living in areas of conflict, have improved general psychological health and coping (Ager and others 2011; Jordans and others 2010; Khamis, Macy, and Coignez 2004; Qouta and others 2012). However, these effects are contingent on individual variables, such as age and gender, as well as contextual variables, such as conflict, displacement, and family functioning (Tol and others 2014), and may be better suited for children with less severe risks and difficulties (Fazel and others 2014). Box 10.3 describes a case study of the impact of a classroom, community, and camp–based intervention for children in economies at war and with complex emergencies. The intervention was taken to scale in the West Bank and Gaza (Khamis, Macy, and Coignez 2004).

Economic analyses from HICs indicate that SEL interventions in schools are cost-effective, resulting in savings from better health outcomes, as well as reduced expenditures in the criminal justice system (McCabe 2007).

The cost of implementing school-based SEL interventions in LMICs has not yet been estimated. An attempt is made in chapter 12 in this volume (Levin and Chisholm 2015) on the basis of a psychosocial intervention to prevent depression in adolescents ages 12 to 16 years in Mauritius (Rivet-Duval, Heriot, and Hunt 2011). The findings suggest that school-based SEL interventions represent a low-cost strategy to promote adolescent mental health. Universal and targeted school-based SEL interventions are considered as best-practice interventions for LMICs.

Identification and Case Detection

Many MNS disorders have their onset during childhood and adolescence, and these early difficulties are likely to be present in the school context. Teachers have a critical role in identifying emerging problems and taking

---

Box 10.2

The HealthWise Program in South Africa

HealthWise combines leisure, life skills, and sexuality education into a 12-lesson program for students in grade eight, with six booster sessions in grade nine delivered by teachers during life orientation, with the aim of reducing health risk behaviors. The lessons cover socio-emotional skills building, such as decision making, self-awareness, and anxiety and anger management, as well as the positive use of free time and attitudes, knowledge, and skills building to reduce substance use and sexual risk behaviors.

An efficacy trial involving 2,383 participants from a low-income community in Cape Town demonstrated that HealthWise had a moderately positive effect on alcohol use. It was also effective in increasing awareness of condom availability and perceived condom self-efficacy. The program is being expanded to 56 schools in the Cape Town area to assess the effects of fidelity issues, namely, enhanced teacher training; enhanced teacher support, structure, and supervision; and enhanced school environment on outcomes.

Source: Caldwell and others 2012.

Classroom, Community, and Camp–Based Intervention in the West Bank and Gaza

Classroom, community, and camp–based intervention provides structured expressive-behavioral group activities over 15 sessions to reduce traumatic stress reactions and strengthen children's resiliency to cope with the stress of ongoing violence and trauma. The program was delivered by trained school counselors and other social workers to more than 100,000 children in the West Bank and Gaza. A randomized control trial involving 664 children ages 6–16 years found that the program improved psychological functioning and coping in young boys and girls (ages 6–11 years), as well as in adolescent girls (ages 12–16 years), enabling them to function as other children would in relation to family, school, and peers. However, this effect was not the case with adolescent boys (ages 12–16 years), who demonstrated an increased tendency to use avoidance of cognitions and feelings as a defense mechanism, which may relate to their greater exposure to violence.

Source: Khamis, Macy, and Coignez 2004.

Teacher Training Program, Brazil

An exploratory study in São Paulo, Brazil, tested the effectiveness of an educational strategy to build teachers' capacity to identify students with possible mental health problems and subsequently make appropriate referrals. Teacher training involved two two-hour sessions that included a lecture followed by theoretical and practical exercises. Teachers were evaluated on their ability to identify and refer students with mental health problems in a hypothetical vignette scenario. When assessing responses specifically among teachers who did not initially respond correctly to the vignettes, researchers found at least 50 percent had learned to identify and make referrals of problematic cases following the training, and 60 percent learned to identify normal adolescent behaviors. The study suggests that brief training can increase teachers' capacity to identify mental health problems and make appropriate referrals, especially among those who initially struggled to do so.

Source: Vieira and others 2014.

appropriate action. RCTs from HICs provide evidence for training in indicated screening of developmental and behavioral disorders in schools. Programs such as Mental Health First Aid for High School Teachers have been tested using a cluster RCT (Jorm and others 2010).

Data from LMICs are limited. However, evidence supports the feasibility and reliability of identifying and assessing MNS disorders in primary and secondary school students (Becker and others 2010a, 2010b; Opoliner and others 2013; Vieira and others 2014) (box 10.4). In Haiti, a 2.5 day training program for secondary school teachers focused on recognizing, responding to, and referring students at risk for MNS disorders following the earthquake in 2010.

The intervention was associated with improvements in knowledge, attitudes, and recognition of MNS disorders (Eustache, Becker, and Wozo 2014). In Chandigarh city, India, a one-off educational intervention package improved teachers' knowledge, attitudes, and skills regarding epilepsy immediately after the intervention, and at the three-month follow-up. However, it was noted that further workshops would likely be required for long-term benefit (Goel and others 2014).

Given sufficient evidence from HICs, as well as emerging promising evidence from LMICs, the identification and case detection in schools of children with MNS disorders are recommended as good practice. Further research adapting and developing, validating, and piloting screening tools that are culturally sensitive, user friendly, and easy to administer in LMICs is proposed.

Treatment, Care, and Rehabilitation

There is sufficient evidence of the effective treatment and management of some MNS disorders in schools in HICs. A meta-analysis that examined the effectiveness of various types of school-based CBT for young people with anxiety and depression showed significant reductions in symptoms overall (Mychailyszyn and others 2012). School-based interventions for attention-deficit hyperactivity disorder (ADHD) have been found to be promising in younger children but less so for adolescents; these interventions lack robust long-term program effectiveness data, as well as cost-effectiveness data (Kutcher and Wei 2012). Effective ADHD interventions that improve academic and behavioral outcomes involve contingency management, academic intervention, and cognitive-behavioral interventions (DuPaul, Eckert, and Vilardo 2012). For neurological disorders, a classroom-based headache prevention program in Germany found a small but significant reduction in reported tension-type headaches seven months following the intervention (Albers and others 2015).

Evidence from HICs also indicates that children with emotional and behavioral disorders benefit from classroom environments that are predictable and consistent, with clear structures and rules; such settings are associated with improved classroom and peer behavior and enhanced learning (Simpson, Peterson, and Smith 2011). A classroom strategy focused on punishment is likely to increase aggression and other behavioral problems (Kennedy and Jolivette 2008). Some research indicates the benefits of academic supports; however, there are significant limitations in the current evidence base, as many of these studies used single-subject designs and lacked measures of fidelity, that is, whether the intervention was implemented as intended; most did not include minorities (Mooney and others 2003). Interventions that use direct instruction, peer tutoring, and behaviorally based procedures—such as time delay prompting, trial and error, and differential reinforcement—hold promise (Rivera, Al-Otaiba, and Koorland 2006).

Evidence from LMICs for treatment, care, and rehabilitation for children with MNS disorders is limited and equivocal. An RCT of a universal school-based intervention for reducing depressive symptoms was conducted in Chile. It used CBT techniques delivered by nonspecialists and comprised 11 one-hour weekly sessions and two booster classroom sessions. Although it was a universal intervention, the study analyzed subgroups of young people with high depression scores. The analysis showed no clinically significant difference between the intervention and control groups and no evidence of effect modification by severity of symptoms (Araya and others 2013).

A few CBI trials have incorporated cognitive behavioral techniques and creative expressive elements to help children with depressive, anxiety, and post-traumatic stress disorder (PTSD) symptoms in complex emergencies in LMICs (Jordans and others 2010; Tol and others 2008; Tol and others 2012; Tol and others 2014). The emerging evidence on the effectiveness of treatment of PTSD and depressive symptoms is inconsistent; CBI has more consistent prevention benefits, particularly when the risks are less severe. Accordingly, CBI cannot be recommended for treatment of these conditions in conflict-affected children (Fazel and others 2014). Given the equivocal evidence from LMICs, further research generating positive outcomes for treatment, care, and rehabilitation for children with MNS disorders in schools is required before recommendations can be made.

Neighborhood and Community Groups

Primary Prevention and Promotion

An array of primary prevention and promotion interventions is delivered at the neighborhood level or through community groups. These interventions include programs on early childhood enrichment and preschool educational programs, community-based parenting, and gender and economic empowerment interventions.

Early Childhood Enrichment and Preschool Educational Programs. Robust evidence from HICs demonstrates the effectiveness and cost-effectiveness of early childhood enrichment and preschool educational programs on social and emotional well-being, cognitive skills, problem behaviors, and school readiness (Anderson and others 2003; Nelson, Westhues, and MacLeod 2003; Tennant and others 2007). There is also evidence of long-term effects on school attainment, social gains, and occupational status in HICs (Schweinhart and others 2005).

The evidence from LMICs is promising (Aboud 2006; Cueto and others 2009; Kagitcibasi, Sunar, and Bekman 2001; Kagitcibasi and others 2009). Evidence of the long-term benefits of early childhood enrichment and preschool educational programs is provided by the Turkish early childhood enrichment project. Long-term follow-up of a cohort of 131 participants found that children who received a home-based educational intervention, preschool education, or both, achieved higher educational attainment and occupational status and obtained employment earlier that those participants who received neither (Kagitcibasi and others 2009). These interventions are therefore considered to represent good practice.

Parenting Interventions. There is sufficient evidence from LMICs of the effectiveness and feasibility of parenting programs to enhance mother-child interaction during infancy for these interventions to be considered good practice (Cooper and others 2009; Jin and others 2007; Mejia, Calam, and Sanders 2012; Rahman and others 2009; Walker and Chang 2013; Wendland-Carro, Piccinini, and Millar 1999). Many interventions are delivered at health centers or utilize a home visitation program and may overlap with interventions delivered at the first-level facilities described in chapter 11 in this volume (Shidhaye, Lund, and Chisholm 2015).

The effectiveness of community parenting programs for the prevention of internalizing and externalizing disorders in children who are preschool and school age has been demonstrated in HICs (e.g., Kaminski and others 2008), with promising evidence from LMICs (Fayyad and others 2010; Oveisi and others 2010; Vasquez and others 2010; Wendland-Carro, Piccinini, and Millar 1999); these are also considered as good practice.

Gender Equity and Economic Empowerment Interventions. A growing body of research indicates the feasibility and benefits for vulnerable adolescents and adults of gender equity and economic empowerment programs in LMICs (Balaji and others 2011; Brady and others 2007; Jewkes and others 2008; Kermode and others 2007; Kim and others 2009; Pronyk and others 2006; Ssewamala, Han, and Neilands 2009). For poor people in Sub-Saharan Africa, microfinance (micro-credit and microsavings) schemes that incorporate gender empowerment, health, and educational training components are more effective in terms of mental health benefits over standalone programs (Lund and others 2011; Stewart and others 2010). Further evidence is, however, required before these programs can be recommended as good practice.

Identification and Case Detection
Mental health first aid training at the community level involves training community members to identify when a person is developing a mental disorder, is suicidal, or is in crisis; to know how to manage the situation; and to know where to refer the person appropriately (Jorm 2012).

Evidence for feasible and effective identification training programs for non-mental health workers is particularly robust for police officers and community health workers in HICs and LMICs (Chibanda and others 2011;

Hansson and Markstrom 2014; Krameddine and others 2013; Teller and others 2006; Watson and others 2008). Given that community health workers may operate from health centers or utilize a home visitation program, these interventions may overlap with interventions delivered at the first-level facility platform described in chapter 11 in this volume (Shidhaye, Lund, and Chisholm 2015).

With respect to neurological disorders, research from HICs suggests that trained community health workers can facilitate early detection of dementia in resource-poor communities (Han and others 2013). Moreover, if screening leads to early intervention within a year of detection, it could be associated with cost savings through reduced health care costs in the long run (Saito and others 2014). Mental health first aid training of community members generally has been found to increase knowledge, reduce stigma, and increase help-seeking behavior in HICs. Although mental health first aid training is being rolled out in several LMICs, evidence of effectiveness is still lacking (Jorm and others 2004). Given sufficient evidence from HICs, as well as emerging promising evidence from LMICs, for training non-mental health workers and community members in identification and case detection, it is recommended as good practice. Further research on the impact of such interventions on increasing access to mental health care in LMICs is required.

Treatment, Care, and Rehabilitation
Policy shifts to deinstitutionalize and decentralize care in many LMICs are heightening the need for community-based treatment and rehabilitation for mental disorders. These interventions are generally delivered through health care platforms and are described in detail in chapter 11 in this volume (Shidhaye, Lund, and Chisholm 2015).

CONCLUSIONS

This chapter has reviewed the evidence on population- and community-level interventions that improve mental health in LMICs.

Population-Level Interventions

Interventions at the population platform have a broad reach, promoting and protecting the mental health of the entire population through legislation, regulations, and public campaigns. Legislation and regulations to control alcohol demand can reduce consumption in LMICs at minimal cost; and taxation on alcohol products is recommended as best practice.

Laws and regulations restricting access to lethal means of suicide that are region specific can reduce suicide rates in LMICs and are also recommended as best practice. Mental health laws aligned with international standards for human rights protection are recommended as good practice on the assumption that they are likely to help to curb violations in mental health and social care facilities. Child protection laws and improved control of neurocysticercosis are recommended as good practice, given the emerging evidence of their health and safety benefits in LMICs.

Legislative changes are relatively low cost, but they can be difficult to implement, with adaptation and implementation requiring the buy-in and cooperation of multiple sectors. With respect to alcohol legislation in particular, unregulated markets, easy access to home brews, and access to the black market in LMICs may limit the success of this strategy. LMICs are also likely to encounter opposition from local and international alcohol producers, with the latter increasingly targeting emerging markets. Strong political will and advocacy work, within and outside governments, are necessary to garner public and political support for legislation to reduce the demand for alcohol. National and international nongovernmental organizations and the media can play an important role. International cooperation and regulation-related legislation to help prevent illicit trade and cross-border advertising, promotion of alcohol consumption, and sponsorship have been suggested as important, particularly for emerging markets struggling to enter the global economy (Casswell and Thamarangsi 2009).

Suicide prevention through restricting access to the means of suicide may encounter challenges in regulating access to certain means of suicide, such as by hanging or self-immolation, and this may also limit the success of this strategy.

For mass information and awareness campaigns for promoting mental health literacy and reducing stigma as a public health strategy at the population level, some small-scale but promising evidence from LMICs indicates the potential effectiveness of mass public awareness campaigns; they are recommended as good practice.

Community-Level Interventions

Interventions at the community platform have less broad reach but more depth and intensity. This chapter reviewed the evidence for interventions delivered in the workplace, at schools, and in neighborhoods and community groups. In the workplace, integrating mental health promotion strategies, such as stress reduction and awareness of alcohol and drug misuse, into occupational health and safety policies is recommended as good practice, based on emerging evidence in LMICs.

Stronger evidence exists in LMICs for schools as a delivery channel for interventions across primary prevention and promotion and identification. There is robust evidence of life skills training in schools to promote social and emotional competencies. This is recommended as best practice. There is promising evidence for the identification of mental disorders in schools, which is recommended as good practice.

Emerging promising evidence supports the delivery of neighborhood and community group interventions in LMICs. In primary prevention and promotion programs, parenting programs, particularly during infancy, are recommended as good practice. Evidence is emerging on the long-term benefits of early childhood enrichment and preschool educational programs, and these are recommended as good practice. Emerging evidence also suggests the mental health benefits of gender and economic empowerment programs, but is still insufficient to recommend as good practice. For identification and treatment, care, and rehabilitation, the training of gatekeepers to identify people with mental illness is recommended as good practice, based on emerging promising evidence in LMICs.

Many MNS disorders have their onset during childhood and adolescence (Kessler and others 2005; WHO 2013b); early difficulties are likely to present at the community platform in schools and neighborhoods. Interventions along the continuum of care described in this chapter are particularly important to prevent the onset and reduce the severity of the course of MNS disorders. However, community-level interventions require strong intersectoral engagement, as well as buy-in to task-sharing. Teachers, social workers, police, community health workers, and community members can provide first-line mental health care with sufficient training and support. To enable collaborative arrangements with different departments, as well as community-based groups, including nongovernmental organizations, spiritual leaders, and traditional healers, Skeen and others (2010) suggest the formalization of these arrangements through legislation of intersectoral forums for mental health from the national to the local levels. Such forums can facilitate awareness of mental health as a public health priority in other sectors, illuminate the role these other sectors can play, and clarify the roles and responsibilities and referral pathways between sectors (Skeen and others 2010).

Although much attention has historically been paid to platforms within the health sector for the delivery of mental health services, it is increasingly clear that greater consideration of population- and community-level platforms is necessary for the delivery of prevention and promotion interventions, as well as for the early identification of mental disorders, particularly in children and adolescents.

The annex to this chapter is as follows. It is available at www.dcp-3.org/mentalhealth.

- Annex 10A. Evidence of Interventions at the Population- and Community-Level Platforms

NOTES

Disclaimer: Dan Chisholm is a staff member of the World Health Organization. The author alone is responsible for the views expressed in this publication, and they do not necessarily represent the decisions, policy, or views of the World Health Organization.

This chapter was previously published in an article by M. Semrau, S. Evans-Lacko, A. Alem, J. L. Ayuso-Mateos, D. Chisholm, O. Gureje, C. Hanlon, M. Jordans, F. Kigozi, H. Lempp, C. Lund, I. Petersen, R. Shidhaye, and G. Thornicroft, titled "Strengthening Mental Health Systems in Low- and Middle-Income Countries: The Emerald Programme." *BMC Medicine*, 2015; 13 (79). doi:10.1186/s12916-015-0309-4. <http://bmcmedicine.biomedcentral.com/articles/10.1186/s12916-015-0309-4>.

World Bank Income Classifications as of July 2014 are as follows, based on estimates of gross national income (GNI) per capita for 2013:

- Low-income countries (LICs) = US$1,045 or less
- Middle-income countries (MICs) are subdivided:
  a) lower-middle-income = US$1,046 to US$4,125
  b) upper-middle-income (UMICs) = US$4,126 to US$12,745
- High-income countries (HICs) = US$12,746 or more.

REFERENCES

Aboud, F. E. 2006. "Evaluation of an Early Childhood Preschool Program in Rural Bangladesh." *Early Childhood Research Quarterly* 21: 46–60.

Ager, A., B. Akesson, L. Stark, E. Flouri, B. Okot, and others. 2011. "The Impact of the School-Based Psychosocial Structured Activities (PSSA) Program on Conflict-Affected Children in Northern Uganda." *Journal of Child Psychology and Psychiatry* 52 (11): 1124–33.

Albers, L., F. Heinen, M. Landgraf, A. Straube, B. Blum, and others. 2015. "Headache Cessation by an Educational Intervention in Grammar Schools: A Cluster Randomized Trial." *European Journal of Neurology* 22 (2): 270–76, e22.

Anderson, L. M., C. Shinn, M. T. Fullilove, S. C. Scrimshaw, J. E. Fielding, and others. 2003. "The Effectiveness of Early Childhood Development Programs. A Systematic Review." *American Journal of Preventive Medicine* 24 (Suppl. 3): 32–46.

Andreasen, A. 2006. *Social Marketing in the 21st Century*. Thousand Oaks, CA: Sage Publications.

Araya, R., R. Fritsch, M. Spears, G. Rojas, V. Martinez, and others. 2013. "School Intervention to Improve Mental Health of Students in Santiago, Chile: A Randomized Clinical Trial." *JAMA Pediatrics* 167 (11): 1004–10.

Balaji, M., T. Andrews, G. Andrew, and V. Patel. 2011. "The Acceptability, Feasibility, and Effectiveness of a Population-Based Intervention to Promote Youth Health: An Exploratory Study in Goa, India." *Journal of Adolescent Health* 48 (5): 453–60.

Barry, M. M., A. M. Clarke, R. Jenkins, and V. Patel. 2013. "A Systematic Review of the Effectiveness of Mental Health Promotion Interventions for Young People in Low and Middle Income Countries." *BMC Public Health* 13 (1): 835.

Becker, A. E., J. J. Thomas, A. Bainivualiku, L. Richards, K. Navara, and others. 2010a. "Adaptation and Evaluation of the Clinical Impairment Assessment to Assess Disordered Eating Related Distress in an Adolescent Female Ethnic Fijian Population." *International Journal of Eating Disorders* 43 (2): 179–86. doi:10.1002/eat.20665.

———. 2010b. "Validity and Reliability of a Fijian Translation and Adaptation of the Eating Disorder Examination Questionnaire." *International Journal of Eating Disorders* 43 (2): 171–78. doi:10.1002/eat.20675.

BOHRF (British Occupational Health Research Foundation). 2005. *Workplace Interventions for People with Common Mental Health Problems: Evidence Review and Recommendations*. London: BOHRF.

Brady, M., R. Assaad, B. Ibrahim, A. Salem, and R. Salem. 2007. "Providing New Opportunities to Adolescent Girls in Socially Conservative Settings: The Ishraq Program in Rural Upper Egypt." Population Council, New York.

Caldwell, L. L., E. A. Smith, L. M. Collins, J. W. Graham, M. Lai, and others. 2012. "Translational Research in South Africa: Evaluating Implementation Quality Using a Factorial Design." *Child Youth Care Forum* 41 (2): 119–36. doi:10.1007/s10566-011-9164-4.

Carter, R., C. Stone, T. Vos, J. Hocking, C. Mihalopoulos, and others. 2000. *Trial of Program Budgeting and Marginal Analysis (PBMA) to Assist Cancer Control Planning in Australia*. Canberra: Commonwealth Department of Health and Aged Care.

Casswell, S., and T. Thamarangsi. 2009. "Reducing Harm from Alcohol: Call to Action." *The Lancet* 373 (9682): 2247–57.

Cheng, S.-T., L. C. W. Lam, L. C. K. Chan, A. C. B. Law, A. W. T. Fung, and others. 2011. "The Effects of Exposure to Scenarios about Dementia on Stigma and Attitudes toward Dementia Care in a Chinese Community." *International Psychogeriatrics* 23 (09): 1433–41.

Chibanda, D., P. Mesu, L. Kajawu, F. Cowan, R. Araya, and others. 2011. "Problem-Solving Therapy for Depression and Common Mental Disorders in Zimbabwe: Piloting a Task-Shifting Primary Mental Health Care Intervention in a Population with a High Prevalence of People Living with HIV." *BMC Public Health* 11 (1): 828.

Clarke, G. N., W. Hawkins, M. Murphy, L. B. Sheeber, P. M. Lewinsohn, and J. R. Seeley. 1995. "Targeted Prevention of Unipolar Depressive Disorder in an At-Risk Sample of High School Adolescents: A Randomized Trial of a Group Cognitive Intervention." *Journal of the American Academy of Child and Adolescent Psychiatry* 34 (3): 312–21.

Clement, S., F. Lassman, E. Barley, S. Evans-Lacko, P. Williams, and others. 2013. "Mass Media Interventions for Reducing Mental Health–Related Stigma." *Cochrane Database of Systematic Reviews* 7: CD009453. doi:10.1002/14651858 .CD009453.pub2.

Clement, S., A. van Nieuwenhuizen, A. Kassam, C. Flach, A. Lazarus, and others. 2012. "Filmed v. Live Social Contact Interventions to Reduce Stigma: Randomised Controlled Trial." *British Journal of Psychiatry* 201 (1): 57–64.

Cooper, P. J., M. Tomlinson, L. Swartz, M. Landman, C. Molteno, and others. 2009. "Improving Quality of Mother-Infant Relationship and Infant Attachment in Socioeconomically Deprived Community in South Africa: Randomised Controlled Trial." *BMJ* 338: b974. doi: http:// dx.doi.org/10.1136/bmj.b974.

Corker, E., S. Hamilton, C. Henderson, C. Weeks, V. Pinfold, and others. 2013. "Experiences of Discrimination among People Using Mental Health Services in England 2008–2011." *British Journal of Psychiatry* 55: s58–63. doi:10.1192/bjp .bp.112.112912.

Corrigan, P. W., S. B. Morris, P. J. Michaels, J. D. Rafacz, and N. Rusch. 2012. "Challenging the Public Stigma of Mental Illness: A Meta-Analysis of Outcome Studies." *Psychiatric Services* 63 (10): 963–73.

Crowther, R. E., M. Marshall, G. R. Bond, and P. Huxley. 2001. "Helping People with Severe Mental Illness to Obtain Work: Systematic Review." *British Medical Journal* 322: 204–08.

Cueto, S., G. Guerrero, J. Leon, A. Zevallos, and C. Sugimaru. 2009. "Promoting Early Childhood Development through a Public Programme: Wawa Wasi in Peru." Working Paper 51, Department of International Development, Oxford, U.K.

Degenhardt, L., E. Stockings, J. Strang, J. Marsden, and W. D. Hall. 2015. "Illicit Drug Dependence." In *Disease Control Priorities* (third edition): Volume 4, *Mental, Neurological, and Substance Use Disorders,* edited by V. Patel, D. Chisholm, T. Dua, R. Laxminarayan, and M. E. Medina-Mora. Washington, DC: World Bank.

De Villiers, M., and H. van den Berg. 2012. "The Implementation and Evaluation of a Resiliency Programme for Children." *South African Journal of Psychology* 42 (1): 93–102.

Dickson, K., and D. Gough. 2008. "Supporting People in Accessing Meaningful Work: Recovery Approaches in Community-Based Adult Mental Health Services." SCIE Knowledge Review 21, Social Care Institute for Excellence, London.

Dugan, L. 2003. "Domestic Violence Legislation: Exploring Its Impact on the Likelihood of Domestic Violence, Police Involvement, and Arrest." *Criminology and Public Policy* 2 (2): 283–312.

Dunion, L., and L. Gordon. 2005. "Tackling the Attitude Problem. The Achievements to Date of Scotland's 'See Me' Anti-Stigma Campaign." *Mental Health Today (Brighton, UK)* March: 22–25.

DuPaul, G. J., T. Eckert, and B. Vilardo. 2012. "The Effects of School-Based Interventions for Attention Deficit Hyperactivity Disorder: A Meta-Analysis 1996–2010." *School Psychology Review* 41: 387–412.

Durlak, J. A., R. P. Weissberg, A. B. Dymnicki, R. D. Taylor, and K. B. Schellinger. 2011. "The Impact of Enhancing Students'

Social and Emotional Learning: A Meta-Analysis of School-Based Universal Interventions." *Child Development* 82 (1): 405–32. doi:10.1111/j.1467-8624.2010.01564.x.

Eustache, E., A. E. Becker, and E. Wozo. 2014. "Developing Research Capacity for Mental Health Interventions for Youth in Haiti." In *Frontiers in Neuroscience for Global Health/Tenth Anniversary of Brain Disorders in the Developing World: Research across the Lifespan.* Bethesda, MD: National Institutes of Health.

Evans-Lacko, S., C. Henderson, G. Thornicroft, and P. McCrone. 2013. "Economic Evaluation of the Anti-Stigma Social Marketing Campaign in England 2009–2011." *British Journal of Psychiatry* Suppl. 55: s95–101. doi:10.1192 /bjp.bp.112.113746.

Evans-Lacko, S., J. London, S. Japhet, N. Rusch, C. Flach, and others. 2012. "Mass Social Contact Interventions and Their Effect on Mental Health Related Stigma and Intended Discrimination." *BMC Public Health* 12: 489. doi:10.1186/1471-2458-12-489.

Evans-Lacko, S., E. Malcolm, K. West, D. Rose, J. London, and others. 2013. "Influence of Time to Change's Social Marketing Interventions on Stigma in England 2009–2011." *British Journal of Psychiatry* Suppl. 55: s77–88.

Fayyad, J. A., L. Farah, Y. Cassir, M. M. Salamoun, and E. G. Karam. 2010. "Dissemination of an Evidence-Based Intervention to Parents of Children with Behavioral Problems in a Developing Country." *European Child and Adolescent Psychiatry* 19 (8): 629–36. doi:10.1007 /s00787-010-0099-3.

Fazel, M., V. Patel, S. Thomas, and W. Tol. 2014. "Mental Health Interventions in Schools in Low-Income and Middle-Income Countries." *The Lancet Psychiatry* 1 (5): 388–98.

Fernald, L. C. H., and M. R. Gunnar. 2009. "Poverty-Alleviation Program Participation and Salivary Cortisol in Very Low-Income Children." *Social Science and Medicine* 68 (12): 2180–89.

Finkelstein, J., O. Lapshin, and E. Wasserman. 2008. "Randomized Study of Different Anti-Stigma Media." *Patient Education and Counseling* 71 (2): 204–14. doi:10.1016/j.pec.2008.01.002.

Fluke, J. D., P. S. Goldman, J. Shriberg, S. D. Hillis, K. Yun, and others. 2012. "Systems, Strategies, and Interventions for Sustainable Long-Term Care and Protection of Children with a History of Living Outside of Family Care." *Child Abuse and Neglect* 36 (10): 722–31. doi:10.1016/j .chiabu.2012.09.005.

Godard, C., A. Chevalier, Y. Lecrubier, and G. Lahon. 2006. "APRAND Programme: An Intervention to Prevent Relapses of Anxiety and Depressive Disorders: First Results of a Medical Health Promotion Intervention in a Population of Employees." *European Psychiatry* 21 (7): 451–59.

Goel, S., N. Singh, V. Lal, and A. Singh. 2014. "Evaluating the Impact of Comprehensive Epilepsy Education Programme for School Teachers in Chandigarh City, India." *Seizure* 23 (1): 41–46.

Graveling, R. A., J. O. Crawford, H. Cowie, C. Amati, and S. Vohra. 2008. *A Review of Workplace Interventions That*

Promote Mental Wellbeing in the Workplace. Edinburgh: Institute of Occupational Medicine.

Grime, P. R. 2004. "Computerized Cognitive Behavioural Therapy at Work: A Randomized Controlled Trial in Employees with Recent Stress-Related Absenteeism." *Occupational Medicine* 54 (5): 353–59.

Gunnell, D., R. Fernando, M. Hewagama, W. D. Priyangika, F. Konradsen, and M. Eddleston. 2007. "The Impact of Pesticide Regulations on Suicide in Sri Lanka." *International Journal of Epidemiology* 36 (6): 1235–42.

Han, H.-R., S.-Y. Park, H. Song, M. Kim, K. B. Kim, and others. 2013. "Feasibility and Validity of Dementia Assessment by Trained Community Health Workers Based on Clinical Dementia Rating." *Journal of the American Geriatrics Society* 61 (7): 1141–45.

Hansson, L., and U. Markstrom. 2014. "The Effectiveness of an Anti-Stigma Intervention in a Basic Police Officer Training Programme: A Controlled Study." *BMC Psychiatry* 14: 55. doi:10.1186/1471-244X-14-55.

Henderson, C., E. Corker, E. Lewis-Holmes, S. Hamilton, C. Flach, and others. 2012. "England's Time to Change Antistigma Campaign: One-Year Outcomes of Service User-Rated Experiences of Discrimination." *Psychiatric Services* 63 (5): 451–57. doi:10.1176/appi.ps.201100422.

Hess, S. G., T. S. Cox, L. C. Gonzales, E. A. Kastelic, S. P. Mink, and others. 2004. "A Survey of Adolescents' Knowledge about Depression." *Archives of Psychiatric Nursing* 18 (6): 228–34.

Hill, D., D. Lucy, C. Tyers, and L. L James. 2007. *What Works at Work? Review of Evidence Assessing the Effectiveness of Workplace Interventions to Prevent and Manage Common Health Problems.* Leeds, U.K.: Health Work and Wellbeing Delivery Unit.

Jaycox, L. H., K. J. Reivich, J. Gillham, and M. E. P. Seligman. 1994. "Prevention of Depressive Symptoms in School Children." *Behaviour Research and Therapy* 32 (8): 801–16.

Jewkes, R., M. Nduna, J. Levin, N. Jama, K. Dunkle, and others. 2008. "Impact of Stepping Stones on Incidence of HIV and HSV-2 and Sexual Behaviour in Rural South Africa: Cluster Randomised Controlled Trial." *BMJ* 337: a506.

Jin, X., Y. Sun, F. Jiang, J. Ma, C. Morgan, and X. Shen. 2007. "'Care for Development' Intervention in Rural China: A Prospective Follow-Up Study." *Journal of Developmental and Behavioral Pediatrics* 28 (3): 213–18. doi:10.1097 /dbp.0b013e31802d410b.

Jordans, M. J. D., I. H. Komproe, W. A. Tol, B. A. Kohrt, N. P. Luitel, and others. 2010. "Evaluation of a Classroom-Based Psychosocial Intervention in Conflict-Affected Nepal: A Cluster Randomized Controlled Trial." *Journal of Child Psychology and Psychiatry* 51 (7): 818–26.

Jorm, A. F. 2012. "Mental Health Literacy: Empowering the Community to Take Action for Better Mental Health." *American Psychologist* 67 (3): 231–43. doi:10.1037 /a0025957.

Jorm, A. F., H. Christensen, and K. M. Griffiths. 2005. "The Impact of Beyondblue: The National Depression Initiative on the Australian Public's Recognition of Depression and Beliefs about Treatments." *Australian and New Zealand Journal of Psychiatry* 39 (4): 248–54. doi:10.1111/j.1440-1614.2005.01561.x.

Jorm, A. F., B. A. Kitchener, R. O'Kearney, and K. B. Dear. 2004. "Mental Health First Aid Training of the Public in a Rural Area: A Cluster Randomized Trial [Isrctn53887541]." *BMC Psychiatry* 4: 33. doi:10.1186/1471-244X-4-33.

Jorm, A. F., B. A. Kitchener, M. G. Sawyer, H. Scales, and S. Cvetkovski. 2010. "Mental Health First Aid Training for High School Teachers: A Cluster Randomized Trial." *BMC Psychiatry* 10: 51. doi:10.1186/1471-244X-10-51.

Kagitcibasi, C., D. Sunar, and S. Bekman. 2001. "Long-Term Effects of Early Intervention: Turkish Low-Income Mothers and Children." *Journal of Applied Developmental Psychology* 22 (4): 333–61.

Kagitcibasi, C., D. Sunar, S. Bekman, N. Baydar, and Z. Cemalcilar. 2009. "Continuing Effects of Early Enrichment in Adult Life: The Turkish Early Enrichment Project 22 Years Later." *Journal of Applied Developmental Psychology* 30 (6): 764–79.

Kaminski, J. W., L. A. Valle, J. H. Filene, and C. L. Boyle. 2008. "A Meta-Analytic Review of Components Associated with Parent Training Program Effectiveness." *Journal of Abnormal Child Psychology* 36 (4): 567–89. doi:10.1007 /s10802-007-9201-9.

Kennedy, C., and K. Jolivette. 2008. "The Effects of Positive Verbal Reinforcement on the Time Spent Outside the Classroom for Students with Emotional and Behavioral Disorders in a Residential Setting." *Behavioural Disorders* 33 (4): 211–21.

Kermode, M., H. Herrman, R. Arole, J. White, R. Premkumar, and V. Patel. 2007. "Empowerment of Women and Mental Health Promotion: A Qualitative Study in Rural Maharashtra, India." *BMC Public Health* 7 (1): 225.

Kessler, R. C., P. Berglund, O. Demler, R. Jin, K. R. Merikangas, and others. 2005. "Lifetime Prevalence and Age-of-Onset Distributions of DSM-IV Disorders in the National Comorbidity Survey Replication." *Archives of General Psychiatry* 62 (6): 593–602.

Khamis, V., R. Macy, and V. Coignez. 2004. "The Impact of the Classroom/Community/Camp-Based Intervention (CBI) Program on Palestinian Children." Save the Children USA West Bank/Gaza Field Office, Jerusalem.

Kim, J., G. Ferrari, T. Abramsky, C. Watts, J. Hargreaves, and others. 2009. "Assessing the Incremental Effects of Combining Economic and Health Interventions: The Image Study in South Africa." *Bulletin of the World Health Organization* 87 (11): 824–32.

Kitchener, B. A., and A. F. Jorm. 2004. "Mental Health First Aid Training in a Workplace Setting: A Randomized Controlled Trial." *BMC Psychiatry* 4: 23.

Krameddine, Y. I., D. DeMarco, H. Robert, and P. H. Silverstone. 2013. "A Novel Training Program for Police Officers That Improves Interactions with Mentally Ill Individuals and Is Cost-Effective." *Frontiers in Psychiatry* 4 (9): 1–10. doi:10.3389/fpsyt.2013.00009.

Kutcher, S., and Y. F. Wei. 2012. "Mental Health and the School Environment: Secondary Schools, Promotion and Pathways to Care." *Current Opinion in Psychiatry* 25 (4): 311–16.

Levin, C., and D. Chisholm. 2015. "Cost and Cost-Effectiveness of Interventions, Policies, and Platforms for the Prevention and Treatment of Mental, Neurological, and Substance Use Disorders." In *Disease Control Priorities* (third edition): Volume 4, *Mental, Neurological, and Substance Use Disorders*, edited by V. Patel, D. Chisholm, T. Dua, R. Laxminarayan, and M. E. Medina-Mora. Washington, DC: World Bank.

Lister-Sharp, D., S. Chapman, S. Stewart-Brown, and A. Sowden. 1999. "Health Promoting Schools and Health Promotion in Schools: Two Systematic Reviews." *Health Technology Assessment* 3 (22): 1–207.

Lund, C., M. De Silva, S. Plagerson, S. Cooper, D. Chisholm, and others. 2011. "Poverty and Mental Disorders: Breaking the Cycle in Low-Income and Middle-Income Countries." *The Lancet* 378 (9801): 1502–14.

McCabe, C. 2007. "A Systematic Review of Cost-Effectiveness Analyses of Whole School Interventions to Promote Children's Mental Health." Leeds Institute of Health Sciences, Leeds, U.K.

McCrone, P., M. Knapp, M. Henri, and D. McDaid. 2010. "The Economic Impact of Initiatives to Reduce Stigma: Demonstration of a Modelling Approach." *Epidemiologia e Psichiatria Sociale* 19 (2): 131–39.

McDaid, D. 2008. "Mental Health in Workplace Settings". Consensus Paper, European Communities, Luxembourg.

Medina, M. T., R. L. Aguilar Estrada, A. Alvarez, R. M. Durón, L. Martínez, and others. 2011. "Reduction in Rate of Epilepsy from Neurocysticercosis by Community Interventions: The Salama, Honduras Study." *Epilepsia* 52 (6): 1177–85.

Medina-Mora, M. E., M. Monteiro, R. Room, J. Rehm, D. Jernigan, D. Sánchez-Moreno, and T. Real. 2015. "Alcohol Use and Alcohol Use Disorders." In *Disease Control Priorities* (third edition): Volume 4, *Mental, Neurological, and Substance Use Disorders*, edited by V. Patel, D. Chisholm, T. Dua, R. Laxminarayan, and M. E. Medina-Mora. Washington, DC: World Bank.

Mejia, A., R. Calam, and M. R. Sanders. 2012. "A Review of Parenting Programs in Developing Countries: Opportunities and Challenges for Preventing Emotional and Behavioral Difficulties in Children." *Clinical Child and Family Psychology Review* 15 (2): 163–75. doi:10.1007/s10567-012-0116-9.

Mongini, F., A. Evangelista, C. Milani, L. Ferrero, G. Ciccone, and others. 2012. "An Educational and Physical Program to Reduce Headache, Neck/Shoulder Pain in a Working Community: A Cluster-Randomized Controlled Trial." *PloS One* 7 (1): e29637.

Mooney, P., M. H. Epstein, R. Reid, and J. R. Nelson. 2003. "Status of and Trends in Academic Intervention Research for Students with Emotional Disturbance." *Remedial and Special Education* 24 (5): 273–87.

Mueller, J., C. Alie, B. Jonas, E. Brown, and L. Sherr. 2011. "A Quasi-Experimental Evaluation of a Community-Based Art Therapy Intervention Exploring the Psychosocial Health of Children Affected by HIV in South Africa." *Tropical Medicine and International Health* 16 (1): 57–66.

Mychailyszyn, M. P., D. M. Brodman, K. L. Read, and P. C. Kendall. 2012. "Cognitive-Behavioral School-Based Interventions for Anxious and Depressed Youth: A Meta-Analysis of Outcomes." *Clinical Psychology Science and Practice* 52 (11): 1124–33.

Nelson, G., A. Westhues, and J. MacLeod. 2003. "A Meta-Analysis of Longitudinal Research on Preschool Prevention Programs for Children." *Prevention and Treatment* 6 (1).

NICE (National Institute for Health and Care Excellence). 2009. "Social and Emotional Wellbeing in Secondary Education." NICE Public Health Guidance 20, NICE, London.

Nigam, A, N. Reykar, M. Majumder, and D. Chisholm. 2015. "Self-Harm in India: Cost-Effectiveness Analysis of a Proposed Pesticide Ban." Disease Control Priorities Working Paper Series. No. 15. http://dcp-3.org/resources/self-harm-india-cost-effectiveness-analysis-proposed-pesticide-ban.

Ntsiea, M. V. 2013. "The Effect of a Workplace Intervention Programme on Return to Work after Stroke." Faculty of Health Sciences, University of the Witwatersrand, Johannesburg.

Nytro, K., P. O. Saksvik, A. Mikkelsen, P. Bohle, and M. Quinlan. 2000. "An Appraisal of Key Factors in the Implementation of Occupational Stress Interventions." *Work and Stress* 14 (3): 213–25.

Opoliner, A., D. Blacker, G. Fitzmaurice, and A. Becker. 2013. "Challenges in Assessing Depressive Symptoms in Fiji: A Psychometric Evaluation of the Ces-D." *International Journal of Social Psychiatry* 60 (4): 367–76. doi:10.1177/0020764013490871.

Oveisi, S., H. E. Ardabili, M. R. Dadds, R. Majdzadeh, P. Mohammadkhani, and others. 2010. "Primary Prevention of Parent-Child Conflict and Abuse in Iranian Mothers: A Randomized-Controlled Trial." *Child Abuse and Neglect* 34 (3): 206–13. doi:10.1016/j.chiabu.2009.05.008.

Page, M. J., L. C. Paramore, D. Doshi, and M. F. T. Rupnow. 2009. "Evaluation of Resource Utilization and Cost Burden before and after an Employer-Based Migraine Education Program." *Journal of Occupational and Environmental Medicine* 51 (2): 213–20.

Patel, V., C. Lund, S. Hatherill, S. Plagerson, J. Corrigall, M. Funk, and others. 2010. "Mental Disorders: Equity and Social Determinants." In *Equity, Social Determinants and Public Health Programmes*, edited by E. Blas and A. S. Kurup, 115–34. Geneva: World Health Organization.

Petersen, I., M. Barry, A. Bhana, and C. Lund. 2014. "Mental Health Promotion and Prevention of Mental Disorders." In *Global Mental Health*, edited by H. Minas, V. Patel, M. Cohen, and M. Prince, 245–75. London: Oxford University Press.

Pinfold, V., H. Toulmin, G. Thornicroft, P. Huxley, P. Farmer, and others. 2003. "Reducing Psychiatric Stigma and Discrimination: Evaluation of Educational Interventions in UK Secondary Schools." *British Journal of Psychiatry* 182 (4): 342–46.

Probst, T. M., D. Gold, and J. Caborn. 2008. "A Preliminary Evaluation of SOLVE: Addressing Psychosocial Problems at Work." *Journal of Occupational Health Psychology* 13 (1): 32–42. doi:10.1037/1076-8998.13.1.32.

Pronyk, P. M., J. R Hargreaves, J. C. Kim, L. A. Morison, G. Phetla, and others. 2006. "Effect of a Structural Intervention for the Prevention of Intimate-Partner Violence and HIV in Rural South Africa: A Cluster Randomised Trial." *The Lancet* 368 (9551): 1973–83.

Qouta, S. R., E. Palosaari, M. Diab, and R.-L. Punamäki. 2012. "Intervention Effectiveness among War-Affected Children: A Cluster Randomized Controlled Trial on Improving Mental Health." *Journal of Traumatic Stress* 25 (3): 288–98.

Rahman, A., Z. Iqbal, C. Roberts, and N. Husain. 2009. "Cluster Randomized Trial of a Parent-Based Intervention to Support Early Development of Children in a Low-Income Country." *Child: Care, Health and Development* 35 (1): 56–62. doi:10.1111/j.1365-2214.2008.00897.x.

Rahman, A., M. H. Mubbashar, R. Gater, and D. Goldberg. 1998. "Randomised Trial of Impact of School Mental-Health Programme in Rural Rawalpindi, Pakistan." *The Lancet* 352 (9133): 1022–25.

Rehm, J., D. Chisholm, R. Room, and A. Lopez. 2006. "Alcohol." In *Disease Control Priorities in Developing Countries*, 2nd ed., edited by D. T. Jamison, J. G. Breman, A. R. Measham, G. Alleyne, M. Claeson, D. B. Evans, P. Jha, A. Mills, and P. Musgrove, 887–906. Washington, DC: World Bank and Oxford University Press.

Rivera, M. O., S. Al-Otaiba, and M. A. Koorland. 2006. "Reading Instruction for Students with Emotional and Behavioral Disorders and at Risk of Antisocial Behaviors in Primary Grades: Review of Literature." *Behavioural Disorders* 31 (3): 323–37.

Rivet-Duval, E., S. Heriot, and C. Hunt. 2011. "Preventing Adolescent Depression in Mauritius: A Universal School-Based Program." *Child and Adolescent Mental Health* 16 (2): 86–91.

Rota, E., A. Evangelista, G. Ciccone, L. Ferrero, A. Ugolini, and others. 2011. "Effectiveness of an Educational and Physical Program in Reducing Accompanying Symptoms in Subjects with Head and Neck Pain: A Workplace Controlled Trial." *Journal of Headache and Pain* 12 (3): 339–45.

Saito, E., B. K. Nakamoto, M. F. Mendez, B. Mehta, and A. McMurtray. 2014. "Cost Effective Community Based Dementia Screening: A Markov Model Simulation." *International Journal of Alzheimer's Disease* 103138. doi:10.1155/2014/103138.

Sartorius, N. 2010. "Short-Lived Campaigns Are Not Enough." *Nature* 468 (7321): 163–65.

Schneider, W. J., A. P. Furth, T. H. Blalock, and T. A. Sherrill. 1999. "A Pilot Study of a Headache Program in the Workplace: The Effect of Education." *Journal of Occupational and Environmental Medicine* 41 (3): 202–09.

Schweinhart, L. J., J. Montie, Z. Xiang, W. S. Barnett, C. R. Belfield, and others. 2005. *Lifetime Effects: The High/Scope Perry Preschool Study through Age 40*. Ypsilanti, MI: HighScope Press.

Scott, J. G., C. Mihalopoulos, H. E. Erskine, J. Roberts, and A. Rahman. 2015. "Child Developmental and Mental Disorders." In *Disease Control Priorities* (third edition): Volume 4, *Mental, Neurological, and Substance Use Disorders*, edited by V. Patel, D. Chisholm, T. Dua, R. Laxminarayan, and M. E. Medina-Mora. Washington, DC: World Bank.

Seymour, L. 2010. *Common Mental Health Problems at Work: What We Now Know about Successful Interventions. A Progress Review*. London: Sainsburys Centre for Mental Health.

Shidhaye, R., C. Lund, and D. Chisholm. 2015. "Health Care Delivery Platforms." In *Disease Control Priorities* (third edition): Volume 4, *Mental, Neurological, and Substance Use Disorders*, edited by V. Patel, D. Chisholm, T. Dua, R. Laxminarayan, and M. E. Medina-Mora. Washington, DC: World Bank.

Shucksmith, J., C. Summerbell, S. Jones, and V. Whittaker. 2007. "Mental Wellbeing of Children in Primary Education (Targeted/Indicated Activities)." Report, University of Teesside, Middlesbrough, U.K.

Simpson, R. L., R. L. Peterson, and C. R. Smith. 2011. "Critical Educational Program Components for Students with Emotional and Behavioral Disorders: Science, Policy, and Practice." *Remedial and Special Education* 32 (3): 230–42.

Sjögren, T., K. J. Nissinen, S. K. Järvenpää, M. T. Ojanen, H. Vanharanta, and others. 2005. "Effects of a Workplace Physical Exercise Intervention on the Intensity of Headache and Neck and Shoulder Symptoms and Upper Extremity Muscular Strength of Office Workers: A Cluster Randomized Controlled Cross-over Trial." *Pain* 116 (1): 119–28.

Skeen, S., S. Kleintjes, C. Lund, I. Petersen, A. Bhana, and others. 2010. "Mental Health Is Everybody's Business': Roles for an Intersectoral Approach in South Africa." *International Review of Psychiatry* 22 (6): 611–23.

Smith, E. A., L.-A. Palen, L. L. Caldwell, A. J. Flisher, J. W. Graham, and others. 2008. "Substance Use and Sexual Risk Prevention in Cape Town, South Africa: An Evaluation of the HealthWise Program." *Prevention Science* 9 (4): 311–21.

Srikala, B., and K. V. Kishore. 2010. "Empowering Adolescents with Life Skills Education in Schools—School Mental Health Program: Does It Work?" *Indian Journal of Psychiatry* 52 (4): 344.

Ssewamala, F. M., C. K. Han, and T. B. Neilands. 2009. "Asset Ownership and Health and Mental Health Functioning among AIDS-Orphaned Adolescents: Findings from a Randomized Clinical Trial in Rural Uganda." *Social Science and Medicine* 69 (2): 191–98. doi:10.1016/j.socscimed.2009.05.019.

Stewart, R., C. van Rooyen, K. Dickson, M. Majoro, and Thea de Wet. 2010. "What Is the Impact of Microfinance on Poor People? A Systematic Review of Evidence from Sub-Saharan Africa." Evidence for Policy and Practice, Information and Co-ordinating Centre, Social Science Research Unit, Institute of Education, University of London.

Stuart, H. 2008. "Fighting the Stigma Caused by Mental Disorders: Past Perspectives, Present Activities, and Future Directions." *World Psychiatry* 7 (3): 185–88.

Swartz, K. L., E. A. Kastelic, S. G. Hess, T. S. Cox, L. C. Gonzales, and others. 2010. "The Effectiveness of a School-Based Adolescent Depression Education Program." *Health Education and Behavior* 37 (1): 11–22.

Tansella, M., and G. Thornicroft. 2009. "Implementation Science: Understanding the Translation of Evidence into Practice." *British Journal of Psychiatry* 195 (4): 283–85. doi:10.1192/bjp.bp.109.065565.

Teller, J. L., M. R. Munetz, K. M. Gil, and C. Ritter. 2006. "Crisis Intervention Team Training for Police Officers Responding to Mental Disturbance Calls." *Psychiatric Services* 57 (2): 232–73. doi:10.1176/appi.ps.57.2.232.

Tennant, R., C. Goens, J. Barlow, C. Day, and S. Stewart-Brown. 2007. "A Systematic Review of Reviews of Interventions to Promote Mental Health and Prevent Mental Health Problems in Children and Young People." *Journal of Public Mental Health* 6 (1): 25–32.

Thakur, K. T., E. Albanese, P. Giannakopoulos, N. Jette, M. Linde, M. J. Prince, T. J. Steiner, and T. Dua. 2015. "Neurological Disorders." In *Disease Control Priorities* (third edition): Volume 4, *Mental, Neurological, and Substance Use Disorders*, edited by V. Patel, D. Chisholm, T. Dua, R. Laxminarayan, and M. E. Medina-Mora. Washington, DC: World Bank.

Thornicroft, C., A. Wyllie, G. Thornicroft, and N. Mehta. 2014. "Impact of the 'Like Minds, Like Mine' Anti-Stigma and Discrimination Campaign in New Zealand on Anticipated and Experienced Discrimination." *Australian and New Zealand Journal of Psychiatry* 48 (4): 360–70. doi:10.1177/0004867413512687.

Thornicroft, G. 2000. "National Service Framework for Mental Health." *Psychiatric Bulletin* 24 (6): 203–06.

Thornicroft, G., A. Alem, R. A. Santos, E. Barley, R. E. Drake, and others. 2010. "WPA Guidance on Steps, Obstacles and Mistakes to Avoid in the Implementation of Community Mental Health Care." *World Psychiatry* 9 (2): 67–77.

Thornicroft, G., N. Mehta, S. Clement, S. Evans-Lacko, M. Doherty, and others. 2015. "Evidence for Effective Interventions to Reduce Mental Health Related Stigma and Discrimination: Narrative Review." *The Lancet* pii:S0140-6736(15)00298-6. doi:10.1016/S0140-6736(15)00298-6.

Tol, W. A., I. H. Komproe, M. J. D. Jordans, A. Ndayisaba, P. Ntamutumba, and others. 2014. "School-Based Mental Health Intervention for Children in War-Affected Burundi: A Cluster Randomized Trial." *BMC Medicine* 12 (1): 56.

Tol, W. A., I. H. Komproe, M. J. D. Jordans, A. Vallipuram, H. Sipsma, and others. 2012. "Outcomes and Moderators of a Preventive School-Based Mental Health Intervention for Children Affected by War in Sri Lanka: A Cluster Randomized Trial." *World Psychiatry* 11 (2): 114–22.

Tol, W. A., I. H. Komproe, D. Susanty, M. J. D. Jordans, R. D. Macy, and others. 2008. "School-Based Mental Health Intervention for Children Affected by Political Violence in Indonesia: A Cluster Randomized Trial." *Journal of the American Medical Association* 300 (6): 655–62.

van der Feltz-Cornelis, C. M., M. Sarchiapone, V. Postuvan, D. Volker, S. Roskar, and others. 2011. "Best Practice Elements of Multilevel Suicide Prevention Strategies: A Review of Systematic Reviews." *Crisis* 32 (6): 319–33. doi:10.1027/0227-5910/a000109.

van der Klink, J. J., R. W. Blonk, A. H. Schene, and F. J. van Dijk. 2001. "The Benefits of Interventions for Work-Related Stress." *American Journal of Public Health* 91 (2): 270–76.

Vasquez, M., L. Meza, O. Almandarez, A. Santos, R. C. Matute, and others. 2010. "Evaluation of a Strengthening Families (Familias Fuertes) Intervention for Parents and Adolescents in Honduras." *Southern Online Journal of Nursing Research* 10 (3): 1–25.

Vieira, M. A., A. A. Gadelha, T. S. Moriyama, R. A. Bressan, and I. A. Bordin. 2014. "Evaluating the Effectiveness of a Training Program That Builds Teachers' Capability to Identify and Appropriately Refer Middle and High School Students with Mental Health Problems in Brazil: An Exploratory Study." *BMC Public Health* 14 (1): 210. doi:10.1186/1471-2458-14-210.

Walker, S., and S. M. Chang. 2013. "Effectiveness of Parent Support Programmes in Enhancing Learning in the Under-3 Age Group." *Early Childhood Matters* 120: 45–49.

Warner, R. 2005. "Local Projects of the World Psychiatric Association Programme to Reduce Stigma and Discrimination." *Psychiatric Services* 56 (5): 570–75.

Watson, A. C., M. S. Morabito, J. Draine, and V. Ottati. 2008. "Improving Police Response to Persons with Mental Illness: A Multi-Level Conceptualization of CIT." *International Journal of Law and Psychiatry* 31 (4): 359–68. doi:10.1016/j.ijlp.2008.06.004.

Watson, A. C., E. Otey, A. L. Westbrook, A. L. Gardner, T. A. Lamb, and others. 2004. "Changing Middle Schoolers' Attitudes about Mental Illness through Education." *Schizophrenia Bulletin* 30 (3): 563–72.

Weare, K., and M. Nind. 2011. "Mental Health Promotion and Problem Prevention in Schools: What Does the Evidence Say?" *Health Promotion International* 26 (Suppl. 1): i29–69. doi:10.1093/heapro/dar075.

Wells, J., J. Barlow, and S. Stewart-Brown. 2003. "A Systematic Review of Universal Approaches to Mental Health Promotion in Schools." *Health Education* 103 (4): 197–220.

Wendland-Carro, J., C. A. Piccinini, and W. S. Millar. 1999. "The Role of an Early Intervention on Enhancing the Quality of Mother-Infant Interaction." *Child Development* 70 (3): 713–21.

Williams, O., A. DeSorbo, J. Noble, M. Shaffer, and W. Gerin. 2012. "Long-Term Learning of Stroke Knowledge among Children in a High-Risk Community." *Neurology* 79 (8): 802–06.

WHO (World Health Organization). 2000. *Mental Health and Work: Impact, Issues and Good Practices.* Geneva: WHO.

———. 2008. *mhGAP: Mental Health Gap Action Programme: Scaling up Care for Mental, Neurological and Substance Use Disorders.* Geneva: WHO.

———. 2011a. *Scaling Up Action against Noncommunicable Diseases: How Much Will It Cost?* Geneva: WHO.

———. 2011b. *WHO Handbook for Guideline Development.* Geneva: WHO.

———. 2012. *WHO QualityRights Toolkit to Assess and Improve Quality and Human Rights in Mental Health and Social Care Facilities.* Geneva: WHO. http://apps.WHO.int/iris/bitstream/10665/70927/3/9789241548410_eng.Pdf.

———. 2013a. *Suicide Prevention (SUPRE).* Geneva: WHO.

———. 2013b. *Mental Health Action Plan 2013–2020.* Geneva: WHO.

———. 2014. *Preventing Suicide: A Global Imperative.* Geneva: WHO.

Yang, L., A. Kleinman, B. G. Link, J. Phelan, S. Lee, and others. 2007. "Culture and Stigma: Adding Moral Experience to Stigma Theory." *Social Science and Medicine* 64: 1521–35.

Chapter 11

Health Care Platform Interventions

Rahul Shidhaye, Crick Lund, and Dan Chisholm

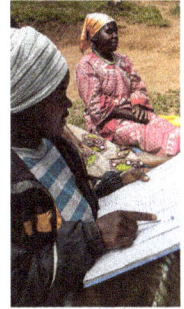

INTRODUCTION

Evidence-based interventions often fail to achieve their goal, not so much because of an inherent flaw in the interventions, but because of the unpredictable behavior of the system around them. Every intervention, from the simplest to the most complex, has an effect on the overall system, and the overall system has an effect on every intervention (Savigny and Adam 2009). As a result of this, the current *Disease Control Priorities* series has shifted its focus from a strictly disorder-oriented intervention analysis (vertical approach) to a more horizontal approach focusing on health system strengthening.

This chapter seeks to identify cost-effective interventions that can be appropriately packaged for one or more specific mental, neurological, and substance use (MNS) disorders, as well as for different levels or platforms of the health or welfare system. A platform is the level of the health or welfare system at which interventions can be appropriately, effectively, and efficiently delivered. A particular platform is defined on the basis of *where* the intervention will be delivered (the setting) and *who* will deliver the intervention (service provider). There are essentially three major platforms for the provision of interventions: population, community, and health care. A specific delivery channel—such as a school—can be the vehicle for the delivery of a particular intervention on a specified platform (the community platform). Similarly, a primary health care center is the delivery channel for a specified platform (the health

care platform). Identifying the set of interventions that fall within a particular delivery channel will help decision makers to identify potential opportunities, synergies, and efficiencies. This identification will also reflect how resources are often allocated in practice, for example, to schools or primary health care services, rather than to specific interventions or disorders.

Chapter 10 of this volume (Petersen and others 2015) considers the evidence relating to interventions that improve mental health at the population and community levels. This chapter outlines the main elements and features of a health care platform and its delivery channels, namely, informal health care, primary health care, and specialized services. We consider evidence-based interventions that can be delivered in general health care settings and mental health care settings, as well as broader health system–strengthening strategies for more effective and efficient delivery of services on this platform.

ELEMENTS OF A MENTAL HEALTH CARE DELIVERY PLATFORM

Health care services as a delivery platform for improving population mental health consist of three interlinked service delivery channels:

- Self-care and informal health care
- Primary health care
- Specialist health care.

Corresponding author: Rahul Shidhaye, Centre for Chronic Conditions and Injuries, Public Health Foundation of India, rahul.shidhaye@phfi.org.

These three key delivery channels map well onto the commonly cited *Service Organization Pyramid for an Optimal Mix of Services for Mental Health* supported by the World Health Organization (WHO) (figure 11.1) (WHO 2003a). At each subsequent level of the pyramid, the mental health needs of individuals become greater and require more intensive professional assistance, usually resulting in higher costs of care. In certain settings beset with conflict, natural disaster, or other emergencies, a further channel for delivering much-needed mental health care is humanitarian aid and emergency response.

Self-Care and Informal Health Care

The foundation of the health care delivery platform rests on self-care and emphasizes health worker–patient partnerships. Persons with MNS disorders and their family and friends play a central role in the management of mental health problems. The role of individuals may range from collaborative decision-making concerning their treatment, to actively adhering to prescribed medication, to changing health-related behaviors, such as drug and alcohol use, stress management, and identification of seizure triggers and avoiding them for seizure control.

Self-care is important for MNS disorders, but it is also important for the prevention and treatment of physical health problems (WHO 2003a). Self-care is most effective when it is supported by populationwide health promotion programs and formal

Figure 11.1 World Health Organization Service Organization Pyramid for an Optimal Mix of Services for Mental Health

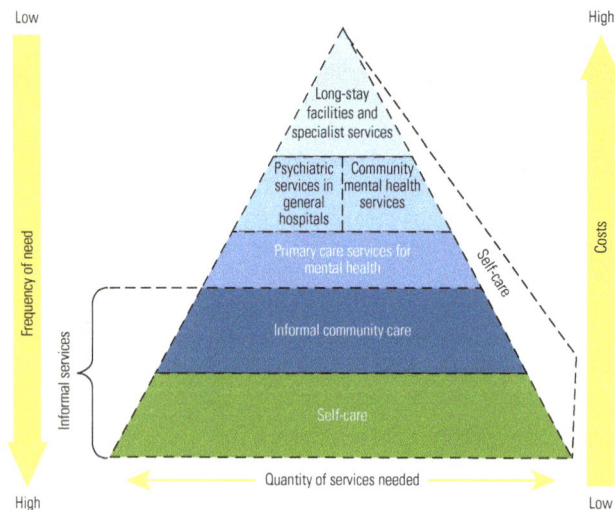

Source: Reprinted from *Mental Health Policy and Service Guidance Package*, World Health Organization (WHO), "Organization of Services for Mental health," page 34, WHO 2003a. Reprinted with permission.

health care services. Health promotion interventions delivered at the population level can be important in improving mental health literacy by helping people to recognize problems or illnesses, increasing their knowledge about the causes of disorders and options for treatment, and informing them about where to go to get help (see chapter 10 in this volume, Petersen and others 2015).

Informal health care comprises service providers who are not part of the formal health care system, such as traditional healers, village elders, faith-based organizations, peers, user and family associations, and lay people (WHO 2003a). Traditional and religious healers are of particular significance, as populations throughout East Asia and Pacific, South Asia, Latin America and the Caribbean, and Sub-Saharan Africa often use traditional medicine to meet their health needs (WHO 2002). In many parts of the world, making contact with such informal providers represents the initial pathway to care (Bekele and others 2009); these service providers are typically very accessible and more acceptable because they are integral members of the local community. Given the widespread presence of traditional and religious healers and the shortage of human resources in mainstream biomedical services, it is imperative that primary health and other formal care services establish strong links with informal health care providers, especially traditional healers (Patel 2011). It is also critical to note that the evidence base regarding the effectiveness of services provided by traditional and religious healers is limited. Nevertheless, it is essential to engage with them, as they provide accessible, acceptable, and affordable care, and efforts need to be made to ensure that their practices do not harm the patients.

Peers are another key human resource at this level of health care. Peer-led education and behavioral interventions have been effective with target populations and health issues in low- and middle-income countries (LMICs) (Manandhar and others 2004; Medley and others 2009; Tripathy and others 2010). Peers are more numerous, may be perceived as more approachable, and may be able to identify with other community members, as they share similar characteristics, experiences, and health conditions with members of the target population (Simoni and others 2011).

Mental health self-help groups form another key component of informal community care. Mental health self-help groups may be defined as "any mutual support oriented initiative directed by people with [MNS disorders] or their family members" (Brown and others 2008, 105). Participation in mental health self-help groups has a positive impact on the clinical and social outcomes of patients with MNS disorders (Pistrang, Barker, and Humphreys 2008). Some of these self-help groups are primarily concerned with the provision of peer support, while others may devote their efforts toward changing public policies and, more broadly, changing public attitudes. Still others may focus on self-empowerment, including monitoring and critiquing the mental health services they are receiving (Cohen and others 2012). Social support also plays an important role in self-management of epilepsy (Jayalakshmi and others 2014; Walker and others 2014). However, informal community care should not be viewed as a substitute for publicly funded, evidence-based mental health care.

Stigmatization of and discrimination against people with MNS disorders is common in all sections of society, from community to schools, workplace, and even health care settings. Stigma and discrimination present formidable barriers to social inclusion for affected people and their families, and to access to appropriate health care (Shidhaye and Kermode 2013). This is particularly important in the area of self-care and informal care services, which are relatively less regulated and less subject to quality review or policy oversight. Interventions at the community level to address negative attitudes toward people with MNS disorders and improve health care utilization are covered in chapter 10 in this volume (Petersen and others 2015).

Primary Health Care

Delivery of mental health services through primary health care is a fundamental component of a mental health care delivery platform, since it serves as the first level of care within the formal health care system. The strong emphasis on primary health care is due to the fact that the services provided at this level of the health system are generally accessible, affordable, and acceptable for individuals, families, and communities (WHO 2003a). Where the provision of mental health care is integrated into these services, access is improved, MNS disorders are more likely to be identified and treated, and comorbid physical and mental health problems can be managed more seamlessly.

Specialist Health Care

Psychiatric Services in First-Level Hospitals and Community Mental Health Services

People with severe MNS disorders may require hospitalization at some point. First-level hospitals provide an accessible and acceptable location for 24-hour medical care for people with acute worsening of disorders, in the same way that these facilities manage acute exacerbations of physical health conditions (WHO 2003a).

The mental health services provided in first-level hospitals also enable 24-hour access to services for any physical health problems that might arise during the course of inpatient stays. Ideally, first-level hospitals will have wards dedicated to the treatment of MNS disorders; these wards will have floor plans that support good observation and care, minimizing the risk of neglect and suicide. To minimize the risk of human rights violations, facilities should adhere to clear policies and guidelines that support the treatment and management of MNS disorders within a framework that promotes human dignity and uses evidence-based clinical practice.

In addition, specialist mental health services are needed in the community for severe cases that cannot be managed by generalists. Examples include assertive community treatment teams and community outreach teams, which provide support to service users to enable them to continue to function in the community without requiring admission, and close liaison with general primary care services and other social and criminal justice services (WHO 2003a).

Extended-Stay Facilities and Specialist Psychiatric Services

A small minority of people with MNS disorders requires specialist care (WHO 2003a). For example, people with treatment-resistant or complex presentations may need to be referred to specialized centers for further testing and treatment. In LMICs with meager resources, the demand of the population and the emphasis of the public health system is to treat persons with severe MNS disorders. These aspects of care provision along with services for vulnerable populations—such as individuals living in abject poverty; women, especially in childbearing age; children facing abuse; and elderly persons—should not be overlooked when designing programs.

Because of their severe mental disorders or intellectual disabilities and lack of family support, many of these individuals may occasionally require ongoing care in community-based residential facilities. Unfortunately, very scarce resources are allocated to these services. The vulnerable populations require particular attention, from a mental health care perspective and a financial risk protection perspective. The final part of this volume addresses the issue of financial risk protection at length. Forensic psychiatry is another type of specialist service in this category. The need for referral to specialist and extended-stay services is reduced when first-level hospitals are staffed with highly specialized health workers, such as psychiatrists and psychologists.

Emergency Mental Health Care

The traumas, personal losses, and other consequences of armed conflict and disasters place affected populations at an increased risk of mental and behavioral problems; these consequences can overwhelm the local capacity to respond, particularly if the existing infrastructure or health system is already weak. Moreover, the local health care system may have been rendered dysfunctional as a result of the emergency situation, placing further limits on access to key resources, such as mental health professionals or essential psychotropic medicines. There is a heightened need to identify and allocate resources to provide mental health and psychosocial support in these humanitarian settings, for those with mental or behavioral problems induced by emergencies and those with preexisting illness. International humanitarian aid and emergency response at the national level can be a channel for rapidly enabling or supporting the availability of and access to basic or specialist care. In many countries, such emergencies have provided opportunities for systemic change or service reform in public mental health (WHO 2013a). Emergency response or relief efforts are essentially concerned with setting up, organizing, and rebuilding services for local populations; the central principles and standard practice of care, including what evidence-based interventions should be prioritized, remain unchanged.

Relationships among Different Delivery Channels

No single service delivery channel can meet all mental health needs. For example, on the one hand, primary mental health care must be complemented by specialist care services that primary health workers can use for referrals, support, and supervision; on the other hand, primary mental health care needs to promote and support self-care and informal community care that encourages the involvement of people in their own recovery. Support of self-care and management can be provided via routine primary care visits or via group sessions led by health or lay workers in health care settings or community venues. Another increasingly accessible option for the effective support of self-care and management is telephone- or Internet-based programs. In short, the potential of the health care system as a delivery platform for enhanced mental health and well-being can only be fully realized if genuine continuity and collaboration of care occur across the three service delivery channels; continuity and collaboration, in turn, rely on an appropriate flow of support, supervision, information-sharing, and education.

EVIDENCE-BASED INTERVENTIONS FOR HEALTH CARE DELIVERY PLATFORMS

A strong evidence base supports integrated services across the different delivery channels of the health care platform. This evidence has been synthesized in several publications, including the *mhGAP Intervention Guide* (WHO 2010b); a series of papers on packages of care for MNS disorders in LMICs, published in *PLoS Medicine* (Patel and Thornicroft 2009); and a report on mental health in primary health care (WHO and WONCA 2008). Earlier disagreement and controversy over emergency mental health care has given way to emerging consensus on key social and mental health intervention strategies and principles, as exemplified by the Inter-Agency Standing Committee's *Guidelines on Mental Health and Psychosocial Support in Emergency Settings* (IASC 2007); the inclusion of a mental and social aspects of health standard in the handbook on minimal standards in disaster response (Sphere 2011); and the report on sustainable mental health care after emergencies, *Building Back Better* (WHO 2013a).

For each of the delivery channels, interventions may be categorized as follows:

- Promotion and primary prevention
- Identification and case detection
- Treatment, care, and rehabilitation.

Table 11.1 summarizes the evidence base for interventions by various delivery channels. The interventions are intended as examples rather than as recommendations.

SYSTEM-STRENGTHENING STRATEGIES FOR INTEGRATED HEALTH CARE DELIVERY

The availability of evidence-based interventions does not ensure their translation into practice. In this section, we address the question of how to integrate evidence-based mental health care interventions into primary care and self-care delivery channels and how to link this integration to specialist care.

A comprehensive and multifaceted approach that contains the following elements is essential for the successful integration of mental health into health care systems:

- A *whole-of-government approach* involves the promotion, pursuit, and protection of health through concerted action by many sectors of government.

Table 11.1 Examples of Evidence-Based Interventions Relating to the Mental Health Care Delivery Platform, by Various Delivery Channels

Delivery channel	Promotion and primary prevention	Identification and case detection	Treatment, care, and rehabilitation
Self-care and informal health care	• Adoption of a healthy lifestyle, including diet and physical activity • Self-monitoring of high-risk behaviors, such as substance abuse	• Self-detection of depression and anxiety disorders	• Web-based psychological therapy for depression and anxiety disorders • Self-managed treatment of migraine • Self-identification and management of seizure triggers • Improved adherence to anti-epileptic treatment by intensive reminders and implementation intention interventions
Primary health care	• Parent skills training for internalizing and externalizing problems in child and parental mental health	• Screening for developmental delays in children • Screening and brief interventions for alcohol use disorders by trained primary health care staff • Community-based case-finding of psychosis and severe depression • Diagnosis of depression, anxiety disorders, maternal depression, alcohol use disorders, dementia, headaches, and epilepsy	• Management—pharmacological and psychosocial interventions—of depression, anxiety, psychosis, alcohol use disorders, epilepsy, dementia, and drug use based on mhGAP Intervention Guidelines • Cognitive behavioral therapy–based interventions for anxiety disorders in children • Cognitive behavioral therapy–based interventions for depression and anxiety disorders in adults and mothers in the perinatal period • Management of alcohol withdrawal in conjunction with motivational interviewing and motivation enhancement involving family and friends • Interventions for caregivers of patients with psychosis and dementia
Specialist health care		• Diagnosis of complex childhood mental disorders • Diagnosis of severe psychosis and depression • Diagnosis of secondary causes of headache	• Electroconvulsive therapy for severe refractory depression • Surgical interventions for refractory epilepsy • Pharmacological management of dementia (cholinesterase inhibitors and memantine) • Methadone maintenance therapy for opioid dependence, buprenorphine as opioid substitution therapy • Management of refractory psychosis using clozapine • Management of severe alcohol withdrawal • Management of severe maternal depression using antidepressants • Stimulant medication for severe cases of attention-deficit hyperactivity disorder • Cognitive behavioral therapy–based interventions and anger control training for adolescents with disruptive behavioral disorders

Note: The list of evidence-based interventions in the table is for illustration. mhGAP = Mental Health Gap Action Programme (WHO 2010b).

These include ministries of planning and development, finance, law and justice, labor, education, and social welfare. The health system cannot tackle the health, social, and economic determinants and consequences of MNS disorders alone.

- A **public health approach** stresses the establishment of partnerships between patients and service providers, as well as equitable access for the whole population (Lund and others 2012). This approach requires the integration of care at the patient level. Services should be person centered and coordinated across diseases and settings. Collaborative, coordinated, and continuing care, within a framework of evidence-based interventions, provides the foundation of the public health approach. This means providing good quality, accessible services to those in need, as well as preventing the onset of disease and promoting mental health and well-being over the entire life course (WHO 2010a). Priority setting and provision of interventions based on the needs of the population under consideration are also an integral part of the public health approach, which is also central to the work undertaken by the Disease Control Priorities Network.

Table 11.2 summarizes the key features of a public mental health approach.

- A **systems approach** to integrated service planning and development encompasses the critical ingredients of a health system—good governance, appropriate resourcing, timely information, and the actual delivery of health services or technologies—that need to be in place for desired health outcomes or program goals to be realized. Effective governance, strong leadership, and cogent policy making merit particular mention, since they provide the framework for appropriate action and subsequent service development. Indeed, a well-articulated mental health policy, along with a clear mental health implementation plan and budget, can be a strong driver for change and can appreciably

boost efforts to deliver mental health services at the primary care level (WHO and WONCA 2008).

How to operationalize the public health, whole-of-government, and systems approaches to integrate service delivery for MNS disorders is a major challenge. In South Africa, some important steps have been taken toward intersectoral collaboration, particularly at the national level, such as a national forum on forensic psychiatry convened by the Department of Health, with the South African Police Service (SAPS), the Department of Justice, and the Department of Correctional Services. The Departments of Education and Correctional Services have developed policies regarding mental health, and SAPS has developed a standing order that sets out roles and responsibilities for police in relation to mental health. At the provincial level, there are formal collaborations between the government department responsible for mental health and other departments and agencies in most provinces across a range of sectors. Some provinces have also established intersectoral forums for mental health, and intersectoral collaboration is a standing item on the agenda of the quarterly meetings of the provincial mental health coordinators. However, at the district level, such intersectoral collaboration is not common. A policy brief prepared by the Mental Health and Poverty Project provides specific recommendations for shared responsibilities in policy and program development among sectors, such as education, social development, housing, justice and constitutional development, correctional services, labor, local government, public works, and mental health (MHaPP 2008).

Many evidence-based interventions fail to translate into practice because key decision makers, especially in LMICs, are merely seen as targets for dissemination of study results by academicians and researchers. To address this challenge, it is imperative to understand that research should be concerned with the users of the research and not purely the production of knowledge. The users may include managers and teams using

Table 11.2 Key Characteristics of a Public Health Approach to MNS Disorder Prevention and Management

Prevention essentials	Management essentials
Promotion of healthy behaviors	Person-centered care and support
Prevention of exposure to adverse events and risks	Family and community support
Early detection	Coordinated, holistic care
Intersectoral collaboration	Continuity of care and proactive follow-up
Life course approach	

Source: WHO and Calouste Gulbenkian Foundation 2014.
Note: MNS = mental, neurological, and substance use.

research findings, executive decision makers seeking advice for specific decisions, policy makers who need to be informed about particular programs, practitioners who need to be convinced to use interventions that are based on evidence, people who are influenced to change their behavior to have a healthier life, or communities that are conducting the research and taking action through the research to improve their conditions. It is critical to involve these actors in the identification, design, and conduct phases of research and program implementation (Peters and others 2013).

Within the three broad approaches, specific strategies can be identified for integrated health care delivery.

Strategy 1: Improving the Organization and Delivery of Services through Collaborative Stepped Care

Collaborative care is an evidence-based approach to improve the management of MNS disorders at the primary care level. The overall aim of collaborative care is to enhance the quality of care and quality of life, consumer satisfaction, and system efficiency for patients with complex, long-term problems (Kodner and Spreeuwenberg 2002). Collaborative care has been used successfully for the management of common mental disorders, such as depression, as well as for comorbidities cutting across multiple services, providers, and settings (Katon and others 2010). Collaborative care is closely related to a stepped care approach; some programs describe themselves as *collaborative stepped care*, in that they incorporate aspects of each approach within their interventions (Patel and others 2010). In the stepped care approach, patients typically start treatment with low-intensity, low-cost interventions. Treatment results are monitored systematically, and patients move to a higher-intensity treatment only if necessary. Programs seek to maximize efficiency by deploying available human resources according to need, reserving the most specialized and intensive resources for those with the most complex or severe problems.

The essential element of collaborative care is a multidisciplinary team approach that seeks to integrate primary care professionals and specialists. Collaborative care rests primarily on the presence of a case manager with enhanced responsibilities for integration of care across comorbid conditions. It starts with systematic identification of those in need, followed by close involvement of patients in joint decision-making regarding their care. It continues with the design of a holistic care plan that includes medication management and psychological interventions and, where appropriate, social care, with a streamlined referral pathway that allows patients to move easily from one service to another.

There is provision for regular and planned monitoring of patients and systematic caseload reviews and consultation with mental health specialists regarding patients who do not show clinical improvement (WHO and Calouste Gulbenkian Foundation 2014).

Collaborative care is the best-evaluated model for treating common mental disorders in primary care. A recent Cochrane Collaboration review of 79 randomized controlled trials concluded that collaborative care for depression is consistently more effective than usual care; it has also been shown to be effective in a range of MNS disorders—anxiety disorders and post-traumatic stress disorder—and for improving general health outcomes. The evidence base for collaborative care is mostly from high-income countries (HICs), although evidence from LMICs is growing (Archer and others 2012). It might be very difficult to replicate these case studies directly in low-income settings, but it is possible to extract the lessons from these experiences and contextualize them for a particular setting. There is absolutely no one-size-fits-all strategy for the heterogeneous settings across and within the countries. It is critical to test rigorously and generate evidence around the contextualization of these strategies in low-resource settings. The Balanced Care Model provides guidelines for the inclusion of program components that are appropriate for the available resources (Thornicroft and Tansella 2013).

Mental health programs can be designed on the basis of these guiding principles, drawing on the following case studies.

- The MANAS (MANashanti Sudhar Shodh, or project to promote mental health) study in Goa, India, is the largest mental health care trial to date in that country. The study showed that a lay counselor–led collaborative stepped care intervention for depression and anxiety disorders in primary health care settings led to substantial reductions in the prevalence of these disorders, suicidal behaviors, and days of work lost, compared with usual care. The trial also evaluated the economic impact of the intervention and found that the overall health system costs were lower in the intervention arm, despite the intervention costs, because patients recovered sooner and had lower overall health care costs (Patel and others 2010).
- The Home Care Program for elderly people affected by dementia, led by the Dementia Society of Goa, evaluated a community-based collaborative care model led by lay counselors. The model showed benefits in reducing caregiver burden and improving caregiver mental health (Dias and others 2008).
- In Chile, a multicomponent intervention lasting three months and comprising nine weekly sessions

of psychoeducational groups, structured and systematic follow-up, and pharmacotherapy for women with severe depression, and led by nonmedical health workers, demonstrated that at the six-month follow-up, 70 percent of the stepped care group had recovered, compared with 30 percent in the usual-care group (Araya and others 2003). The program is being rolled out across Chile. A similar program was subsequently tested among low-income mothers in postnatal primary care clinics in Santiago, Chile. The program demonstrated significant improvement in the intervention group (Rojas and others 2007).

- In Ibadan, Nigeria, a pilot study evaluated the usefulness of a stepped care intervention for depression. The intervention was delivered by non-physician primary health workers, with support and supervision by physicians and psychiatrists, as needed, using mobile phones. The intervention was based on WHO's mhGAP guidelines, adapted for the Nigerian health system. Recovery at follow-up, defined as no longer meeting the *Diagnostic and Statistical Manual of Mental Disorders: DSM-IV-TR*, 4th edition (APA 2000), major depression criteria at six months, was achieved by 73.0 percent of the participants in the intervention group and 51.6 percent in the usual-care group, representing a risk difference of 21.4 percent. A fully powered study is being implemented to determine the effectiveness and cost-effectiveness of the package (WHO and Calouste Gulbenkian Foundation 2014).

- The Headache Management Trial assessed the effect of a coordinated headache management program in general clinical practice. Patients in the intervention arm received a headache management program consisting of a class specifically designed to inform them about headache types, triggers, and treatment options; diagnosis and treatment by a professional specially trained in headache care; and proactive follow-up by a case manager. This trial demonstrated that a systematic approach to headache care is practical and achievable in a general clinical setting and effectively reduced headache disability in a wide range of patients (Matchar and others 2008).

These case studies primarily focused on evidence generation and were conducted in controlled settings. There are also several case studies from LMICs.

- In the city of Sobral, Brazil, primary care practitioners conducted physical and mental health assessments for all patients as part of integrated primary care for mental health. Primary care practitioners treat patients if they are able, or request an assessment from a specialist mental health team, which makes regular visits to family health centers. Joint consultations are undertaken among mental health specialists, primary care practitioners, and patients. This model ensures good-quality mental health care, and it serves as a training and supervision tool whereby primary care practitioners gain skills that enable greater competence and autonomy in managing mental disorders (WHO and WONCA 2008).

- A similar model is being practiced as part of the District Mental Health Programme in Thiruvananthapuram district, Kerala, India. Trained medical officers diagnose and treat mental disorders as part of their general primary care functions. A multidisciplinary district mental health team provides outreach clinical services, including direct management of complex cases and in-service training and support of the trained medical officers and other workers in the primary care centers. The primary care centers have incrementally assumed responsibility for independently operating mental health clinics with minimal support from the mental health team (WHO and WONCA 2008).

- In the Moorreesburg district of Western Cape province, South Africa, the role of primary care practitioners is filled by general primary care nurses, who provide basic mental health services in the primary health clinic. They are supported by specialist mental health nurses and a psychiatrist, who visits the clinic intermittently to manage complex cases and provide supervision (WHO and WONCA 2008).

- The European Headache Federation and Lifting the Burden: the Global Campaign against Headache (Steiner and others 2011) has proposed a collaborative care model for the management of headache disorders. In this model, 90 percent of people consulting for migraine and tension-type headaches can be diagnosed and managed by staff at the primary care level. In the case of the remaining 10 percent of the patients, common primary and secondary headache disorders can be recognized but not necessarily managed; these can be referred to the next level, where physicians can provide more advanced care. Finally, specialists can provide advanced care to approximately 1 percent of patients first seen at the first-level and second-level facilities, and can focus on the diagnosis and management of the underlying causes of all secondary headache disorders. There is a demonstrational intervention project based on this model in Yekaterinburg, Sverdlovsk Oblast, Russian Federation (Lebedeva and others 2013). Headache services in China have been designed on this model (Yu and others 2014).

The collaborative stepped care approach relies heavily on the introduction of additional human resources, identification of core competencies, adequate training to ensure that these core competencies are fulfilled, and specialist support to maintain these competencies. The next section describes this critical component of mental health system strengthening in more detail.

Strategy 2: Strengthening Human Resources for Mental Health through Task-Sharing

One of the main reasons for the substantial treatment gap for MNS disorders is the lack of a skilled workforce. In HICs, the number of mental health workers is often inadequate; in LMICs, the situation is dramatically worse, with an estimated shortage of 1.18 million workers (Kakuma and others 2011). The collaborative stepped care approach can be implemented only if skilled human resources are available at the different levels of service delivery.

Task-Sharing Approach

Task-sharing is a human resource innovation in which the skills to deliver specific mental health care tasks are transferred to appropriately trained and supervised general health workers. This process helps in improving access to evidence-based mental health care and leads to more efficient use of the limited resources. This approach has been evaluated for mental health service delivery, and its efficacy has been established using rigorous evaluation methodologies (Araya and others 2003; Patel and others 2010; Rahman and others 2008). Task-sharing is implemented through a collaborative care framework with four key human resources: the community health worker or case manager; the person with a mental health problem and family members; the primary or general health care physician; and the mental health professional (Bower and Gilbody 2005). The overall shortage of human resources can be addressed by introducing newly skilled nonspecialist health workers at the community level; reorienting medical officers and paramedical staff to integrate mental health interventions; and redefining the role of specialists from service providers to leaders, trainers, and supervisors of mental health programs.

The task-sharing approach is at the heart of establishing the collaborative stepped care model of care; the most crucial element in this approach is the availability of a case manager. The results of the MANAS trial clearly indicate the effectiveness of a lay health counselor or case manager leading the collaborative stepped care intervention for common mental disorders in public primary health care facilities in India (Patel and others 2010). Several global case studies have found that primary care for mental health is usually most effective where a mental health coordinator or case manager is responsible for overseeing integration (WHO and WONCA 2008). These case managers can play a crucial role in screening; engaging; educating patients and family members; maintaining close follow-up; tracking adherence and clinical outcomes; and delivering targeted, evidence-based, psychological interventions, such as motivational interviewing, behavioral activation, problem solving, or interpersonal therapy (Patel and others 2013). The case managers can serve as the link between the primary care and self-care platforms, and can work under the close supervision of the medical officers. The evidence base for psychological interventions delivered using a task-sharing approach is set out in box 11.1.

A recent multi-site, qualitative study as part of the PRogramme for Improving Mental health carE (PRIME) investigated the acceptability and feasibility of task-sharing mental health care in five LMICs. The study examined the perceptions of primary care service providers (physicians, nurses, and community health workers), community members, and service users (Mendenhall and others 2014). Task-sharing mental health services is feasible as long as the following key conditions are met:

- Increased numbers of human resources and better access to medications
- Ongoing structured supportive supervision at the community and primary care levels
- Adequate training and compensation for health workers involved in task-sharing.

Competency-Based Education

Primary care workers function best when their tasks related to mental health service delivery are limited and achievable. The most common reasons for failure to integrate mental health care into primary care programs are the lack of adequate assessment and the overly ambitious target-setting without the necessary customization of the detailed activities, and a full and explicit agreement on the targets and activities needed to achieve them (Patel and others 2013). A shift away from knowledge-based education to competency-based education is needed. This approach mainly focuses on the skills of providers, with the ultimate goal of improving patient outcomes. *Competency* is defined as an attribute of an individual human resource and the ability of that worker to deliver an intervention to a desired performance standard based on the acquired knowledge and skills.

The Institute of Medicine's (IOM) Forum on Neuroscience and Nervous System Disorders convened a workshop to discuss and identify core competencies that specialized and nonspecialized primary care providers

Box 11.1

Clinical and Functional Outcomes of Psychological Interventions Delivered Using a Task-Sharing Approach

- Recovery of adults suffering from depression or anxiety, or both, at 7–12 months following the intervention
- Reduction in symptoms for mothers with perinatal depression symptoms
- Reduction in the prevalence and the symptoms of adults with post-traumatic stress disorder over six months
- Improvement in symptoms of people with dementia

- Improvement in the mental well-being, burden, and distress of caregivers of people with dementia
- Decrease in the amount of alcohol consumed by people with alcohol-use disorders
- Reduction in functional impairment of children affected by post-traumatic stress disorder at six and 12 months following the intervention.

Sources: Clarke, King, and Prost 2013; van Ginneken and others 2013.

might need to help ensure the effective delivery of services for depression, psychosis, epilepsy, and alcohol use disorders in Sub-Saharan Africa (IOM 2013). Table 11.3 lists the steps to strengthen human resource competencies for MNS disorders; the core competencies for all service providers across MNS disorders are listed in table 11.4. In addition to the common competencies for all service providers, the IOM framework also focuses on a diverse range of cadre-specific competencies.

Pre-service and in-service training of primary care workers on mental health issues is an essential prerequisite for the integration of mental health into primary care platforms. The training, to the extent possible, should happen in primary care or community mental health care facilities, to ensure that practical experience is gained and that ongoing training and support are facilitated (WHO and WONCA 2008). The effects of training are nearly always short lived if health workers do not practice newly learned skills and receive ongoing specialist supervision. A trial from Kenya did not find any impact of the training program of medical officers on improvement in diagnostic rates of mental disorders (Jenkins and others 2013). A quasi-experimental study from Brazil had similar findings and noted that wider changes in the system of care may be required to augment training and encourage reliable changes in clinical practice (Goncalves and others 2013). Ongoing support and supervision from mental health specialists are essential. Case studies from Australia, Brazil, and South Africa have demonstrated that a collaborative stepped care approach, in which joint consultations and interventions occur between primary care workers and

mental health specialists, increases the skills of primary care workers and builds mental health networks (WHO and WONCA 2008).

Specialist Transitioning

Specialists, especially in LMICs, are usually engaged in service delivery. It is imperative to make a transition from providing clinical services to training and supervising the primary health care staff and providing direct clinical interventions judiciously and sparingly. In separate projects focusing on integrated primary care for mental health in the city of Sobral, Brazil, and the Sembabule district of Uganda, specialists together with medical officers in primary care visited primary care settings and assessed patients. Over time, psychiatrists started taking less active roles, while general practitioners assumed added responsibilities, under the supervision of the psychiatrists. Specialists can interact with primary care staff via referral and back-referral (WHO and WONCA 2008).

Planning and Consultation

Involving primary health care staff in the overall program planning and rollout process enhances ownership and commitment to achieve the planned outcomes within agreed timelines (Patel and others 2013). Consultations with general practitioners have been demonstrated to be one of the key factors in the success of the new mental health services in Australia (WHO and WONCA 2008). Decisions need to be made after careful consideration of local circumstances; this requires consultation with policy makers as well as users of mental health services and their families and the primary care staff.

Table 11.3 Steps to Strengthen Human Resource Competencies for MNS Disorders

Step 1:	Understand the tasks necessary for delivering evidence-based interventions.
Step 2:	Define the candidate core competencies needed to perform those tasks to an expected standard, acknowledging that there might be limits to what a particular human resource category may be able to do, or is permitted to do in a particular context.
Step 3:	Define how individual health care workers can acquire and maintain these competencies and how to evaluate them.

Source: IOM 2013.
Note: MNS = mental, neurological, and substance use.

Table 11.4 Core Competencies for All Service Providers across MNS Disorders

Competency

Screening and identification

- Demonstrate awareness of common signs and symptoms of MNS disorders
- Recognize the potential for risk to self and others
- Demonstrate basic knowledge of causes
- Provide the patient and community with awareness and education
- Demonstrate cultural competence
- Demonstrate knowledge of other MNS disorders

Formal diagnosis and referral

- Demonstrate knowledge of when to refer to the next level of care or other providers
- Demonstrate knowledge of providers for specialized care within the community

Treatment and care

- Provide support for patients and families while in treatment and care
- Identify and assist patients and families in overcoming barriers to successful treatment and recovery, for example, adherence, stigma, finances, accessibility, and access to social support
- Demonstrate ability to monitor mental status
- Demonstrate knowledge of how to offer emergency first aid
- Initiate and participate in community-based treatment, care, and prevention programs
- Demonstrate knowledge of treatment and care resources in the community
- Promote mental health literacy, for example, to minimize the impact of stigma and discrimination
- Communicate to the public about MNS disorders
- Monitor for adherence to regimens and side effects of medication
- Practice good therapeutic patient interactions, for example, communication, relationship, and attitude
- Provide links between patients and community resources
- Identify available resources to support patients, for example, rehabilitation and medication supplies
- Promote activities to raise awareness and improve the uptake of interventions and the use of services
- Protect patients and identify vulnerabilities, for example, human rights
- Demonstrate respect, compassion, and responsiveness to patient needs
- Demonstrate knowledge and skills to use information technology to improve treatment and care.

Source: IOM 2013.
Note: MNS = mental, neurological, and substance use.

Psychotropic Medications

It is important to ensure that primary care staff members have the appropriate permission to prescribe psychotropic medications, and they must be adequately trained to perform this task. In many countries, nurses and even general physicians are not permitted to prescribe psychotropic medications. If access to psychotropic medications is to be improved, then initiatives to allow primary care nurses to prescribe psychotropic medications need to be promoted and undertaken, provided appropriate training and supervision is conducted. In Belize, psychiatric nurse practitioners have been given additional prescription rights. In Uganda, general primary care nurses are permitted to prescribe psychotropic medication to patients who require continued medication on the recommendation of a mental health professional (WHO and WONCA 2008).

Strategy 3: Integrating Mental Health into Existing Health Programs

MNS disorders frequently occur throughout the course of many noncommunicable diseases and infectious diseases, such as HIV/AIDS and tuberculosis, increasing morbidity and mortality (Prince and others 2007). People with comorbid disorders risk poor outcomes for both disorders. To achieve the desired outcomes for priority programs in the health sector, it is crucial to manage MNS disorders, pursue synergies in the health system, and deliver interventions through integrated approaches to care. Expansion and integration of mental health services in primary health care can be achieved by using existing service delivery for maternal and child health, noncommunicable diseases, and HIV/AIDS and tuberculosis (Collins and others 2013). Patients with severe MNS disorders often do not receive appropriate care for their general health conditions because of the negative attitudes of service providers, resulting in reductions of 10–25 years in life expectancy compared with the general population. Integration of MNS services within other health care platforms is essential.

Maternal and Child Health Programs

Maternal depression is the second leading cause of disease burden in women worldwide, following infections and parasitic diseases (Rahman and others 2013). Systematic reviews from HICs provide evidence of the effectiveness of psychological therapies—including cognitive behavioral therapy (CBT) and interpersonal therapy that can be delivered in individual or group format—and pharmacotherapy in the treatment of maternal depression (Rahman and others 2013). Promising evidence

suggests the benefits of the integration of maternal mental health into maternal and child health (MCH) programs. Examples of community-based trials with a maternal mental health component integrated into an MCH program, and a case study demonstrating that the screening and management of maternal mental disorders can be integrated successfully into an existing health system at a facility level, build a strong case for the integration of mental health care into MCH programs (Rahman and others 2013). The Thinking Healthy Programme in Pakistan is a simple and culturally appropriate intervention for integrating depression care into an MCH program. The intervention is child centered, ensuring buy-in from the families and avoiding stigmatization. It is woven into the routine work of the community health workers, so it is not perceived as an additional burden. The Thinking Healthy Programme has been further adapted so that it can be used universally for all women rather than only depressed women (Rahman and others 2013).

The Perinatal Mental Health Project in the Western Cape Province in South Africa developed a stepped care intervention for maternal mental health that is integrated into antenatal care in three primary care midwife obstetric units (Honikman and others 2012). Midwives are trained to screen women routinely during their antenatal visits for maternal mood and anxiety disorders. Women who screen positive for anxiety or depression are referred to onsite counselors who also act as case managers. Women are referred to an onsite psychiatrist when specialist intervention is indicated. The Perinatal Mental Health Project works directly with facility managers and health workers through collaborative partnerships, focusing on problem solving and capacity development in the primary health care system. Over a three-year period, 90 percent of all women attending antenatal care in the maternity clinic were offered mental health screening, with 95 percent uptake. Of those screened, 32 percent qualified for referral; of these, 47 percent received counseling through the program. This case study clearly demonstrates that onsite, integrated mental health services can increase access for women who have scarce resources and competing health, family, and economic priorities (Honikman and others 2012).

Parenting skills training aims to enhance and support the parental role through education and skills enhancement, thereby improving emotional and behavioral outcomes for children. Primary health care workers can play a significant role in this training. The use of scarce professional resources to train parents is a cost-effective use of resources. Several systematic reviews have shown parent skills training to be effective for reducing internalizing and externalizing problems in children (Furlong and others 2012; Kaminski and others 2008), as well as reducing the risk of unintentional childhood injuries (Kendrick and others 2013) and improving the mental health of parents (Barlow and others 2014). Individual and group parent training have been beneficial. Four components of parenting skills training have been found to be most effective:

- Increasing positive parent-child interactions
- Teaching parents how to communicate emotionally with their children
- Teaching parents the use of time-out as a means of discipline
- Supporting parents to respond in a consistent manner to their children's behavior (Kaminski and others 2008).

Noncommunicable Disease Programs

Existing service delivery platforms for noncommunicable diseases are also promising entry points for the integration of mental health into primary care. The collaborative care models discussed demonstrate a strong evidence base for integration in primary care settings.

In North America, TEAMcare USA and TEAMcare Canada provide team-based primary care for diabetes, coronary heart disease, and depression. TEAMcare trains primary care staff to work in collaborative teams that deliver care in a clinic and by phone. Each service user is assigned a TEAMcare care manager, usually a medically supervised nurse, who serves as the conduit for the consultation team, the primary care team, and the service user. The program takes a treat-to-target approach, modifying treatment as needed to ensure improvement in symptoms. The program teaches self-care skills to service users to control illnesses and encourages behaviors that enhance the quality of life. About 1,400 people have received TEAMcare, with a trial showing improvements in medical disease control and depression symptoms (Katon and others 2012). In the United Kingdom, 3 Dimensions of Care for Diabetes uses a team consisting of a psychiatrist and a social worker from a nongovernmental organization embedded in the diabetes care team to integrate medical, psychological, and social care for people with diabetes and mental health problems, and social problems, such as housing and debt (Parsonage, Fossey, and Tutty 2012).

The National Depression Detection and Treatment Program in Chile integrated depression care with more traditional primary care programs for the management of hypertension and diabetes within a network of 520 primary care clinics. The program follows a collaborative stepped care approach and is led by psychologists, with additional support from physicians and specialists for severe depression (Araya and others 2012). In Myanmar and several other LMICs, epilepsy has been included as part of the process of local adaptation and implementation of WHO's package of essential noncommunicable disease interventions in primary care (WHO and Calouste Gulbenkian Foundation 2014).

Care for patients with dementia can be well integrated with health care for noncommunicable diseases. Patients with dementia need to be assessed for behavioral and psychosocial symptoms, in addition to a careful physical assessment to monitor hearing and visual impairments, pain, constipation, urinary tract infections, and bed sores that may explain some exacerbation of psychological symptoms. Monitoring and effective treatment of vascular risk factors and diseases, including high blood pressure, hypercholesterolemia, smoking, obesity, and diabetes, to improve secondary prevention of cerebrovascular events, are an integral component of care. A well-conducted clinical trial of cognitive stimulation (reality orientation, games, and discussions based on information processing rather than knowledge) conducted in the United Kingdom as a group intervention and a small pilot trial from Brazil suggest that cognitive benefits from this intervention are similar to the benefits from pharmacological management of dementia using cholinesterase inhibitors (Prince and others 2009). Cognitive rehabilitation, an individualized therapy designed to enhance residual cognitive skills and cope with deficits, showed promise in uncontrolled case series undertaken in HICs. A large body of literature attests to the benefits of caregiver interventions in dementia. These include psychoeducational interventions, often caregiver training; psychological therapies such as CBT and counseling; caregiver support; and respite care (Chapter 5 in this volume, Thakur and others 2015). Many interventions combine several of these elements. Interventions targeting the caregiver may have small, but significant, beneficial effects on the behavior of the person with dementia.

HIV/AIDS and Tuberculosis Programs

WHO's Integrated Management of Adult and Adolescent Illness (IMAI) is a broadly disseminated health care strategy that addresses the overall health of patients with HIV/AIDS and co-occurring tuberculosis; clear opportunities exist for the integration of mental health in this program. IMAI promotes the inclusion of mental health in the overall care model for HIV/AIDS, as the mental health needs of many persons living with HIV/AIDS can be largely addressed with little duplication or waste, while improving program outcomes, such as antiretroviral drug adherence (WHO 2013b). Interventions for substance use disorders can be integrated with HIV/AIDS interventions. This delivery channel can be used to identify individuals who use injectable drugs, as well as those with dependence on opioids, cannabis, and cocaine. The evidence base supports the efficacy of brief interventions on harm from drug use and the overall pattern of drug consumption, including drug abstinence. The brief intervention constitutes a single session of 5–30 minutes, incorporating individualized feedback and advice on reducing or stopping cannabis/psychostimulant consumption, and the offer of follow-up (NICE 2008).

In South Africa, the government has published integrated guidelines for all primary health workers, including HIV/AIDS; major noncommunicable diseases; and a range of mental health problems, including depression, anxiety, mania, substance abuse, and psychosis. These guidelines, called Primary Care 101 (PC101) (DOH 2012), are used by the national Department of Health as part of a primary care revitalization program to deliver integrated care within a chronic disease management framework (Asmall and Mahomed 2013). This approach includes consolidating care for all patients with chronic diseases into a single care delivery point at the facility level and strengthening clinical decision support for nurses. PC101 provides a set of clinical algorithms using a pragmatic signs-and-symptoms approach and integrates detection and management of MNS disorders with other chronic conditions. The guidelines include training materials delivered in a cascaded train-the-trainer format and ongoing support for primary care practitioners from trainers at the district and subdistrict levels. At the community level, outreach teams of community health workers are trained to support clinically stable patients and self-care.

QUALITY OF CARE FOR MNS DISORDERS

Quality in health care has been defined by the IOM as the degree to which health care services for individuals and populations increase the likelihood of desired health outcomes and are consistent with current professional knowledge (IOM 2001). Good-quality care is effective, efficient, equitable, timely, person centered, and safe, and delivers a positive patient experience (IOM 2001).

Despite the strong and growing knowledge base for delivery of mental health services, the treatment gap for MNS disorders remains unacceptably large, with over 90 percent of people with mental disorders in LMICs going without treatment (Kohn and others 2004). This treatment gap is not just a quantitative phenomenon; it also contains an important quality

of care dimension. There is a significant gap between what is known about effective treatment and what is actually provided to and experienced by consumers in routine care (Proctor and others 2009). In the language of universal health coverage, it is the difference between contact coverage and effective coverage; that is, substantial improvement in access to care needs to be accompanied by improvement in the quality of service delivery. The inadequacy of resources and low priority given to MNS disorders might suggest that consideration of the quality of care is subservient to the quantity of available and accessible services. However, quality improvement (QI) mechanisms ensure that available resources are well-utilized, in the sense that those in contact with services actually derive appropriate benefit from evidence-based interventions.

Moreover, good-quality services help to build people's confidence in making use of mental health care interventions, increasing the likelihood of seeking the care that they need (Funk and others 2009). Low-quality services lead people with MNS disorders to experience human rights violations and discrimination in health care settings. In many countries, the quality of care in inpatient and outpatient facilities is poor or even harmful and can actively hinder recovery (The Health Foundation 2013).

QI methods have been shown to be effective for sustained scale-up and adaptation of standardized treatment packages for Millennium Development Goal health priority areas. QI could be included as a routine part of mental health implementation and customization (Patel and others 2013). Quality assurance (QA) involves the use of tools and logic to assess quality performance. QI is the use of methods to enhance quality performance. QA/QI is an integrative process for identifying current levels of quality and improving the quality of performance. QA/QI plays an important role in monitoring and improving the implementation of evidence-based practices; it also helps to monitor and improve the quality of training and supervision required for the delivery of services. Some important QI approaches are continuous quality improvement, Lean, Six Sigma, Plan Do Study Act, Statistical Process Control, and Total Quality Management (The Health Foundation 2013).

QI frameworks and guidelines for LMICs have been developed in the form of a WHO guidance package for QI in mental health services (WHO 2003b). The package provides an integrated resource for the planning and refining of mental health systems on a national scale (Funk and others 2009). In a quality framework, standards and criteria are important tools for assessment and improvement. A standard is a broad statement of the desired and achievable level of performance against which actual performance can be measured. The criteria are measurable elements of service provision. Criteria relate to the desired outcome or performance of staff or services. The standard is achieved when all criteria associated with it are met.

Protection of human rights is a critical aspect of the quality of mental health care. The treatment provided in health care settings is often intended to keep people and their conditions under control rather than to enhance their autonomy and improve their quality of life. People can be seen as objects of treatment rather than human beings with the same rights and entitlements as everybody else. They often are not consulted on their care or recovery plans; many receive treatment against their wishes. The situation in inpatient facilities is often far worse: people may be locked away for weeks, months, and even years in psychiatric hospitals or social care homes, where they can be subject to dehumanizing, degrading treatment, including violence and abuse (WHO 2003b).

WHO developed the QualityRights Toolkit to assess and improve the quality of life and human rights of people with MNS disorders receiving treatment in mental health and social care facilities (WHO 2012). People living in these facilities are isolated from society and have little or no opportunity to lead normal, fulfilling lives in the community. WHO recommends that countries progressively close down this type of facility and instead establish community-based services and integrate mental health into primary care services and the services offered by general hospitals. Although this tool does not endorse long-stay facilities as an appropriate setting for treatment and care, as long as these types of facilities continue to exist all over the world, there is a need to promote the rights of those residing in them.

The QualityRights Toolkit covers the following five themes drawn from the United Nations Convention on the Rights of Persons with Disabilities:

- Right to an adequate standard of living and social protection
- Right to enjoyment of the highest attainable standard of physical and mental health
- Right to exercise legal capacity and the right to personal liberty and security of person
- Freedom from torture or cruel, inhuman, or degrading treatment or punishment and from exploitation, violence, and abuse
- Right to live independently and be included in the community.

A comprehensive assessment of facilities based on these themes can help to identify problems in existing health care practices and to plan effective means to ensure that the services are of good quality, respectful of human rights, and responsive to the users' requirements, and promote the users' autonomy, dignity, and right to self-determination.

CONCLUSIONS

This chapter has described the health care delivery platform and its delivery channels and evidence-based interventions. The key points for effective and efficient delivery of mental health services are as follows:

- To deliver interventions for MNS disorders, the focus needs to move from vertical programs to horizontal health service platforms.
- The WHO pyramid framework of self-care, primary care, and specialist care continues to provide a useful approach for understanding potential delivery channels.
- A set of evidence-based interventions within this framework can be identified for promotion and prevention; identification and case detection; and treatment, care, and rehabilitation interventions.
- The delivery of these interventions requires an approach that embraces public health, systems, and whole-government principles.
- The key strategies for this delivery are implementing collaborative stepped care, strengthening human resources, and integrating mental health into general health care.
- Finally, it is important not only to improve access to health services, but also to focus on improving the quality of care delivered.

Recommendations for policy makers include adopting these principles and strategies using a platformwide approach. Policy makers need to engage with a wide range of stakeholders in this process and make use of the best available evidence in a transparent manner.

NOTE

Disclaimer: Dan Chisholm is a staff member of the World Health Organization. The author alone is responsible for the views expressed in this publication, and they do not necessarily represent the decisions, policy, or views of the World Health Organization.

This chapter was previously published as an article by R. Shidhaye, C. Lund, and D. Chisholm, titled "Closing the Treatment Gap for Mental, Neurological, and Substance Use Disorders by Strengthening Existing Health Care Platforms: Strategies for Delivery and Integration of Evidence-Based Interventions." *International Journal of Mental Health Systems*, 2015: 9 (40). doi:10.1186/s13033-015-0031-9.

World Bank Income Classifications as of July 2014 are as follows, based on estimates of gross national income (GNI) per capita for 2013:

- Low-income countries (LICs) = US$1,045 or less
- Middle-income countries (MICs) are subdivided:
  a) Lower-middle-income = US$1,046 to US$4,125
  b) Upper-middle-income(UMICs)=US$4,126 to US$12,745
- High-income countries (HICs) = US$12,746 or more.

REFERENCES

APA (American Psychiatric Association). 2000. *Diagnostic and Statistical Manual of Mental Disorders: DSM-IV-TR*. 4th ed., text revision. Washington, DC: APA.

Araya, R., R. Alvarado, R. Sepulveda, and G. Rojas. 2012. "Lessons from Scaling Up a Depression Treatment Program in Primary Care in Chile." *Revista Panamericana de Salud Publica* 32 (3): 234–40.

Araya, R., G. Rojas, R. Fritsch, J. Gaete, M. Rojas, and others. 2003. "Treating Depression in Primary Care in Low-Income Women in Santiago, Chile: A Randomised Controlled Trial." *The Lancet* 361 (9362): 995–1000. doi:10.1016/S0140-6736(03)12825-5.

Archer, J., P. Bower, S. Gilbody, K. Lovell, D. Richards, and others. 2012. "Collaborative Care for Depression and Anxiety Problems." *Cochrane Database of Systematic Reviews* 10: CD006525. doi:10.1002/14651858.CD006525.pub2.

Asmall, S., and O. H. Mahomed. 2013. *The Integrated Chronic Disease Management Manual*. Pretoria, South Africa: Department of Health.

Barlow, J., N. Smailagic, N. Huband, V. Roloff, and C. Bennett. 2014. "Group-Based Parent Training Programmes for Improving Parental Psychosocial Health." *Cochrane Database of Systematic Reviews* 5: CD002020. doi:10.1002/14651858.CD002020.pub4.

Bekele, Y. Y., A. J. Flisher, A. Alem, and Y. Baheretebeb. 2009. "Pathways to Psychiatric Care in Ethiopia." *Psychological Medicine* 39 (3): 475–83. doi:10.1017/S0033291708003929.

Bower, P., and S. Gilbody. 2005. "Managing Common Mental Health Disorders in Primary Care: Conceptual Models and Evidence Base." *BMJ* 330 (7495): 839–42. doi:10.1136/bmj.330.7495.839.

Brown, L. D., M. D. Shepherd, S. A. Wituk, and G. Meissen. 2008. "Introduction to the Special Issue on Mental Health Self-Help." *American Journal of Community Psychology* 42 (1–2): 105–09. doi:10.1007/s10464-008-9187-7.

Clarke, K., M. King, and A. Prost. 2013. "Psychosocial Interventions for Perinatal Common Mental Disorders Delivered by Providers Who Are Not Mental Health Specialists in Low- and Middle-Income Countries: A Systematic Review and Meta-Analysis." *PLoS Medicine* 10 (10): e1001541. doi:10.1371/journal.pmed.1001541.

Cohen, A., S. Raja, C. Underhill, B. P. Yaro, A. Y. Dokurugu, and others. 2012. "Sitting with Others: Mental Health Self-Help Groups in Northern Ghana." *International Journal of Mental Health Systems* 6 (1): 1. doi:10.1186/1752-4458-6-1.

Collins, P. Y., T. R. Insel, A. Chockalingam, A. Daar, and Y. T. Maddox. 2013. "Grand Challenges in Global Mental Health: Integration in Research, Policy, and Practice." *PLoS Medicine* 10 (4): e1001434. doi:10.1371/journal.pmed.1001434.

Dias, A., M. E. Dewey, J. D'Souza, R. Dhume, D. D. Motghare, and others. 2008. "The Effectiveness of a Home Care Program for Supporting Caregivers of Persons with Dementia in Developing Countries: A Randomised Controlled Trial from Goa, India." *PLoS One* 3 (6): e2333.

DOH (Department of Health). 2012. "Primary Care 101." DOH, Pretoria, South Africa.

Funk, M., C. Lund, M. Freeman, and N. Drew. 2009. "Improving the Quality of Mental Health Care." *International Journal for Quality in Health Care* 21 (6): 415–20. doi:10.1093/intqhc/mzp048.

Furlong, M., S. McGilloway, T. Bywater, J. Hutchings, S. M. Smith, and others. 2012. "Behavioural and Cognitive-Behavioural Group-Based Parenting Programmes for Early-Onset Conduct Problems in Children Aged 3 to 12 Years." *Cochrane Database of Systematic Reviews* 2: CD008225. doi:10.1002/14651858.CD008225.pub2.

Goncalves, D. A., S. Fortes, M. Campos, D. Ballester, F. B. Portugal, and others. 2013. "Evaluation of a Mental Health Training Intervention for Multidisciplinary Teams in Primary Care in Brazil: A Pre- and Posttest Study." *General Hospital Psychiatry* 35 (3): 304–08. doi:10.1016/j.genhosppsych.2013.01.003.

Honikman, S., T. van Heyningen, S. Field, E. Baron, and M. Tomlinson. 2012. "Stepped Care for Maternal Mental Health: A Case Study of the Perinatal Mental Health Project in South Africa." *PLoS Medicine* 9 (5): e1001222. doi:10.1371/journal.pmed.1001222.

IASC (Inter-Agency Standing Committee). 2007. *Guidelines on Mental Health and Psychosocial Support in Emergency Settings*. Geneva: IASC.

IOM (Institute of Medicine). 2001. *Crossing the Quality Chasm: A New Health System for the 21st Century*. Washington, DC: National Academies Press.

———. 2013. "Strengthening Human Resources through Development of Candidate Core Competencies for Mental, Neurological, and Substance Use Disorders in Sub-Saharan Africa: Workshop Summary." National Academies Press, Washington, DC.

Jayalakshmi, S., G. Padmaja, S. Vooturi, A. Bogaraju, and M. Surath. 2014. "Impact of Family Support on Psychiatric Disorders and Seizure Control in Patients with Juvenile Myoclonic Epilepsy." *Epilepsy and Behavior* 37: 7–10. doi:10.1016/j.yebeh.2014.05.020.

Jenkins, R., C. Othieno, S. Okeyo, D. Kaseje, J. Aruwa, and others. 2013. "Short Structured General Mental Health in Service

Training Programme in Kenya Improves Patient Health and Social Outcomes But Not Detection of Mental Health Problems—A Pragmatic Cluster Randomised Controlled Trial." *International Journal of Mental Health Systems* 7 (1): 25. doi:10.1186/1752-4458-7-25.

Kakuma, R., H. Minas, N. van Ginneken, M. R. Dal Poz, K. Desiraju, and others. 2011. "Human Resources for Mental Health Care: Current Situation and Strategies for Action." *The Lancet* 378 (9803): 1654–63. doi:10.1016/S0140-6736(11)61093-3.

Kaminski, J. W., L. A. Valle, J. H. Filene, and C. L. Boyle. 2008. "A Meta-Analytic Review of Components Associated with Parent Training Program Effectiveness." *Journal of Abnormal Child Psychology* 36 (4): 567–89. doi:10.1007/s10802-007-9201-9.

Katon, W. J., E. H. Lin, M. Von Korff, P. Ciechanowski, E. J. Ludman, and others. 2010. "Collaborative Care for Patients with Depression and Chronic Illnesses." *New England Journal of Medicine* 363 (27): 2611–20. doi:10.1056/NEJMoa1003955.

Katon, W., J. Russo, E. H. Lin, J. Schmittdiel, P. Ciechanowski, and others. 2012. "Cost-Effectiveness of a Multicondition Collaborative Care Intervention: A Randomized Controlled Trial." *Archives of General Psychiatry* 69 (5): 506–14. doi:10.1001/archgenpsychiatry.2011.1548.

Kendrick, D., C. A. Mulvaney, L. Ye, T. Stevens, J. A. Mytton, and others. 2013. "Parenting Interventions for the Prevention of Unintentional Injuries in Childhood." *Cochrane Database of Systematic Reviews* 3: CD006020. doi:10.1002/14651858.CD006020.pub3.

Kodner, D. L., and C. Spreeuwenberg. 2002. "Integrated Care: Meaning, Logic, Applications, and Implications: A Discussion Paper." *International Journal of Integrated Care* 2: e12.

Kohn, R., S. Saxena, I. Levav, and B. Saraceno. 2004. "The Treatment Gap in Mental Health Care." *Bulletin of the World Health Organization* 82 (11): 858–66.

Lebedeva, E. R., J. Olesen, V. V. Osipova, L. I. Volkova, G. R. Tabeeva, and others. 2013. "The Yekaterinburg Headache Initiative: An Interventional Project, within the Global Campaign against Headache, to Reduce the Burden of Headache in Russia." *Journal of Headache Pain* 14: 101. doi:10.1186/1129-2377-14-101.

Lund, C., M. Tomlinson, M. De Silva, A. Fekadu, R. Shidhaye, and others. 2012. "PRIME: A Programme to Reduce the Treatment Gap for Mental Disorders in Five Low- and Middle-Income Countries." *PLoS Medicine* 9 (12): e1001359.

Manandhar, D. S., D. Osrin, B. P. Shrestha, N. Mesko, J. Morrison, and others. 2004. "Effect of a Participatory Intervention with Women's Groups on Birth Outcomes in Nepal: Cluster-Randomised Controlled Trial." *The Lancet* 364 (9438): 970–79. doi:10.1016/S0140-6736(04)17021-9.

Matchar, D. B., L. Harpole, G. P. Samsa, A. Jurgelski, R. B. Lipton, and others. 2008. "The Headache Management Trial: A Randomized Study of Coordinated Care." *Headache* 48 (9): 1294–310. doi:10.1111/j.1526-4610.2007.01148.x.

Medley, A., C. Kennedy, K. O'Reilly, and M. Sweat. 2009. "Effectiveness of Peer Education Interventions for HIV Prevention in Developing Countries: A Systematic Review and Meta-Analysis." *AIDS Education and Prevention* 21 (3): 181–206. doi:10.1521/aeap.2009.21.3.181.

Mendenhall, E., M. J. De Silva, C. Hanlon, I. Petersen, R. Shidhaye, and others. 2014. "Acceptability and Feasibility of Using Non-Specialist Health Workers to Deliver Mental Health Care: Stakeholder Perceptions from the PRIME District Sites in Ethiopia, India, Nepal, South Africa, and Uganda." *Social Science and Medicine* 118C: 33–42. doi:10.1016/j.socscimed.2014.07.057.

MHaPP (Mental Health and Poverty Project). 2008. "Inter-Sectoral Collaboration for Mental Health in South Africa." World Health Organization, Geneva. http://www.who.int/mental_health/policy/development/MHPB5.pdf.

NICE (National Institute for Health and Care Excellence). 2008. "Drug Misuse: Psychosocial Interventions." National Clinical Practice Guideline 51, NICE, London.

Parsonage, M., M. Fossey, and C. Tutty. 2012. *Liaison Psychiatry in the Modern NHS*. London: Centre for Mental Health.

Patel, V. 2011. "Traditional Healers for Mental Health Care in Africa." *Global Health Action* 4. doi:10.3402/gha.v4i0.7956.

Patel, V., G. S. Belkin, A. Chockalingam, J. Cooper, S. Saxena, and others. 2013. "Grand Challenges: Integrating Mental Health Services into Priority Health Care Platforms." *PLoS Medicine* 10 (5): e1001448. doi:10.1371/journal.pmed.1001448.

Patel, V., and G. Thornicroft. 2009. "Packages of Care for Mental, Neurological, and Substance Use Disorders in Low- and Middle-Income Countries: PLoS Medicine Series." *PLoS Medicine* 6 (10): e1000160.

Patel, V., H. A. Weiss, N. Chowdhary, S. Naik, S. Pednekar, and others. 2010. "Effectiveness of an Intervention Led by Lay Health Counsellors for Depressive and Anxiety Disorders in Primary Care in Goa, India (MANAS): A Cluster Randomised Controlled Trial." *The Lancet* 376 (9758): 2086–95.

Peters, D. H., T. Adam, O. Alonge, I. A. Agyepong, and N. Tran. 2013. "Implementation Research: What It Is and How to Do It." *BMJ* 347: f6753. doi:10.1136/bmj.f6753.

Petersen, I., S. Evans-Lacko, M. Semrau, M. Barry, D. Chisholm, P. Gronholm, C. Egbe, and G. Thornicroft. 2015. "Population- and Community-Level Platforms." In *Disease Control Priorities* (third edition): Volume 4, *Mental, Neurological, and Substance Use Disorders*, edited by V. Patel, D. Chisholm, T. Dua, R. Laxminarayan, and M. E. Medina-Mora. Washington, DC: World Bank.

Pistrang, N., C. Barker, and K. Humphreys. 2008. "Mutual Help Groups for Mental Health Problems: A Review of Effectiveness Studies." *American Journal of Community Psychology* 42 (1–2): 110–21. doi:10.1007/s10464-008-9181-0.

Prince M., D. Acosta, E. Castro-Costa, J. Jackson, and K. Shaji. 2009. "Packages of Care for Dementia in Low- and Middle-Income Countries." *PLoS Medicine* 6 (11): e1000176.

Prince, M., V. Patel, S. Saxena, M. Maj, J. Maselko, and others. 2007. "No Health without Mental Health." *The Lancet* 370 (9590): 859–77.

Proctor, E. K., J. Landsverk, G. Aarons, D. Chambers, C. Glisson, and others. 2009. "Implementation Research in Mental Health Services: An Emerging Science with Conceptual, Methodological, and Training Challenges." *Administration and Policy in Mental Health* 36 (1): 24–34. doi:10.1007/s10488-008-0197-4.

Rahman, A., A. Malik, S. Sikander, C. Roberts, and F. Creed. 2008. "Cognitive Behaviour Therapy–Based Intervention by Community Health Workers for Mothers with Depression and Their Infants in Rural Pakistan: A Cluster-Randomised Controlled Trial." *The Lancet* 372 (9642): 902–09.

Rahman, A., P. J. Surkan, C. E. Cayetano, P. Rwagatare, and K. E. Dickson. 2013. "Grand Challenges: Integrating Maternal Mental Health into Maternal and Child Health Programmes." *PLoS Medicine* 10 (5): e1001442. doi:10.1371/journal.pmed.1001442.

Rojas, G., R. Fritsch, J. Solis, E. Jadresic, C. Castillo, and others. 2007. "Treatment of Postnatal Depression in Low-Income Mothers in Primary-Care Clinics in Santiago, Chile: A Randomised Controlled Trial." *The Lancet* 370 (9599): 1629–37. doi:10.1016/S0140-6736(07)61685-7.

Savigny, D., and T. Adam, eds. 2009. *Systems Thinking for Health Systems Strengthening.* Geneva: World Health Organization.

Shidhaye, R., and M. Kermode. 2013. "Stigma and Discrimination as a Barrier to Mental Health Service Utilization in India." *International Health* 5 (1): 6–8. doi:10.1093/inthealth/ihs011.

Simoni, J. M., J. C. Franks, K. Lehavot, and S. S. Yard. 2011. "Peer Interventions to Promote Health: Conceptual Considerations." *American Journal of Orthopsychiatry* 81 (3): 351–59. doi:10.1111/j.1939-0025.2011.01103.x.

Sphere. 2011. *Humanitarian Charter and Minimum Standards in Disaster Response.* Geneva: Sphere Project.

Steiner, T. J., F. Antonaci, R. Jensen, M. J. Lainez, M. Lanteri-Minet, and others. 2011. "Recommendations for Headache Service Organisation and Delivery in Europe." *Journal of Headache Pain* 12 (4): 419–26. doi:10.1007/s10194-011-0320-x.

Thakur, K., E. Albanese, P. Giannakopoulos, N. Jette, M. Linde, M. Prince, T. Steiner, and T. Dua. 2015. "Neurological Disorders." In *Disease Control Priorities* (third edition): Volume 4, *Mental, Neurological, and Substance Use Disorders,* edited by V. Patel, D. Chisholm, T. Dua, R. Laxminarayan, and M. E. Medina-Mora. Washington, DC: World Bank.

The Health Foundation. 2013. *Quality Improvement Made Simple.* London: The Health Foundation.

Thornicroft, G., and M. Tansella. 2013. "The Balanced Care Model for Global Mental Health." *Psychological Medicine* 43 (4): 849–63. doi:10.1017/S0033291712001420.

Tripathy, P., N. Nair, S. Barnett, R. Mahapatra, J. Borghi, and others. 2010. "Effect of a Participatory Intervention with Women's Groups on Birth Outcomes and Maternal Depression in Jharkhand and Orissa, India: A Cluster-Randomised Controlled Trial." *The Lancet* 375 (9721): 1182–92.

van Ginneken, N., P. Tharyan, W. Lewin, G. N. Rao, S. M. Meera, and others. 2013. "Non-Specialist Health Worker Interventions for the Care of Mental, Neurological and Substance-Abuse Disorders in Low- and Middle-Income Countries." *Cochrane Database of Systematic Reviews* 11: CD009149. doi:10.1002/14651858.CD009149.pub2.

Walker, E. R., C. Barmon, R. E. McGee, G. Engelhard, C. E. Sterk, and others. 2014. "Perspectives of Adults with Epilepsy and Their Support Persons on Self-Management Support." *Qualitative Health Research* 24 (11): 1553–66. doi:10.1177/1049732314548880.

WHO (World Health Organization). 2002. *Traditional Medicine: Growing Needs and Potential.* Geneva: WHO.

———. 2003a. "Organization of Services for Mental Health." In *Mental Health Policy and Service Guidance Package.* Geneva: WHO.

———. 2003b. "Quality Improvement for Mental Health." In *Mental Health Policy and Service Guidance Package.* Geneva: WHO.

———. 2010a. *The World Health Report 2010: Health Systems Financing: The Path to Universal Coverage.* Geneva: WHO.

———. 2010b. *mhGAP Intervention Guide for Mental, Neurological and Substance Use Disorders in Non-Specialized Health Settings: Mental Health Gap Action Programme (mhGAP).* Geneva: WHO.

———. 2012. *WHO QualityRights Toolkit.* Geneva: WHO.

———. 2013a. *Building Back Better: Sustainable Mental Health Care after Emergencies.* WHO: Geneva.

———. 2013b. "HIV Service Delivery [Internet]." http://www.who.int/hiv/topics/capacity/imai/en/index.html.

WHO and Calouste Gulbenkian Foundation. 2014. *Integrating the Response to Mental Disorders and Other Chronic Diseases in Health Care Systems.* Geneva: WHO.

WHO and WONCA (World Organization of Family Doctors). 2008. *Integrating Mental Health in Primary Care: A Global Perspective.* Geneva: WHO.

Yu, S., M. Zhang, J. Zhou, R. Liu, Q. Wan, and others. 2014. "Headache Care in China." *Headache: The Journal of Head and Face Pain* 54 (4): 601–09. doi:10.1111/head.12330.

Chapter 12

Cost-Effectiveness and Affordability of Interventions, Policies, and Platforms for the Prevention and Treatment of Mental, Neurological, and Substance Use Disorders

Carol Levin and Dan Chisholm

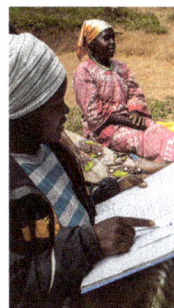

INTRODUCTION

Since the turn of the millennium, considerable progress has been made in developing an evidence base on which interventions are effective and feasible for improving mental health in low- and middle-income countries (LMICs). Such evidence provides a critical input to the formulation of plans and priorities to address the large and growing burden of mental, neurological, and substance use (MNS) disorders. However, for successful and sustainable scale-up of effective interventions and innovative service delivery strategies, decision makers require not only evidence of an intervention's impact on health and other outcomes, such as equity or poverty, but also evidence of its cost and cost-effectiveness. Cost data provide information relevant to the financial planning and implementation of prioritized, evidence-based strategies; cost-effectiveness analysis indicates the relative efficiency or value for money associated with interventions or innovations.

The application of economic evaluation to MNS disorders has largely focused on the assessment of a specific intervention's costs and health outcomes, relative to some comparator, which may be treatment as usual, another innovation, or no intervention.

Such assessments have often been conducted alongside clinical trials, enabling health economic researchers to add resource use questions to study protocols, generate estimates of each trial participant's health care costs, and relate these costs to primary outcome measures in the form of cost-effectiveness ratios. We review this type of economic evidence over the course of this chapter, with a particular focus on studies that have been successfully carried out in LMICs. However, the number of completed studies remains small and insufficient to inform resource allocation decisions in all the national settings where cost-effectiveness information would be valuable, including the many countries where informal or traditional health care represents the predominant model of service availability. This paucity of economic evidence reflects the overall lack of resources and infrastructure for mental health services in LMICs, including research capacity.

Partly to address the paucity of cost-effectiveness trials, as well as their intrinsic specificity to the setting in which they are conducted, a broader, modeling-based approach has also been used to build up economic evidence for international mental health policy and planning. This approach includes the earlier editions of the Disease Control Priorities (DCP) project and

Corresponding author: Carol Levin, Department of Global Health, University of Washington, Seattle, WA, United States; clevin@uw.edu.

the World Health Organization's (WHO) CHOosing Interventions that are Cost-Effective (CHOICE) project. Such model-based studies rely on existing data, as well as several analytical assumptions; these studies have adopted an epidemiological, population-based approach that identifies the expected costs and health impacts of delivering evidence-based interventions at scale in the population as a whole, whether a specific country or an entire region. We also review this form of economic evidence and comment on important gaps in the current evidence base, as well as the relative strengths and limitations of this approach.

One important limitation of conventional cost-effectiveness analysis—whether garnered through trial-based or model-based approaches—is that it is restricted to consideration of the specific implementation costs and health-related outcomes of an intervention; it does not typically extend to the nonhealth or wider economic or social value of investing in mental health innovation and service scale-up. In particular, cost-effectiveness analysis in its conventional form has little to say about the equitable distribution of costs and health gains across different groups of the target population. Incorporation of such concerns into economic evaluation represents a major objective of extended cost-effectiveness analysis, which is explored and addressed specifically in chapter 13 in this volume (Chisholm, Johansson, and others 2015).

In this chapter, we review the available cost-effectiveness evidence for the different levels and underpinning strategies of the mental health care system, with a focus on information generated in or for LMICs. Based on the overall analytical framework and priority intervention matrices developed for this volume, the remainder of the chapter is presented as follows. First, we consider the economic evidence for mental health prevention and protection at the population and community levels of the health and welfare system, including legislative, regulatory, and informational measures at the public policy level (population platform), as well as school-, workplace-, and community-based programs (community platform). We then examine the economic evidence relating to the identification and treatment of MNS disorders (health care platform), focusing on the relative cost-effectiveness or efficiency of treatment programs implemented in nonspecialized versus more specialized health care settings. Finally, we assess the financial costs and budgetary implications of implementing or scaling up a set of prioritized, cost-effective interventions.

Our review is based on available, published literature. A systematic search of the literature for LMICs was undertaken in PubMed to find articles published since 2000 in English. The search combined terms for specific mental health interventions with economic terms such as "cost," "cost-effectiveness," or "quality-adjusted life year (QALY)," as well as the names of all LMICs and their respective regions (see annex 12A for a list of search terms used to identify relevant literature). Where little or no literature was found for LMICs on interventions of potential importance, this systematic search was augmented by selective searches of the literature available since 1995 for high-income countries (HICs); however, these results are not included in the figures or tables. Annex 12B provides the search statistics.

Articles included in the review were graded using the checklist of Drummond and others (2005) to generate a quality score for each article, with most studies graded between 7 and 10. Annex 12C provides a list of studies that were used to generate the tables and figures presented in this chapter. It presents detailed information on the intervention characteristics and comparators, target population group, geographic location, methodology, results, and quality scores. All cost-effectiveness results are presented in 2012 US$ except where noted otherwise. Consistent with earlier iterations of DCP, reported regional estimates refer to the World Bank's categorization of countries by income.

COST-EFFECTIVENESS OF MENTAL HEALTH PROMOTION AND PROTECTION MEASURES AT THE POPULATION AND COMMUNITY LEVELS

Economic evaluation has yet to be extensively applied to mental health promotion, largely because of the challenges associated with using conventional methods and principles of cost-effectiveness analysis in the context of such programs, in particular, the limitations of experimental study design; the multifaceted, complex, and long-term nature of anticipated program benefits; and the shortage of sensitive or suitable outcome measures (Petticrew and others 2005). Moreover, many of the determinants of poor mental health and mental health inequalities lie outside the health sector, thereby requiring an evaluation of intersectoral action. Certain mental health promotion strategies are not amenable to controlled studies, because it is not feasible or ethical to exclude a segment of the target population from exposure to the intervention in question. Since cost-effectiveness is by definition a relative concept, this limitation makes estimation of the relative or comparative efficiency of one strategy over another problematic. Where such comparisons are not possible, prospective observational studies, time-series analyses, or ecological studies within a single population can still be conducted and may provide a sufficient basis for decision making. An alternative approach is via modeling studies, which attempt to simulate empirical studies on the basis of publicly available data sources.

Chapter 10 of this volume (Petersen and others 2015) identifies a number of good and best practices for protecting mental health at the population and community levels, including the following:

- Laws and regulations to reduce harmful alcohol use
- Laws and regulations to reduce access to lethal means of suicide
- School-based social emotional learning programs to prevent the onset of mental disorders and promote mental health in children and adolescents
- Community-based parenting programs, particularly during infancy and early childhood
- Training programs to help gatekeepers to identify people with mental illness.

We consider the economic evidence for each of these policy options. Clearly, there are other potential approaches that can be tested and adopted that can help to promote and protect mental health. For example, cash transfers and microfinance have been used to support the health of women and children in several settings and have the potential to improve mental health outcomes such as cognitive development in young children. Better understanding of the impact and costs of cash transfers and other social programs, such as microfinance, is essential for addressing the cycle of poverty and mental disorders (Lund and others 2011).

Laws and Regulations to Reduce Harmful Alcohol Use

Population-based measures for reducing the demand for or access to alcohol include fiscal instruments (excise taxes), legal limits (minimum drinking age, maximum blood alcohol content levels when driving), and regulation (advertising bans and restricted access to retail outlets). Within the category of pricing policies, consistent evidence shows that the consumption of alcohol is responsive to an increase in final prices, and this can be effectuated via higher excise taxes on alcoholic beverages. Tax increases of 20 percent or even 50 percent represent a highly cost-effective response in countries with a high prevalence of heavy drinking, defined as greater than 5 percent of adults. For example, Rehm and others (2006) estimated that in LMICs in Europe and Central Asia, Latin America and the Caribbean, and Sub-Saharan Africa, a disability-adjusted life year (DALY) can be averted for US$200–US$400, equivalent to 2,500–5,000

DALYs averted per US$1 million expenditure (reported values have been updated to 2012 price levels).

In lower-prevalence contexts, such as East Asia and Pacific and South Asia, population-level effects drop off and cost-effectiveness ratios rise accordingly. The impact of alcohol tax increases stands to be mitigated by illegal production, tax evasion, and illegal trading, which account for approximately 30 percent of all consumption in European and Latin American subregions and up to 80 percent in certain parts of Sub-Saharan Africa. Reducing this unrecorded consumption by 20–50 percent via concerted tax enforcement efforts by law enforcement and excise officers is estimated to cost 50–100 percent more than a tax increase, but it produces similar levels of health gain in the population (Anderson, Chisholm, and Fuhr 2009). In settings with higher levels of unrecorded production and consumption, such as India, increasing the proportion of consumption that is taxed may be a more effective pricing policy than simply increasing the excise tax; excise tax increases may only encourage further illegal production, smuggling, and cross-border purchases (Patel and others 2011).

The impact of reducing access to retail outlets for specified periods of the week to limit the availability and implementing a comprehensive advertising ban to limit the marketing of alcoholic beverages have the potential to be very cost-effective countermeasures, but only if they are fully enforced; compared with doing nothing, each DALY averted costs between US$200 and US$1,200 (Rehm and others 2006). For impaired-driving policies and countermeasures, there is good evidence from HICs on the effectiveness of impaired-driving laws and their enforcement via roadside breath testing and checkpoints. The estimated cost-effectiveness of such countermeasures in LMICs ranges from US$800 to US$3,000 per DALY averted. However, the applicability—and by extension, the cost-effectiveness—of such measures may be limited in settings where large segments of the population do not drive or where noncommercial alcoholic home brews represent the predominant form of consumption.

Country-level information on the cost-effectiveness of legislation to control alcohol use is limited, with only one study conducted in a low-income setting. A country contextualization study of the WHO-CHOICE model in Nigeria, a lower-middle-income country, showed that alcohol taxation does generate appreciable health gains. However, these gains did not result in a significant improvement in cost-effectiveness, because it was expected that an increase in taxes would lead to a rise in the amount of illicit and untaxed consumption of alcohol. The study did find that implementation of random roadside breath testing for alcohol could potentially generate considerably more healthy life years than could other interventions and would do so at a lower cost (Gureje and others 2007).

Laws to Restrict Access to Means of Self-Harm and Suicide

There is a paucity of robust economic studies to inform policy makers about the budgetary requirements and return on investment associated with scaled-up efforts to prevent self-harm or suicide (Zechmeister and others 2008). A recent WHO review of suicide prevention strategies that included cost as a parameter of interest, however, showed that two-thirds of the strategies assessed as being effective or promising were categorized as low cost; low cost was also closely associated with universal or selective, as opposed to more indicated or targeted, prevention approaches (WHO 2010). Australia's ACE-Prevention (Assessing Cost-Effectiveness in Prevention) project assessed the cost-effectiveness of reducing access to means via revised legislation for gun ownership and estimated that the cost per healthy life year gained would exceed US$57,000; guidelines for more responsible media reporting would cost US$30,800 per healthy life year gained if at least one suicide is averted (Vos and others 2010).

Partly to address this paucity of available evidence, an extended cost-effectiveness analysis was undertaken for this volume relating to a pesticide ban in India to prevent self-harm and suicide, based on the experience of Sri Lanka's ban on pesticides in the 1990s (Nigam and others 2015). The authors estimated that 3,750 deaths could be averted per year if 80 percent of the population no longer had access to endosulfan, a commonly used Class II pesticide. Implementation of the ban plus hospital treatment for self-harm cases was estimated to cost US$0.10 per capita, yielding a cost-effectiveness ratio of close to US$1,000 per life-year gained (Nigam and others 2015). However, the analysis did not take into account costs potentially falling to other sectors or agents as a result of the ban, or potential substitution effects.

School-Based Social Emotional Learning Programs

Integrated mental health promotion programs in schools targeting children and adolescents have long-term benefits, including improved emotional and social functioning and academic achievement (Tennant and others 2007; Weare and Nind 2011). Furthermore, economic analyses from HICs indicate that social emotional learning (SEL) interventions in schools are cost-effective, resulting in savings from better health outcomes, as well as reduced expenditure in the criminal justice system

(Knapp and others 2011; McCabe 2007). Although such life skills programs seem to represent good value for money, there is a need to ascertain this via formal cost-effectiveness studies on specific early childhood development and classroom-based educational strategies, even in HICs (Barry and others 2009; Mihalopoulos and others 2011).

A recent randomized control trial (RCT) on classroom-based cognitive behavioral therapy (CBT) for reducing symptoms of depression in adolescents found that despite high levels of fidelity and adherence, a universally provided CBT depression prevention program was not cost-effective, in part because of the relatively high cost per student and the marginal gain in health outcomes (Anderson and others 2014). In Chile, an HIC, a similar school-based RCT was implemented that compared a CBT depression prevention program with usual care with enhanced counseling; the results indicated that the program was not effective compared with usual care (Araya and others 2011). In India, peer education and teacher training in educational institutions that was provided as part of a multicomponent, population-based youth health promotion intervention had limited feasibility and effect because of several logistical and financial barriers (Balaji and others 2011). In Mauritius, evaluation of a school-based prevention program for adolescent depression showed short-term benefits to depression, hopelessness, coping skills, and self-esteem, but its sustainability has yet to be ascertained (Rivet-Duval, Heriot, and Hunt 2011).

These study findings can offer insights about which interventions are most likely to be acceptable and feasible as well as effective in the long term. In particular, it seems that the cost-effectiveness of more intensive, individual-based approaches such as CBT can be adversely affected by the cost of their implementation.

Community-Based Parenting Programs

Systematic reviews show that early child development and parenting skills training are effective in enhancing the cognitive and social skills of children under age five years, and the training promotes mental and social development (Mejia, Calam, and Sanders 2012; Merry and others 2012). Such programs are provided on a group, individual, or self-administered basis in a variety of settings, including health clinics, community centers, and schools, by different types of providers, such as health visitors, social workers, and psychologists. These differences influence the cost and cost-effectiveness of parenting programs. Studies in the United Kingdom indicate little difference between community-based and hospital-based implementations of this kind of program (Cunningham, Bremner, and Boyle 1995; Harrington and others 2000).

Cost-effectiveness studies in LMICs have yet to be conducted, but analyses in HICs indicate that such programs are cost-effective and pay for themselves if the averted costs of future ill-health are taken into account. In Australia, for example, Mihalopoulos and others (2007) assessed the costs and benefits of a stepped, multidisciplinary preventative family intervention called Positive Parenting Program (Triple P). The intervention is designed to prevent behavioral disorders in children by increasing parenting knowledge and skills and fostering emotional competence in children; the researchers found that the intervention costs less than the amount it saves, until the reduction in prevalence of conduct disorder falls below 7 percent, at which point net costs become positive. Similarly, in the United Kingdom, parenting programs are expected to be cost saving, with gross savings exceeding the average cost of the intervention by a factor of 8 to 1 (Knapp, McDaid, and Parsonage 2011). Since studies from HICs show such promise, it will be important to determine the feasibility, impact, and costs of these programs in lower-resourced settings.

Programs to Train Gatekeepers to Identify People with Mental Illness

As discussed in chapter 10 in this volume (Petersen and others 2015), mental health first aid training is commonly used at the community level to promote identification and case detection. For example, training of police officers can reduce stigma and improve care for people with MNS disorders (Krameddine and others 2013). There are no studies of the cost-effectiveness of such programs in LMICs; however, a study from Canada showed that a one-day training course significantly increased the recognition of mental health issues, improved efficiency in dealing with mental health issues, and decreased the use of weapons or physical interactions with individuals who were mentally ill. The training cost was US$120 per officer but led to significant cost savings of more than US$80,000 in the following six months (Krameddine and others 2013).

COST-EFFECTIVENESS OF CARE AND TREATMENT FOR MENTAL, NEUROLOGICAL, AND SUBSTANCE USE DISORDERS

Chapter 11 in this volume (Shidhaye, Lund, and Chisholm 2015) discusses health care services as a delivery platform for improving population mental health via three key delivery channels: self-care and informal health care; primary health care; and specialist health care. Chapter 11 also identifies several core strategies for strengthening the capacity of mental health systems through collaborative care, task sharing, and integration with existing health programs. The cost-effectiveness literature relating to care and treatment for MNS disorders is reviewed here in terms of these delivery channels and health system–strengthening strategies.

Self-Care and Informal Health Care

The evidence base on innovative methods that provide an alternative to facility-based services and have the potential to increase access to cost-effective treatment and care in LMICs remains relatively sparse. Yet such innovation will be essential to overcome the inadequate supply of and access to mental health specialists (Patel and others 2010). With the greater support for and diffusion of global mental health research and innovation in alternative models, such as case detection by community members and self-care via e-health or other technologies, greater awareness of the potential impact of such innovations is emerging (http://mhinnovation.net).

Evidence on the known effectiveness, feasibility, or cost-effectiveness remains limited for the purposes of informing program design. Even in HICs where systematic reviews of the efficacy, acceptability, and affordability of these approaches have been conducted, cost-effectiveness has not received significant attention. For example, despite a growing number of e-health and self-help randomized clinical trials conducted in HICs in the past decade, most studies fail to provide information on long-term clinical benefits, acceptability, or cost-effectiveness. This lack limits the usefulness of the studies for LMICs, which have more fragmented access to web-based information (Lewis, Pearce, and Bisson 2012; Martinez and others 2014; van Boeijen and others 2005). An example of the kind of information that can be garnered from economic evaluation of these technologies is a Swedish cost-effectiveness trial of Internet- versus group-based CBT for persons with social anxiety disorders (Hedman and others 2011). The study found that both interventions reduced overall societal costs appreciably and delivered similar health benefits to the target population; however, because the Internet-based CBT is less costly, it is the more cost-effective option.

The relative cost-effectiveness of traditional and complementary systems of medicine in the treatment of MNS disorders, vis-a-vis established biopsychosocial models of care, has not been evaluated, despite the fact that such systems of care are widely available and used in LMICs (Gureje and others 2015). This lack of evaluation reflects the highly heterogeneous nature of the practices undertaken, as well as a lack of established efficacy for them. Estimation of the costs and outcomes associated with a collaborative model of care involving the liaison between traditional and allopathic systems of medicine represents an important if challenging research question, especially in countries or regions where the practice of traditional medicine prevails.

Primary Health Care

With the increasing attention to mental health care in LMICs and growing evidence that improvements can be achieved with limited resources and impoverished populations, there has been a rise in country-level economic evaluations. Most of the economic analyses to date have been directed to the treatment of mental disorders in health care settings, particularly for mood (affective) disorders, such as depression, and nonaffective psychotic disorders, such as schizophrenia; trial-based and model-based evaluations have been undertaken.

A summary of country-level cost-effectiveness studies that report on the cost per healthy life year gained is shown in figure 12.1 and annex 12D.

National Studies

One of the first depression trials to include an economic dimension in LMICs was a stepped care, multicomponent program in Chile. The program comprised group intervention, monitoring of clinical progress and medication compliance, and coordinating of further management with primary care physicians (Araya and others 2006). The program was implemented by trained non-physician health care workers and assessed the cost-effectiveness of a task-shifting, stepped care approach to treatment. The results indicated that the innovative program was significantly more effective than the usual care of physician consultations combined with the prescription of antidepressants only and the program was achieved at a modest cost increase; it is now a nationally supported program.

In India, a study of a task-shifting approach to the treatment of depression and/or anxiety (MANAS trial)

Figure 12.1 Country-Specific Cost-Effectiveness of MNS Interventions
(cost per disability-adjusted life year averted or healthy life year gained, 2012 US$)

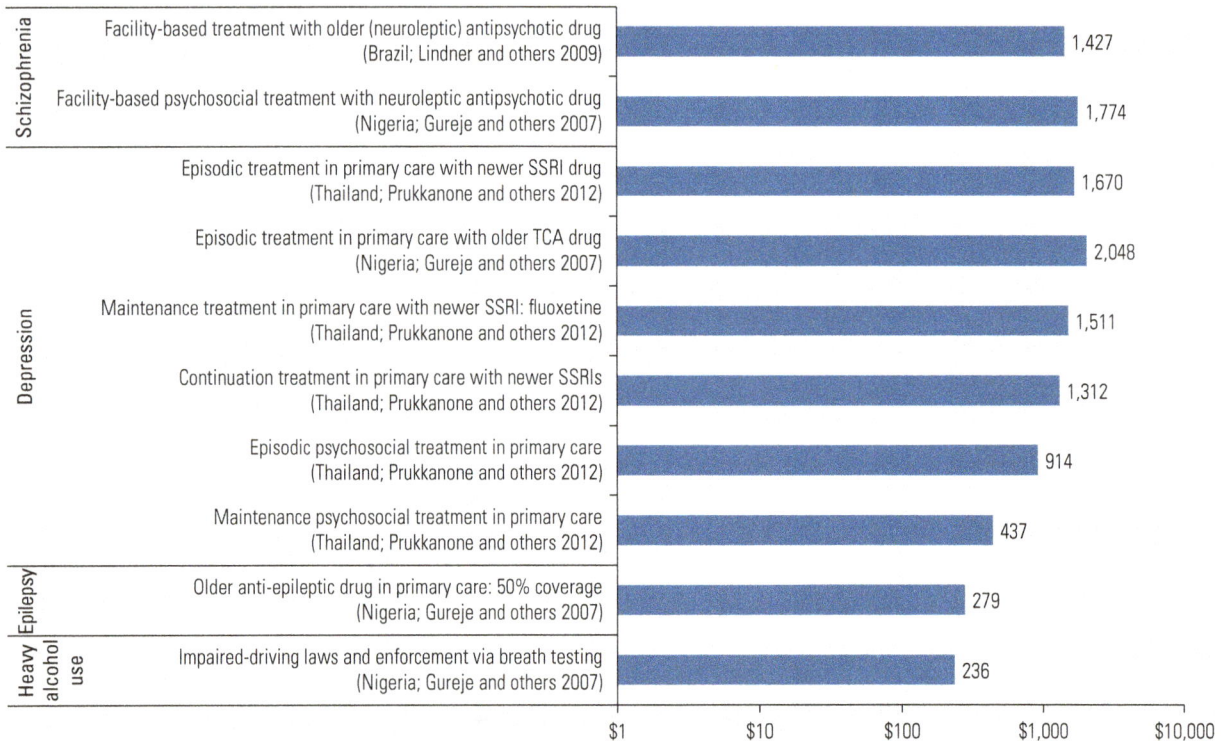

Note: ** = effects measured in quality-adjusted life years gained; all other effect estimates are measured as disability-adjusted life years averted; MNS = mental, neurological, and substance use; SSRI = selective serotonin reuptake inhibitor; TCA = tricyclic antidepressant. All reported cost-effectiveness estimates have been converted to 2012 US$.

involved trained lay health workers to provide psychosocial interventions as part of primary care. The intervention was found to be cost-effective and cost saving, and it overcame barriers posed by a shortage of mental health professionals (Buttorff and others 2012).

In other country studies, a modeling approach has been used to inform decisions on priority setting and resource allocation. In Thailand, lower cost yet equally effective generic antidepressants and CBT were found to be cost-effective interventions in the acute, continuation, and maintenance treatment phases of depression up to five years after its onset (Prukkanone and others 2012). Maintenance treatment using CBT was the single-most cost-effective strategy, but this finding has to be balanced against the shortage of trained mental health personnel available to deliver psychotherapy services. Applying the same methodological approach to schizophrenia, Phanthunane and others (2011) showed that despite the higher costs of including family psychoeducation, the inclusion of this psychosocial support element increases adherence to and outcomes from medication and is the most cost-effective option. Analysis of these factors helped Thailand to prioritize a strategy to use generic newer drugs as the first-line treatment, ideally in combination with family interventions, to increase health gains and lower hospitalization costs (Phanthunane and others 2011).

In Brazil, where differences in unit prices between older and newer drugs are more marked than in HICs and hospitalization costs are relatively low, cost-effectiveness and budget impact analyses have been conducted to select the most feasible and affordable drug therapy for the treatment of schizophrenia and depression. The use of newer atypical antipsychotic drugs for schizophrenia reduces the probability of hospitalization. But the analysis for Brazil found older neuroleptic drugs to be the more cost-effective strategy overall (Lindner and others 2009). For depression, drug costs represent a smaller share of the economic cost and did not affect the cost-effectiveness across competing alternatives. A budget impact analysis suggested that the addition of serotonin-norepinephrine reuptake inhibitors (SNRIs) for treating depression could generate cost savings to the health care system, given the overall lower average cost per patient treated (Machado and others 2007).

In Colombia, a cost-effectiveness analysis of three classes of antidepressants showed that the older tricyclic antidepressants had greater effectiveness and lower costs compared with the newer selective serotonin reuptake inhibitors and SNRIs. Colombia's lower hospitalization costs compared with Brazil's were the more important cost driver, and in this setting, the drug costs had a minimal impact. In summary, the cost-effectiveness of

antidepressants depends on the relative effectiveness of the choice of drugs, but it is likely determined by budget constraints, pricing policies, and relative hospital costs (Machado and others 2008).

In Nigeria, treating schizophrenia had higher costs per treated case; however, given the larger proportion of the population suffering from depression, the total costs for treating depression were higher (Gureje and others 2007). Cost-effective treatment options for schizophrenia include community-based interventions that combine older antipsychotic drugs with psychosocial treatment or case management. The use of newer atypical antipsychotic drugs without supportive psychosocial therapy was found to be the least cost-effective treatment strategy.

The literature offers very little guidance for what may be cost-effective for other MNS disorders in LMICs, such as dementia, drug use disorders, and childhood disorders. The limited economic evaluations for dementia have been conducted in HICs, focusing on burden and mood, with only a few studies capturing health gains expressed as QALYs (Jones, Edwards, and Hounsome 2012). In the United Kingdom, for example, a manual-based coping strategy program for promoting the mental health of caregivers of people with dementia was found to be cost-effective in cost per QALY terms (Livingston and others 2014). For attention-deficit hyperactivity disorder (ADHD), consistent evidence from HICs demonstrates that drug therapy is cost-effective compared with no treatment or behavioral therapy. None of the cost-effectiveness studies were relevant for adults, in whom ADHD is a growing concern, or for long-term cost-effectiveness beyond six months (King and others 2006; Wu and others 2012).

Very little evidence is available for parent training and education programs for childhood disorders, although these may also offer cost-effective solutions for conduct disorder (Dretzke and others 2005). ADHD and dementia are characterized by a high economic burden on care systems and caregivers of children, adolescents, and the elderly. Evidence shows there is an increase in the indirect costs to caregivers in terms of increased absenteeism and lost productivity associated with managing a family member's care (Matza, Paramore, and Prasad 2005). Findings from HICs are not necessarily transferable to LMICs, given the differences in the recognition, diagnosis, and health care system costs. Yet, as demographic and economic transitions occur, dementia and disorders in childhood and adolescence are likely to rise in prominence (Albanese and others 2011).

There is also a dearth of economic evidence to guide and support drug policy and resource allocation decisions. Even in HICs, evidence is restricted to one or two studies of specific treatment modalities, such as substitution or maintenance treatment of opioid dependence. In Australia, for example, methadone maintenance treatment and buprenorphine maintenance treatment were found to lead to appreciable increases in heroin-free days at an acceptable and not significantly different level of cost-effectiveness (Doran 2005; Harris, Gospodarevskaya, and Ritter 2005). In countries where the spread of HIV is being fueled by injecting drug users, methadone maintenance programs can also be an effective and cost-effective strategy for HIV prevention, as evidenced by a study undertaken in Belarus, where the average cost per averted HIV infection was projected at less than US$500 (Kumaranayake and others 2004).

International Studies

Cost-effectiveness modeling has also been conducted at the regional and international levels. Although these levels lack specificity to a national decision-making context, they can inform priority-setting agendas at the national and international levels, including investment decisions by donors and nongovernmental organizations.

The primary source of evidence for MNS disorders to date comes from the WHO-CHOICE program (Chisholm 2005; Chisholm and Saxena 2012; Hyman and others 2006). An advantage of the WHO-CHOICE approach is its application of a consistent methodology, which enables like-with-like comparisons to be made between different disorders and geographical regions. Table 12.1 shows the comparative cost-effectiveness of a range of interventions for addressing MNS disorders in different regions of the world, relative to a situation of no intervention. Because each intervention is compared with a situation of no treatment, the resulting metric is called an average, as opposed to incremental, cost-effectiveness ratio.

The results are reported for six geographically distinct groupings of LMICs that are used by the World Bank for reporting purposes. Inevitably, such country groupings contain substantial sociocultural as well as economic heterogeneity, which limits their applicability to particular contexts or populations. Previously published and updated findings (Chisholm and Saxena 2012; Hyman and others 2006) have been converted here to 2012 US$ values, based on International Monetary Fund inflation estimates, to enable comparison with other cost and cost-effectiveness information presented in this and other DCP-3 volumes. The exception to this price conversion process relates to newer psychotropic medications, such as fluoxetine for depression or risperidone for

psychotic disorders, which are now produced in several countries under nonbranded, generic licenses and can be purchased for approximately 10 times less than a decade ago.

As long as these lower, generic prices of newer antidepressant and antipsychotic medications are sought out and applied, the previously demonstrated cost-effectiveness superiority of interventions using older drugs for treating schizophrenia and depression essentially disappears, meaning that there is little reason to choose between them on efficiency grounds (see table 12.1). What remains clear, however, is that drug treatment alone does not constitute the most cost-effective option for treating mental disorders; rather, it is the combination of pharmacological and psychosocial treatment that leads to the best overall balance of cost and health outcome for severe mental disorders.

Across the six regions considered, the average cost per healthy life year gained for such a combination strategy—the most cost-effective of the strategies considered—ranges from US$3,300 to US$14,000 for schizophrenia and bipolar disorder. For depression, treatment in primary health care on an episodic basis costs between US$800 and US$3,500 per healthy life year gained; for a little more cost, as well as more overall health gain in the population, treatment on a proactive, maintenance basis is also a cost-effective alternative, because so many persons experience recurrent episodes (US$1,300–US$4,900 per healthy life year gained). Differences in cost per healthy life year gained are largely driven by the cost of labor and contacts with the health care system (relatively higher in Latin America and the Caribbean and relatively lower in Sub-Saharan Africa and South Asia).

Other disorders that can be appropriately managed in nonspecialist health care settings and that have been subjected to economic evaluation cover neurological disorders (epilepsy and migraine) and substance use disorders (harmful alcohol use). WHO-CHOICE analyses conducted for these disorders, again updated to 2012 prices, indicate that they are at least as cost-effective to treat as the aforementioned mental disorders (Chisholm 2005; Linde, Chisholm, and Steiner 2015; Rehm and others 2006). Table 12.1 indicates that a year of healthy life can be obtained for less than US$1,000 by offering brief interventions to persons with alcohol use disorders, and for between US$600 and US$2,500 by treating epilepsy with first-line anti-epileptic drugs. For migraine, a recent multicountry study using WHO-CHOICE methods has been completed and is highlighted in box 12.1.

Table 12.1 Regional Cost-Effectiveness of Interventions for MNS Disorders
(cost per disability-adjusted life year averted or healthy life year gained, 2012 US$)

Disorder: intervention	World Bank region					
	Sub-Saharan Africa	Latin America and the Caribbean	Middle East and North Africa	Europe and Central Asia	South Asia	East Asia and Pacific
Schizophrenia						
SCZ-1: community-based treatment with older (neuroleptic) antipsychotic drug	8,390	20,465	21,263	13,799	4,915	5,688
SCZ-2: community-based treatment with newer (atypical) antipsychotic drug	7,978	18,961	19,755	12,891	4,718	5,414
SCZ-3: community-based treatment with older antipsychotic drug + psychosocial treatment	6,005	13,858	14,413	11,396	3,490	3,865
SCZ-4: community-based treatment with newer antipsychotic drug + psychosocial treatment	6,014	13,649	14,192	11,233	3,523	3,890
Bipolar disorder						
BIP-1: community-based treatment with older mood stabilizer drug (lithium)	4,571	14,261	12,120	9,999	3,392	4,402
BIP-2: community-based treatment with newer mood stabilizer drug (valproate)	7,930	16,470	13,911	12,339	5,047	5,839
BIP-3: community-based treatment with older mood stabilizer drug + psychosocial care	4,516	13,292	11,440	9,329	3,281	4,136
BIP-4: community-based treatment with newer mood stabilizer drug + psychosocial care	7,583	15,287	13,094	11,426	4,784	5,434
Depression						
DEP-1: episodic treatment in primary care with older antidepressant drug (TCAs)	1,410	3,491	3,171	2,668	786	899
DEP-2: episodic treatment in primary care with newer antidepressant drug (SSRIs)	1,395	3,361	3,057	2,456	788	894
DEP-3: episodic psychosocial treatment in primary care	2,189	4,838	4,594	2,724	1,161	1,223
DEP-4: episodic psychosocial treatment + older antidepressant	2,083	4,427	4,232	2,722	1,128	1,178
DEP-5: episodic psychosocial treatment + newer antidepressant	2,144	4,477	4,285	2,660	1,167	1,218
DEP-6: maintenance psychosocial treatment + older antidepressant	2,461	4,866	4,783	3,225	1,315	1,373
DEP-7: maintenance psychosocial treatment + newer antidepressant	2,532	4,927	4,847	3,137	1,367	1,425
Alcohol use disorders						
ALC-8: brief physician advice in primary care	407	878	—	494	684	332
Epilepsy						
EPI-1: older anti-epileptic drug in primary care	694	1,511	1,450	2,516	600	1,057
EPI-2: newer anti-epileptic drug in primary care	1,884	2,854	2,877	4,115	1,639	2,249

Sources: Chisholm and Saxena 2012; Hyman and others 2006.
Note: MNS = mental, neurological, and substance use; TCAs = tricyclic antidepressants; SSRIs = selective serotonin reuptake inhibitors; — = not available.

Cost-Effectiveness of Interventions for Migraine

A WHO-CHOICE (World Health Organization–CHOosing Interventions that are Cost-Effective) analysis was conducted for a selected core set of interventions for migraine in four countries: China, India, the Russian Federation, and Zambia. The analysis included first-line analgesics, such as acetylsalicylic acid 1,000 milligrams (mg), and second-line medications, such as sumatriptan 50 mg, for acute treatment of attacks. It was assumed that the latter would be used only by nonresponders to first-line medications (a stepped care treatment paradigm). The analysis included prophylactic drugs, such as amitriptyline 100 mg daily. The expected consequences of adding consumer education, in the form of posters and leaflets in pharmacies explaining how to acquire and use these medications, and training for health care providers were also modeled. Compared with no treatment, the cost per healthy

life year gained ranged from less than US$100 for acute management with simple analgesics to thousands or even tens of thousands of US$ for treatment of analgesic nonresponders with triptans.

The most cost-effective strategy by far is acute management with simple analgesics; it was less than US$100 per disability-adjusted life year averted and therefore represents a highly cost-effective use of resources for health. Adding consumer education and improving adherence has a small upward influence on cost-effectiveness. Compared with no treatment at all, this strategy is less than US$150 per healthy life year gained; compared with use of simple analgesics without consumer education, the incremental cost to be paid to obtain one extra healthy life year rises to US$600.

Source: Linde, Chisholm, and Steiner 2015.

Specialist Health Care

Specialized mental health care covers hospital-based outpatient and inpatient care for acute and severe episodes or cases of mental disorder. In many LMICs, mental hospitals absorb a disproportionate share of the government mental health budget—over 70 percent in many cases—yet such institutions are commonly associated with isolation, human rights violations, and poor outcomes. Such expenditure patterns also curb the development of more equitable and cost-effective community-based services.

The dramatic deinstitutionalization observed in most HICs in recent decades has been accompanied by a certain amount of economic research into the costs, needs, and outcomes of persons relocated into community-based care. Such research has shown that community-based care is certainly associated with better health and social outcomes, and it is not inherently more costly than institutions, once account is taken of individuals' needs and the quality of care (Knapp and others 2011). New community-based care arrangements could be more expensive than long-stay hospital care, but they may still be seen as more cost-effective because, when appropriately set up and managed, they deliver better health and economic outcomes. Accordingly, such a process of deinstitutionalization should not be predicated on

the basis of expected cost savings; inadequate expenditure on community-based care is quite likely to result in poor outcomes for the individuals and families concerned (Knapp and others 2011).

Detailed analysis of this kind has not been conducted in the context of ongoing efforts to relocate services in LMICs. However, a simple comparison of the cost of a community-based versus hospital-based service model has been carried out as part of the WHO-CHOICE analysis for schizophrenia and bipolar affective disorder. For schizophrenia, the costs of the hospital-based service model exceeded those of the community-based service model by 33–50 percent, reflecting greater use of resource-intensive services, such as acute and long-term psychiatric inpatient care (Chisholm 2005; Chisholm and others 2008). Even if one assumes no improved outcomes for persons treated under the community-based service model, there is a clear difference in terms of cost-effectiveness; the costs of the community-based service model are 25–40 percent lower.

Relocating services and resources away from long-stay mental hospitals toward nonspecialized health settings is a key financing issue for mental health systems. Efforts to change the balance of mental health care are often hindered by a lack of appropriate transitional funding. Transitional or dual funding is required over a period of time to build up appropriate community-based services before residents of long-term institutions can be relocated. It is crucial to present an evidence-based case for relocating the locus of care, not only on the grounds of equity, human rights, and user satisfaction, but also on the grounds of financial feasibility over a defined transitional period.

AFFORDABILITY: COSTS OF INTERVENTION SCALE-UP

The finding that interventions for the prevention and treatment of a range of MNS disorders have been cost-effective in LMICs does not necessarily translate into their affordability, especially given very low budget allocations for mental health. In addition to evidence on the effectiveness and cost-effectiveness of different policy or treatment options, therefore, information is also needed on the feasibility and acceptability of interventions, including their financial feasibility or affordability. In this section, we provide estimates of the expected costs of scaling up the delivery of a set of cost-effective policies and intervention strategies, including demand reduction measures for harmful alcohol use at the population level, school-based mental health promotion at the community level, and treatment of priority MNS disorders in nonspecialized health care settings.

Demand Reduction Strategies for Harmful Alcohol Use

The economic evidence presented earlier in this chapter indicates that the most cost-effective strategy for reducing alcohol consumption is raising taxes or prices on alcohol products, followed by banning alcohol advertising, restricting access to alcohol, and enforcing drinking and driving legislation. Analysis of the costs of scaling up these interventions in LMICs was undertaken by the WHO in preparation for the High-Level Meeting on Non-communicable Diseases (WHO 2011). The overall annual cost per capita of implementing the constituent elements of an alcohol demand reduction strategy was estimated for countries with low versus middle incomes. The median cost ranges from less than US$0.10 per capita for low-income countries (LICs) and lower-middle-income countries to around US$0.25 for upper-middle-income countries (figure 12.2). These costs are driven by human resource needs for program management and enforcement of alcohol-related laws and policies, as well as media-related expenses.

The variability around the median cost of implementation results from large intercountry differences in the prevalence of alcohol use. Application of the same costing

Figure 12.2 Cost of Scaling Up Population-Based Alcohol Control Measures in Low- and Middle-Income Countries

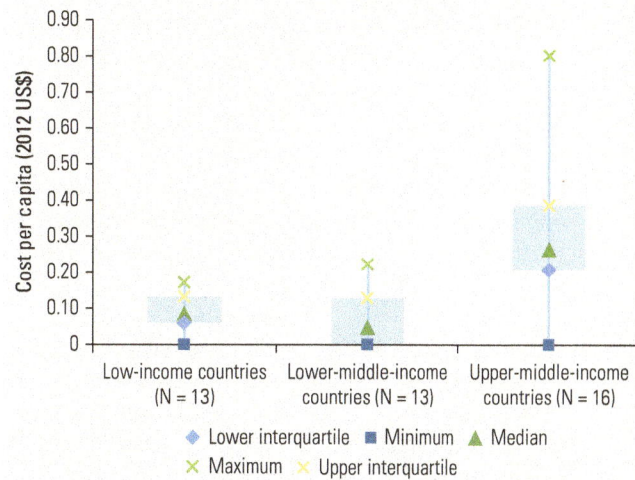

Source: WHO 2011.
Note: N = number.

methods to three illustrative countries from these different income strata—Ethiopia, India, and Mexico—yields similar results (US$0.06, US$0.10, and US$0.24, respectively). Although such per capita costs indicate that these strategies are inherently affordable, total costs can add up quickly. This is particularly the case in larger countries, such as Nigeria, where government policies that increase taxation on alcohol are expected to cost US$13 million per year, and policies such as roadside breath testing are expected to cost even more (US$25 million per year at 80 percent coverage) (Gureje and others 2007).

Social Emotional Learning Programs

As documented in chapter 10 in this volume (Petersen and others 2015), sufficient evidence exists from LMICs and HICs to consider universal and targeted SEL programs as best practice policies for countries to implement. This finding is particularly true when teachers and school counselors can be trained to deliver these interventions by integrating social and emotional learning and life skills development in life orientation curricula.

The cost of implementing school-based SEL interventions in the context of LMICs has not yet been estimated, so an analysis was undertaken for the specific purpose of this volume for a selection of countries—Ethiopia, India, Mauritius, and Mexico—using methods already developed for micro-costing of population-based alcohol control strategies (WHO 2011). In addition, the analysis used data from a psychosocial intervention to prevent depression in adolescents ages 12 to 16 years in Mauritius (Rivet-Duval, Heriot, and Hunt 2011). The Resourceful

Adolescent Programme–Adolescent version (RAP-A) showed that 11 hourly psychosocial sessions led to short-term benefits to depression, hopelessness, coping skills, and self-esteem; benefits to coping skills and self-esteem were sustained at follow-up after six months.

For costing this intervention, we assessed the annual budgetary impact associated with the implementation of the program among all 12-year-olds in the local population, who make up 0.8–1.4 percent of the total population in the selected countries. The health educators, who are teachers, are assumed to work full-time on this program, visiting and delivering the intervention at different schools within municipalities or districts (six sessions per day). If teachers deliver the RAP-A program on a part-time basis, training costs—which include training of trainers at the national level and subnational courses each year for the health educators—will be higher. For every set of 20 health educators, we included one supervisor; central administration and program management costs were also included.

Based on 220 school days per year and 20 students per session, 1.7–2.8 full-time health educators would be needed to deliver the intervention at scale for a district of one million persons (table 12.2). Country-specific unit cost estimates taken from the WHO-CHOICE database (http://www.who.int/choice/costs) were used to place a monetary value on these various resource inputs. The resulting cost of implementing this program at full scale (100 percent coverage) ranges from US$0.03 per head of population in Ethiopia and India to US$0.11 in Mexico and US$0.24 in Mauritius, reflecting higher salary and other input costs. These findings indicate that school-based SEL interventions represent a low-cost strategy for promoting adolescent mental health. More information about and evaluation of the long-term effectiveness of programs such as RAP-A is needed.

Mental Health Care in Nonspecialized Treatment Settings

Successful scaling up of mental health services involves putting together a range of human, physical, and other resource inputs to deliver interventions and services capable of improving mental health and related outcomes. Accordingly, an essential element of evidence-based mental health service planning and scale-up relates to an assessment of what resources are required to deliver services to the population in need and to meet program goals. However, the lack of complete or reliable local epidemiological and resource data has often thwarted such efforts in many countries, although that is changing with the generation of national mental health profiles (see, for example, WHO's mental health ATLAS database, http://apps.who.int/globalatlas).

Empirical studies offer insights into average treatment costs for depression and schizophrenia, when using medication alone or in combination with psychotherapy (annex 12E). Using older antidepressant drugs and providing stepped care tailored to the needs of patients has relatively low annual costs per case of depression, from US$107 in India to less than US$200 in Nigeria (Buttorff and others 2012; Gureje and others 2007). Similarly, the annual cost per treated case of epilepsy is relatively low; in Nigeria, older anti-epileptic drugs are less than US$100 per patient per year. Schizophrenia is generally more expensive to treat per person, using drug therapy alone, than either depression or epilepsy. Schizophrenia treatment costs are more likely to vary widely across countries, depending on the combination of inpatient and outpatient treatment and the antipsychotic medications used.

In Nigeria, treating schizophrenia with older antipsychotic drugs falls between US$200 and US$300; newer antipsychotic drugs cost more than US$6,000 per year. In Brazil, treatment with older, first-generation antipsychotic drugs is as low as US$120 per patient per year; second-generation drugs cost more than US$4,000 per person annually (Lindner and others 2009). In Thailand, direct medical costs for drug treatment in combination with family interventions are US$764 per patient per year. The variability in costs per person treated is in part due to the small number of studies that have explored the costs of different combinations of interventions and are not necessarily comparable. Accordingly, the studies are not particularly useful for estimating the total cost of an essential package of mental health services. Total costs also

Table 12.2 Cost of Implementing Resourceful Adolescent Programme–Adolescent Version in Four Countries

Cost item	Ethiopia	India	Mexico	Mauritius
Total population age 12 years (%)	1.4	1.1	1.0	0.8
Health educators needed per 1 million population (at 100% coverage)	2.8	2.3	2.1	1.7
Cost per head of population at 100% coverage (US$)	0.03	0.03	0.11	0.24

Source: World Health Organization, CHOICE (database), http://www.who.int/choice/costs.

vary considerably among countries, given their different epidemiological mental health profiles, national policies, and access to health care.

Analytical tools and methods for financial planning have been developed for many disease areas and programs; these have been used to estimate the cost of significantly scaling up the delivery of a specified package of mental health care in LMICs (Chisholm, Lund, and Saxena 2007). These authors carried out a financial analysis to estimate the expenditures needed to scale up over a 10-year period the delivery of a specified mental health care package, comprising pharmacological and/or psychosocial treatment for schizophrenia, bipolar disorder, depression, and hazardous alcohol use. Current service levels in 12 selected LMICs were established using the WHO-AIMS (Assessment Instrument for Mental Health Systems) assessment tool.

The analysis estimated the costs to meet the specified target coverage levels of 80 percent of cases with psychosis and bipolar disorder, and 25–33 percent of cases with depression and risky drinking. Spending for this package would need to be approximately US$2.00 per capita in LICs (compared with current spending of US$0.10–US$0.20), and US$3.00–US$4.00 in middle-income countries. For a middle-income country of 50 million people, total annual spending on the package would amount to between US$150 million and US$200 million. A subsequent, updated assessment of the comparative cost-effectiveness analysis of 44 neuropsychiatric interventions in two WHO subregions (one in Sub-Saharan Africa, the other in South Asia) estimated that the annual cost of delivering a defined package of interventions for schizophrenia, depression, epilepsy, and alcohol use disorders would be US$3–US$4 per capita (Chisholm and Saxena 2012).

This approach to service costing has been applied more recently to the subnational context of scaling up mental health services in LMICs, as part of the PRogramme for Improving Mental health carE (PRIME) study being conducted at the district level in Ethiopia, India, Nepal, South Africa, and Uganda (Lund and others 2012). The costing analysis was carried out to inform local PRIME country teams about the expected resource implications and financial feasibility associated with the implementation of their respective district mental health care plans (Chisholm, Burman-Roy, and others 2015). The results indicated that, starting from a generally very low base of mental health service coverage and expenditure, the cost of scaled-up provision in nonspecialist health care settings of an evidence-based package of care that included psychosis, depression, alcohol use disorders and, in some countries, epilepsy, range from US$0.25 to US$0.70 per capita in four of the five districts

assessed (figure 12.3). For a district with a total population of one million persons, therefore, an annual outlay of US$250,000–US$700,000 would be required to reach the specified target coverage levels. The outlier is South Africa, where the prevailing price and quantity of health care service inputs are much higher. The cost per capita of delivering the specified care package at target coverage levels in the South African district approaches US$2.50 per capita; this is higher than in the other countries but relatively low in the context of current health spending levels in South Africa.

Getting to target levels of annual spending in each district would necessitate a steady budgetary increase, estimated at US$0.02–US$0.11 extra per head of population per year if a 10-year period is used. Extending the cost estimation to take into account program management and some utilization of specialist, hospital-based services by the district population increases these baseline cost projections, substantially so in India and South Africa (by at least 100 percent) and modestly so in the other three sites (by approximately 20 percent). These upper cost estimates amount to only 1 percent of total current health spending per capita in South Africa and up to 7 percent in Ethiopia.

A limitation of the costing methods used for this recent analysis is that they are unable to take proper account of critical health system constraints to service scale-up, such as midterm expenditure caps, supply-side bottlenecks in recruiting staff or accessing essential medicines, and inadequate referral and supervision mechanisms. Such constraints can substantially alter the actual level of program implementation or achievement. Even if such supply-side factors were managed successfully, there is the additional concern that demand for and actual uptake of available services do not match the desired levels of effective coverage, for example because of the influence on help-seeking behaviors of stigma around mental illness. Broader environmental and political factors can likewise impact the success or efficiency of implemented strategies of care or prevention.

CONCLUSIONS

This chapter reviewed the available evidence concerning the cost and cost-effectiveness of interventions for the protection, prevention, and treatment of MNS disorders. The review has shown that there is a considerably greater economic evidence base now than there was when *Disease Control Priorities in Developing Countries,* first edition, was published (Jamison and others 1993). Seminal clinical trials of the treatment of common mental disorders in LMICs have included a cost-effectiveness component. Country- and regional-level economic

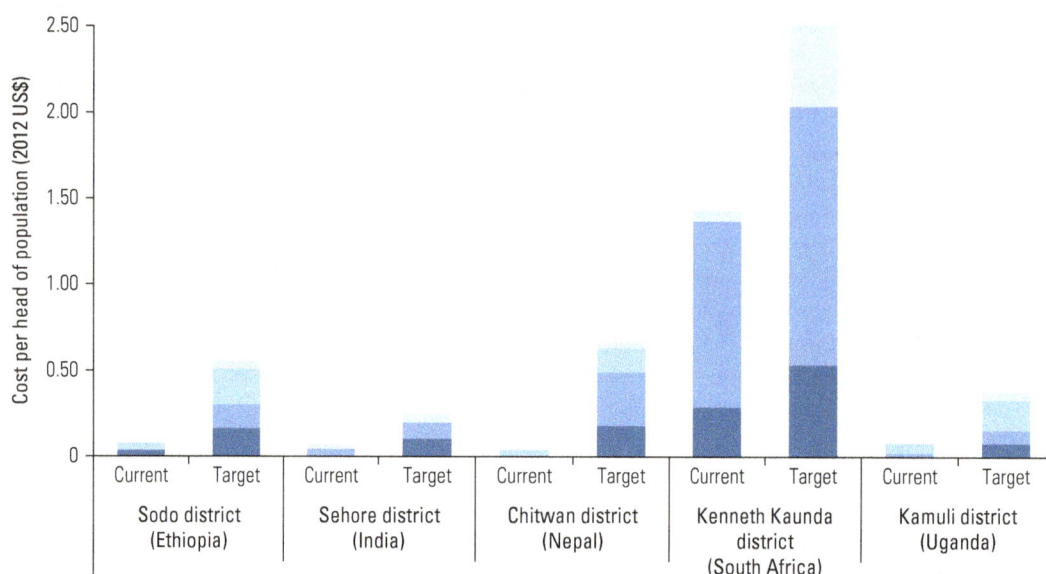

Figure 12.3 Costs of Scaling Up a Mental Health Care Package in Nonspecialized Health Care Settings in Five Low- and Middle-Income Country Districts

| | Sodo district (Ethiopia) | | Sehore district (India) | | Chitwan district (Nepal) | | Kenneth Kaunda district (South Africa) | | Kamuli district (Uganda) | |
	Current	Target	Current	Target	Current	Target	Current	Target	Current	Target
Alcohol use disorders	$0.006	$0.052	$0.023	$0.057	$0.002	$0.035	$0.061	$0.477	$0.003	$0.054
Epilepsy	$0.036	$0.210	$0	$0	$0.028	$0.136	$0	$0	$0.062	$0.184
Psychosis	$0.017	$0.144	$0.030	$0.098	$0.007	$0.317	$1.081	$1.505	$0.011	$0.072
Depression	$0.024	$0.155	$0.014	$0.097	$0.006	$0.178	$0.284	$0.530	$0.007	$0.073

Source: Chisholm, Burman-Roy, and others 2015.

modeling studies have been conducted for a range of disorders, permitting comparison of relative cost-effectiveness with other DCPs. Arguably, there is now sufficient evidence to counteract or debunk the overgeneralized claim that treatment of mental disorders is not a cost-effective use of scarce health care resources.

As with any other area of health, the reality is that the range of possible interventions varies a great deal with respect to their cost-effectiveness. An analysis of 500 single and combined interventions assessed by the WHO-CHOICE project for the prevention and control of noncommunicable diseases and injuries in two LMIC regions found that costs differed by at least three orders of magnitude (from a few cents to more than US$10 per capita), as did cost-effectiveness (from US$10 to more than US$100,000 per healthy life year gained) (Chisholm and others 2012).

In the economic analysis for MNS disorders in this series, Chisholm and Saxena (2012) found a very substantial range of cost-effectiveness, with alcohol control measures, drug treatment for epilepsy, and depression treatment identified as offering the best value for money in the two WHO subregions assessed (one in Sub-Saharan

Africa, the other in South-East Asia). This wide range of cost-effectiveness points to the importance of carefully evaluating and choosing an appropriate set of interventions for scaled-up investment and implementation; selecting an inefficient set will waste money and limit potential health gains. Unfortunately, however, a high proportion of mental health budgets is being used in the provision of the least cost-effective interventions, such as long-term inpatient treatment of severe mental disorders in mental hospitals. Very little is invested in more cost-effective strategies, including the community-based provision of adjuvant psychosocial treatment for severe mental disorders, and measures to reduce access to or marketing of alcohol.

Ultimately, policies are enacted and resources allocated at the level of individual countries. It is important that more economic evidence be generated alongside clinical trials or other evaluations at the national level, rather than relying on international estimates that may lack sensitivity to local priorities or health system characteristics. Our review highlighted several cost-effectiveness studies from high as well as lower-income country settings to show the informational and policy value of such evaluations. Such studies are particularly needed in areas where there is currently a dearth of evidence, including prevention and treatment of childhood disorders, drug use disorders, community-based parenting programs, suicide prevention, and dementia care. The use of comparable costing methods and outcome measurements, that should ideally also incorporate the impact of interventions on income, employment, or poverty, will greatly serve to build up a cogent international evidence base for greater investment in the care and prevention of MNS disorders.

Similarly, the use and application of available tools and methods for costing interventions can help to articulate in budgetary terms the scaling-up or universal coverage goals that a country has set for itself and place financial planning on a firmer footing. Costing analysis to date, including that presented in this chapter, has indicated that significantly scaled-up delivery of a prioritized, evidence-based set of interventions is actually far from being unaffordable in absolute terms. What remains strikingly high is the funding gap between what is needed and what is available, and it is this fact that can make the *relative* increase in budgetary allocations appear daunting in many LICs. Scaling up needs time, not only to build human resource and system capacity, but also to allow for the reallocation of resources away from less efficient uses (including mental hospitals) and the allocation of new domestic or international resources for mental health system development.

ANNEXES

Annexes to this chapter are as follows. They are available at http://www.dcp-3.org/mentalhealth.

- Annex 12A. List of Search Terms
- Annex 12B. Flow Chart and Search Statistics of Identification, Screening, and Eligibility of Included Studies for Mental, Neurological, and Substance Use Disorders
- Annex 12C. List of Studies for Costs and Cost-Effectiveness
- Annex 12D. Cost-Effectiveness Results by Intervention
- Annex 12E. Cost Estimates by Intervention

NOTES

Disclaimer: Dan Chisholm is a staff member of the World Health Organization. The author alone is responsible for the views expressed in this publication, and they do not necessarily represent the decisions, policy, or views of the World Health Organization.

World Bank Income Classifications as of July 2014 are as follows, based on estimates of gross national income (GNI) per capita for 2013:

- Low-income countries (LICs) = US$1,045 or less
- Middle-income countries (MICs) are subdivided:
  a) lower-middle-income = US$1,046 to US$4,125
  b) upper-middle-income (UMICs) = US$4,126 to US$12,745
- High-income countries (HICs) = US$12,746 or more.

REFERENCES

Albanese, E., Z. Liu, D. Acosta, M. Guerra, Y. Huang, and others. 2011. "Equity in the Delivery of Community Healthcare to Older People: Findings from 10/66 Dementia Research Group Cross-Sectional Surveys in Latin America, China, India and Nigeria." *BMC Health Services Research* 11: 153.

Anderson, P., D. Chisholm, and D. Fuhr. 2009. "Effectiveness and Cost-Effectiveness of Policies and Programmes to Reduce the Harm Caused by Alcohol." *The Lancet* 373: 2234–46.

Anderson, R., O. Ukoumunne, K. Sayal, R. Phillips, J. Taylor, and others. 2014. "Cost-Effectiveness of Classroom-Based Cognitive Behaviour Therapy in Reducing Symptoms of Depression in Adolescents: A Trial-Based Analysis." *Journal of Child Psychology and Psychiatry* 55 (12): 1390–77.

Araya, R., T. Flynn, G. Rojas, R. Fritsch, and G. Simon. 2006. "Cost-Effectiveness of a Primary Care Treatment Program for Depression in Low-Income Women in Santiago, Chile." *American Journal of Psychiatry* 163 (8): 1379–87.

Araya, R., A. Montgomery, R. Fritsch, D. Gunnell, P. Stallard, and others. 2011. "School-Based Intervention to Improve the Mental Health of Low-Income, Secondary School Students in Santiago, Chile (YPSA): Study Protocol for a Randomized Controlled Trial." *Trials* 12 (49): 49.

Balaji, M., T. Andrews, G. Andrew, and V. Patel. 2011. "The Acceptability, Feasibility, and Effectiveness of a Population-Based Intervention to Promote Youth Health: An Exploratory Study in Goa, India." *Journal of Adolescent Health* 48 (5): 453–60.

Barry, M., R. Canavan, A. Clarke, C. Dempsey, and M. O'Sullivan. 2009. *Review of Evidence-Based Mental Health Promotion and Primary/Secondary Prevention.* Report prepared for the Department of Health, London. Galway, Ireland: Health Promotion Research Centre, National University of Ireland.

Buttorff, C., R. Hock, H. Weiss, S. Naik, R. Araya, and others. 2012. "Economic Evaluation of a Task-Shifting Intervention for Common Mental Disorders in India." *Bulletin of the World Health Organization* 90: 813–21.

Chisholm, D. 2005. "Choosing Cost-Effective Interventions in Psychiatry: Results from the CHOICE Programme of the World Health Organization." *World Psychiatry* 4: 37–44.

Chisholm, D., R. Baltussen, D. Evans, G. Ginsberg, J. Lauer, and others. 2012. "What Are the Priorities for Prevention and Control of Non-Communicable Diseases and Injuries in

Sub-Saharan Africa and South East Asia?" *British Medical Journal* 344: e586.

Chisholm, D., S. Burman-Roy, A. Fekadu, T. Kathree, D. Kizza, and others. 2015. "Estimating the Cost of Implementing District Mental Health Care Plans in Five Low- and Middle-Income Countries: The PRIME Study." *British Journal of Psychiatry* doi:10.1192/bjp.bp.114.153866.

Chisholm, D., O. Gureje, S. Saldivia, M. Villalón Calderón, R. Wickremasinghe, and others. 2008. "Schizophrenia Treatment in the Developing World: An Interregional and Multinational Cost-Effectiveness Analysis." *Bulletin of the World Health Organization* 86: 542–51.

Chisholm, D., K. A. Johansson, N. Raykar, I. Megiddo, A. Nigam, and others. 2015. "Moving Toward Universal Health Coverage for Mental, Neurological, and Substance Use Disorders: An Extended Cost-Effectiveness Analysis." In *Disease Control Priorities* (third edition): Volume 4, *Mental, Neurological, and Substance Use Disorders*, edited by V. Patel, D. Chisholm, T. Dua, R. Laxminarayan, and M. E. Medina-Mora. Washington, DC: World Bank.

Chisholm, D., C. Lund, and S. Saxena. 2007. "Cost of Scaling Up Mental Healthcare in Low- and Middle-Income Countries." *British Journal of Psychiatry* 191 (6): 528–35.

Chisholm, D., and S. Saxena. 2012. "Cost Effectiveness of Strategies to Combat Neuropsychiatric Conditions in Sub-Saharan Africa and South East Asia: Mathematical Modelling Study." *British Medical Journal* 344: e609.

Cunningham, C. E., R. Bremner, and M. Boyle. 1995. "Large Group Community-Based Parenting Programs for Families of Preschoolers at Risk for Disruptive Behaviour Disorders: Utilization, Cost-Effectiveness and Outcome." *Journal of Child Psychology and Psychiatry* 36: 1141–59.

Doran, C. M. 2005. "Buprenorphine, Buprenorphine/Naloxone and Methadone Maintenance: A Cost-Effectiveness Analysis." *Expert Review of Pharmacoeconomics and Outcomes Research* 5 (5): 583–91. doi:http://dx.doi.org/10.1586/14737167.5.5.583.

Dretzke, J., E. Frew, C. Davenport, J. Barlow, S. Stewart-Brown, and others. 2005. "The Effectiveness and Cost-Effectiveness of Parent Training/Education Programmes for the Treatment of Conduct Disorder, Including Oppositional Defiant Disorder in Children." *Health Technology Assessment* 9 (50): iii, ix-x, 1–233.

Drummond, M. F., M. Sculpher, G. W. Torrance, B. O'Brien, and G. L. Stoddart. 2005. *Methods for the Economic Evaluation of Health Care Programmes*, 3rd ed. New York: Oxford University Press.

Gureje, O., D. Chisholm, L. Kola, V. Lasebikan, and S. Saxena. 2007. "Cost-Effectiveness of an Essential Mental Health Intervention Package in Nigeria." *World Psychiatry* 6: 42–48.

Gureje, O., G. Nortje, V. Makanjuola, B. Oladeji, S. Seedat, and others. 2015. "The Role of Global Traditional and Complementary Systems of Medicine in the Treatment of Mental Health Disorders." *The Lancet Psychiatry* 2: 168–177.

Harrington, R., S. Peters, J. Green, S. Byford, J. Woods, and others. 2000. "Randomised Comparison of the Effectiveness and Costs of Community and Hospital Based Mental Health Services for Children with Behavioural Disorders." *British Medical Journal* 321: 1047.

Harris, A. H., E. Gospodarevskaya, and A. J. Ritter. 2005. "A Randomised Trial of the Cost Effectiveness of Buprenorphine as an Alternative to Methadone Maintenance Treatment for Heroin Dependence in a Primary Care Setting." *Pharmacoeconomics* 23: 77–91.

Hedman, E., E. Andersson, B. Ljótsson, G. Andersson, C. Rück, and others. 2011. "Cost-Effectiveness of Internet-Based Cognitive Behavior Therapy vs. Cognitive Behavioral Group Therapy for Social Anxiety Disorder: Results from a Randomized Controlled Trial." *Behaviour Research and Therapy* 49 (11): 729–36.

Hyman, S., D. Chisholm, R. Kessler, V. Patel, and H. Whiteford. 2006. "Mental Disorders." In *Disease Control Priorities in Developing Countries*, 2nd ed., edited by D. T. Jamison, J. G. Breman, A. R. Measham, G. Alleyne, M. Claeson, D. B. Evans, P. Jha, A. Mills, and P. Musgrove, 605–26. Washington, DC: World Bank and Oxford University Press.

Jamison, D. T., W. H. Mosley, A. R. Measham, and J. L. Bobadilla, eds. 1993. *Disease Control Priorities in Developing Countries*. Washington, DC: World Bank.

Jones, C., R. T. Edwards, and B. Hounsome. 2012. "Health Economics Research into Supporting Careers of People with Dementia: A Systematic Review of Outcome Measures." *Health Quality Life Outcomes* 10: 142.

King, S., S. Griffin, Z. Hodges, H. Weatherly, C. Asseburg, and others. 2006. "A Systematic Review and Economic Model of the Effectiveness and Cost-Effectiveness of Methylphenidate, Dexamfetamine and Atomoxetine for the Treatment of Attention Deficit Hyperactivity Disorder in Children and Adolescents." *Health Technology Assessment* (Winchester, England) 10 (23): Iii–Iv, Xiii–146.

Knapp, M., J. Beecham, D. McDaid, T. Matosevic, and M. Smith. 2011. "The Economic Consequences of Deinstitutionalisation of Mental Health Services: Lessons from a Systematic Review of European Experience." *Health and Social Care in the Community* 19: 113–25.

Knapp, M. R. J., D. McDaid, and M. Parsonage, eds. 2011. *Mental Health Promotion and Mental Illness Prevention: The Economic Case*. London: Department of Health.

Krameddine, Y. I., D. DeMarco, R. Hassel, and P. H. Silverstone. 2013. "A Novel Training Program for Police Officers That Improves Interactions with Mentally Ill Individuals and Is Cost-Effective." *Frontiers in Psychiatry* 4: 9. doi:10.3389/fpsyt.2013.00009.

Kumaranayake, L., P. Vickerman, D. Walker, S. Samoshkin, V. Romantzov, and others. 2004. "The Cost-Effectiveness of HIV Preventive Measures among Injecting Drug Users in Svetlogorsk, Belarus." *Addiction* 99 (12): 1565–76. doi:10.1111/j.1360-0443.2004.00899.x.

Lewis, C., J. Pearce, and J. Bisson. 2012. "Efficacy, Cost-Effectiveness and Acceptability of Self-Help Interventions for Anxiety Disorders: Systematic Review." *British Journal of Psychiatry* 200: 15–21. doi:10.1192/Bjp.Bp.110.084756.

Linde, M., D. Chisholm, and T. Steiner. 2015. "Cost-Effectiveness Analysis of Interventions for Migraine in Four Low- and Middle-Income Countries." *Journal of Headache and Pain* 16: 15.

Lindner, L. M., A. C. Marasciulo, M. R. Garias, and G. E. M. Grohs. 2009. "Economic Evaluation of Antipychotic Drugs for Schizophrenia Treatment within the Brazilian Healthcare System." *Revista de Saúde Pública* 43 (Suppl. 1): 1–7.

Livingston, G., J. Barber, P. Rapaport, M. Knapp, M. Griffin, and others. 2014. "START (STrAtegies for RelaTives) Study: A Pragmatic Randomised Controlled Trial to Determine the Clinical Effectiveness and Cost-Effectiveness of a Manual-Based Coping Strategy Programme in Promoting the Mental Health of Careers of People with Dementia." *Health Technology Assessment* 18 (61): 1–242.

Lund, C., M. De Silva, S. Plagerson, S. Cooper, D. Chisholm, and others. 2011. "Poverty and Mental Disorders: Breaking the Cycle in Low-Income and Middle-Income Countries." *The Lancet* 378 (9801): 1502–14.

Lund, C., M. Tomlinson, M. De Silva, A. Fekadu, R. Shidhaye, and others. 2012. "PRIME: A Programme to Reduce the Treatment Gap for Mental Disorders in Five Low- and Middle-Income Countries." *PLoS Medicine* 9: E1001359. doi:10.1371/Journal.Pmed.1001359.

Machado, M., M. Iskedjian, I. A. Ruiz, and T. R. Einarson. 2007. "The Economic Impact of Introducing Serotonin-Noradrenaline Reuptake Inhibitors into the Brazilian National Drug Formulary: Cost-Effectiveness and Budget-Impact Analyses." *Pharmacoeconomics* 25 (11): 979–90.

Machado, M., M. M. Lopera, J. Diaz-Rojas, L. E. Jaramillo, T. R. Einarson, and others. 2008. "Pharmacoeconomics of Antidepressants in Moderate-to-Severe Depressive Disorder in Colombia." *Revista Panamericana de Salud Pública* (4): 233–39.

Martinez, V., P. Martinez, P. A. Vohringer, R. Araya, and G. Rojas. 2014. "Computer-Assisted Cognitive-Behavioral Therapy for Adolescent Depression on Primary Care Clinics in Santiago, Chile (YPSA-M): Study Protocol for a Randomized Controlled Trial." *Trials* 15: 309.

Matza, L. S., C. Paramore, and M. Prasad. 2005. "A Review of the Economic Burden of ADHD." *Cost Effectiveness and Resource Allocation* 3: 5.

McCabe, C. 2007. *A Systematic Review of Cost-Effectiveness Analyses of Whole School Interventions to Promote Children's Mental Health.* Leeds: Leeds Institute of Health Sciences.

Mejia, A., R. Calam, and M. R. Sanders. 2012. "A Review of Parenting Programs in Developing Countries: Opportunities and Challenges for Preventing Emotional and Behavioral Difficulties in Children." *Clinical Child and Family Psychology Review* 15 (2): 163–75.

Merry, S. N., S. E. Hetrick, G. R. Cox, T. Brudevold-Iversen, J. J. Bir, and others. 2012. "Psychological and Educational Interventions for Preventing Depression in Children and Adolescents (Review)." *Cochrane Review Journal* 7 (5): 1409–1685.

Mihalopoulos, C., M. R. Sanders, K. M. Turner, M. Murphy-Brennan, and R. Carter. 2007. "Does the Triple P-Positive Parenting Program Provide Value for Money?" *Australian and New Zealand Journal of Psychiatry* 41 (3): 239–46.

Mihalopoulos, C., T. Vos, J. Pirkis, and R. Carter. 2011. "The Economic Analysis of Prevention in Mental Health Programs." *Annual Review of Clinical Psychology* 7: 169–201.

Nigam, A., N. Reykar, M. Majumder, and D. Chisholm. 2015. "Self-Harm in India: Cost-Effectiveness Analysis of a Proposed Pesticide Ban." *Disease Control Priorities* Working Paper No. 15. http://dcp-3.org/resources/self-harm-india-cost-effectiveness-analysis-proposed-pesticide-ban.

Patel, V., S. Chatterji, D. Chisholm, S. Ebrahim, G. Gopalakrishna, and others. 2011. "Chronic Diseases and Injuries in India." *The Lancet* 377: 413–28.

Patel, V., M. Maj, A. J. Flisher, M. J. De Silva, M. Koschorke, and others. 2010. "Reducing the Treatment Gap for Mental Disorders: A WPA Survey." *World Psychiatry* 9 (3): 169–76.

Petersen, I., S. Evans-Lacko, M. Semrau, M. Barry, D. Chisholm, and others. 2015. "Population and Community Platforms." In *Disease Control Priorities*, (third edition): Volume 4, *Mental, Neurological, and Substance Use Disorders*, edited by V. Patel, D. Chisholm, T. Dua, R. Laxminarayan, and M. E. Medina-Mora. Washington, DC: World Bank.

Petticrew, M., D. Chisholm, H. Thomson, and E. Jané-Llopis. 2005. "Evidence: The Way Forward." In *Promoting Mental Health: Concepts, Emerging Evidence, and Practice*, edited by H. Herrman, S. Saxena, and R. Moodie, 203–15. Melbourne, Australia: World Health Organization, University of Melbourne, and Victorian Health Promotion Foundation.

Phanthunane, P., T. Vos, H. Whiteford, and M. Bertram. 2011. "Cost-Effectiveness of Pharmacological and Psychosocial Interventions for Schizophrenia." *Cost Effectiveness and Resource Allocation* 9 (6): 1–9.

Prukkanone, B., T. Vos, M. Bertram, and S. Lim. 2012. "Cost-Effectiveness Analysis for Antidepressants and Cognitive Behavioral Therapy for Major Depression in Thailand." *Value Health* 15 (Suppl. 1): S3–8.

Rehm, J., D. Chisholm, R. Room, and A. Lopez. 2006. "Alcohol." In *Disease Control Priorities in Developing Countries*, 2nd ed., edited by D. T. Jamison, J. G. Breman, A. R. Measham, G. Alleyne, M. Claeson, D. B. Evans, P. Jha, A. Mills, and P. Musgrove, 887–906. Washington, DC: World Bank and Oxford University Press.

Rivet-Duval, E., S. Heriot, and C. Hunt. 2011. "Preventing Adolescent Depression in Mauritius: A Universal School-Based Program." *Child and Adolescent Mental Health* 16 (2): 86–91.

Shidhaye, R., C. Lund, and D. Chisholm. 2015. "Health Care Delivery Platforms." In *Disease Control Priorities in Developing Countries* (third edition): Volume 4, *Mental, Neurological, and Substance Use Disorders,* edited by V. Patel, D. Chisholm, T. Dua, R. Laxminarayan, and M. E. Medina-Mora. Washington, DC: World Bank.

Tennant, R., C. Goens, J. Barlow, C. Day, and S. Stewart-Brown. 2007. "A Systematic Review of Reviews of Interventions to Promote Mental Health and Prevent Mental Health Problems in Children and Young People." *Journal of Public Mental Health* 6 (1): 25–32.

van Boeijen, C. A., A. J. Van Balkom, P. Van Oppen, N. Blankenstein, A. Cherpanath, and others. 2005. "Efficacy of Self-Help Manuals for Anxiety Disorders in Primary Care: A Systematic Review." *Family Practice* 22: 192–96.

Vos, T., R. Carter, J. Barendregt, C. Mihalopoulos, J. Veerman, and others. 2010. *Assessing Cost-Effectiveness in Prevention (ACE–Prevention): Final Report.* Melbourne: University of Queensland, Brisbane and Deakin University.

Weare, K., and M. Nind. 2011. "Mental Health Promotion and Problem Prevention in Schools: What Does the Evidence Say?" *Health Promotion International* 26 (Suppl. 1): I29–69.

WHO (World Health Organization). 2010. *Towards Evidence-Based Suicide Prevention Programmes.* Western Pacific Regional Office. Manila: WHO.

———. 2011. *Scaling Up Action against Noncommunicable Diseases: How Much Will It Cost?* Geneva: WHO.

Wu, E. Q., P. Hodgkins, R. Ben-Hamadi, J. Setyawan, J. Xie, and others. 2012. "Cost Effectiveness of Pharmacotherapies for Attention-Deficit Hyperactivity Disorder." *CNS Drugs* 26 (7): 581–600.

Zechmeister, I., R. Kilian, D. McDaid, and the MHEEN Group. 2008. "Is It Worth Investing in Mental Health Promotion and Prevention of Mental Illness? A Systematic Review of the Evidence from Economic Evaluations." *BMC Public Health* 8: 20.

Chapter 13

Universal Health Coverage for Mental, Neurological, and Substance Use Disorders: An Extended Cost-Effectiveness Analysis

Dan Chisholm, Kjell Arne Johansson, Neha Raykar,
Itamar Megiddo, Aditi Nigam, Kirsten Bjerkreim Strand,
Abigail Colson, Abebaw Fekadu, and Stéphane Verguet

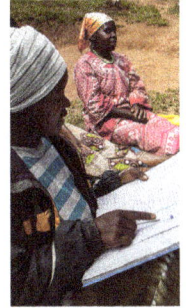

INTRODUCTION

Universal Health Coverage and Mental, Neurological, and Substance Use Disorders

Health System Goals

Health systems are complex entities, involving the development of appropriate policies and legal frameworks, mobilization and allocation of resources, organization, and actual delivery of services, as well as the timely evaluation of these components. Ultimately, the goal of such a system and each of its parts is to improve the mental and physical health of the population it seeks to serve, revealed in terms of enhanced well-being or declining rates of morbidity and mortality.

Earlier chapters in this volume showed the extent of global health losses associated with a range of mental, neurological, and substance use (MNS) disorders— and how the implementation of evidence-based, cost-effective treatment and prevention strategies can mitigate these losses. This chapter goes further by considering important attributes of health systems other than health improvement itself, namely, equity and financial protection. Equitable access to care, fair financing, service quality, and human rights protection represent other important goals; a well-functioning health system should deliver high-quality services to all people, whenever and wherever they need those services (WHO 2010a). A health system functions fully only if it protects the right to health for everyone, including people with MNS disorders. That right to health includes physical or geographical access to essential services, as well as financial access, so that those in need can use and benefit from services without risking financial hardship.

Toward Universal Health Coverage for Mental, Neurological, and Substance Use Disorders

MNS disorders pose several service and financial access challenges. First, persons with these disorders are too often subjected to discrimination and stigmatization, which can reduce their willingness to seek care. Second, individuals may be unaware of their condition and not seek or know about appropriate treatment. Third, MNS disorders are typically chronic and require ongoing treatment. Yet health care and treatment for MNS disorders are often excluded from essential packages of care or insurance schemes. Without such coverage, people with MNS disorders and their families face a difficult choice: pay out-of-pocket (OOP) for treatment

Corresponding author: Dan Chisholm, Department of Health System Financing, World Health Organization; chisholmd@who.int.

by private providers of variable and sometimes poor quality—often by cutting other household spending and investment, or by liquidating assets or savings—or go without treatment altogether.

Either way, MNS disorders pose a direct threat to the well-being of households. In India, for example, the National Sample Survey Organization found that in 2004, national OOP expenditures for treatment of psychiatric disorders amounted to nearly Rs 7 billion (US$280 million in 2012 US$), half of which was borrowed, and a further 40 percent drawn from household income or savings (Mahal, Karan, and Engelgau 2010). Another study, conducted in the Indian state of Goa, found that 15 percent of women with common mental disorders, such as depression or anxiety, spent more than 10 percent of household income on health-related care (Patel and others 2007).

The high, potentially catastrophic cost to households of securing needed health services and goods is a fundamental concern underlying the drive toward universal health coverage (UHC). Direct OOP payments represent a regressive form of health financing—penalizing those least able to afford care—and are an obvious channel through which impoverishment may occur or deepen. Prepayment mechanisms, such as national or social insurance, more equitably safeguard at-risk populations from the adverse financial consequences of mental disorders. Accordingly, ongoing efforts to move toward UHC focus on increasing (1) the proportion of the population covered by some form of financial protection; (2) the proportion of total costs covered by some form of prepayment, such as health insurance; and (3) the depth of coverage (the range of services or interventions available to insured persons) (WHO 2010a).

Current coverage of essential health care and treatment services for MNS disorders is limited, in terms of access and financial protection or benefit inclusion. Efforts to scale up community-based public health services for these conditions can contribute strongly to greater equality of access, because such services will serve more people in need, with less reliance on direct OOP spending. This chapter explores the veracity of this claim through an innovative approach to economic evaluation called extended cost-effectiveness analysis (ECEA) (Verguet, Laxminarayan, and Jamison 2015; Verguet and others 2015).

ECEA goes beyond conventional cost-effectiveness analysis (CEA) not only by considering the distribution of costs and outcomes across different socioeconomic groups in the population, but also by explicitly examining the extent to which interventions or policies protect households against the financial risk of medical impoverishment. We apply this ECEA approach to a range of MNS disorders in two distinct geographical and health system contexts: India and Ethiopia. India is a very large, lower-middle-income country in South Asia; Ethiopia is a large, low-income country in East Africa. We selected these two countries for in-depth analysis because both have recently articulated ambitious plans to enhance mental health service quality and coverage, as well as to extend financial protection or health insurance for their citizens.

Extended Cost-Effectiveness Analysis: Principles and Practice

Objectives and Components

In addition to health gains, a potential nonhealth benefit of specific interventions or policies, such as public financing, is the value that some form of health insurance bestows on households that would otherwise pay privately for health services and goods. Because OOP spending for the care and treatment of MNS disorders can be considerable and enduring, the reduction or elimination of such expenditures can represent major savings or even financial salvation for affected households. Public financing of health service costs can also increase the use of services, especially for those whose incomes are so low that they do not access services in the first place.

Our application of ECEA to MNS disorders focuses on public financing as an instrument for financial risk protection (FRP). Public financing provides FRP benefits to households by shielding them from the OOP costs and impoverishment-related consequences of the covered health care services (Verguet and others 2015). Our approach to the measurement of FRP is described in box 13.1.

Another essential component of ECEA is its examination of the distribution of health and economic benefits by population subgroup, for example, by geographical location, care setting, or income quintile. Such an analysis enables policy makers to understand how an intervention or a policy such as public financing would affect different segments of the population, particularly those with low incomes or high vulnerability.

In short, ECEA provides a tool to amplify understanding of the extent and distribution of health and financial benefits associated with health policies and interventions. Elucidation and enumeration of these benefits provides a more holistic assessment of the expected returns on health service investments while providing new, evidence-based insights to the national policy makers responsible for setting priorities and allocating resources within and beyond the health sector.

Box 13.1

Measuring the Financial Risk Protection Effects of Health Policies

Several metrics can be used to quantify the financial risk protection (FRP) benefits of health policies. One approach is to estimate the amount of households' private out-of-pocket (OOP) expenditures averted by the policy; another is to estimate the number of cases of poverty averted by counting the number of individuals no longer falling under a poverty line/threshold because of substantial OOP medical expenditures. In this study, we used as FRP metric the money-metric value of insurance provided by public financing (Verguet, Laxminarayan, and Jamison 2015), which quantifies insurance risk premiums; it reflects risk aversion, in which individuals would prefer the certainty of insurance over the uncertainty/risk of possible OOP expenditures, and hence are willing to pay a certain amount of money to avoid that risk.

To estimate the FRP, we first estimated the individual's expected income before public financing, which depends on treatment coverage and associated OOP costs. We then estimated the individual's certainty equivalent by assigning individuals a utility function that specifies their risk aversion, which is equivalent to calculating their willingness to pay for insurance against the risk of medical expenditures. Finally, we derived a money-metric value of the insurance provided by public financing (risk premium) as the difference between the expected value of income and the certainty equivalent (Verguet, Laxminarayan, and Jamison 2015). Aggregating the money-metric value of insurance with the income distribution of the population—with a proxy based on the country's gross domestic product per capita and Gini coefficient—yielded a dollar value of FRP at the societal level.

Application to Mental, Neurological, and Substance Use Disorders

ECEA is applicable to many interventions to prevent or treat MNS disorders, whether considered separately or in combination. However, since this approach to economic analysis is new and yet to be tried in the context of MNS disorders, our first goal was to test its applicability and assess its internal validity. We accomplished this by constructing a series of equation-based ECEA models that employed the same epidemiological and treatment cost-outcome input data used in previous CEA studies, such as the treatment of psychosis, bipolar disorder, and depression with psychosocial treatment and psychotropic medication, which Chisholm and Saxena (2012) already examined in the contexts of Sub-Saharan Africa and South-East Asia. Additional information output from the ECEA model—particularly the estimated value of FRP arising from public financing of health care costs—could then be readily interpreted with reference to this earlier published work.

We combined the results of these intervention-specific analyses to evaluate the impact of defined packages of care. Future applications of the ECEA approach could focus more on prevention, including the prevention of childhood behavioral disorders as part of a community

health worker care package, and the prevention of common mental disorders and substance use disorders as part of a school-based intervention package.

These analyses focus on establishing the distributional consequences and the value of FRP resulting from increased levels of publicly financed interventions. Because the availability and use of mental health services in most low- and middle-income countries is very low, however, the economic benefit associated with a switch from private to public payment for services would be correspondingly small. Accordingly, we assess the impacts of increased FRP and increased service coverage.

TOWARD UNIVERSAL HEALTH COVERAGE: TWO COUNTRY ANALYSES

Although analysis has only been conducted for the two countries presented, the insights and lessons from it have a far broader applicability that can be confirmed through further country-based work using the methods and models developed for this chapter. Analysis of this kind can be of particular informational value to other countries planning to reform their mental health programming and public health financing policies.

India

India's health sector is undergoing a rapid and stark transition, not only in epidemiological terms as the deaths and disabilities from chronic diseases and injuries take an ever-higher toll, but also in systemic terms as efforts to improve service quality and expand financial protection take effect (Patel and others 2011). In particular, there is a strong push to move toward universal public finance (UPF)—the government finances an intervention irrespective of who is delivering or receiving it—to reverse decades of high, often impoverishing OOP health care expenditures and to allocate resources more equitably.

This subsection estimates the expected health and economic benefits of scaling up services for the treatment of three prominent contributors to the burden of MNS disorders: epilepsy, schizophrenia, and depression. All monetary values are expressed in 2012 US$.

Enhanced Financial and Service Coverage of Epilepsy Treatment

Fewer than half of the estimated 6 million to 10 million individuals with epilepsy in India receive any treatment (Meyer and others 2010). To counter this health and financial burden, the Ministry of Health is considering a national epilepsy program that could increase access to, and utilization of, treatment through three interventions (Tripathi and others 2012): public awareness campaigns, better training of health workers, and UPF for first- and second-line anti-epilepsy drugs (AEDs) and epilepsy surgery. The ECEA that follows examines UPF—a policy intervention that would also address the financial risk posed by OOP spending on epilepsy treatment. The incremental impacts of three UPF interventions were assessed: UPF for first-line AEDs (intervention 1); UPF for first- and second-line AEDs (intervention 2); and UPF for first- and second-line AEDs and epilepsy surgery (intervention 3).

First-line AEDs include carbamazepine, phenytoin, and valproate, as well as phenobarbital; the second-line AED is lamotrigine. Seventy percent of patients are expected to respond to first-line AEDs; the remaining 30 percent are allocated equally to three groups: those receiving second-line AED treatment, those receiving surgery, and refractory cases who do not respond to any treatment.

Each intervention increases access to the treatment provided by UPF to 80 percent (from less than 50 percent without UPF). We estimate that 70 percent of all treatment costs—including outpatient visits, inpatient visits, and drugs—are paid OOP in the baseline and that the interventions reduce OOP expenditures for the covered services to zero. Relative to the full model and detailed results presented by Megiddo and others (2016), we

make several simplifying assumptions so that the results are comparable to the ECEAs presented for schizophrenia and depression treatment. For example, treatment-seeking costs, such as travel expenses, were omitted. The analysis by Megiddo and others (2016) also employs differing government and consumer costs, but here we assume the costs of a given service to be equal, regardless of the purchaser.

Prevalence and other epidemiological parameters came from the Global Burden of Disease (GBD) 2010 study estimates for South Asia (Whiteford and others 2013). For calculation of healthy life-years, we applied the following disability weights: 0.072 for seizure-free patients, 0.319 for patients with seizures, and 0.420 for untreated individuals with epilepsy (IHME 2012). For each scenario, we estimated the policy's impact on population health (healthy life-years gained), direct government expenditures, OOP expenditures averted, and the FRP provided.

The results, presented in table 13.1, relate to a population of one million persons in the general population, divided into equal household income quintiles of 200,000 persons. The model is dynamic, and the values change over time (meaning that the data for each point in time are needed to replicate the results exactly): here we present the results for the average year. The estimated disease burden associated with epilepsy amounts to 2,200 lost years of healthy life per one million population. Current intervention efforts lead to 503 healthy life-years gained (23 percent of the total estimated disease burden); the three enhanced-coverage intervention scenarios result in gains of between 1,118 and 1,251 healthy life-years, equivalent to more than 50 percent of the measured disease burden. Public financing of second-line AEDs as well as first-line AEDs to 80 percent of those in need (intervention 2) generates 90 more healthy life-years than intervention 1 alone; the addition of surgery (intervention 3) adds a further 44 healthy life-years per one million population. Intervention health benefits are distributed equitably across income quintiles.

The total cost of implementing intervention 1 is US$0.16 per capita, rising to US$0.30 for intervention 3 (table 13.1). Compared with no intervention, the cost per healthy life-year gained for all three intervention scenarios falls below US$200 (range: US$112–US$181). Relative to the current situation, the incremental cost-effectiveness of intervention 1 is US$70 per healthy life-year gained; intervention 3 is the next most cost-effective (incremental cost-effectiveness ratio US$850).

UPF coverage would avert more than US$100,000 in OOP expenditures per one million population under intervention 1, and US$190,000 and US$208,000 under interventions 2 and 3, respectively. Finally, the

Table 13.1 Extended Cost-Effectiveness Analysis of Publicly Financed Epilepsy Treatment in India

Outcome	Income quintile					Total (per one million persons)
	I	II	III	IV	V	
Averted disease burden[a]						
Current burden (healthy life-years lost)	448	440	442	432	435	2,197
Current-coverage averted burden (healthy life-years gained)	89	95	99	112	108	503
Intervention 1 averted burden (healthy life-years gained)	221	219	224	229	225	1,118
Intervention 2 averted burden (healthy life-years gained)	238	237	242	245	245	1,207
Intervention 3 averted burden (healthy life-years gained)	248	247	250	254	252	1,251
Cost of care ($)[b]						
Current-coverage total costs	19,738	21,120	21,167	23,393	22,864	108,283
Current-coverage private expenditures averted (under UPF)	13,817	14,784	14,817	16,375	16,005	75,798
Intervention 1 total costs	32,930	33,132	33,431	33,536	33,608	166,636
Intervention 1 private expenditures averted (under UPF)	23,051	23,192	23,401	23,475	23,526	116,645
Intervention 2 total costs	53,830	53,893	54,578	54,757	54,976	272,033
Intervention 2 private expenditures averted (under UPF)	37,681	37,725	38,204	38,330	38,483	190,423
Intervention 3 total costs	58,980	59,121	59,421	59,810	59,381	296,714
Intervention 3 private expenditures averted (under UPF)	41,286	41,385	41,595	41,867	41,567	207,699
Insurance value ($)[c]						
Intervention 1	778	484	408	253	176	2,098
Intervention 2	4,096	2,699	1,925	1,490	899	11,109
Intervention 3	4,096	2,699	1,925	1,490	1,200	11,410

Source: Megiddo and others 2016.

Note: UPF = universal public financing for 80 percent of the population in need. Intervention 1 = UPF for first-line anti-epileptic drugs (AEDs). Intervention 2 = UPF for first- and second-line AEDs. Intervention 3 = UPF for first- and second-line AEDs and epilepsy surgery. First-line AEDs include carbamazepine, phenytoin, and valproate, as well as phenobarbital. The second-line AED is lamotrigine. Results are based on a population of one million people, with intervention benefits equally divided among income quintiles of 200,000 persons each (quintile I having the lowest household income and quintile V the highest). All monetary values are expressed in 2012 US$.

a. The estimated disease burden, expressed as healthy life-years lost or gained, is drawn from the Global Burden of Disease 2010 study for South Asia (Whiteford and others 2013). Healthy life-years lost are based on the prevalence of individuals with active epilepsy: seizure-free patients (disability weight [DW] 0.072), patients with seizures (DW 0.319), and untreated individuals with seizures (DW 0.420).

b. Total costs = (direct government expenditures) + (private expenditures, including out-of-pocket costs). The costs and expenditures are based on the number of prescriptions and surgeries, which are dependent on the prevalence of epilepsy and the coverage of treatment.

c. Insurance value = financial risk protection provided, based on current coverage.

monetized value of insurance was found to amount to US$11,000 per one million population for interventions 2 and 3, with evidence of a clear trend for it to decrease with wealth. For example, the poorest quintile derives 37 percent of the total insurance value, compared with 8 percent for the wealthiest.

The primary conclusion from this analysis is that intervention 1 is the most cost-effective and least costly strategy to implement from a public payer perspective, but intervention 3—increased service and financial coverage of first- *and* second-line AEDs, as well as surgery—would generate the greatest level of health gain and offer the greatest level of financial protection at the population level.

Enhanced Financial and Service Coverage of Schizophrenia Treatment

Schizophrenia poses a considerable public health and social policy challenge because of its severity, its often catastrophic effect on the welfare and income of family members, and the significant risk that patients will suffer severe human rights violations. Here we analyze the impact of enhanced public financing and provision of schizophrenia treatment on health and financial outcomes, including increased uptake of treatment (leading to more health gains), reduced OOP treatment costs, and greater insurance against catastrophic health expenses (Raykar, Nigam, and Chisholm 2015).

In this model, all persons treated for schizophrenia in nonspecialized health care settings receive a combination of first-generation antipsychotic drugs, such as haloperidol or chlorpromazine, as well as basic—or, for a small proportion, intensive—psychosocial treatment. Fifteen percent of cases are expected to require short-term inpatient psychiatric care; 2 percent are assumed to be long-term residential patients in community-based facilities; and 50 percent receive hospital outpatient care (Chisholm and others 2008).

The resulting cost per treated case is US$177 per year. Given that OOP spending as a share of total health expenditure amounts to at least 70 percent for noncommunicable diseases in India (Mahal, Karan, and Engelgau 2010), we estimate that the annual expected cost to households would be US$124. Treatment improves the average level of functioning or disability by an estimated 24 percent (Chisholm and others 2008); adherence to treatment was set at 76 percent (Chatterjee and others 2014). The estimated proportion of total cases currently receiving treatment in India is 40 percent (Murthy 2011), to which we applied a socioeconomic gradient to account for increased detection and health care utilization rates among wealthier groups (ranging from 30 percent in the poorest income group to 50 percent in the richest). Target coverage for all income groups was set at 80 percent, meaning that 80 percent of those needing treatment would receive publicly financed care.

Schizophrenia prevalence rates for South Asia were taken from the GBD 2010 study (Whiteford and others 2013), stratified by region, age, and gender, but not by income. To derive prevalence rates by income group, these estimates were applied to the household survey in India (District Level Household and Facility Survey-3); this showed a higher prevalence among higher-income groups, which could reflect better detection, greater health service uptake, or both. Disability weights, which are necessary for the calculation of healthy life-years lost or gained, are 0.576 and 0.756 for residual and acute cases, respectively (IHME 2012). A composite disability weight of 0.612 was used, based on a weighted average of acute (20 percent) and residual (80 percent) cases.

The results, displayed in table 13.2, indicate that the current public health burden of schizophrenia amounts to 1,700 lost healthy life-years per one million population. Treatment of schizophrenia with a combination of psychosocial treatment and antipsychotic medication generates 126 healthy life-years at current levels of

Table 13.2 Extended Cost-Effectiveness Analysis of Publicly Financed Schizophrenia Treatment in India

Outcome	Income quintile					Total (per one million persons)
	I	II	III	IV	V	
Averted disease burden[a]						
Current burden (healthy life-years lost)	307	316	333	354	394	1,704
Current-coverage averted burden (healthy life-years gained)	17	20	24	29	36	126
Target-coverage averted burden (healthy life-years gained)	45	46	49	52	57	249
Cost of care ($)[b]						
Current-coverage total costs	26,721	32,042	38,666	46,156	57,059	200,644
Current-coverage private expenditures averted (under UPF)	18,705	22,429	27,066	32,309	39,942	140,451
Target-coverage total costs	71,257	73,238	77,331	82,055	91,295	395,176
Target-coverage private expenditures averted (under UPF)	49,880	51,267	54,132	57,439	63,906	276,623
Insurance value ($)[c]	7,282	5,587	4,972	4,302	2,439	24,582

Source: Raykar, Nigam, and Chisholm 2015.

Note: UPF = universal public financing for 80 percent of the population in need. Results are based on a population of one million people, with intervention benefits equally divided among income quintiles of 200,000 persons each (quintile I having the lowest household income and quintile V the highest). Target coverage of UPF for schizophrenia treatment for all income groups was set at 80 percent. All monetary values are expressed in 2012 US$.

a. The estimated disease burden, expressed as healthy life-years lost or gained, is drawn from the Global Burden of Disease 2010 study for South Asia (Whiteford and others 2013).

b. Total costs = (direct government expenditures) + (private expenditures, including out-of-pocket costs).

c. Insurance value = financial risk protection provided, based on current coverage.

coverage in the population, and 249 at target coverage rates, equivalent to 7.4 percent and 14.6 percent of the current disease burden, respectively (Raykar, Nigam, and Chisholm 2015). Each healthy life-year would be gained at a cost of approximately US$1,600.

Public financing of the 70 percent of treatment costs incurred by households would remove US$140,000 of OOP spending per one million population at current coverage, and US$277,000 at target coverage (US$0.28 per capita). On top of the share already financed publicly (30 percent), this would take the total government cost to US$0.39 per capita. The health impacts of healthy life-years gained and averted OOP spending would be higher for higher-income groups; however, UPF would still flatten the distribution of public health spending appreciably away from today's regressive pattern to a more equitable allocation of resources, as shown in figure 13.1 and Mahal, Karan, and Engelgau (2010). Moreover, analysis of the insurance value indicates that increasing service and financial coverage for schizophrenia treatment in India would have a clear pro-poor effect: 30 percent

of the total insurance value (estimated at US$24,582) is bestowed on the poorest quintile of the population, compared with 10 percent for the richest quintile.

Enhanced Financial and Service Coverage of Depression Treatment

As the single-largest contributor to the burden of mental and behavioral disorders, depression presents major public health and economic challenges to India. Using the same methods and data sources as those applied to schizophrenia, we assess the consequences of scaled-up service and financial coverage for depression.

In this model, all cases of depression receive basic psychosocial treatment, advice, and follow-up in non-specialized health care settings; 20 percent receive more intensive psychological treatment (an average of eight sessions); and 70 percent are prescribed a generic selective serotonin reuptake inhibitor (SSRI) antidepressant (fluoxetine). Hospital-based outpatient and inpatient services are used by 20 and 2 percent of cases, respectively. The mean cost per treated episode is estimated to

Figure 13.1 Distribution of Public Spending and Insurance Value of UPF for Schizophrenia Treatment in India, by Income Quintile

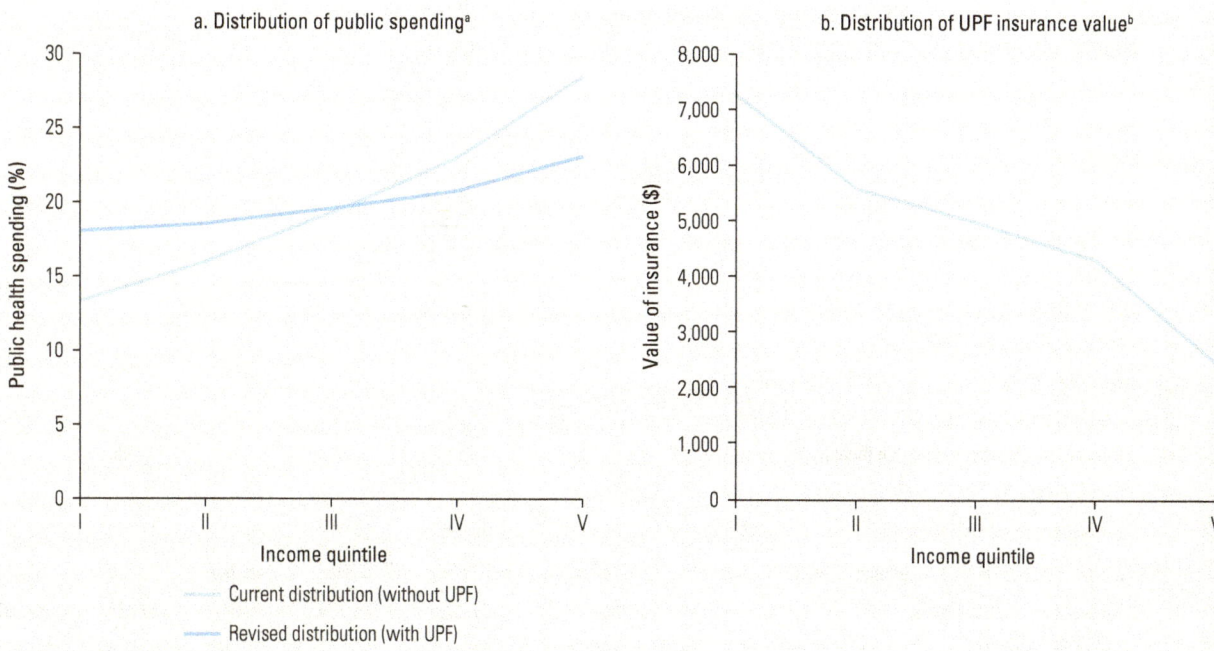

a. Distribution of public spending[a]

b. Distribution of UPF insurance value[b]

Current distribution (without UPF)

Revised distribution (with UPF)

Source: Raykar, Nigam, and Chisholm 2015.
Note: UPF = universal public finance. Results are based on a population of one million people, with intervention benefits equally divided among income quintiles of 200,000 persons each (quinti..
having the lowest household income and quintile V the highest). All monetary values are expressed in 2012 US$.
a. Target coverage of UPF for schizophrenia treatment for all income groups was set at 80 percent. Current coverage ranges from 30 percent in the poorest income group to 50 percent in the rich..
This panel shows the distribution of public health spending across income quintiles before and after the introduction of UPF.
b. Insurance value is the financial risk protection provided by UPF for those in contact with services. This panel shows the distribution of final protection benefits across income quintiles resultin..
from a policy of UPF; the value of insurance is per income quintile (each with 200,000 persons).

be close to US$35 (Chisholm and Saxena 2012; Patel and others 2011), of which 70 percent (US$25) is projected to be paid by households. Treatment affects the duration of a depressive episode and is expressed here as an improvement in the remission rate by 35 percent, subsequently adjusted downward to reflect expected rates of nonadherence of 70 percent (Chisholm and Saxena 2012). We modeled the impact of moving from current coverage (ranging from an estimated 10 percent for the lowest-income quintile to 30 percent for the highest) to a target coverage of 50 percent for all income groups.

As shown in table 13.3, the public health burden of depression is considerable (more than 14,000 healthy life-years lost per one million population). At current coverage rates in the population, treatment is estimated to generate 729 healthy life-years (equivalent to only 5 percent of current disease burden) per million population. With coverage scaled up to 50 percent, close to 1,800 healthy life-years would be gained, equivalent to 12 percent of the current disease burden; as a proportion of current burden, the impact is similar to that of schizophrenia treatment, but because of the higher prevalence of depression, the absolute amount of avertable health gain in the population is at least five times greater.

As in the case of schizophrenia treatment, health benefits are distributed much more evenly across income groups at the assumed scaled-up coverage level of 50 percent among all income groups than under current coverage, which is skewed in favor of the richer quintiles. The total cost of providing this elevated level of service coverage approaches US$700,000 per one million population per year, or US$0.70 per head of population, compared with US$0.28 now. Publicly financing this scaled-up treatment will avert more than US$477,000 of OOP spending per one million population, shared fairly equally among income quintiles. The overall insurance value is approximately US$5,400, much lower than that of schizophrenia treatment because of the lower coverage rate and cost of treatment, and also much flatter (there is no clear income gradient between quintiles I–IV).

Combination Package
Combining the results of these analyses of UPF for the treatment of epilepsy, schizophrenia, and depression, several findings become apparent. First, over 90 percent of the total avertable burden of disease, in healthy life-years gained per one million population, is attributable to UPF of treatment for depression and epilepsy; UPF of treatment for schizophrenia accounts for only 7 percent of the 3,683 healthy life-years. Second, UPF for treatment of depression also accounts for the greatest share of averted OOP spending at specified target-coverage levels—half in this instance (US$477,000 of a total of US$962,000 per one million population). Both of these findings reflect the larger number of prevalent cases

Table 13.3 Extended Cost-Effectiveness Analysis of Publicly Financed Depression Treatment in India

Outcome	Income quintile					Total (per one million persons)
	I	II	III	IV	V	
Averted disease burden[a]						
Current-coverage burden (healthy life-years lost)	2,754	2,817	2,914	2,996	3,153	14,633
Current-coverage averted burden (healthy life-years gained)	67	104	143	184	232	729
Target-coverage averted burden (healthy life-years gained)	337	345	357	367	386	1,793
Cost of care ($)[b]						
Current-coverage total costs	25,669	39,385	54,318	69,821	88,178	277,371
Current-coverage private expenditures averted (under UPF)	17,968	27,569	38,023	48,875	61,725	194,160
Target-coverage total costs	128,346	131,282	135,795	139,642	146,964	682,028
Target-coverage private expenditures averted (under UPF)	89,842	91,897	95,056	97,750	102,875	477,420
Insurance value ($)[c]	1,101	1,167	1,232	1,183	717	5,400

Note: UPF = universal public financing for 50 percent of the population in need. Results are based on a population of one million people, with intervention benefits equally divided among income quintiles of 200,000 persons each (quintile I having the lowest household income and quintile V the highest). Target coverage of UPF for depression treatment for all income groups was set at 80 percent. All monetary values are expressed in 2012 US$.
a. The estimated disease burden, expressed as healthy life-years lost or gained, is drawn from the Global Burden of Disease 2010 study for South Asia (Whiteford and others 2013).
b. Total costs = (direct government expenditures) + (private expenditures, including out-of-pocket costs).
c. Insurance value = financial risk protection provided, based on current coverage.

in the population. By contrast, by far the largest share of the composite value of insurance is associated with UPF of schizophrenia treatment (77 percent of the total US$32,000 per one million population).

Comparing these results by income quintile rather than by disease shows that, at target coverage levels, the averted disease burden and averted OOP expenditures are shared more or less equally across income groups (not shown). However, the value of insurance is markedly skewed toward the poorer income groups (figure 13.2).

Ethiopia

Ethiopia is one of many low-income countries in Sub-Saharan Africa that is facing a severe shortage of skilled workers and other resources for addressing the burden of MNS disorders; for example, there are only 0.4 psychiatrists per one million population in Ethiopia, compared with a global average of more than 10. However, the Ethiopian government has launched a National Mental Health Strategy to scale up mental health services over the next decade (Federal Democratic Republic of Ethiopia 2012). The strategy explicitly recognizes the

importance of an efficient, equitable scale-up of mental health care within a broader, ongoing effort to increase levels of health insurance in the general population (Federal Democratic Republic of Ethiopia 2010).

This section on the ECEA of UHC for MNS disorders assesses the health, distributional, and financial impacts of scaling up a publicly financed mental health program in Ethiopia. Unlike the Indian analysis, which considered each disease in turn before assessing the combined effect, the primary interest here was in the cumulative impact of a defined package of care. In addition, this Ethiopian analysis includes an assessment of the potential productivity effects of scaling up for depression.

Enhanced Financial and Service Coverage of a Mental and Neurological Health Care Package

The basic scale-up scenario in the National Mental Health Strategy targets treatment for depression, schizophrenia, bipolar disorder, and epilepsy—all of which are priority disorders in the World Health Organization's (WHO) Mental Health Gap Action Programme (mhGAP) *Intervention Guide* (WHO 2010b). We included for this analysis the most cost-effective interventions for each disease category, identified through a recent contextualized

Figure 13.2 Composite Value of Insurance through UPF for Treatment of MNS Disorders in India, by Illness and Income Quintile

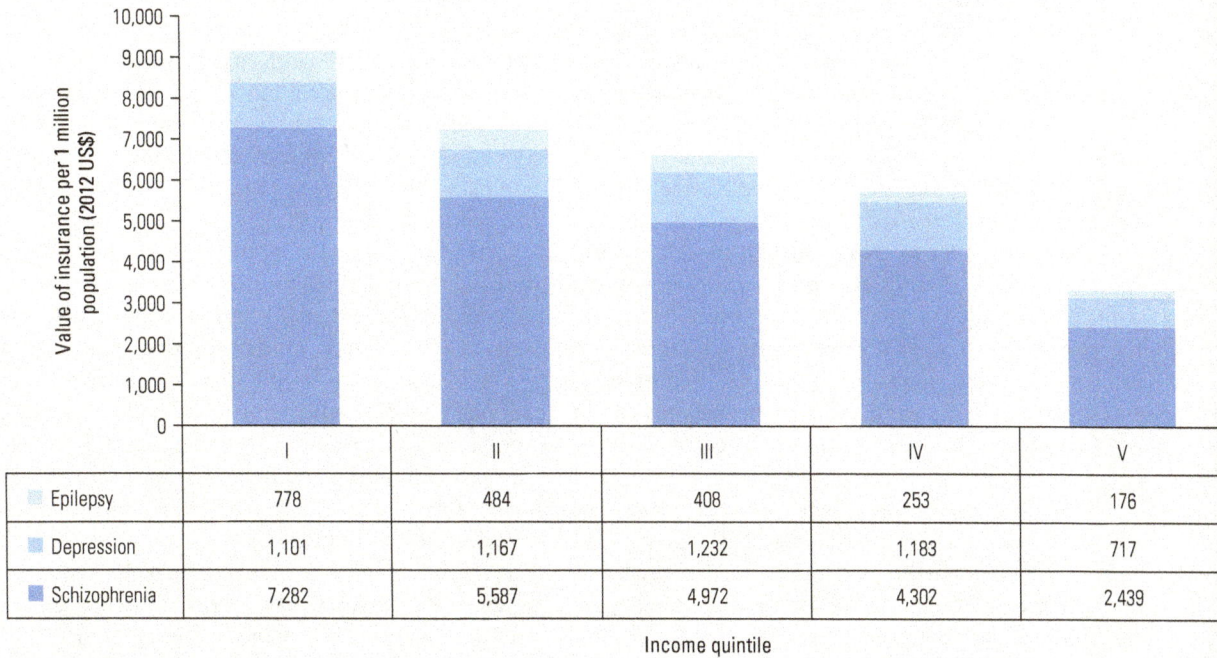

	I	II	III	IV	V
Epilepsy	778	484	408	253	176
Depression	1,101	1,167	1,232	1,183	717
Schizophrenia	7,282	5,587	4,972	4,302	2,439

Income quintile

Note: MNS = mental, neurological, and substance use; UPF = universal public finance. Value of insurance = financial risk protection provided at current coverage. Results are based on a population of one million people, equally divided into income quintiles of 200,000 persons each (quintile I having the lowest household income and quintile V the highest). Results assume target coverage levels of 80 percent for all income groups.

CEA of the National Mental Health Strategy (Bjerkreim Strand and others 2015). The selected interventions include phenobarbital for epilepsy, fluoxetine combined with cognitive therapy and proactive case management for depression, valproate combined with psychosocial therapy for bipolar affective disorder, and first-line antipsychotic medication (haloperidol or chlorpromazine) plus psychosocial treatment for schizophrenia.

As with the Indian analyses, the ECEA splits the population into five income quintiles and runs the analytical model for each income group with quintile-specific prevalence rates. The average age-specific disease prevalence rates used in the standard CEA (Bjerkreim Strand and others 2015) were distributed into income-quintile-specific prevalence rates, using a population-based prevalence study conducted in Ethiopia (n = 1,497) (Fekadu and others 2014).[1] Disease-specific mortality, intervention coverage, and intervention effectiveness were held constant in each income group. Estimates of the efficacy of interventions were drawn from systematic reviews, meta-analyses, and randomized controlled trials (full details can be found in Bjerkreim Strand and others 2015).

Current treatment coverage for all disorders is less than 5 percent (Bjerkreim Strand and others 2015). Following the introduction of UPF, and in line with the National Mental Health Strategy, coverage for all income groups is modeled to reach 75 percent for treatment of schizophrenia and epilepsy, 50 percent for treatment of bipolar disorder, and 30 percent for treatment of depression (Federal Democratic Republic of Ethiopia 2012). Target coverage for depression is lower than the other disorders because of its higher prevalence and lower detectability.

A significant proportion of total health spending in Ethiopia is from OOP expenditures, varying between 30 and 40 percent of the total over the past 10 years (World Bank 2014). This analysis assumes a current household contribution of 34 percent toward the cost of treatment; the government covers the remaining 66 percent. To estimate the amount of household OOP expenditures averted by UPF, we quantified what households would pay for illness-related treatment cost at current service delivery levels.

For the country as a whole, which had a population of 94.6 million in 2012 (United Nations 2015), the expected annual cost of implementing the defined mental and neurological health care package at specified target coverage levels is approximately US$153 million, equivalent to a little more than US$1.60 per capita (Johansson and others 2015). The return on this investment, in total population health gain, exceeds 155,000 healthy life-years, the majority of which derives from treatment of

depression and epilepsy. The costs and health benefits of the intervention package are estimated to be higher for the lowest-income groups (table 13.4) based on the higher prevalence and treatment gap among those groups. Similarly, the measured value of insurance is highest among the lowest-income group. Although UPF would reduce household private expenditures for those with current access to care, the averted OOP expenditures would be extremely low, given the very low current access to and coverage of treatment services (less than 5 percent), particularly among the lower-income quintiles (Bjerkreim Strand and others 2015). In other words, the FRP of UPF is extremely low because of the low current level of private spending on mental health care in Ethiopia, a direct consequence of the very low coverage of services.

Findings from this ECEA indicate that investing in UPF of public mental health will create substantial health benefits, but it will most likely produce a low degree of FRP. Accordingly, while the ECEA approach captures FRP and equity in the economic evaluation of mental health policy, the FRP benefits are less relevant when the current utilization and spending on care is low, as they are in Ethiopia. Nevertheless, we expect that many families experience impoverishing loss of income because of mental disorders.

Productivity Impact of Scaled-Up Depression Treatment

Owing to low levels of current investment, OOP spending averted and FRP conferred as a result of switching to a publicly financed model of mental health care are modest. However, implementation of the National Mental Health Strategy can lead to other important welfare gains, in particular, productivity at the household and societal levels.

Therefore, we also explored the expected productivity gains from scaling up the provision of depression care and treatment. We focused only on depression because the disease burden of depression is high, and evidence indicates that depression has a substantial impact on productivity (Clark and others 2009; Goetzel and others 2004). Between 1 and 3 percent of the adult Ethiopian population is estimated to have a depressive episode at any given time, with an average duration of 8.4 months (Bjerkreim Strand and others 2015). Productivity is lost during such episodes because of increased absence from work (absenteeism) and decreased work performance when present at work (presenteeism). Depression treatment programs have been shown to improve rates of employment by up to 5 percent in the United Kingdom (Clark and others 2009); in the United States, costs associated with

Table 13.4 Extended Cost-Effectiveness Analysis of a Publicly Financed Mental and Neurological Health Care Package in Ethiopia

Outcome	Income quintile					Total (per one million persons)
	I	II	III	IV	V	
Healthy life-years gained (at target coverage)[a]						
Schizophrenia	26	22	19	16	12	95
Bipolar disorder	58	50	43	35	28	214
Depression	173	152	130	108	86	649
Epilepsy	187	163	140	115	77	682
Total cost of care (at target coverage)[b]						
Schizophrenia ($)	75,900	66,100	56,300	46,400	36,600	281,200
Bipolar disorder ($)	109,300	95,100	81,000	66,800	52,600	404,800
Depression ($)	159,200	139,000	118,600	98,100	77,600	592,500
Epilepsy ($)	92,500	80,500	69,900	56,600	37,200	336,600
Private expenditures averted (at current coverage)[c]						
Schizophrenia ($)	380	330	280	230	180	1,420
Bipolar disorder ($)	1,140	990	840	700	550	4,220
Depression ($)	760	660	610	5870	470	2,840
Epilepsy ($)	2,610	2,280	1,980	1,600	1,600	9,520
Insurance value (at current coverage)[d]						
Schizophrenia ($)	0.08	0.03	0.01	0.01	0.01	0.14
Bipolar disorder ($)	3.2	1.1	0.6	0.6	0.3	5.7
Depression ($)	9.5	3.4	1.9	1.8	0.8	17.3
Epilepsy ($)	70.7	22.9	13.0	11.9	3.6	122.1

Source: Johansson and others 2015.

Note: Results are based on a population of one million people, equally divided into income quintiles of 200,000 persons (quintile I has the lowest household income and quintile V the highest). Target coverage associated with enhanced public financing for all income groups was set at 30 percent for depression treatment, 50 percent for bipolar disorder, and 75 percent for the other two disorders. All monetary values are expressed in 2012 US$.

a. The estimated disease burden, expressed as healthy life-years gained, is drawn from the Global Burden of Disease 2010 study for Eastern Sub-Saharan Africa (Whiteford and others 2013).

b. Total cost of care = direct government expenditure associated with public financing at target coverage.

c. Private expenditures averted = out-of-pocket spending that is eliminated by switching to public financing.

d. Insurance value = financial risk protection provided, based on current coverage.

presenteeism have been estimated to be higher than the costs of treatment (Goetzel and others 2004).

To estimate the productivity impact across income groups from scaling up treatment of depression in Ethiopia, we first adapted the Goetzel and others (2004) approach to presenteeism to the context of Ethiopia. We used epidemiological, demographic, efficacy, and cost data from the contextualized CEA of mental health care in Ethiopia by Bjerkreim Strand and others (2015). It was estimated that treatment led to an average reduction in the duration of a depressive episode of 2.9 months (8.4 months * efficacy of 0.35). Second, this reduction in duration was converted to reduction in absenteeism.

Disability days (per month) because of depression are estimated to be 2.9 in low-income settings (Alonso and others 2011). Hence, we assumed treatment would reduce the number of disability days by 8.7 days in total (2.9 days * 2.9 months). Subsequently, the population with depression, target coverage (30 percent), and average daily income (per wealth quintile in the productive age groups [ages 15–60 years]) were multiplied by this change in absenteeism (8.7 days) to derive an estimate of the potential productivity gains in Ethiopia. In addition, persons with depression have been found to have 3.7 days with partial disability per month in low-income countries (Bruffaerts and others 2012). Partial disability means that on-the-job productivity is reduced because of disease; it was estimated that patients with depression had 1.2 full days lost per month because of presenteeism, based on the assumption that each partial day is equivalent to one-third of a full lost day. Subsequently, the associated productivity gain was estimated using the same method as for absenteeism.[2]

The results shown in table 13.5 indicate that scaled-up depression treatment at 30 percent coverage could lead to total productivity gains of close to US$40 million per year. The largest benefits accrue to the wealthier quintiles because of their higher average income level (Johansson and others 2015). Our estimates indicate that the expected productivity gain from scaled-up treatment of depression is likely to reduce the expected governmental cost of the treatment program by 71 percent.

We acknowledge that it is problematic to apply a high-income country method to an agrarian economy like Ethiopia to estimate productivity losses. Nevertheless, calculations of productivity impact, based on presenteeism and absenteeism, are applied to illustrate how such information may be an important supplement to information on the expected FRP of mental health care in a low-income context. Appropriate measures of presenteeism and absenteeism need to be contextualized and found for each particular setting. More conceptual and empirical work on this issue is needed.

CONCLUSIONS AND RECOMMENDATIONS

This chapter employed a novel approach to the economic analysis of mental health care interventions, with a view to gaining insights into intervention or policy impacts other than health gain itself. Assessment of the health and nonhealth impacts of scaled-up treatment

by income group, for example, provides an important equity dimension that has so far been largely absent from conventional economic evaluation methods (including the WHO's CHOICE [CHOosing Interventions that are Cost-Effective] project and earlier editions of *Disease Control Priorities*). Identification of the averted OOP spending associated with a move to UPF usefully complements other research related to UHC, such as estimation of the costs of scaling up services.

We found ECEA to be a feasible approach and a useful addition to the methodological toolbox available to analysts, particularly since it can be incorporated into existing cost-effectiveness modeling frameworks. The main additional data requirement is to be able to break down epidemiological and other key input parameters by income group, the source of which would typically be nationally representative demographic and health surveys. Static and more dynamic approaches to ECEA modeling have been developed and employed; for MNS disorders with long-term impacts, or for other interventions, a dynamic, agent-based approach to modeling can be used that requires more data as well as analytical expertise, but may be better able to capture sociodemographic changes and disease interactions over time.

Whichever approach is used, both are subject to the inherent uncertainty surrounding population-level projections of intervention costs, impacts, and consequences, consideration of which is contained in the primary analyses underlying the base case findings reported in this chapter (Johansson and others 2015; Megiddo and others 2016; Raykar, Nigam, and Chisholm 2015). These uncertainty analyses indicate that results for FRP—as well as overall costs and health effects—are sensitive to assumptions around target coverage rates to be achieved in the population, the proportion of total

Table 13.5 Productivity Impact of Scaled-Up Depression Treatment in Ethiopia

| Cost/outcome | Income quintile | | | | | Total population |
	I	II	III	IV	V	
Government cost of depression treatment program ($, millions)	−15.1	−13.2	−11.2	−9.3	−7.3	−56.1
Productivity gain from scaled-up depression treatment ($, million)[a]						
Caused by absenteeism	3.0	4.9	5.9	6.6	7.9	28.3
Caused by presenteeism	1.2	2.0	2.4	2.7	3.3	11.6
Net societal cost of depression treatment program ($, million)[b]	−10.9	−6.3	−2.9	−0.0	3.9	−16.2

Source: Johansson and others 2015.
Note: Results are based on the total Ethiopian population, with intervention costs equally divided among income quintiles of the population (quintile I having the lowest household income and quintile V the highest). All monetary values are expressed in 2012 US$.
a. Total societal income/wealth in productive ages (15–60 years) (2012) in Ethiopia is US$879: by quintile (Q), US$281 for QI, US$536 for QII, US$772 for QIII, US$1,072 for QIV, and US$1,732 for QV.
b. Net societal cost = (governmental cost) − (productivity gain).

spending that is OOP, and the estimated cost per treated case. Our initial findings from the application of ECEA to MNS disorders need to be interpreted with a due degree of caution.

A primary aim of the preceding analysis was to ascertain the extent to which scaled-up and publicly funded mental health services can contribute to greater equality of access to care and fairness in financial contributions as well as health gains. Across the two geographical settings and multiple disorders considered (table 13.6), and after allowing for uncertainty, it is clear that enhanced coverage of effective treatment leads to significant improvements in population health (1,500 and 3,000 healthy life-years per one million population in Ethiopia and India, respectively, when the three disorders are considered together) and that this can be achieved at a very reasonable cost

Table 13.6 Comparative Results of Extended Cost-Effectiveness in India and Ethiopia

Disease/outcome	Per one million population	
	India	Ethiopia
Schizophrenia		
Current treatment coverage (target coverage) (%)	40 (80)	1 (75)
Avertable burden (at target coverage)[a]	249	95
Treatment cost (at target coverage, in $, millions)[b]	0.40	0.28
Averted OOPs (at current coverage, in $, millions)[c]	0.140	0.001
Insurance value (at current coverage, in $)[d]	24,582	0.1
Insurance value, two lowest quintiles (% of total)[e]	52	78
Depression		
Current treatment coverage (target coverage) (%)	20 (50)	1 (30)
Avertable burden (at target coverage)[a]	1,793	649
Treatment cost (at target coverage, in $, millions)[b]	0.68	0.59
Averted OOPs (at current coverage, in $, millions)[c]	0.190	0.003
Insurance value (at current coverage, in $)[d]	5,400	17
Insurance value, two lowest quintiles (% of total)[e]	42	74
Epilepsy		
Current treatment coverage (target coverage) (%)	47 (80)	5 (75)
Avertable burden (at target coverage)[a]	1,251	682
Treatment cost (at target coverage, in $, millions)[b]	0.30	0.34
Averted OOPs (at current coverage, in $, millions)[c]	0.210	0.010
Insurance value (at current coverage, in $)[d]	11,410	122
Insurance value, two lowest quintiles (% of total)[e]	60	77
Combined		
Avertable burden (at target coverage)[a]	3,293	1,425
Treatment cost (at target coverage, in $, millions)[b]	1.37	1.21
Averted OOPs (at current coverage, in $, millions)[c]	0.540	0.014
Insurance value (at current coverage, in $)[d]	41,392	139
Insurance value, two lowest quintiles (% of total)[e]	51	76

Note: Results are based on a population of one million people. All monetary values are expressed in 2012 US$. OOP = out-of-pocket.

a. Averted disease burden is expressed as healthy life-years gained and is drawn from the Global Burden of Disease 2010 study for Eastern Sub-Saharan Africa (Whiteford and others 2013).

b. Total cost of care = direct government expenditure associated with public financing at target coverage.

c. Private expenditures averted = out-of-pocket spending that is eliminated by switching to public financing.

d. Insurance value = financial risk protection provided, based on current coverage.

e. Proportion of total insurance value that accrues to the two lowest income quintile groups (the poorest 40 percent of households).

(US$1.21 per capita in Ethiopia and US$1.37 in India). Furthermore, a UPF policy can lead to a more equitable allocation of public health resources across income groups, and benefit the lowest-income groups most in terms of the value of insurance, used here as a measure of financial protection: the poorest 40 percent of households receive over 50 percent of the combined value of insurance in India, and 76 percent in Ethiopia.

It should be pointed out, however, that because existing treatment coverage is low (especially in Ethiopia, where it is 5 percent or less), averted OOP expenditures arising from a switch to public finance of treatment costs will be correspondingly low (table 13.6). This again points to the substantial shortage of appropriate mental health services in Ethiopia. It should also be noted that private expenditures on complementary or traditional remedies would not be covered by such public financing, and this might continue to be a significant drain on the income or resources of some household groups.

Only when a substantial increase in service coverage is modeled does one see the true scale of the private expenditures that would pertain in the absence of UPF. It is vital that increased financial protection goes hand in hand with enhanced coverage of an essential package of care. Improved service access without commensurate financial protection will lead to inequitable rates of service uptake and outcomes, but improved financial protection without appropriate service scale-up will bring little improvement at all. In short, a concerted, multidimensional effort is needed if the much-needed move toward UHC for MNS disorders is to be realized.

ACKNOWLEDGMENT

The authors thank Ramanan Laxminarayan for his comments on an earlier draft of this chapter.

NOTES

Disclaimer: Dan Chisholm is a staff member of the World Health Organization. The authors alone are responsible for the views expressed in this publication, and they do not necessarily represent the decisions, policy, or views of the World Health Organization.

This chapter was previously published as "Health and Economic Benefits of Public Financing of Epilepsy Treatment in India: An Agent-Based Simulation Model." I. Megiddo, A. Colson, D. Chisholm, T. Dua, A. Nandi, and R. Laxminarayan. *Epilepsia*. 2016. Epub January 14. doi:10.1111/epi.13294.

World Bank Income Classifications as of July 2014 are as follows, based on estimates of gross national income (GNI) per capita for 2013:

- Low-income countries (LICs) = US$1,045 or less
- Middle-income countries (MICs) are subdivided:
  a) Lower-middle-income = US$1,046–US$4,125
  b) Upper-middle-income (UMICs) = US$4,126–US$12,745
- High-income countries (HICs) = US$12,746 or more.

1. For each disorder, based on data extracted from Fekadu and others (2014), we extract a prevalence ratio between income quintiles using a risk index by income quintile (Q) (QI, 1.4; QII, 1.2; QIII, 1; QIV, 0.8; and QV, 0.6) applied to the mean prevalence of each disorder (Johansson and others 2015).

2. The total gain in productivity by wealth quintile i due to absenteeism averted is given by: $Prod\_A_i = AP * Income_i * Dur_{dis} * Eff * Pop_i * Cov$, where AP is the number of days of absenteeism prevented (8.7 days); $Income_i$ is the average daily income in each wealth quintile i; Dur_{dis} is the average duration of a depressive episode (8.4 months); Eff is the efficacy of the intervention (SSRI + cognitive therapy + proactive case management = 0.35); Pop_i is the number of people with depression in each wealth quintile i; and Cov is the target coverage of treatment (0.30). The total gain in productivity by wealth quintile i due to presenteeism averted is given by: $Prod\_P_i = PP * Income_i * Dur_{dis} * Eff * Pop_i * Cov$, where PP is the number of full days of presenteeism prevented by going from depressed to nondepressed (1.2); and the other variables are identical to those in $Prod\_A_i$. The estimated annual number of people with depression (ages 15–60 years) per quintile (Q) is QI, 900,000; QII, 771,000; QIII, 641,000; QIV, 511,000; and QV, 381,000.

REFERENCES

Alonso, J., M. Petukhova, G. Vilagut, S. Chatterji, S. Heeringa, and others. 2011. "Days Out of Role Due to Common Physical and Mental Conditions: Results from the WHO World Mental Health Surveys." *Molecular Psychiatry* 16: 1234–46.

Bjerkreim Strand, K. B., D. Chisholm, A. Fekadu, and K. A. Johansson. 2015. "Scaling-Up Essential Neuropsychiatric Services in Ethiopia: A Cost-Effectiveness Analysis." *Health Policy and Planning* doi:10.1093/heapol/czv093.

Bruffaerts, R., G. Vilagut, K. Demyttenaere, J. Alonso, A. Alhamzawi, and others. 2012. "Role of Common Mental and Physical Disorders in Partial Disability around the World." *British Journal of Psychiatry* 200: 454–61.

Chatterjee, S., S. Naik, S. John, H. Dabholkar, M. Balaji, and others. 2014. "Effectiveness of a Community-Based Intervention for People with Schizophrenia and Their Caregivers in India (COPSI): A Randomized Controlled Trial." *The Lancet* 383 (9926): 1385–94.

Chisholm, D., O. Gureje, S. Saldivia, M. V. Calderon, R. Wickremasinghe, and others. 2008. "Schizophrenia Treatment in the Developing World: An Interregional and Multinational Cost-Effectiveness Analysis." *Bulletin of the World Health Organization* 86 (7): 497–576.

Chisholm, D., and S. Saxena. 2012. "Cost Effectiveness of Strategies to Combat Neuropsychiatric Conditions in Sub-Saharan Africa and South East Asia: Mathematical Modelling Study." *BMJ* 344: e609.

Clark, D. M., R. Layard, R. Smithies, D. A. Richards, E. Suckling, and others. 2009. "Improving Access to Psychological Therapy: Initial Evaluation of Two UK Demonstration Sites." *Behaviour Research and Therapy* 47 (11): 910–20.

Federal Democratic Republic of Ethiopia. 2010. "Social Health Insurance Proclamation No. 690/2010." Federal Negarit Gazeta, Federal Democratic Republic of Ethiopia, Addis Ababa.

———. 2012. "National Mental Health Strategy 2012/13–2015/16." Public policy document, Federal Democratic Republic of Ethiopia, Addis Ababa. http://www.centreforglobalmentalhealth.org/sites/www.centreforglobalmentalhealth.org/files/uploads/documents/ETHIOP~2.pdf.

Fekadu, A., G. Medhin, A. Selamu, M. Hailemariam, A. Alem, and others. 2014. "Population Level Mental Distress in Rural Ethiopia." *BMC Psychiatry* 14: 194.

Goetzel, R. Z., S. R. Long, R. J. Ozminkowski, K. Hawkins, S. Wang, and others. 2004. "Health, Absence, Disability, and Presenteeism Cost Estimates of Certain Physical and Mental Health Conditions Affecting U.S. Employers." *Journal of Occupational and Environmental Medicine* 46 (4): 398–412.

IHME (Institute for Health Metrics and Evaluation). 2012. "Global Burden of Disease Study 2010. Disability Weights." Dataset, IHME, Seattle. http://ghdx.healthdata.org/record/global-burden-disease-study-2010-gbd-2010-disability-weights.

Johansson, K. J., K. Bjerkreim Strand, A. Fekadu, and D. Chisholm. 2015. "Health Gains and Financial Protection Provided by the Ethiopian Mental Health Strategy." *Disease Control Priorities* (third edition), Working Paper 16, World Bank, Washington, DC. http://www.dcp-3.org/resources/health-gains-and-financial-risk-protection-provided-ethiopian-mental-health-strategy.

Mahal, A., A. Karan, and M. Engelgau. 2010. "The Economic Implications of Non-Communicable Disease for India." Health, Nutrition and Population (HNP) Discussion Paper, World Bank, Washington, DC.

Megiddo, I., A. Colson, D. Chisholm, T. Dua, A. Nandi, and R. Laxminarayan. 2016. "Health and Economic Benefits of Public Financing of Epilepsy Treatment in India: An Agent-Based Simulation Model." *Epilepsia* Epub January. doi:10.1111/epi.13294.

Meyer, A.-C., T. Dua, J. Ma, S. Saxena, and G. Birbeck. 2010. "Global Disparities in the Epilepsy Treatment Gap: A Systematic Review." *Bulletin of the World Health Organization* 88 (4): 260–66.

Murthy, R. S. 2011. "Mental Health Initiatives in India (1947–2010)." *The National Medical Journal of India* 24 (2): 98–107.

Patel, V., S. Chatterji, D. Chisholm, S. Ebrahim, G. Gopalakrishna, and others. 2011. "Chronic Diseases and Injuries in India." *The Lancet* 377 (9763): 413–28.

Patel, V., D. Chisholm, B. R. Kirkwood, and D. Mabey. 2007. "Prioritizing Health Problems in Women in Developing Countries: Comparing the Financial Burden of Reproductive Tract Infections, Anaemia and Depressive Disorders in a Community Survey in India." *Tropical Medicine and International Health* 12 (1): 130–39.

Raykar, N., A. Nigam, and D. Chisholm. 2015. "An Extended Cost-Effectiveness Analysis of Schizophrenia Treatment in India under Universal Public Finance." *Disease Control Priorities* (third edition), Working Paper 17, World Bank, Washington, DC. http://www.dcp-3.org/resources/extended-cost-effectiveness-analysis-schizophrenia-treatment-india-under-universal-public.

Tripathi, M., D. C. Jain, M. Gourie Devi, S. Jain, V. Saxena, and others. 2012. "Need for a National Epilepsy Control Program." *Annals of Indian Academy of Neurology* 15 (2): 89–93.

United Nations. 2015. *World Population Prospects: The 2015 Revision.* Custom data acquired via website, Department of Economic and Social Affairs, Population Division, United Nations, New York.

Verguet, S., R. Laxminarayan, and D. T. Jamison. 2015. "Universal Public Finance of Tuberculosis Treatment in India: An Extended Cost-Effectiveness Analysis." *Health Economics* 24 (3): 318–32.

Verguet, S., Z. Olson, J. B. Babigumira, D. Desalegn, K. A. Johansson, and others. 2015. "Health Gains and Financial Risk Protection Afforded by Public Financing of Selected Interventions in Ethiopia: An Extended Cost-Effectiveness Analysis." *The Lancet Global Health* 3 (5): e288–96.

Whiteford, H., L. Degenhardt, J. Rehm, A. J. Baxter, A. J. Ferrari, and others. 2013. "Global Burden of Disease Attributable to Mental and Substance Use Disorders: Findings from the Global Burden of Disease Study 2010." *The Lancet* 382 (9904): 1575–86.

WHO (World Health Organization). 2010a. *The World Health Report: Health Systems Financing; The Path to Universal Coverage.* Geneva: WHO.

———. 2010b. *mhGAP (Mental Health Gap Action Programme) Intervention Guide.* Geneva: WHO. http://www.who.int/mental_health/publications/mhGAP_intervention_guide/en/.

World Bank. 2014. *World Development Indicators 2014.* Washington, DC: World Bank.

DCP3 Series Acknowledgments

Disease Control Priorities, third edition *(DCP3)* compiles the global health knowledge of institutions and experts from around the world, a task that required the efforts of over 500 individuals, including volume editors, chapter authors, peer reviewers, advisory committee members, and research and staff assistants. For each of these contributions, we convey our acknowledgment and appreciation. First and foremost, we would like to thank our 33 volume editors who provided the intellectual vision for their volumes based on years of professional work in their respective fields, and then dedicated long hours to reviewing each chapter, providing leadership and guidance to authors, and framing and writing the summary chapters. We also thank our chapter authors who collectively volunteered their time and expertise to writing over 160 comprehensive, evidence-based chapters.

We owe immense gratitude to the institutional sponsor of this effort: The Bill & Melinda Gates Foundation. The Foundation provided sole financial support of the Disease Control Priorities Network. Many thanks to Program Officers Kathy Cahill, Philip Setel, Carol Medlin, and (currently) Damian Walker for their thoughtful interactions, guidance, and encouragement over the life of the project. We also wish to thank Jaime Sepúlveda for his longstanding support, including chairing the Advisory Committee for the second edition and, more recently, demonstrating his vision for *DCP3* while he was a special advisor to the Gates Foundation. We are also grateful to the University of Washington's Department of Global Health and successive chairs King Holmes and Judy Wasserheit for providing a home base for the *DCP3* Secretariat, which included intellectual collaboration, logistical coordination, and administrative support.

We thank the many contractors and consultants who provided support to specific volumes in the form of economic analytical work, volume coordination, chapter drafting, and meeting organization: the Center for Disease Dynamics, Economics & Policy; Centre for Chronic Disease Control; Centre for Global Health Research; Emory University; Evidence to Policy Initiative; Public Health Foundation of India; QURE Healthcare; University of California, San Francisco; University of Waterloo; University of Queensland; and the World Health Organization.

We are tremendously grateful for the wisdom and guidance provided by our advisory committee to the editors. Steered by Chair Anne Mills, the advisory committee assures quality and intellectual rigor of the highest order for *DCP3*.

The National Academy of Medicine, in collaboration with the InterAcademy Medical Panel, coordinated the peer-review process for all *DCP3* chapters. Patrick Kelley, Gillian Buckley, Megan Ginivan, and Rachel Pittluck managed this effort and provided critical and substantive input.

The World Bank External and Corporate Relations Publishing and Knowledge division provided exceptional guidance and support throughout the demanding production and design process. We would particularly like to thank Carlos Rossel, the publisher; Mary Fisk, Nancy Lammers, Rumit Pancholi, and Deborah Naylor for their diligence and expertise. Additionally, we thank Jose de Buerba, Mario Trubiano, Yulia Ivanova, and Chiamaka Osuagwu of the World Bank for providing professional counsel on communications and marketing strategies.

Several U.S. and international institutions contributed to the organization and execution of meetings that supported the preparation and dissemination of *DCP3*.

We would like to express our appreciation to the following institutions:

- University of Bergen, consultation on equity (June 2011)
- University of California, San Francisco, surgery volume consultations (April 2012, October 2013, February 2014)
- Institute of Medicine, first meeting of the Advisory Committee to the Editors (March 2013)
- Harvard Global Health Institute, consultation on policy measures to reduce incidence of noncommunicable diseases (July 2013)
- Institute of Medicine, systems strengthening meeting (September 2013)
- Center for Disease Dynamics, Economics & Policy (Quality and Uptake meeting, September 2013; reproductive and maternal health volume consultation, November 2013)
- National Cancer Institute, cancer consultation (November 2013)
- Union for International Cancer Control, cancer consultation (November 2013, December 2014)

Carol Levin provided outstanding governance for cost and cost-effectiveness analysis. Stéphane Verguet added invaluable guidance in applying and improving the extended cost-effectiveness analysis method. Shane Murphy, Zachary Olson, Elizabeth Brouwer, Kristen Danforth, and David Watkins provided exceptional research assistance and analytic assistance. Brianne Adderley ably managed the budget and project processes. The efforts of these individuals were absolutely critical to producing this series, and we are thankful for their commitment.

Series and Volume Editors

VOLUME EDITORS

Vikram Patel

Vikram Patel is Professor of International Mental Health and Wellcome Trust Principal Research Fellow at the London School of Hygiene & Tropical Medicine (LSHTM). He is a psychiatrist whose work focuses on the epidemiology and treatment of mental disorders in low-resource settings. He was the Founding Director of the Centre for Global Mental Health at the LSHTM and is the Co-Director of the Centre for Control of Chronic Conditions at the Public Health Foundation of India. In 2011, Dr. Patel served on the Government of India's Mental Health Policy group, which produced India's first national mental health policy in 2014.

Dan Chisholm

Dan Chisholm is a Health Systems Adviser in the Department of Mental Health and Substance Abuse at the World Health Organization. His main areas of work include development and monitoring of global mental health plans and activities, technical assistance to Member States on mental health system strengthening, and analysis of the costs and cost-effectiveness of strategies for reducing the global burden of mental disorders and other noncommunicable diseases.

Tarun Dua

Tarun Dua is a Medical Officer working in the Evidence, Research and Action on Mental and Brain Disorders unit in the Department of Mental Health and Substance Abuse at the World Health Organization. Dr. Dua serves as the focal point for neurological disorders in the organization.

Ramanan Laxminarayan

Ramanan Laxminarayan is Vice President for Research and Policy at the Public Health Foundation of India, and he directs the Center for Disease Dynamics, Economics & Policy in Washington, DC, and New Delhi. His research deals with the integration of epidemiological models of infectious diseases and drug resistance into the economic analysis of public health problems. He was one of the key architects of the Affordable Medicines Facility–malaria, a novel financing mechanism to improve access and delay resistance to antimalarial drugs. In 2012, he created the Immunization Technical Support Unit in India, which has been credited with improving immunization coverage in the country. He teaches at Princeton University.

María Elena Medina-Mora

María Elena Medina-Mora is the General Director for the National Institute of Psychiatry Ramón de la Fuente Muñiz in Mexico. She is a member of the National System of Researchers. Dr. Medina-Mora is a full researcher of the National Institutes of Health and has a teaching appointment in the National Autonomous University of Mexico and as Adjunct Professor in the Harvard T. H. Chan School of Public Health. She is also member of the World Health Organization's Expert Committee on Addictions.

SERIES EDITORS

Dean T. Jamison

Dean T. Jamison is a Senior Fellow in Global Health Sciences at the University of California, San Francisco, and an Emeritus Professor of Global Health at the University of Washington. He previously held academic appointments at Harvard University and the University of California, Los Angeles; he was an economist on the staff of the World Bank, where he was lead author of the World Bank's *World Development Report 1993: Investing in Health*. He was lead editor of *DCP2*. He holds a PhD in economics from Harvard University and is an elected member of the Institute of Medicine of the National Academy of Sciences. He recently served as Co-Chair and Study Director of *The Lancet's* Commission on Investing in Health.

Rachel Nugent

Rachel Nugent is a Research Associate Professor in the Department of Global Health at the University of Washington. She was formerly Deputy Director of Global Health at the Center for Global Development, Director of Health and Economics at the Population Reference Bureau, Program Director of Health and Economics Programs at the Fogarty International Center of the National Institutes of Health, and senior economist at the Food and Agriculture Organization of the United Nations. From 1991–97, she was Associate Professor and Department Chair in Economics at Pacific Lutheran University. She has advised the World Health Organization, the U.S. government, and nonprofit organizations on the economics and policy environment of noncommunicable diseases.

Hellen Gelband

Hellen Gelband is Associate Director for Policy at the Center for Disease Dynamics, Economics & Policy (CDDEP). Her work spans infectious disease, particularly malaria and antibiotic resistance, and noncommunicable disease policy, mainly in low- and middle-income countries. Before joining CDDEP, then Resources for the Future, she conducted policy studies at the (former) Congressional Office of Technology Assessment, the Institute of Medicine of the National Academies, and a number of international organizations.

Susan Horton

Susan Horton is Professor at the University of Waterloo and holds the Centre for International Governance Innovation (CIGI) Chair in Global Health Economics in the Balsillie School of International Affairs there. She has consulted for the World Bank, the Asian Development Bank, several United Nations agencies,

and the International Development Research Centre, among others, in work carried out in over 20 low- and middle-income countries. She led the work on nutrition for the Copenhagen Consensus in 2008, when micronutrients were ranked as the top development priority. She has served as Associate Provost of Graduate Studies at the University of Waterloo, Vice-President Academic at Wilfrid Laurier University in Waterloo, and interim dean at the University of Toronto Scarborough.

Prabhat Jha

Prabhat Jha is the Founding Director of the Centre for Global Health Research at St. Michael's Hospital and holds Endowed and Canada Research Chairs in Global Health in the Dalla Lana School of Public Health at the University of Toronto. He is Lead Investigator of the Million Death Study in India, which quantifies the causes of death and key risk factors in over two million homes over a 14-year period. He is also Scientific Director of the Statistical Alliance for Vital Events, which aims to expand reliable measurement of causes of death worldwide. His research includes the epidemiology and economics of tobacco control worldwide.

Ramanan Laxminarayan

See the list of Volume Editors.

Charles N. Mock

Charles N. Mock, MD, PhD, FACS, has training as both a trauma surgeon and an epidemiologist. He worked as a surgeon in Ghana for four years, including at a rural hospital (Berekum) and at the Kwame Nkrumah University of Science and Technology (Kumasi). In 2005–07, he served as Director of the University of Washington's Harborview Injury Prevention and Research Center. In 2007–10, he worked at the World Health Organization (WHO) headquarters in Geneva, where he was responsible for developing the WHO's trauma care activities. In 2010, he returned to his position as Professor of Surgery (with joint appointments as Professor of Epidemiology and Professor of Global Health) at the University of Washington. His main interests include the spectrum of injury control, especially as it pertains to low- and middle-income countries: surveillance, injury prevention, prehospital care, and hospital-based trauma care. He is President (2013–15) of the International Association for Trauma Surgery and Intensive Care.

Contributors

Emiliano Albanese
Department of Psychiatry, University of Geneva, Geneva, Switzerland

Margaret Barry
National University of Ireland Galway, Galway, Ireland

Amanda J. Baxter
School of Public Health, University of Queensland, Brisbane, Queensland, Australia; Queensland Centre for Mental Health Research, Wacol, Queensland, Australia

Vladimir Carli
Swedish National Center for Suicide Research and Prevention, Karolinska Institutet, Stockholm, Sweden

Fiona J. Charlson
School of Public Health, University of Queensland, Herston, Queensland, Australia; Institute for Health Metrics and Evaluation, University of Washington, Seattle, Washington, United States

Pamela Y. Collins
U.S. National Institute of Mental Health, Bethesda, Maryland, United States

Abigail Colson
Center for Disease Dynamics, Economics & Policy, Washington, DC, United States; Department of Management Science, University of Strathclyde, Glasgow, Scotland

Louisa Degenhardt
National Drug and Alcohol Research Centre, University of New South Wales Australia, Sydney, New South Wales, Australia; Melbourne School of Population and Global Health, University of Melbourne, Victoria, Australia; Institute for Health Metrics and Evaluation, University of Washington, Seattle, Washington, United States

Catherine O. Egbe
University of KwaZulu-Natal, Durban, South Africa; Center for Tobacco Control Research and Education, University of California San Francisco, San Francisco, California, United States

Holly E. Erskine
School of Public Health, University of Queensland, Herston, Queensland, Australia; Institute for Health Metrics and Evaluation, University of Washington, Seattle, Washington, United States

Sara Evans-Lacko
Centre for Global Mental Health, Institute of Psychiatry, Psychology, and Neuroscience, King's College London, London, United Kingdom

Valery Feigin
National Institute for Stroke and Applied Neurosciences, Auckland University of Technology, Auckland, New Zealand

Abebaw Fekadu
Addis Ababa University, Addis Ababa, Ethiopia

Alize J. Ferrari
School of Public Health, University of Queensland, Herston, Queensland, Australia; Institute for Health Metrics and Evaluation, University of Washington, Seattle, Washington, United States

Panteleimon Giannakopoulos
Department of Psychiatry, University of Geneva, Geneva, Switzerland

Petra Gronholm
Centre for Global Mental Health, Institute of Psychiatry, Psychology, and Neuroscience, King's College London, London, United Kingdom

David Gunnell
University of Bristol, Bristol, United Kingdom

Wayne D. Hall
Centre for Youth Substance Abuse Research, University of Queensland, Brisbane, Queensland, Australia

Steven Hyman
Stanley Center for Psychiatric Research, Broad Institute of MIT and Harvard and Department of Stem Cell and Regenerative Biology, Harvard University, Cambridge, Massachusetts, United States

David Jernigan
Johns Hopkins Bloomberg School of Public Health, Johns Hopkins University, Baltimore, Maryland, United States

Nathalie Jette
University of Calgary, Calgary, Alberta, Canada

Kjell Arne Johansson
University of Bergen, Bergen, Norway

Carol Levin
Department of Global Health, University of Washington, Seattle, Washington, United States

Mattias Linde
Department of Neuroscience, Norwegian University of Science and Technology, Trondheim, Norway; Norwegian Advisory Unit on Headaches, St. Olavs Hospital, Trondheim, Norway

Crick Lund
Department of Psychiatry and Mental Health, Alan J. Flisher Centre for Public Mental Health, University of Cape Town, Cape Town, South Africa; Centre for Global Mental Health, Institute of Psychiatry, Psychology, and Neuroscience, King's College London, London, United Kingdom

John Marsden
National Addiction Centre, King's College London, London, United Kingdom

Itamar Megiddo
Center for Disease Dynamics, Economics & Policy, Washington, DC, United States; Department of Management Science, University of Strathclyde, Glasgow, Scotland

Cathrine Mihalopoulos
Deakin University, Melbourne, Victoria, Australia

Maristela Monteiro
Pan American Health Organization, Washington DC, United States

Aditi Nigam
Center for Disease Dynamics, Economics & Policy, Washington, DC, United States

Rachana Parikh
Public Health Foundation of India, New Delhi, India

Inge Petersen
University of KwaZulu-Natal, Durban, South Africa

Michael R. Phillips
Shanghai Mental Health Center, Shanghai Jiao Tong University School of Medicine, Shanghai, China; Departments of Psychiatry and Global Health, Emory University, Atlanta, Georgia, United States

Martin J. Prince
Institute of Psychiatry, Psychology, and Neuroscience, King's College London, London, United Kingdom

Atif Rahman
University of Liverpool, Liverpool, United Kingdom

Neha Raykar
Public Health Foundation of India, New Delhi, India

Tania Real
National Institute of Psychiatry Ramón de la Fuente Muñiz, Mexico City, Mexico

Jürgen Rehm
Centre for Addiction and Mental Health, Toronto, Ontario, Canada

Jacqueline Roberts
Autism Centre of Excellence, Griffith University, Brisbane, Queensland, Australia

Robin Room
Centre for Alcohol Policy Research, La Trobe University, Melbourne, Victoria, Australia; Centre for Social Research on Alcohol and Drugs, Stockholm University, Stockholm, Sweden

Diego Sánchez-Moreno
Ministry of Health, Mexico City, Mexico

James G. Scott
University of Queensland Centre for Clinical Research, Brisbane, Queensland, Australia; Metro North Mental Health, Royal Brisbane and Women's Hospital, Brisbane, Queensland, Australia

Maya Semrau
Centre for Global Mental Health, Institute of Psychiatry, Psychology, and Neuroscience, King's College London, London, United Kingdom

Rahul Shidhaye
Public Health Foundation of India, New Delhi, India; CAPHRI School for Public Health and Primary Care, Maastricht University, Maastricht, the Netherlands

Morton M. Silverman
Suicide Prevention Resource Center, Education Development Center, Waltham, Massachusetts, United States, The University of Colorado Denver School of Medicine, Aurora, Colorado, United States; The Jed Foundation, New York, New York, United States

Timothy J. Steiner
Norwegian University of Science and Technology, Trondheim, Norway; Imperial College London, London, United Kingdom

Emily Stockings
National Drug and Alcohol Research Centre, University of New South Wales, Sydney, Australia

Kirsten Bjerkreim Strand
University of Bergen, Bergen, Norway

John Strang
National Addiction Centre, King's College London, London, United Kingdom

Kiran T. Thakur
Columbia University College of Physicians and Surgeons, New York, New York, United States

Graham Thornicroft
Centre for Global Mental Health, Institute of Psychiatry, Psychology, and Neuroscience, King's College London, United Kingdom

Stéphane Verguet
Department of Global Health and Population, Harvard T. H. Chan School of Public Health, Boston, Massachusetts, United States

Lakshmi Vijayakumar
SNEHA, Voluntary Health Services, Chennai, India; Centre for Youth Mental Health, University of Melbourne, Melbourne, Victoria, Australia

Theo Vos
Institute for Health Metrics and Evaluation, University of Washington, Seattle, Washington, United States

Harvey A. Whiteford
School of Public Health, University of Queensland, Herston, Queensland, Australia; Queensland Centre for Mental Health Research, Wacol, Queensland, Australia; Institute for Health Metrics and Evaluation, University of Washington, Seattle, Washington, United States

Advisory Committee to the Editors

Carol Medlin
Senior Health and Nutrition Specialist,
Health, Nutrition, and Population Global Practice,
World Bank, Washington, DC, United States

Alvaro Moncayo
Researcher, Universidad de los Andes, Bogotá,
Colombia

Jaime Montoya
Executive Director, Philippine Council for Health
Research and Development, Taguig City, the
Philippines

Ole Norheim
Professor, University of Bergen, Bergen, Norway

Folashade Omokhodion
Professor, University College Hospital, Ibadan,
Nigeria

Toby Ord
President, Giving What We Can, Oxford,
United Kingdom

K. Srinath Reddy
President, Public Health Foundation of India,
New Delhi, India

Sevkat Ruacan
Dean, Koç University School of Medicine, Istanbul,
Turkey

Jaime Sepúlveda
Executive Director, Global Health Sciences, University
of California, San Francisco, San Francisco, California,
United States

Richard Skolnik
Lecturer, Health Policy Department, Yale School of
Public Health, New Haven, Connecticut, United States

Stephen Tollman
Professor, University of the Witwatersrand,
Johannesburg, South Africa

Jürgen Unutzer
Professor, Department of Psychiatry, University of
Washington, Seattle, Washington, United States

Damian Walker
Senior Program Officer, Bill & Melinda Gates
Foundation, Seattle, Washington, United States

Ngaire Woods
Director, Global Economic Governance Programme,
Oxford University, Oxford, United Kingdom

Nopadol Wora-Urai
Professor, Department of Surgery, Phramongkutklao
Hospital, Bangkok, Thailand

Kun Zhao
Researcher, China National Health Development
Research Center, Beijing, China

Reviewers

Sergio Aguilar-Gaxiola
University of California, Davis, School of Medicine, Sacramento, California, United States

Pierre K. Alexandre
Management Department, College of Business, Florida Atlantic University, Boca Raton, Florida, United States

Peter Anderson
Newcastle University, Institute for Health and Society, Newcastle, United Kingdom

Margaret Barry
National University of Ireland Galway, School of Health Sciences, Galway, Ireland

Angelina Brotherhood
Centre for Public Health, Liverpool John Moores University, Liverpool, United Kingdom

Anja Busse
United Nations Office on Drugs and Crime, Vienna, Austria

Dixon Chibanda
Department of Community Medicine, University of Zimbabwe, Harare, Zimbabwe

Mary De Silva
Centre for Global Mental Health, London School of Hygiene & Tropical Medicine, London, United Kingdom

Tedla W. Giorgis
Office of the Minister, Ministry of Health, Addis Ababa, Ethiopia

Alexander Grinshpoon
Israel Institute of Technology, Haifa, Israel

Yasemin Gürsoy-Özdemir
Department of Neurology, Koç University School of Medicine, Istanbul, Turkey

Murad M. Khan
Aga Khan University, Karachi, Pakistan

Rena Kurs
Sha'ar Menashe Mental Health Center, Sha'ar Menashe, Israel

David Leon
London School of Hygiene & Tropical Medicine, London, United Kingdom

Ron Manderscheid
National Association of County Behavioral Health and Developmental Disability Directors, Washington, DC, United States

Pallab K. Maulik
George Institute for Global Health, India, New Delhi, India

David McDaid
London School of Economics and Political Science, London, United Kingdom

Nicole M. Monteiro
Center for Healing and Development, Washington, DC, United States

Chiadi U. Onyike
The Johns Hopkins Hospital, Baltimore, Maryland, United States

Gregory Simon
Group Health Research Institute, Seattle, Washington, United States

Jürgen Unützer
Department of Psychiatry and Behavioral Sciences, University of Washington, Seattle, Washington, United States

Steven D. Vannoy
University of Massachusetts, Boston, Boston, Massachusetts, United States

Chiu-Wan Ng
Faculty of Medicine, University Malaya, Kuala Lumpur, Malaysia

Index

Boxes, figures, notes, and tables are indicated by b, f, n, and t respectively.

www.ingramcontent.com/pod-product-compliance
Lightning Source LLC
Chambersburg PA
CBHW080606270326
41928CB00016B/2939